I0479134

Biochemical Pharmacology and Toxicology

Biochemical Pharmacology and Toxicology

Edited by Mary Durrant

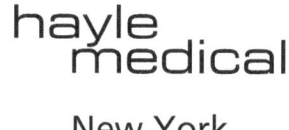

hayle
medical

New York

Hayle Medical,
750 Third Avenue, 9th Floor,
New York, NY 10017, USA

Visit us on the World Wide Web at:
www.haylemedical.com

© Hayle Medical, 2019

This book contains information obtained from authentic and highly regarded sources. Copyright for all individual chapters remain with the respective authors as indicated. All chapters are published with permission under the Creative Commons Attribution License or equivalent. A wide variety of references are listed. Permission and sources are indicated; for detailed attributions, please refer to the permissions page and list of contributors. Reasonable efforts have been made to publish reliable data and information, but the authors, editors and publisher cannot assume any responsibility for the validity of all materials or the consequences of their use.

ISBN: 978-1-63241-534-9

Trademark Notice: Registered trademark of products or corporate names are used only for explanation and identification without intent to infringe.

Cataloging-in-Publication Data

Biochemical pharmacology and toxicology / edited by Mary Durrant.
   p. cm.
Includes bibliographical references and index.
ISBN 978-1-63241-534-9
1. Pharmacology. 2. Biochemical toxicology. 3. Biopharmaceutics. 4. Biochemistry.
5. Pharmaceutical chemistry. I. Durrant, Mary.
RM301.4 .B56 2019
615.1--dc23

Table of Contents

Preface

Pharmacology is a branch of biology. It studies drug action and explores the interactions between living organisms and chemicals that have an influence on normal or abnormal biochemical function. Drugs can be man-made, natural or endogenous. The field of pharmacology studies the design, composition, properties and synthesis of drugs. Toxicology and pharmacology are interrelated areas of study. The field of toxicology studies the adverse reactions of chemical substances on living organisms as well as the diagnosis and treatment of exposures to toxins and toxicants. Dosage, route of exposure, age, sex, species and the environment are significant factors that determine chemical toxicity and its effect. The aim of this book is to present researches that have transformed the disciplines of pharmacology and toxicology and aided their advancement. It also covers in detail some existing theories and innovative concepts of these fields. This book is a vital tool for all researching or studying pharmacology and toxicology as it gives incredible insights into emerging trends and concepts.

The researches compiled throughout the book are authentic and of high quality, combining several disciplines and from very diverse regions from around the world. Drawing on the contributions of many researchers from diverse countries, the book's objective is to provide the readers with the latest achievements in the area of research. This book will surely be a source of knowledge to all interested and researching the field.

In the end, I would like to express my deep sense of gratitude to all the authors for meeting the set deadlines in completing and submitting their research chapters. I would also like to thank the publisher for the support offered to us throughout the course of the book. Finally, I extend my sincere thanks to my family for being a constant source of inspiration and encouragement.

Editor

Phytochemical Screening, Antioxidant Activities and *In Vitro* Anticancer Potential of Egyptian *Capsicum* Spp.

Shaimaa GA[1]*, Mahmoud MS[1], Mohamed MR[2] and Emam AA[2]

[1]*Functional Food and Nutrition Department, Food Technology Research Institute, Agricultural Research Center, Giza 12613, Egypt*
[2]*Biochemistry Department, Cairo University, Giza 12613, Egypt*

Abstract

In the present study, two cultivars of pepper (*Capsicum annuum* and *Capsicum frutescens*) at two maturity stages (green and red) were evaluated for total phenolic and flavonoid content, organic acids, vitamin C, β-carotene, vitamin E, capsaicin and the antioxidant and anticancer activities of their aqueous extracts. Total phenolic content was found to be ranged from 11.09-26.14 mg GAE/g DW, while total flavonoid content was ranged from 2.7 mg to 5.0 mg QE/g DW. Twenty six phenolic and aromatic compounds, twelve flavonoid compounds and eleven organic acids were identified in all samples by using of HPLC. Vitamin C, β-carotene, vitamin E and capsaicin contents were also estimated by HPLC and detected at high levels which were ranged from 500.0-645.5 mg/100 g DW, 6.56-35.69 mg/100 g DW, 10.44-19.36 mg/100 g DW and 37.46-69.90 mg/100 g DW, respectively. Antioxidant activities of pepper samples were carried out by using of both DPPH•-scavenging activity and total antioxidant capacity (ABTS•+) assays and the extracts exhibited high activities which were ranged from 96.95% to 98.64% and from 77.73% to 93.11%, respectively. Finally, the potential anticancer activity of pepper extracts and capsaicin standard was tested against prostate (PC-3) and breast (MCF-7) carcinoma cell lines *in vitro*. The results showed that sweet pepper had a higher anticancer activity against PC-3, in contrast, chilli pepper had a higher against MCF-7.

Keywords: Chilli pepper; Sweet pepper; Capsicum; Phytochemical components; Capsaicin; Antioxidant activities; Anticancer activity

Introduction

Capsicum is a genus of plants from the family of *Solanaceae*. Some species of the genus *Capsicum* are grown for their fruits, which can be consumed fresh (in salads, baked dishes, salsa, pizzas, etc.), cooked, as a dried powder, in a sauce, or processed into oleoresin [1].

Peppers contain phenolics and flavonoids [2], carotenoids [3], vitamin C, vitamin E [4] and alkaloids [5], which play important roles in human health. In other studies, antioxidant activities in peppers were measured by radical-scavenging activity [6,7], inhibition of lipid peroxidation [8] and metal-chelating activity [9]. Capsaicinoids and carotenoids exhibit anticancer [10,11] and antioxidant activities [12-14]. Flavonoids have been shown to act as antioxidants, and they possess anti-inflammatory [15], antiallergic [16], and antibacterial activities [17]. The antioxidant activity of pepper extracts involves bioactive compounds, such as polyphenols, carotenoids, capsaicinoids and ascorbic acid [18-20].

Hot chili peppers that belong to the plant genus *Capsicum* (family, *Solanaceae*) are among the most frequently consumed spices throughout the world. The principal pungent ingredient present in hot red pepper (*Capsicum annuum L.*) and chili pepper (*Capsicum frutescence L.*) is the phenolic substance named capsaicin (*trans*-8-methyl-N-vanillyl-6-non-enamide). The capsaicin content of hot peppers varies from 0.1% to 1%. Capsaicin was subjected to extensive investigations with regard to its possible tumorigenicity and genotoxicity [21,22]. However, the compound has recently attracted considerable attention because of its chemoprotective properties against certain carcinogens and mutagens.

Prostate cancer remains the most commonly diagnosed cancer in men living in the Western world [23]. There is increasing evidence that dietary factors play a role in the development and progression of prostate cancer. It is estimated that at least 30% of all prostate cancer patients use complementary and alternative medicine, which includes the consumption of micronutrient supplements [24]. Many dietary agents have been studied for the protective effects on prostate cancer

[25,26]. Capsaicin has recently emerged as a potent anti-cancer agent, exhibiting anti-proliferative and pro-apoptotic properties in several different prostate cancer model systems [27]. The use of capsaicin *in vitro* had been reported to induce apoptosis through the generation of reactive oxygen species (ROS) [28-30] (Figure 1).

Breast cancer is the leading cause of death among women worldwide. About 63,300 cases of breast carcinoma *in situ* are expected to be newly diagnosed in 2012 [31]. Capsaicin or N-vanillyl-8- methyl-1-nonenamide, the primary pungent and irritating ingredient present in a variety of red peppers of the genus *Capsicum* [32-34], was reported to selectively inhibit the growth of tumor cells [35]. Despite previous discordant results from studies that determined its potential mutagenic and carcinogenic activity [17], subsequent investigations have shown that capsaicin induces apoptosis in a wide variety of tumor cells [29,36-39]. Additional studies reported that capsaicinoids displayed *in vitro* and *in vivo* antitumor activity [40]. In cultured cells, capsaicin blocked the cell migration in breast cancer, while in mice, oral consumption of capsaicin decreased the size of MDAMB 231 breast cancer tumors by 50%, and inhibited the development of pre-neoplastic breast lesions by up to 80%. Also, direct injection of capsaicin led to an 80% reduction in tumor size [39]. Thus, capsaicin can be considered a potential lead against malignant tumors. Capsaicin has been shown to inhibit the growth of ER-positive (MCF-7, T47D, BT-474) and ER-negative (SKBR-3, MDA-MB231) breast cancer cells by causing G0/G1 cell-cycle arrest and apoptosis [41].

*Corresponding author: Shaimaa GA, Functional Food and Nutrition Department, Food Technology Research Institute, Agricultural Research Center, Giza 12613, Egypt, E-mail: shaimaa_amgad2013@yahoo.com

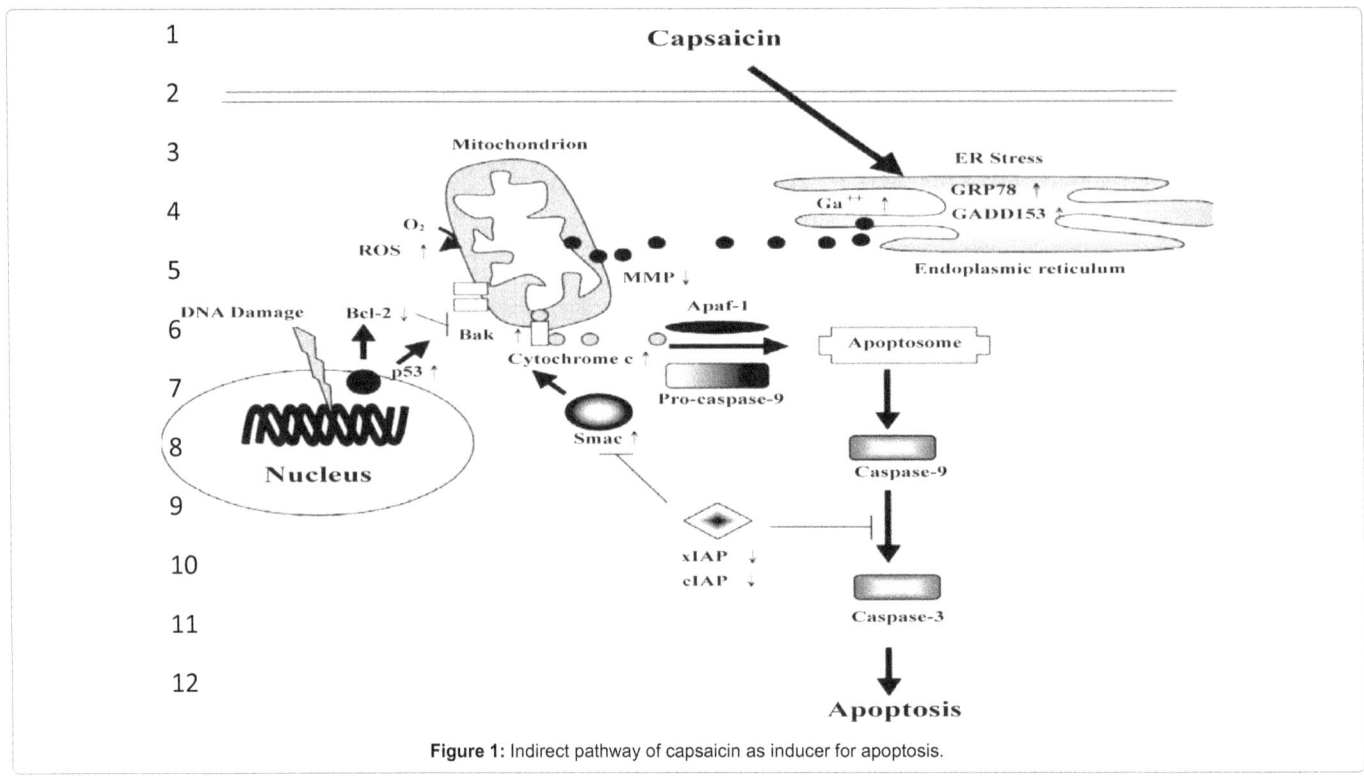

Figure 1: Indirect pathway of capsaicin as inducer for apoptosis.

The aim of the present study was to evaluate the bioactive components, included phenolic and aromatic compounds, flavonoids, organic acids, vitamin C, E, β-carotene and capsaicin in Egyptian dried pepper samples (sweet and chilli) at two ripening stages (green and red). Evaluation was also extended the potential anticancer activity on both prostate and breast carcinoma cell lines *in vitro*.

Materials and Methods

Collection of plant materials and treatment

Fruits of hot chilli pepper (*Capsium frutescens* var. sina) at immature stage (green color) and mature stage (red color) and others of sweet pepper (*Capsium annuum* var. goduion), green and red, were collected from Vegetable Breeding Research Department, Horticultural Research Institute, Agricultural Research Center in September until December 2012 season and were identified at the same institute.

Fresh fruits were washed by using of tap water, seeds were removed and the edible tissues were cut to small pieces which were oven-dried in Lab Companion oven at 55°C for 48 h.

Chemicals and drugs

All the utilized chemical materials (solvents, mineral salts, etc.) were purchased from El Gomhoryia, El Allamyia, El Nasr and Middle East Pharmaceutical Chemical companies, Egypt and the solvents were purified before using. Chemicals, solvents and all standard materials which were used for fractionation and identification by HPLC, purchased from Sigma/Aldrich Chemical Company, USA.

Carcinoma cell lines

Prostate carcinoma cell line (PC-3) and breast carcinoma cell line (MCF-7) test kits were obtained from Pharmacology Unit, Cancer Biology Department, National Cancer Institute, Egypt.

Preparation of extracts

Ten g of dried pepper samples were extracted with 100 ml distilled water (1:10) (i.e., 10 g/100 ml) to produce the aqueous extracts. The extracts were placed in ultrasonic instrument (BANDELIN SONOREX SUPER RK 514H) for 30 min, left up to 24 h at 15°C and filtered through a Whatman paper No. 1. The resultant extracts were used to determine total phenolic and flavonoid contents and their HPLC fractionation, antioxidant and anticancer activities *in vitro*.

Determination of total phenolic content

Total phenolic content (TPC) of each sample was determined using a Folin Ciocalteu assay according to the method of Singleton and Rossi [42,43] with slight modification. The reaction mixture contained 1 ml of extract and 0.5 ml of the Folin-Ciocalteu reagent, 1 ml sodium carbonate 7.5% and 7.5 ml of distilled water were added, respectively. After 45 min of reaction at ambient temperature, the absorbance at 765 nm was measured using a UV-visible spectrophotometer (Beckman). A blue color indicated the presence of phenols. A calibration curve was calculated by using of gallic acid standard (0.1 mg/ml). Total phenolic content of samples were determined in triplicates and the results were expressed on dry weight basis (DW) as mg gallic acid equivalents (GAE), per g of each sample.

HPLC analysis of phenolic and aromatic compounds

Phenolic and aromatic compounds were detected by HPLC according to the method of Goupy et al. [44] as follows: the aqueous extracts were centrifuged at 10000 rpm (in ICE Micro-MB Centrifuge/NARP 64606 instrument) for 10 min and the supernatant was filtrated through a 0.2 µm Millipore membrane filter, then 1-3 ml were collected in a vial for injection into HPLC Agilent (Series 1200) equipped with autosampler injector, solvent degasser, ultraviolet (UV) detector set at 280 nm and quaternary HP pump (Series 1100). The column [Agilent

Phytochemical Screening, Antioxidant Activities and In Vitro Anticancer Potential of Egyptian Capsicum Spp.

3

5HC-C18 (2) 250 × 4.6 mm] temperature was maintained at 35°C. Gradient separation was carried out with methanol and acetonitrile as a mobile phase at flow rate of 1 ml/min. Phenolic acid standards from sigma Co. were dissolved in a mobile phase and injected into HPLC. Retention time and peak area of the tested samples were calibrated against standard solutions of different phenolic and aromatic compounds concentration by the data analysis of HEWLLET Packed (HP) software.

Determination of total flavonoid content

Total flavonoid content was measured by $AlCl_3$ colorimetric assay according to the method of Harborne [45] based on slight modification. Briefly, 500 μl of extract and 2 ml of distilled water, 150 μl of 5% sodium nitrate were added. After 5 min, 150 μl of 10% $AlCl_3$ was added. A total of 2000 μl of sodium hydroxide (1 M) were added after 1 min and followed by 1200 μl of distilled water. The mixture was incubated for 30 min. The absorbance was measured at 510 nm against a prepared blank. A yellow color indicated the presence of flavonoids. A calibration curve was calculated using quercetin standard (0.1 mg/ml). Total flavonoid content of samples was determined in triplicates and the results were expressed on dry weight basis (DW) as mg quercetin equivalents (QE), per g of each sample.

HPLC analysis of flavonoid compounds

Flavonoid fractions were also identified by HPLC according to the method of Mattila et al. [46] as follows: the aqueous extracts were centrifuged at 10000 rpm (in ICE Micro-MB Centrifuge/NARP 64606 instrument) for 10 min and the supernatant was filtrated through a 0.2 μm Millipore membrane filter, then 1-3 ml were collected in a vial for injection into the previous HPLC Agilent (Series 1200) and HP software were used. The ultraviolet (UV) detector was set at 330 nm and the other conditions were set as that previously used in the fractionation of phenolic compounds.

DPPH•-scavenging activity assay

Free radical scavenging activity was determined using the free radical generator DPPH• assay based on slight modifications [47]. One ml of the pepper extract was added to 1 ml of 0.002% methanol solution of DPPH•. The mixture was thoroughly mixed using BioCote/Stuart vortex instrument and kept in the dark for 30 min. The absorbance, using a spectrophotometer, was measured at 517 nm against a blank of methanol without DPPH•.

Total antioxidant capacity assay

Total antioxidant capacity assay was carried out by the improved ABTS•+ method according to the method of Re et al. [48]. ABTS•+ radical cation was generated by reacting 7 mM ABTS•+ and 2.45 mM potassium persulfate after incubation at room temperature (23°C) in the dark for 16 h. The ABTS•+-solution was diluted with 80% ethanol to an absorbance of 0.700 ± 0.005 at 734 nm. 0.1 ml of the tested samples was added to 3.9 ml of ABTS•+ solution and mixed thoroughly. The reactive mixture was allowed to stand at room temperature for 6 min and the absorbance was immediately recorded at 734 nm against a blank of 80% ethanol using a spectrophotometer. The inhibition percent was calculated in both methods (DPPH• and ABTS•+) as follows:

[A control – A extract/A control] × 100

HPLC analysis of organic acids

Organic acid fractionation was conducted according to the method of Wodecki et al. [49]. One g of dried pepper samples were mixed with 50 ml deionized water, placed in the ultrasonic instrument for 30 min and centrifuged at 10000 rpm for 10 min, the supernatant was filtrated through a 0.2 μm Millipore membrane filter then 1 ml was collected in a vial for injection using of HPLC Agilent (Series 1200) equipped with autosampler injector, solvent degasser, ultraviolet (UV) detector (set at 210 nm) and quaternary HP pump (Series 1090). The column [OA-1000 Column S/N: 5927915] temperature was maintained at 55°C. Gradient separation was carried out with methanol and ethanol as a mobile phase.

HPLC analysis of vitamin C: Vitamin C was determined according to the method of Romeu-Nadal et al. [50]. One g of dried pepper samples were mixed with 0.3% metaphosphoric acid solution and centrifuged at 10000 rpm for 10 min and the supernatant was filtrated through a 0.2 μm Millipore membrane filter then 1-3 ml were collected in a vial for injection into HPLC Agilent (Series 1200) equipped with autosampler injector, solvent degasser, ultraviolet (UV) detector (set at 254 nm) and quaternary HP pump (Series 3365). The column [Agilent 5HC-C18 (2) 250 × 4.6 mm] temperature was maintained at 25°C. Ascorbic acid was identified by comparing the retention time of the sample peak with that of the ascorbic standard at 254 nm.

HPLC analysis of β-carotene

β-carotene was determined according to the method of Pupin et al. [51]. Dried (5 g) pepper samples were extracted with ethyl acetate (3 × 50 ml) containing BHT (0.004%). The organic phase was transferred through anhydrous sodium sulfate (50 g) and collected in an ambered round-bottom flask. The dried extract was transferred quantitatively to a 10 ml volumetric flask using portions of 1.5 ml of mobile phase (acetonitrile: methanol: 1,2-dichloromethane, 60:35:5, v/v/v). A vial was injected into HPLC Agilent (Series 1200) equipped with autosampler injector, solvent degasser, ultraviolet (UV) detector (set at 280 nm) and quaternary HP pump (Series 1100). The column [Agilent Hypersil ODS 5 μm 4.0 × 250 mm] temperature was maintained at 35°C.

HPLC analysis of vitamin E

Vitamin E was determined according to the method of Pyka and Sliwiok [52]. Dried (5 g) pepper samples were extracted with hexane (3 × 50 ml) containing BHT (0.004%). The organic phase was transferred through potassium hydroxide (50 g) and collected in an ambered round-bottom flask. The solution was well mixed and further extracted with hexane and petroleum ether (75 and 25 ml, respectively, containing 0.004% BHT). The pooled hexane was evaporated to dryness in a rotary evaporator at 40°C. The extract was transferred quantitatively to a 10 ml methanol. A vial was injected into HPLC Agilent (Series 1200) equipped with autosampler injector, solvent degasser, ultraviolet (UV) detector (set at 290 nm) and quaternary HP pump (Series 1100). Gradient separation was carried out with methanol and water (9:1, v/v) as a mobile phase at a flow rate of 1.5 ml/min. The column [Agilent Hypersil ODS 5 μm 4.0 × 250 mm] temperature was maintained at 35°C. The injection volume was 20 ml of a standard of vitamin E in ethanol.

HPLC analysis of capsaicin

Capsaicin content was determined according to Collins et al. [53]. One g of dried pepper samples was added to 10 ml acetonitrile and placed in 120 ml glass bottles. Bottles were capped, placed in an 80°C water bath for 4 h and then they were swirled manually every hour. After cooling at room temperature, 2 ml of supernatant were taken and filtered (0.45 filter syringe) into a 2 ml glass sample vial, capped, and stored at 5°C until analyzed by HPLC Agilent (Series 1200) equipped with autosampler injector, solvent degasser, ultraviolet (UV) detector set at 280 nm and quaternary HP pump (Series 1100).

The column [Agilent 5HC-C18 (2) 250 × 4.6 mm] temperature was maintained at 35°C. The mobile phase was methanol: water (30%:70%). Standard solution of capsaicin 50% standard was prepared in methanol by dilution of a 2 mg stock solution. Capsaicin was identified by comparing the retention time of the sample peak with that of the CAP standard at 280 nm.

Anticancer activity (Cytotoxicity)

Preparation of the tested samples: Aqueous extracts of dried pepper, which were freeze dried by using of Freeze Dryer Lab Conco USA at -50°C/vacuum, and also capsaicin 50% standard were both tested against prostate (PC-3) and breast (MCF-7) carcinoma cell lines.

In vitro cytotoxicity: The percentage of cell death was estimated by Sulfo-Rhodamine B (SRB) assay. Potential cytotoxicity of both aqueous extracts of dried pepper samples and capsaicin standard (50% capsaicin) was tested using the method of Skehan et al. [54]. Different concentrations of the compounds under test (5, 12.5, 25 and 50 µg/ml DMSO) were added to the cell monolayer triplicate wells which were prepared for each individual dose. Monolayer cells were incubated with the compounds for 48 h at 37°C and in atmosphere of 5% CO_2. After 48 h, cells were fixed, washed and stained with Sulfo-Rhodamine-B stain. Color intensity was measured by ELISA reader (TCAL).

Statistical analysis: All results were expressed as means ± standard deviation. Statistical Analysis System SAS 9.1 software package was used to analysis of data and significant differences between mean values were determined by least significant difference (LSD) test at P > 0.05.

Results and Discussion

Total phenolic content of dried pepper samples and HPLC of their fractionation

Data in Table 1 show that total phenolic content ranged from 19.26-36.87 mg GAE/g DW and sweet peppers were significantly higher than chilli peppers. The resulted data are in accordance with Aliakbarlu et al. [55] who showed that total phenolic content in red pepper was 34 mg GAE/g DW. But they are higher than those found by Rodríguez-Maturino et al. [56] who found that the Habanero pepper had significantly higher total phenolic content (5.92 mg GAE /g DW) than the Chiltepin pepper (4.85 mg GAE/g DW). The obtained data also show that the total phenolic content was increased with maturation from green to red color. This is in agreement with Howard et al. [57] who found that total phenolics were ranged from 2656-5788 mg/kg FW and total phenols increased with maturation. In contrast, Ghasemnezhad et al. [58] reported that phenolic content decreased with maturity and following ripening. Lin and Tang [59] also observed that total phenols in green, yellow and red pepper were 206.0, 191.2 and 180.3 mg GAE/100g FW, respectively.

Data of the phenolic and aromatic compounds show that 3-hydroxy tyrosol, chlorogenic, catechol, E-vanillic and benzoic acids were detected at higher levels than other phenolic acids (Table 1). Pyrogallol is only detected in GRS sample and ellagic acid only in GGS sample. Coumarin not only found in GRS sample. All of α-coumaric, E-vanillic, caffeine and oleuropein were not found in GGS sample. Other phenolic acids found in all extracts at different contents.

Total flavonoid content of dried pepper samples and HPLC of their fractionation

Data in Table 2 show that total flavonoid content of the dried pepper samples were ranged from 371.7-512.0 mg QE/100 g DW and

Sample	SGC	SRC	GGS	GRS
Total phenolic content (mg GAE/g DW)	19.26[c] ± 0.42	19.48[c] ± 0.46	29.11[b] ± 3.82	36.87[a] ± 4.57
HPLC of phenolic and aromatic compounds (mg/100 g DW)				
Gallic acid	1.31	3.00	2.18	2.12
Pyrogallol	ND	ND	ND	52.90
3-Hydroxy tyrosol	14.00	10.00	25.54	15.62
Benzoic acid	112.45	12.35	38.20	16.22
4-Amino benzoic acid	6.16	8.08	9.86	6.94
Caffeine	0.54	1.77	ND	0.77
Protocatchuic acid	1.28	3.11	7.03	4.42
Catechin	4.42	5.30	1.19	4.18
Chlorogenic acid	25.99	15.74	25.68	20.62
Catechol	12.00	8.57	4.09	9.21
Epicatechin	5.27	7.64	15.21	7.29
P-hydroxy benzoic acid	5.73	5.52	11.48	6.97
Caffeic acid	1.72	1.75	10.30	1.11
Vanillic acid	2.18	3.14	3.94	3.26
Ferulic acid	0.30	0.66	0.70	0.49
Isoferulic acid	0.35	0.54	0.62	0.28
Reverstrol	1.27	0.40	0.16	0.41
Oleuropein	86.37	5.67	ND	ND
Ellagic acid	ND	ND	12.24	ND
E-vanillic acid	15.12	20.15	ND	28.07
O-coumaric acid	0.23	0.12	ND	0.03
3,4,5-methoxy cinnamic	0.11	0.28	0.11	0.10
Coumarin	1.14	0.93	1.23	ND
Salicylic acid	2.69	1.59	1.75	0.45
P-coumaric acid	0.30	0.37	0.81	0.26
Cinnamic acid	3.21	3.06	3.43	2.14

Each value represents the mean ± Standard Deviation; the mean values with different letters (a, b and c) within a specific row indicate significant differences (*P* < 0.05).
SGC: Sina Green Chilli; SRC: Sina Red Chilli; GGS: Godiuon Green Sweet; GRS: Godiuon Red Sweet; ND: Not Detected.

Table 1: Total phenolic content and their HPLC fractionation of dried pepper samples.

Sample	SGC	SRC	GGS	GRS
Total flavonoid content (mg QE/100 g DW)	392.2[de] ± 0.14	439.4[bc] ± 0.12	371.7[def] ± 0.09	512.0[a] ± 0.20
HPLC of flavonoid compounds (mg/100 g DW)				
Naringenin	3.30	1.70	4.75	7.30
Rutin	2.65	3.85	3.76	3.75
Hesperidin	15.35	7.18	11.37	6.67
Rosmarinic	8.11	0.31	1.31	0.34
Quercetrin	71.26	8.87	14.35	7.40
Quercetin	0.18	0.32	0.17	0.09
Naringin	0.15	0.14	0.14	0.11
Kaempferol	0.71	0.40	0.56	0.41
Hesperitin	0.41	0.67	0.44	0.21
Apigenin	0.21	0.18	0.29	0.12
7-hydroxy flavone	0.25	0.35	0.24	0.08
Luteolin	0.02	0.42	0.01	0.35

Each value represents the mean ± Standard Deviation; the mean values with different letters (a, b, c, d, e and f) within a specific row indicate significant differences (*P* < 0.05).
SGC: Sina Green Chilli; SRC: Sina Red Chilli; GGS: Godiuon Green Sweet; GRS: Godiuon Red Sweet.

Table 2: Total flavonoid content and their HPLC fractionation of all dried peppers.

their contents increased with maturation (red samples had a higher content than green samples). In contrast, Tundis et al. [60] showed that the flavonoids content decreased with the maturity. The results are lower than those of Materska and Perucka [61] who revealed that flavonoids ranged from 16.7-40.7 mg/g DW. But they are higher than those found by Lin and Tang [59] who observed that total flavonoids for green, yellow and red pepper were 7.8, 4.1 and 10.4 mg QE/100 g FW, respectively. Perucka and Materska [62] also found that the low flavonoid contents ranged from 81.2-91.0 mg QE/100 g DW were detected.

Data of flavonoid fractionation are also observed in Table 2 and they show that quercetrin, hesperidin, naringenin, rosmarinic and rutin are identified at high contents than other compounds. Some of the detected flavonoid compounds increased with maturation and the others were declined (Table 2). These results are in agreement with Ghasemnezhad et al. [58] who reported that the changes in flavonoids (such as quercetin and catachin) were depended on the pepper cultivars.

HPLC of organic acids

Table 3 shows that all pepper samples contain a wide range of organic acids. Lactic, citric, malic and fumaric acids are the major organic acids detected in the different pepper samples at contents which ranged from 29.11-409.79 mg; 14.03-32.08 mg; 109.83-131.62 mg and 3.62-4.34 mg/100 g DW. On contrary, oxalic and maleic acids were not detected in all pepper samples. Finally, the contents of all of the detected organic acids were decreased with the maturation (from green to red color).

These results are in agreement with Serrano et al. [63] who showed that the main organic acid contributing to pepper acidity was citric acid and other organic acids such as succinic, malic, oxalic and fumaric acids were also detected in pepper fruits although at much lower concentrations which ranged from 20-120 mg/100 g FW. In contrast, Matsufuji et al. [64] found that citric acid was ranged from 155-392 mg/100 g FW in different pepper samples.

Antioxidant activities, vitamin C, β-carotene, vitamin E and capsaicin contents of dried pepper samples

The radical scavenging effects and antioxidant activities are demonstrated in Table 4. All of the tested samples were able to reduce the stable free radical 2,2-diphenyl-1-picrylhydrazyl (DPPH) to the yellow-colored diphenylpicrylhydrazine, with inhibition percent ranged from 96.95% to 98.64%. In contrast the previous components, free radical scavenging activity increased in the immature pepper (green color) than mature (red). The free radical scavenging activity on ABTS•+ showed inhibition percent ranged from 77.73% to 93.11% but they increased in the mature pepper (red samples) and sweet pepper had the highest values. The highest antioxidant activities on DPPH• and ABTS•+ radicals were corresponded to the highest values of total phenolic and flavonoid contents. The data are in agreement with Tripathi and Mishra [65] who found that DPPH-radical scavenging activity of powdered red pepper was 96.78%.

Fresh peppers are the vegetables with the highest vitamin C content. It has been reported that consumption of 100 g FW of peppers provides 100-200% of the RDA (recommended daily administration) of vitamin C [66]. Data in Table 4 show that vitamin C content in all pepper samples ranged from 500.0-645.5 mg/100 g DW. Data also observe that vitamin C contents were higher in sweet peppers than chilli peppers and also increased with the maturation stages. The results are in a good agreement with Howard et al. [57], Mozafar [67], Simonne et al. [68]

and Marín et al. [69] who reported an increment in the level of ascorbic acid (AA) during pepper ripening. It might be related to the light intensity and greater levels of glucose, the precursor of ascorbic acid.

β-carotene contents are also shown in Table 4 and ranged from 7.28-35.69 mg/100 g DW in all pepper samples. The resulted data show that red peppers had higher β-carotene content than the green peppers (i.e., β-carotene increased with maturation). The results are in agreement with Perucka and Materska [62] who showed that the contents of β-carotene in red pepper fruits were ranged from 14.0-39.65 mg/100 g DW in all cultivars. Ozgur et al. [70] found that β-carotene contents were 10.29 and 158.31 mg/kg DW in fresh green and red peppers, respectively and were too increased in dried peppers (173.37 and 2282.45 mg/kg DW, respectively) which disagree with our results of dried peppers.

Results in Table 4 also show that vitamin E contents in dried pepper samples were ranged from 10.44-19.36 mg/100 g DW. These contents increased with maturation and the sweet pepper samples had a higher content than chilli pepper. The data are lower than that found by Perucka and Materska [62] who reported that tocopherole contents in red pepper fruits were ranged from 36.0-68.3 mg/100g DW. Matsufuji et al. [64] also showed that α-tocopherole was ranged from 0.49-5.40 mg/100 g FW. Finally, Isabelle et al. [71] found that α-tocopherole content in *Capsicum annuum* var. grossum, green and red, was 3.06 and 24.76 µg vitamin E/g FW, respectively, and its content in *Capsicum annuum* var. longum, green and red chilli, was 8.50 and 56.46 µg vitamin E/g FW, respectively.

Anticancer activity of aqueous extracts of dried pepper samples and capsaicin standard

Tables 5 and 6 and Figures 2 and 3 show the cytotoxicity of freeze dried aqueous extracts of oven-dried pepper samples and capsaicin standard on prostate carcinoma cell line (PC-3) and breast carcinoma cell line (MCF-7). The resulted data observe that sweet peppers had a high inhibition percent on PC-3 than chilli peppers at concentration 50 µg/ml. In contrast, chilli peppers had a higher cytotoxicity on MCF-7. At the same time, capsaicin standard exhibited the highest anticancer activity against PC-3 and MCF-7 that was 71.9% and 78.3%, respectively, at concentration 25 µg/ml for both cell lines.

Quercetin and quercetrin which were detected in these samples with contents ranged from 0.09 to 0.32 and 7.40-71.26 mg/100 g DW, respectively, had been reported to inhibit prostate cancer colony melanoma growth, and act as pro-apoptotic agent [72]. Similarly, ellagic acid, an oxidation product of gallic acid, catechol, kaempferol and its derivatives, which were detected, had undergone different

Sample	SGC	SRC	GGS	GRS
Acetic	26.40	25.27	ND	ND
Propionic	ND	58.26	187.01	33.99
Succinic	16.46	ND	ND	20.76
Formic	ND	ND	58.02	48.41
Butyric	ND	ND	ND	94.40
Citric	32.08	14.03	23.55	15.89
Maleic	ND	ND	ND	ND
Lactic	42.57	29.11	409.79	399.30
Malic	122.63	122.40	131.62	109.83
Fumaric	4.04	4.03	4.34	3.62
Oxalic	ND	ND	ND	ND

SGC: Sina Green Chilli; SRC: Sina Red Chilli; GGS: Godiuon Green Sweet; GRS: Godiuon Red Sweet; ND: Not Detected.

Table 3: Organic acid contents of all dried pepper samples (mg/100 g DW).

Samples	DPPH• (%) at (100 g/L)	ABTS•+ (%) at (100 g/L)	Vitamin C (mg/100 g DW)	β-carotene (mg/100 g DW)	Vitamin E (mg/100 g DW)	Capsaicin (mg/100 g DW)
SGC	98.64[a] ± 0.20	77.73[d] ± 0.07	500.00	7.28	10.44	69.90
SRC	96.95[c] ± 0.10	84.19[c] ± 0.17	521.21	35.69	13.95	65.98
GGS	98.15[ab] ± 0.11	91.52[b] ± 1.13	619.62	6.56	17.77	51.02
GRS	97.78[bc] ± 0.28	93.11[a] ± 0.44	645.50	35.00	19.35	37.46

Each value represents the mean ± Standard Deviation; the mean values with different letters (a, b, c and d) within a specific column indicate significant differences ($P < 0.05$). ABTS•+ showed inhibition percent ranged.
SGC: Sina Green Chilli; SRC: Sina Red Chilli; GGS: Godiuon Green Sweet; GRS: Godiuon Red Sweet.

Table 4: Antioxidant activities, vitamin C, β-carotene, vitamin E and capsaicin contents in all pepper samples.

Sample No.	Aqueous extract concentrations (µg/ml)							
	5		12.5		25		50	
	% Inhibition*	Available cells	% Inhibition	Available cells	% Inhibition	Available cells	% Inhibition	Available cells
SGC	13	0.87	23.9	0.761	53.3	0.467	76.8	0.232
SRC	16.7	0.833	23.9	0.761	62	0.38	72.8	0.272
GGS	6.5	0.935	16.7	0.833	46.1	0.539	72.1	0.279
GRS	9.4	0.906	14.1	0.859	46.7	0.533	70.3	0.297
CAP	34.8	0.652	39.9	0.601	78.3	0.217	70.7	0.293

*% Inhibition = [(Available cells × 100) – 100].

Table 5: Inhibition percent of aqueous extracts of dried pepper and capsaicin standard on breast carcinoma cell line (MCF-7).

Sample No.	Aqueous extract concentrations (µg/ml)							
	5		12.5		25		50	
	% Inhibition	Available cells	% Inhibition	Available cells	% Inhibition	Available cells	% Inhibition	Available cells
SGC	17.1	0.829	32	0.68	56.2	0.438	54.7	0.453
SRC	7.7	0.923	27.7	0.723	50	0.5	56.5	0.435
GGS	3.8	0.962	26.5	0.735	64.8	0.352	67.9	0.321
GRS	16.1	0.839	24	0.76	62.5	0.375	59.3	0.407
CAP	33.5	0.665	63.3	0.367	71.9	0.281	64.8	0.352

SGC: Sina Green Chilli; SRC: Sina Red Chilli; GGS: Godiuon Green Sweet; GRS: Godiuon Red Sweet.

Table 6: Inhibition percent of aqueous extracts of dried pepper and capsaicin standard on prostate carcinoma cell line (PC-3).

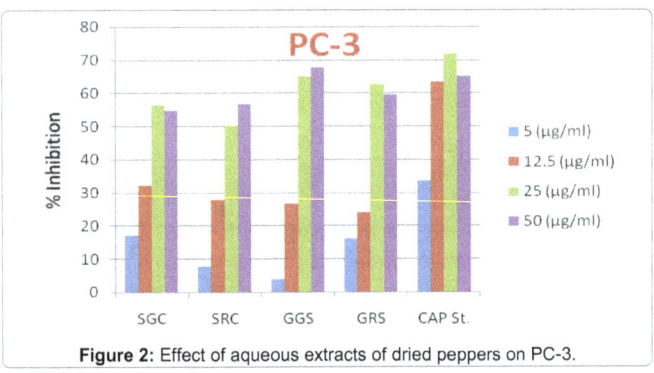

Figure 2: Effect of aqueous extracts of dried peppers on PC-3.

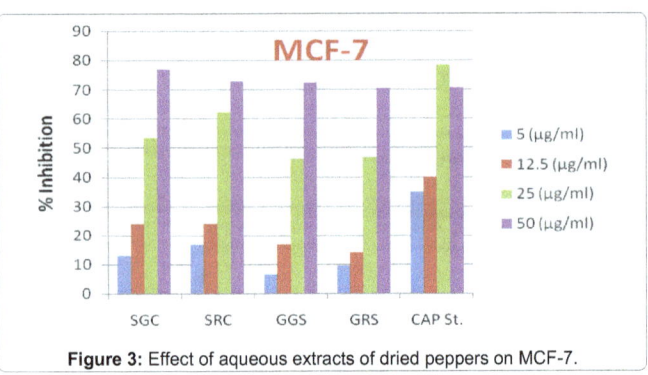

Figure 3: Effect of aqueous extracts of dried peppers on MCF-7.

levels of study as possible prostate cancer chemo-preventive agents, with promising results, including potent anti-mutagenesis, antitumor and anti-metastasis properties [73,74], effects that are also relevant to prostate cancer control and chemoprevention (This paragraph is considered a discussion for the results that were found) [75].

Also, all aqueous extracts of dried pepper samples had luteolin contents ranged from 0.01-0.42 mg/100 g DW. This compound had a strong anticancer activity [18,76,77].

Conclusion

The current study showed that aqueous extracts of Egyptian sweet and hot chilli pepper (in the dried form) at two maturity stages (green and red) have antioxidant and anticancer activities. The results observed that these extracts had high total phenolic and flavonoid contents and contain a wide range of phenolic and flavonoid compounds as well as organic acids. Pepper samples were also rich in vitamin C, β- carotene and vitamin E. Capsaicin, the major bioactive compound presented in pepper plants and responsible for the pungency of pepper, was found in these cultivars at high levels. Therefore, these extracts have antioxidant and anticancer activities against prostate and breast carcinoma cell lines. Treatment of the cancer cells with the aqueous extracts of pepper led to their growth inhibition and the induction of the apoptosis in cancer cells. It is apparent from our study that effective drugs produced from the Egyptian sweet and chilli pepper (Capsicum) tend to support a novel therapeutic methods for treatment of human prostate and breast malignancies.

Phytochemical Screening, Antioxidant Activities and In Vitro Anticancer Potential of Egyptian Capsicum Spp.

7

References

1. Wesolowska A, Jadczak D, Grzeszczuk M (2011) Chemical composition of the pepper fruit extracts of hot cultivars Capsicum annuum L. Acta Sci Pol Hortorum Cultus 10: 171-184.

2. Bae H, Jayaprakasha GK, Jifon J, Patil BS (2012) Variation of antioxidant activity and the levels of bioactive compounds in lipophilic and hydrophilic extracts from hot pepper (Capsicum spp.) cultivars. Food Chem 134: 1912-1918.

3. Ha SH, Kim JB, Park JS, Lee SW, Cho KJ (2007) A comparison of the carotenoid accumulation in Capsicum varieties that show different ripening colours: Deletion of the capsanthin–capsorubin synthase gene is not a prerequisite for the formation of a yellow pepper. J Exp Botany 58: 3135-3144.

4. García-Closas R, Berenguer A, José Tormo M, José Sánchez M, Quirós JR, et al. (2004) Dietary sources of vitamin C, vitamin E and specific carotenoids in Spain. Br J Nutr 91: 1005-1011.

5. Srinivas Ch, Sai Pavan Kumar ChN, China Raju B, Jayathirtha Rao V, Naidu VG, et al. (2009) First stereoselective total synthesis and anticancer activity of new amide alkaloids of roots of pepper. Bioorg Med Chem Lett 19: 5915-5918.

6. Conforti F, Statti AG, Menichini F (2007) Chemical and biological variability of hot pepper fruits (Capsicum annuum var. acuminatum L.) in relation to maturity stage. Food Chem 102: 1096-1104.

7. Oboh G, Ademiluyi AO, Faloye YM, (2011) Effect of combintion on the antioxidant and inhibitory properties of tropical pepper varieties against a-amylase and a-glucosidase activities in vitro. J Med Food 14: 1152-1158.

8. Menichini F, Tundis R, Bonesi M, Loizzo RM, Conforti F, et al. (2009) The influence of fruit ripening on the phytochemical content and biological activity of Capsicum chinense Jacq. cv Habanero. Food Chem 114: 553-560.

9. Ciz M, Cizova H, Denev P, Kratchanova M, Slavov A, et al. (2010) Different methods for control and comparison of the antioxidant properties of vegetables. Food Control 21: 518-523.

10. Aggarwal BB, Kunnumakkara AB, Harikumar KB, Tharakan ST, Sung B, et al. (2008) Potential of spice-derived phytochemicals for cancer prevention. Planta Med 74: 1560-1569.

11. Hwang JT, Lee YK, Shin JI, Park OJ (2009) Anti-inflammatory and anticarcinogenic effect of genistein alone or in combination with capsaicin in TPA-treated rat mammary glands or mammary cancer cell line. Ann N Y Acad Sci 1171: 415-420.

12. Matsufuji H, Nakamura H, Chino M, Takeda M (1998) Antioxidant activity of capsanthin and the fatty acid esters in paprika (Capsicum annuum). J Agric Food Chem 46: 3468-3472.

13. Anandakumar P, Kamaraj S, Jagan S, Ramakrishnan G, Vinodhkumar R, et al. (2008) Capsaicin modulates pulmonary antioxidant defense system during benzo(a)pyrene-induced lung cancer in swiss albino mice. Phytotherapy Res 22: 529-533.

14. Johnson JD (2009) Do carotenoids serve as transmembrane radical channels? Free Radic Biol Med 47: 321-323.

15. Loke WM, Proudfoot JM, Stewart S, McKinley AJ, Needs PW, et al. (2008) Metabolic transformation has a profound effect on anti-inflammatory activity of flavonoids such as quercetin: Lack of association between antioxidant and lipoxygenase inhibitory activity. Biochem Pharmacol 75: 1045-1053.

16. Surh YJ, Lee SS (1995) Capsaicin, a double-edged sword: toxicity, metabolism, and chemopreventive potential. Life Sci 56: 1845-1855.

17. Surh YJ, Lee SS (1996) Capsaicin in hot chili pepper: carcinogen, co-carcinogen or anticarcinogen? Food Chem Toxicol 34: 313-316.

18. Seelinger G, Merfort I, Wölfle U, Schempp CM (2008) Anti-carcinogenic effects of the flavonoid luteolin. Molecules 13: 2628-2651.

19. Hong H, Landauer MR, Foriska MA, Ledney GD (2006) Antibacterial activity of the soy isoflavone genistein. J Basic Microbiol 46: 329-335.

20. Alvarez-Parrilla E, de la Rosa LA, Amarowicz R, Shahidi F (2011) Antioxidant activity of fresh and processed Jalapeño and Serrano peppers. J Agric Food Chem 59: 163-173.

21. Hervert-Hernández D, Sáyago-Ayerdi SG, Gõni I (2010) Bioactive compounds of four hot pepper varieties (Capsicum annuum L.), antioxidant capacity, and intestinal bioaccessibility. J Agric Food Chem 58: 3399-3406.

22. Jeong WY, Jin JS, Cho YA, Lee JH, Park S, et al. (2011) Determination of polyphenols in three Capsicum annuum L. (bell pepper) varieties using high-performance liquid chromatography-tandem mass spectrometry: Their contribution to overall antioxidant and anticancer activity. J Separation Sci 34: 2967-2974.

23. Venier AN, Colquhoun JA, Fleshner EN, Klotz HL, Venkateswaran V (2012) Lycopene enhances the anti-proliferative and pro-apoptotic effects of capsaicin in prostate cancer in vitro. J Can Therapy Res 1: 1-9.

24. Bishop FL, Rea A, Lewith H, Chan YK, Saville J, et al. (2011) Complementary medicine use by men with prostate cancer: a systematic review of prevalence studies. Prostate Cancer Prostatic Diseases 14: 1-13.

25. Venier AN, Klotz HL, Fleshner NE Venkateswaran V (2010) Dietary Agents for Prostate Cancer Chemoprevention: An Overview. Curr Can Therapy Rev 6: 308-316.

26. Venkateswaran V, Klotz LH (2010) Diet and prostate cancer: mechanisms of action and implications for chemoprevention. Nat Rev Urol 7: 442-453.

27. Díaz -Laviada I (2010) Effect of capsaicin on prostate cancer cells. Future Oncol 6: 1545-1550.

28. Kim S, Moon A (2004) Capsaicin-induced apoptosis of H-ras-transformed human breast epithelial cells is Rac-dependent via ROS generation. Arch Pharm Res 27: 845-849.

29. Sánchez AM, Martínez-Botas J, Malagarie-Cazenave S, Olea N, Vara D, et al. (2008) Induction of the endoplasmic reticulum stress protein GADD153/CHOP by capsaicin in prostate PC-3 cells: a microarray study. Biochem Biophys Res Commun 372: 785-791.

30. Zhang R, Humphreys I, Sahu RP, Shi Y, Srivastava SK (2008) In vitro and in vivo induction of apoptosis by capsaicin in pancreatic cancer cells is mediated through ROS generation and mitochondrial death pathway. Apoptosis 13: 1465-1478.

31. Siegel R, Naishadham D, Jemal A (2012) Cancer statistics, 2012. CA Cancer J Clin 62: 10-29.

32. Walpole CSJ, Wrigglesworth R, Bevan S, Campbell EA, Dray A, et al. (1993) Analogues of capsaicin with agonist activity as novel analgesic agents: structure–activity studies. 1. The aromatic "A-region". J Med Chem 36: 2362-2372.

33. Walpole CSJ, Wrigglesworth R, Bevan S, Campbell EA, Dray A, et al. (1993) Analogues of capsaicin with agonist activity as novel analgesic agents: structure-activity studies. 2. The amide bond "B-region". J Med Chem 36: 2373-2380.

34. Walpole CSJ, Wrigglesworth R, Bevan S, Campbell EA, Dray A, et al. (1993) Analogues of capsaicin with agonist activity as novel analgesic agents: structure–activity studies. 3. The hydrophobic side-chain "C-region". J Med Chem 36: 2381-2389.

35. Maity R, Sharma J, Jana NR (2010) Capsaicin induces apoptosis through ubiquitin-proteasome system dysfunction. J Cell Biochem 109: 933-942.

36. Ito K, Nakazato T, Yamato K, Miyakawa Y, Yamada T, et al. (2004) Induction of apoptosis in leukemic cells by homovanillic acid derivative, capsaicin, through oxidative stress: implication of phosphorylation of p53 at Ser-15 residue by reactive oxygen species. Cancer Res 64: 1071-1078.

37. Wu CC, Lin JP, Yang JS, Chou ST, Chen SC, et al. (2006) Capsaicin induced cell cycle arrest and apoptosis in human esophagus epidermoid carcinoma CE 81T/VGH cells through the elevation of intracellular reactive oxygen species and Ca2+ productions and caspase-3 activation. Mutation Res 601: 71-82.

38. Kim JY, Kim EH, Kim SU, Kwon TK, Choi KS (2010) Capsaicin sensitizes malignant glioma cells to TRAIL-mediated apoptosis via DR5 up regulation and surviving downregulation. Carcinogenesis 31: 367-374.

39. Thoennissen NH, O'Kelly J, Lu D, Iwanski GB, La DT, et al. (2010) Capsaicin causes cell-cycle arrest and apoptosis in ER-positive and -negative breast cancer cells by modulating the EGFR/HER-2 pathway. Oncogene 29: 285-296.

40. Oh SH, Kim YS, Lim SC, Hou YF, Chang IY, et al. (2008) Dihydrocapsaicin (DHC), a saturated structural analog of capsaicin, induces autophagy in human cancer cells in a catalase-regulated manner. Autophagy 4: 1009-1019.

41. de-Sá-Júnior LP, Pasqualoto FMK, Ferreira KA, Tavares TM, Damião CM, et al. (2013) RPF101, a new capsaicin-like analogue, which disrupts the microtubule network accompanied by arrest in the G2/M phase, inducing apoptosis and mitotic catastrophe in the MCF-7 breast cancer cells. Toxicol Appl Pharmacol 266: 385-398.

42. Singleton VL, Rossi JA Jr (1965) Colorimetry of total phenolics with phosphomolybdic-phosphotungstic acid reagents. Am J Enol Viticult 16: 144-158.

43. Goupy P, Hugues M, Biovin P, Amiot MJ (1999) Antioxidant composition and activity of barely (Hordeum vulgare) and malt extracts and of isolated phenolic compounds. J Sci Food Agric 79: 1625-1634.

44. Harborne AJ (1998) Phytochemical methods a guide to modern techniques of plant analysis. 3ʳᵈ (Edn) Phytochemical methods 317: 60-65.

45. Mattila P, Astola J, Kumpulainen J (2000) Determination of flavonoids in plant material by HPLC with diode-array and electro-array detections. J Agric Food Chem 48: 5834-5841.

46. Blois MS (1958) Antioxidant determinations by the use of a stable free radical. Nature 181: 1199-1200.

47. Re R, Pellegrini N, Proteggente A, Pannala A, Yang M, et al. (1999) Antioxidant activity applying an improved ABTS radical cation decolorization assay. Free Radic Biol Med 26: 1231-1237.

48. Wodecki JZ, Torlop B, Slebioda M (1991) Chromatographic determination of citric acid for monitoring the mould process. J Chromatogr 558: 302-305.

49. Romeu-Nadal M, Morera-Pons S, Castellote AI, López-Sabater MC (2006) Rapid high-performance liquid chromatographic method for Vitamin C determination in human milk versus an enzymatic method. J Chromatogr B Analyt Technol Biomed Life Sci 830: 41-46.

50. Pupin MA, Dennis JM, Toledo FCM (1999) HPLC analysis of carotenoids in orange juice. Food Chem 64: 269-275.

51. Pyka A, Sliwiok J (2001) Chromatographic separation of tocopherols. J Chromatogr A 935: 71-76.

52. Collins DM, Wasmund ML, Bosland WP (1995) Improved Method for Quantifying Capsaicinoids in Capsicum Using High performance Liquid Chromatography. Hortsci 30: 137-139.

53. Skehan P, Storeng R, Scudiero D, Monks A, McMahon J, et al. (1990) New colorimetric cytotoxicity assay for anticancer-drug screening. J Natl Cancer Inst 82: 1107-1112.

54. Aliakbarlu J, Mohammad S, Khalili S (2014) A study on antioxidant potency and antibacterial activity of water extracts of some spices widely consumed in Iranian diet. J Food Biochem 38: 159-166.

55. Rodríguez-Maturino A, Valenzuela-Solorio A, Troncoso-Rojas R, González-Mendoza D, Grimaldo-Juarez O, et al. (2012) Antioxidant activity and bioactive compounds of Chiltepin (Capsicum annuum var. glabriusculum) and Habanero (Capsicum chinense): A comparative study. J Med Plants Res 6: 1758-1763.

56. Howard LR, Talcott ST, Brenes CH, Villalon B (2000) Changes in phytochemical and antioxidant activity of selected pepper cultivars (Capsicum species) as influenced by maturity. J Agric Food Chem 48: 1713-1720.

57. Ghasemnezhad M, Sherafati M, Payvast GA (2011) Variation in phenolic compounds, ascorbic acid and antioxidant activity of five coloured bell pepper (Capsicum annum) fruits at two different harvest times. J Functional Foods 3: 44-49.

58. Lin YJ, Tang YC (2007) Determination of total phenolic and flavonoid contents in selected fruits and vegetables, as well as their stimulatory effects on mouse splenocyte proliferation. Food Chem 101: 140-147.

59. Tundis R, Menichini F, Bonesi M, Conforti F, Statti G, et al. (2013) Antioxidant and hypoglycaemic activities and their relationship to phytochemicals in Capsicum annuum cultivars during fruit development. Food Sci Technol 53: 370-377.

60. Materska M, Perucka I (2005) Antioxidant activity of the main phenolic compounds isolated from hot pepper fruit (Capsicum annuum L). J Agric Food Chem 53: 1750-1756.

61. Perucka I, Materska M (2003) Antioxidant activity and content of capsaicinoids isolated from paprika fruits. Pol J Food Nut Sci 12/53: 15-18.

62. Serrano M, Zapata JP, Castillo S, Guillén F, Martínez-Romero D, et al. (2010) Antioxidant and nutritive constituents during sweet pepper development and ripening are enhanced by nitrophenolate treatments. Food Chem 118: 497-503.

63. Matsufuji H, Ishikawa K, Nunomura O, Chino M, Takeda M (2007) Antioxidant content of different coloured sweet peppers, white, green, yellow, orange and red (Capsicum annuum L.). Int J Food Sci Technol 42: 1482-1488.

64. Tripathi S, Mishra HN (2009) Nutritional changes in powdered red pepper upon in vitro infection of Aspergillus flavus. Braz J Microbiol 40: 139-144.

65. Lee SK, Kader AA (2000) Preharvest and postharvest factors influencing vitamin C content of horticultural crops. Postharvest Biol Technol 20: 207-220.

66. Mozafar A (1994) Plant vitamins: agronomic, physiological and nutritional aspects. Boca Raton, FL: CRC Press.

67. Simonne AH, Simonne EH, Eitenmiller RR, Mills HA, Green NR (1997) Ascorbic acid and provitamin A contents in unusually colored bell peppers (Capsicum annuum L.). J Food Composition Anal 10: 299-311.

68. Marín A, Ferreres F, Tomás-Barberán FA, Gil MI (2004) Characterization and quantitation of antioxidant constituents of sweet pepper (Capsicum annuum L.). J Agric Food Chem 52: 3861-3869.

69. Ozgur M, Ozcan T, Akpinar-Bayizit A, Yilmaz-Ersan L (2011) Functional compounds and antioxidant properties of dried green and red peppers. Afric J Agric Res 6: 5638-5644.

70. Isabelle M, Lee LB, Lim TM, Koh W, Huang D, et al. (2010) Antioxidant activity and profiles of common vegetables in Singapore. Food Chem 120: 993-1003.

71. Nair HK, Rao KV, Aalinkeel R, Mahajan S, Chawda R, et al. (2004) Inhibition of prostate cancer cell colony formation by the flavonoid quercetin correlates with modulation of specific regulatory genes. Clin Diagn Lab Immunol 11: 63-69.

72. Bell C, Hawthorne S (2008) Ellagic acid, pomegranate and prostate cancer-a mini review. J Pharm Pharmacol 60: 139-144.

73. Lewis JE, Soler- Vilá H, Clark PE, Kresty LA, Allen GO, et al. (2009) Intake of plant foods and associated nutrients in prostate cancer risk. Nutr Cancer 61: 216-224.

74. Atawodi SE (2011) Nigerian foodstuffs with prostate cancer chemopreventive polyphenols. Infect Agent Cancer 6 Suppl 2: S9.

75. Lim do Y, Jeong Y, Tyner AL, Park JH (2007) Induction of cell cycle arrest and apoptosis in HT-29 human colon cancer cells by the dietary compound luteolin. Am J Physiol Gastrointest Liver Physiol 292: G66-G75.

76. Lin Y, Shi R, Wang X, Shen HM (2008) Luteolin, a flavonoid with potential for cancer prevention and therapy. Curr Cancer Drug Targets 8: 634-646.

2

Apoptosis and Differentiation of K562 Cells by Targeting GST-O1 to Inhibit 4-HNE Metabolism

Kathryn Leake[1], Jyotsana Singhal[1], Sharad S Singhal[1] and Sanjay Awasthi[1,2*]

[1]Department of Diabetes, Endocrinology & Metabolism, California, USA
[2]Department of Medical Oncology and Experimental Therapeutics, City of Hope Comprehensive Cancer Center, Duarte, California, USA

Abstract

Bcr-Abl kinase inhibitors are very effective drugs for treatment of chronic myelogenous leukemia (CML), but treatment options are limited and relatively ineffective for patients with de-novo or acquired resistance. The K562 human erythroleukemia cell line, derived from a pleural effusion during blast crisis of a CML patient, is very useful for studying hematopoietic differentiation because it undergoes differentiation and apoptosis in response to chemicals that propagate lipid-peroxidation. 4-hydroxynonenal (4-HNE), a reactive aldehyde produced from peroxidation of polyunsaturated fatty acids, is metabolized primarily by glutathione S-transferases (GSTs). 4-HNE causes differentiation, apoptosis and necrosis in K562 cells, but cannot be used as a drug for resistant CML because of its highly toxic nature. Present studies addressed the possibility of developing an alternative targeted treatment aimed at increasing intracellular 4-HNE through inhibition of GST. Because the major GST-isoenzymes in leukemia cells are also present in normal tissues, we explored the possibility of modulating cellular 4-HNE levels by inhibiting GST isozymes with high activity towards 4-HNE. Our studies identified the presence of the GSTO1 isoenzyme in K562 cells, demonstrated its activity towards 4-HNE, and showed that its depletion causes apoptosis, necrosis and differentiation of these cells. These effects of GSTO1 depletion appear to involve RUNX1 mediated transcriptional regulation of GM-CSF. These findings offer a new target for treatment of resistant CML.

Keywords: K562; Chronic myelogenous leukemia; GST omega; GM-CSF; RUNX1; 4-HNE

Abbreviations: 4-HNE-4-hydroxynonenal; CML-chronic Myelogenous Leukemia; GM-CSF-Granulocyte Macrophage Colony Stimulating Factor; GSTO1-Glutathione S-Transferase Omega1; IL-3-Interleukin-3

Introduction

Bcr-Abl kinase inhibitors are very effective and non-toxic first line therapy for chronic myeloid leukemia (CML), but de-novo as well as acquired resistance occurs in 20-30% of patients for who therapeutic options are limited [1-3]. The K562 human erythroleukemia cell line, isolated during blast crisis from a patient with CML, undergoes erythroid and myeloid differentiation and apoptosis when treated with chemicals that exert oxidative stress and propagate lipid peroxidation [4]. A reactive α, β-unsaturated aldehyde, 4-hydroxy-t-2-nonenal (4-HNE), is quantitatively the major end-product of lipid-peroxidation of eicosanoid lipids. Though 4-HNE can be metabolized further by cytochromes p450, aldehyde dehydrogenases and aldehyde reductases, the quantitatively predominant metabolic pathway for its excretion is through the glutathione S-transferase (GST)-catalyzed formation of a thioether adduct with glutathione (GSH) followed by further metabolism to a mercapturic acid by the kidney [5-8]. GSTs are the rate-limiting enzyme of the mercapturic acid pathway and several GST-isoenzymes display differential catalytic activity against 4-HNE [8-11]. Because they metabolize numerous mutagenic compounds as well as chemotherapy drugs, GSTs play a major role in carcinogenesis and cancer drug-resistance [12-15]. In human CML, they play a role in genetic susceptibility and resistance to Bcr-Abl targeted therapy [16,17]. K562 cells express multiple GST isoenzymes and modulate cell growth and apoptosis in K562 cells [11,18,19]. 4-HNE mediated effects on K562 may be due to effects on several signaling kinases (JNK, MAPK, Akt), apoptotic proteins (Bax, Bcl2) and transcription factors (Myc, Mad, GATA-1, AP-1) are known to be involved with K562 differentiation indicating that multiple simultaneous mechanisms may be operative, but the relative contribution of each or the molecular mechanisms through which 4-HNE exerts these effects are not known [20-27].

Exogenous administration of 4-HNE is not suitable as a pharmacological therapy for treatment of resistant CML because it is quite toxic. However, modulating intracellular 4-HNE by targeting enzymes that metabolize it may be a reasonable approach to consider for patients with resistant CML, and the logical choice for targeted inhibition are the GSTs. We have previously reported that K562 cells contain two quantitatively predominant cytosolic GST isoenzymes belonging to the P- and M-classes.A third low-abundance isoenzyme with pI 5.8 was also identified and shown to be immunologically cross-reactive with alpha-class GSTs (GSTA) and displayed high specific activity towards 4-HNE, but its molecular identity could not be confirmed because of its low abundance [18]. The purpose of the present studies was to reexamine the GSTs of K562 cells to identify the previously observed 4-HNE metabolizing GST and to determine whether its targeted depletion could modulate intracellular 4-HNE levels to exert differentiating or pro-apoptotic effects on K562 cells.

Materials and Methods

Reagents

4-HNE (4-hydroxy-t-2-nonenal) was obtained from

---

*Corresponding author: Sanjay Awasthi, Department of Medical Oncology and Experimental Therapeutics, City of Hope Comprehensive Cancer Center, Duarte, California, E-mail: sawasthi@coh.org

Cayman Chemicals, Chicago, IL. MTT and CDNB (1-chloro-2, 4-dinitrobenzene) were procured from Sigma Chemical Co. Primary antibodies against Bax, Bcl2, JNK, pJNK, β-actin, Akt, pAkt, and cleaved PARP were purchased from Cell Signaling Technology, Inc. (Boston, MA). GSTO1 and AML1 (RUNX1) antibodies were purchased from Abcam (Cambridge, MA). Secondary antibodies goat anti-rabbit and goat anti-mouse were purchased from Cell Signaling Technology. The hGSTO1 siRNA CCUGAGUGGUUCUUUAAGAdTdT were synthesized by City of Hope Core facility, Duarte, CA. OxiSelect HNE Adduct ELISA kit was purchased from Cell Bio Labs, Inc (San Diego, CA).

Cell lines

The K562 erythroleukemia cells were obtained as frozen stock from the ATCC. The culture medium was RPMI1640 supplemented with 10% fetal bovine serum and 1% penicillin/ streptomycin; cells were grown in a 5% CO_2 humidified incubator at 37°C. After 5 medium exchanges over the first two weeks, aliquots of cells were frozen. These aliquots were subsequently thawed and used for each of the studies. Mycoplasma contamination was monitored at 4 week intervals by the Mycotect kit. Doubling time was measured to determine the interval of log-phase growth and drug-treatments were performed on cells in log phase growth at a starting density of 2×10^4 cells /well (96-well plate). Karyotyping was performed using standard methodology in the Cytogenetics Core at City of Hope. All experiments were done with cells in log-phase growth.

Transient transfection with small interfering RNA (siRNA)

In order to knockdown the endogenous GSTO1, transient transfection was performed using Lipofectamine RNAiMAX (Invitrogen). K562 cells were centrifuged at 400xg for 5 min and resuspended in RPMI 1640 medium with 10% FBS. Then, cells were transfected with GSTO1 or scrambled control siRNA (40 nM). After 24 h, Western Blots and RT-PCR were performed to check suppression of GSTO1 protein and mRNA, respectively.

MTT assay

The MTT assay was performed using 96-well plates with 8 replicates per drug concentration and repeated on 3 separate occasions. Cell viability was assessed using trypan-blue staining and initial viable cell density was 2×10^4 cells per well. Treatment with 4-HNE or GSTO1 siRNA was started 12 h after inoculation of cells into wells and MTT was added to wells after 24 h exposure to either 4-HNE or GSTO1 siRNA. The assay reagents and conditions were identical to those described previously [11] and plates were read 570 nm on a Bio-Tek ELx800 ELISA plate reader.

Morphological analysis of K562 differentiation

K562 cells were inoculated into 6-well plates at 2×10^4 cells /mL and treated with the differentiating agent or medium alone followed by 24 h incubation at 37°C prior to cytospin on L-lysine coated slides using a CytoPro centrifuge at 400 rpm for 5 min. Wright-Giemsa stained slides were examined using an Olympus AX70 microscope with photographs at 400x magnification by a hematopathologist blinded to the treatments.

Effect of 4-HNE on apoptosis by TUNEL assay

Six-well plates were inoculated with K562 cells (2×10^5 /mL) in log-phase growth and treated with 20 μM 4-HNE for 24 h at 37°C. Apoptosis was determined by the labeling of DNA fragments with terminal deoxynucleotidyl-transferase dUTP nick-end labeling (TUNEL) assay using Promega (Madison, WI) apoptosis detection system according to the manufacturer's protocol.

Chromatin immunoprecipitation assay

Cells were seeded in 100-mm plates at the density of 5×10^5/mL. Twenty four hours after 20 μM 4-HNE treatment, formaldehyde was added into culture media to a final concentration of 1% and the cells were incubated at room temperature for 10 min. SDS lysis buffer (1% SDS, 10 mM EDTA, 50 mM Tris, pH 8.0 and PMSF) was added to the cell pellet to isolate chromatin, and the lysates were sonicated to shear DNA to an average length of 200-500 base-pairs. Input was prepared by treating aliquots of chromatin with proteinase-K, and heating at 65°C for 6 h, followed by ethanol precipitation. Pellets were re-suspended, and the resulting DNA was quantified on a NanoDrop spectrophotometer. After overnight incubation with primary antibody (AML1/RUNX1 from Abcam) at 4°C, protein G agarose beads were added to isolate immune complexes. Complexes were washed and eluted from the beads with elution buffer (1% SDS and 0.1 M $NaHCO_3$). Cross-links were reversed by incubating at 65°C, and ChIP-DNA was purified by phenol-chloroform extraction and ethanol precipitation. PCR reactions were performed using specific primers with ChIP-bound and input DNA. Results were visualized on a 1.5% agarose gel.

Western blot analyses

K562 cells were treated with differentiating agents (4-HNE and/ or GSTO1 siRNA) for 24 h followed by homogenization using a Vibra-Cell-Sonics CV188 sonicator with 3s pulses×3 at 45W. Aliquots containing 30 μg were boiled with 4x NuPAGE loading sample buffer (Life Technologies) for 5 min, resolved by NuPAGE 4-12% Bis-Tris gel and transferred to a nitrocellulose membrane. Primary antibodies were against PARP, JNK, pJNK, AKT, pAKT, Bax, Bcl2, and GSTO1 at a dilution of 1:1000. The secondary antibodies were horseradish peroxidase conjugated anti-mouse or anti-rabbit goat, and blots were developed with SuperSignal West Femto Substrate (Thermo). The loading control was β-actin (Cell Signaling Technologies, Boston, MA).

Flow cytometry

4-HNE or GSTO1 siRNA treatment was performed on log-phase cells growing at a density (5×10^5 cells/mL) and flow-cytometry was performed after 24 h incubation at 37°C. FITC-anti-hemoglobin anti-hemoglobin antibodies were used to detect intracellular hemoglobin on ethanol fixed cell and cell-surface glycophorin was detected using FITC-anti-glycophorin antibodies (anti-CD235a) on live un-fixed cells. For cell cycle distribution, cells fixed in 70% ethanol, re-suspended in 500 μl of annexin binding buffer containing 2.5 μl of RNase (stock 20 mg/ml) at 37°C for 30 min after which they were treated with 10 μl of propidium iodide (stock 1 mg/ml) solution and then incubated at room temperature for 30 min in the dark. Dual Annexin-V and propidium iodide (PI) staining was performed on live un-fixed cells. Cells were washed once with PBS and resuspended in 400 μl of cold annexin binding buffer containing 5 μl of Annexin V-fluorescein isothiocyanate for 15 min and 5 μl of 0.1 mg/ml propidium iodide for 15 min in the dark. The stained cells were analyzed using the Beckman Coulter CyAn-ADP and results were processed using ModFit Lt and Summit 4.3 Software.

Mass spectroscopic analysis of purified total cytosolic GST fraction

Total cytosolic GSTs were purified using GSH-affinity chromatography. Purity was examined by Coomassie-stained SDS-PAGE and Western-blotting using antibodies to each GST-isoenzyme as described previously [28]. An aliquot containing 200 μg total purified GST protein was subjected to reduction and alkylation of cysteine using 2.5 mM dithiothreitol and 7 mM idoacetamide followed by trypsin digestion and solid phase extraction using a C_{18} cartridge (Supelco, Bellefonte, PA). The digested peptides were analyzed using reverse-phase liquid chromatography-tandem mass spectrometry analysis using a hybrid Linear ion trap (LTQ)–Fourier transform ion cyclotron resonance (FTICR, 7T) mass spectrometer (LTQFT; Thermo, San Jose, CA), which is equipped with nanospray ionization source and operated by X-Calibur [version 2.2] data acquisition software using protocols described previously [29]. Extracted ion chromatograms (areas under the corresponding chromatographic peaks) of isoform-specific doubly or triply charged tryptic peptides from the full-scan high-resolution mass spectra were then used as quantitative measures of respective GST isoenzyme expression levels.

Cloning and sequencing of hGSTO1 from K562 cells

Cells were treated with thymidine 2 mM for 24 h to synchronize them in G1/S. The homogenate was prepared by sonication of cells at 6 h after release from cell-cycle block for isolation of RNA. GSTO1 cDNA was amplified by PCR using GSTO1 specific forward primer (5'TATTTATCCATGGATGTCCGGGGAGTCA3') and reverse primer (5'GATAAATAAGTCGACTCAGAGCCCATAGTC3') (Biosynthesis, Lewisville, TX). Human GSTO1 cDNA was purified and cloned into T-Vector (Retrogen, Inc. San Diego, CA). The sequence of the putative GSTO1 clone was compared with the NCBI sequence (BioEdit Software, Ibis Biosciences, Carlsbad, CA) and structural and chemical similarities were compared (IBM Multiple Sequence Alignment Engine) between our pET30(a)+ vector BL21 cloned peptide and the published NCBI sequence. The hGSTO1 cDNA cleaved from T-Vector, using Nco1 and BamH1 restriction enzymes was ligated into pET30(a)+prokaryotic expression plasmid with the same restriction enzymes. The hGSTO1 cDNA from K562 in pET30(a)+vector was transfected into BL21 E.coli which were grown in bacterial culture and induced by IPTG to produce hGSTO1. GSTO1 protein was purified by GSH-affinity chromatography from the supernatant of the bacterial lysate. The identity of the purified protein was confirmed by mass-spectrometry.

Glutathione S-transferase activities and kinetics

For comparison of enzyme activity and kinetics of GST-isoenzymes towards 4-HNE as the substrate, we additionally cloned cDNA from GSTO1 (provided by Drs. Anneke Blackburn and Philip Board, John Curtain School of Medical Research, New South Wales, Australia), GSTO1 cloned from K562 cells, and other GST isoenzymes (GSTA1, GSTM1, and GSTP1, provided by Dr. Piotr Zimniak, UAMS, Little Rock, AR) into the pET30(a)+vector. The plasmid was expressed in E.coli-BL21 and the expressed proteins were purified by GSH-affinity chromatography. GST activity assays were performed using CDNB and 4-HNE as substrates spectrophotometrically [28].

Measurement of 4-HNE and total Lipid Hydroperoxides

Following treatment of 4-HNE or transfection with human GSTO1 siRNA or scrambled siRNA, K562 cells were harvested at 24 h and subjected to the 4-HNE adduct assay (OxiSelect HNE Adduct ELISA kit, Cell Bio Labs, Inc. San Diego, CA). The 4-HNE-adduct standard was previously prepared according to the manufacturer's instructions and a standard curve was generated to quantify HNE-adducts.

Quantitative Real-time PCR

Total RNA was isolated from cells using the RNeasy kit (Qiagen, Valencia, CA). The cDNA was prepared using the High Capacity cDNA Reverse Transcription Kit (Life Technologies). Real-time qPCR was performed on an ABI-7500 fast real time PCR system (Life Technologies) using Power SYBR Green master mix. The list of primer pairs used and their sequences are provided in supplemental Table 1. After initial incubation for 2 min at 50°C, the cDNA was denatured at 95°C for 10 min followed by 40 cycles of PCR (95°C for 15 s, 60°C for 60 s). The relative mRNA levels of all genes were quantified with β-actin as an internal control. Analysis of relative gene expression data using real-time quantitative PCR and the 2(-delta deltaC(T)) method.

Statistical analyses

Each experiment was repeated at least thrice to ensure reproducibility of the results. The statistical significance of differences between control and treatment groups was determined by ANOVA followed by multiple comparison tests. Differences were considered statistically significant when the p value was less than 0.05.

Results

Cytogenetic characterization of K562 leukemia cells

The K562 cell line differentiates primarily along the erythroid pathway, though there appears to be co-expression of some megakaryocytic markers consistent with lineage infidelity. To ensure that the behavior of our model system was consistent with prior literature on the subject, we performed karyotype analysis of K562

	M_r [kDA]	Km [mM]	Turnover Number K_{cat} [sec^{-1}]	Catalytic Efficiency [K_{cat}/K_m]
GSTα1	50	1.5	1700	1133
GSTμ1	52	1.1	3145	2859
GSTπ1	47	0.5	6815	13630
GSTO1	55	0.3	5133	17111

[a]Activities of purified GST isoenzymes towards 4-HNE were measured [59]. Values are means of four determinations; the relative standard deviation [where applicable] was less than 8% in all cases.

Table 1: Comparison of Kinetic Properties of GST isoenzymes towards 4-HNE[a]

Gene	Forward	Reverse
GST O1	AGGACGCGTCTAGTCCTGAA	CCAAGGATGGCACCTTAGAA
GM-CSF	TTCCCATGTGTGGCTGATAA	CTGTGTACTGGGCTCACTGG
IL3	CCCATCTCTCATCCTCCTTG	GGCGTCGGAAGGATCTTTAT
GST π	TGAATGACGGCGTGGAG	CCCTCACTGTTTCCCGTTGC
GST μ	GAACTCCCTGAAAAGCTAAAGC	CTTGGGCTCAAATATACGGTGG
CD235 (GYPA)	GAAGAGGAAACCGGAGAAAGG	GCTTTTCTTTATCAGTCGGCG
GAPDH	AAGGTGAAGGTCGGAGTCAA	AATGAAGGGGTCATTGATGG
AML1/ETO Fusion	CCACCTACCACAGAGCCATCA	AGCCTAGATTGCGTCTTCACATC

Supplementary Table 1: PCR primers

cells using G-banding. The modal chromosome number of 66, and multiple other chromosomal abnormalities were identical or similar to those seen in previous detailed karyotypic analyses of K562 cells [30] (Figure 1). Because of the unusual appearance of chromosome 8 was at variance with the reported karyotype, we could not rule out the possibility of t (8:21) a translocation most commonly seen in AML, but it has been previously reported due to clonal evolution in end-stage, treatment resistant CML in blast crisis [31]. It encodes the AML1-ETO (aka RUNX1-ETO) fusion protein, a defective transcription factor that cannot normally enhance the transcription of the differentiation promoting factors, GM-CSF and IL3 [32]. To investigate this possibility, we performed RT-PCR using primers bridging the breakpoints, and confirmed the expression of this fusion mRNA in the cell line used for present studies. Because 4-HNE has been implicated in the regulation of AML1 expression [33], we pursued these finding with additional studies on these differentiation factors, as discussed below

Erythroid differentiation of K562 upon 4-HNE exposure *in-vitro*

Wright-Giemsa stain of K562 cells treated with 0.5 to 20 μM 4-HNE showed a noticeable decrease in nuclear/cytoplasmic ratio and increased perinuclear eosinophilia characteristic of cytoplasmic hemoglobin accumulation in pronormoblasts that form during erythroid differentiation (indicated by arrows). This occurred at the lowest concentration of 4-HNE used and increased in a concentration-dependent manner. Nuclear fragmentation typical of necrosis was also evident at the high concentrations (Figures 2A and B). Erythroid differentiation was substantiated by flow-cytometric detection of cell-surface glycophorin expression in 4-HNE treated cells (Figure 2C). Increased accumulation of cellular 4-HNE was confirmed by ELISA assay for 4-HNE-protein adducts (Figure 3A). MTT assay showed a concentration dependent decrease in cell proliferation upon exposure to 4-HNE at concentrations between 1 and 20 μM (Figure 3B). The effector phase of apoptosis was also observed by TUNEL assay upon

treatment with 20 μM 4-HNE (Figure 3C). Determination of PARP-cleavage by Western-blot analysis confirmed the effector phase of apoptosis. The pro-apoptotic protein Bax was increased and the anti-apoptotic protein Bcl2 was decreased. The phosphorylation of JNK, a stress-activated kinase, was increased. Activation of AKT, a survival promoting kinase, was reduced upon 4-HNE treatment (Figure 3D). At 24 h after treatment with 4-HNE, the apoptotic population quantified by flow-cytometry using Annexin-V and PI staining was increased in a concentration dependent manner. Cell cycle analysis revealed that the G1 fraction decreased and G2 fraction increased in a concentration-dependent manner with respect to 4-HNE. A dose-dependent increase in cellular debris and naked nuclei (sub-G1 population) was also observed, indicating cell lysis and necrosis (Figures 4A and B).

GST isoenzymes of K562 cells

Total GSTs were purified from K562 cells using conventional GSH-affinity chromatography and Coomassie-stained SDS-PAGE showed the presence of three protein bands at 23, 26 and 27.5 kDA in this fraction. Western-blot analyses using isoenzyme-specific antibodies confirmed our previous findings, identifying that the 23 kDA band as GSTP and the 26 kDA band as GSTM. The 27.5 kDA was cross-reactive with antibodies towards GSTA, but was not recognized by antibodies against GSTA4, an alpha-class human GST isoenzyme with high activity towards 4-HNE. Sequencing of peptides in the total purified GST fraction by MS-MS confirmed the presence of GSTP and GSTM, and showed the presence of GSTO1. GSTO1 specific primers were used to clone full-length GSTO1 from K562 cells and its identity was confirmed by complete sequencing of the cDNA. A novel substitution mutation A140V was identified by DNA sequencing. The hGSTO1 cDNA was cloned into the pET30(a)+ prokaryotic expression plasmid. The GSTO1 clone from K562, the wild-type clones of GSTO1, GSTA1, GSTM1 and GSTP1 were expressed in *E.coli* BL21 and purified. In kinetic studies, the catalytic efficiency (K_{cat}/K_m) of the GSTO isoenzymes towards 4-HNE was greater than the other GST isoenzymes, and the A140V mutation did not affect the activity (Table 1).

Apoptosis and erythroid differentiation of K562 upon depletion of GSTO1

Transfection of GSTO1 siRNA (67 ± 11% transfection efficiency) significantly reduced GSTO1 mRNA (52 ± 7%, p<0.04) as measured by qRT-PCR. Western blot analysis confirmed the concomitant depletion of GSTO1 protein (Figure 5A). GSTP and GSTM mRNA quantified by qRT-PCR were unaffected by GSTO1 siRNA treatment. The expression of GM-CSF and IL3 was slightly, but significantly increased (p<0.05); in contrast, mRNA for the AML1-ETO fusion protein was remarkably decreased (Figures 5B and 6F). GSTO1 depletion caused erythroid differentiation in Wright-Giemsa stains and apoptosis in TUNEL assays. The degree of differentiation assessed by appearance of erythroid pronormoblasts (indicated by arrows) was less than seen with exogenously added 4-HNE (Figures 5C and 5D). Treatment of GSTO1 depleted cells with 4-HNE increased differentiation at 10 μM 4HNE, whereas apoptosis and necrosis predominated at 20 μM (Figures 5E and 5G) as compared with that seen with 4-HNE alone see Figure 2. The apoptotic population by TUNEL assay in cells treated with 20 μM 4-HNE without GSTO1 depletion (44 ± 6%, Figure 3C) was significantly lower than those with GSTO1 depletion (73 ± 9%, with 854 ± 68 cells counted, n=3, p<0.01). GSTO1 depletion also caused the appearance of cytoplasmic hemoglobin and cell-surface glycophorin by flow-cytometry (Figure 6A). MTT assay revealed a 35 ± 7% decrease in cell proliferation upon partial depletion of GSTO1 (Figure 6B). Depletion

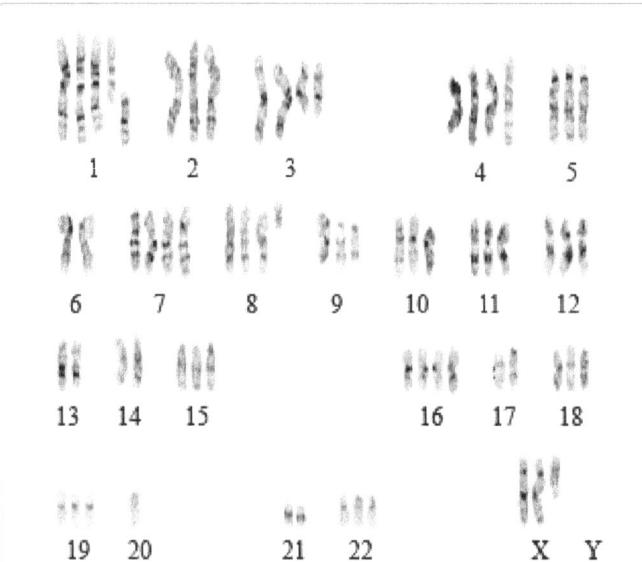

Figure 1: Karyotype of K562 cells The K562 karyotype exhibits tetraploidy in chromosomes 1, 4, 7 and 16. Triploid chromosomes included 2, 5, 8, 9, 10, 11, 12, 15, and 18. Partial additions occur on chromosomes 1, 3, 8, 22, and X while the only deletion occurs on chromosomes 20. Partial deletions are exhibited on chromosomes 21 and 22. The t(9:22) is apparent, however, it differs from typical t(9; 22) translocations in appearance.

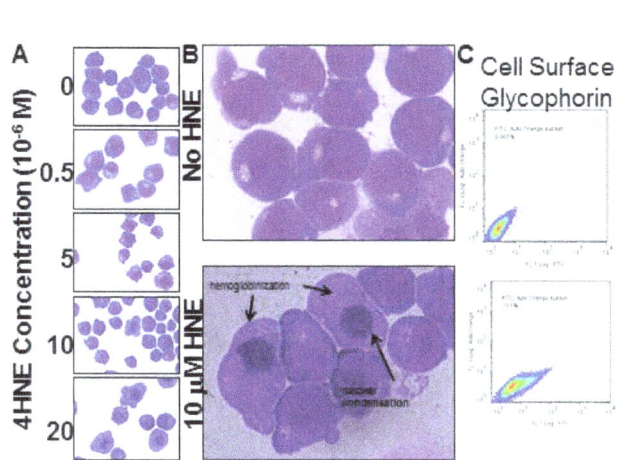

Figure 2: Exogenous addition of 4-HNE induces erythroid differentiation of K562 K562 cells were grown in RPMI 1640 medium and 4-HNE was added 24 h prior to preparation of slides for Wright-Giemsa staining of untreated control and 4-HNE treated cells (A). Higher magnification views are also presented with arrows indicating the appearance of cytoplasmic eosinophilia and nuclear condensation characteristic of erythroid differentiation (B) Flow-cytometric analysis of K562 cells for cell surface glycophorin expression using anti-CD235a antibodies was performed on cells 24 h after treatment with 20 µM 4-HNE. Flow cytometry was performed using a standard protocol in City of Hope Core facilities as described in Materials & Methods. The experiments were repeated three times and representative results are presented. The percent of cell expressing glycophorin were calculated from results of three separate experiments performed under identical conditions; standard deviations were <5%, and p<0.001 (C).

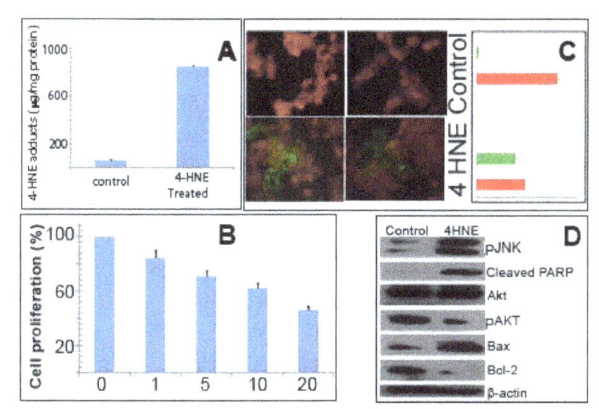

Figure 3: Effects of exogenous 4-HNE addition on K562 cells Total 4-HNE-adducts were measured in the 28,000×g supernatant of homogenate of K562 cells treated with 20 µM 4-HNE for 24 h prior to the assay (A). Cell survival was determined by an MTT assay at 24 h after treatment of cells with varying concentrations of 4-HNE as described in Materials and Methods (B). TUNEL assay was used for apoptosis determination using a Promega fluorescent detection. The percent of apoptotic cells were quantified by Image-J analysis (C). Determination of pJNK, cleaved PARP, AKT, pAKT, Bax, and Bcl2 were performed in Western-blots using commercially available antibodies (D).

4-HNE by the latter treatment.

Effect of 4-HNE on expression of AML1 target genes

The remarkable effects of GSTO1 depletion on the AML1-ETO fusion mRNA led us to examine whether 4-HNE treatment affected the binding of this factor to regulatory elements of GM-CSF and IL3. 4-HNE treatment increased GM-CSF protein (p<0.01) (Figure 6E); IL-3 protein was also increased slightly at the protein level, though the effect was not statistically significant (p<0.1, data not presented). A qRT-PCR analysis revealed that GM-CSF, IL3, and glycophorin (CD-235a) mRNA were increased significantly upon depletion of GSTO1 by siRNA (n=3, p<0.01) (Figure 6F). Since the AML1 transcriptionally regulates both GM-CSF and IL3, a CHiP assay was performed using anti-AML1 antibody for pull-down. Treatment with 4-HNE increased AML-1 (or AML1-ETO) binding to the upstream regulatory sequences of GM-CSF and IL3, though the effect on GM-CSF was greater. Because the precipitating antibodies were to AML1, it cannot be ascertained whether AML1 or the fusion protein were bound to the transcriptional regulatory elements. Control IgG did not pull down either GM-CSF or IL3 regulatory elements (Figure 6G).

Discussion

Results of our studies demonstrated 4-HNE causes concentration-dependent differentiation, apoptosis and necrosis of K562 cells. Our results demonstrated for the first time that these cells express a mutant GSTO1 at aa 140 (A140V), a site at which a different mutation (A140D) is associated with increased risk for pediatric acute lymphoblastic leukemia [60]. GSTO1 displayed high catalytic efficiency towards 4-HNE, unaffected by the mutation. The present results support prior studies showing that genetic instability can give rise to the t(8;21) translocation in cultured K562 cells in a manner similar to that seen in-vivo. Targeted depletion of GSTO1 increased cellular 4-HNE and caused differentiation, apoptosis and necrosis. Treatment with 4-HNE resulted in up-regulation of GM-CSF mRNA and protein, accompanied by down-regulation of the transcriptional repressor, AML1-ETO1. These studies provide new information to develop novel treatment strategies for treatment of resistant CML by targeting the mercapturic acid pathway, and indicate the need for more detailed examination of mechanisms of transcriptional regulation by 4-HNE.

Several lines of evidence supported the therapeutically relevant effects of 4-HNE. Differentiation was evident from cytological studies showing widely accepted cellular changes indicative of hematopoietic differentiation, from cytometric studies of glycophorin expression. These results strengthen our previous findings of increased hemoglobinization of K562 cells upon 4-HNE exposure, and the protective effect of transfection of cells with another 4-HNE metabolizing enzyme, GSTA4 [11]. 4-HNE induced apoptosis was also demonstrated through complementary approaches including cytology, MTT assay, TUNEL assay, flow-cytometry of PI/annexin-V stained cells, changes in cell cycling and accumulation of the sub-G1 population. Discrepancy in the extent of apoptosis between the TUNEL and flow-cytometric assays is characteristic of K562 and other cell types, and is dependent on drug-concentration and time of exposure [34,35]. The observed G2 arrest with 4-HNE in a manner similar to alkylating agent drugs suggests that the effects of 4-HNE may be due to DNA-alkylation [36]. The greater effect on apoptosis of exogenous 4HNE as compared with GSTO1 depletion may be due to an inherent difference in the two techniques for increasing cellular 4-HNE. Because the volume of culture medium is 'infinitely' larger than cell volume, addition of 4-HNE to the medium essentially provides an unlimited

of GSTO1 was accompanied by a 1.7 fold (p<0.01) increase in cellular 4-HNE-adducts (Figure 6C). Western-blot analysis of PARP-cleavage confirmed apoptosis caused by GSTO1 depletion; decreased pAKT, and increased Bax were also apparent (Figure 6D). The apoptotic and necrotic effects of GSTO1 depletion alone were less pronounced than with 20 µM HNE alone, consistent with a greater increase in cellular

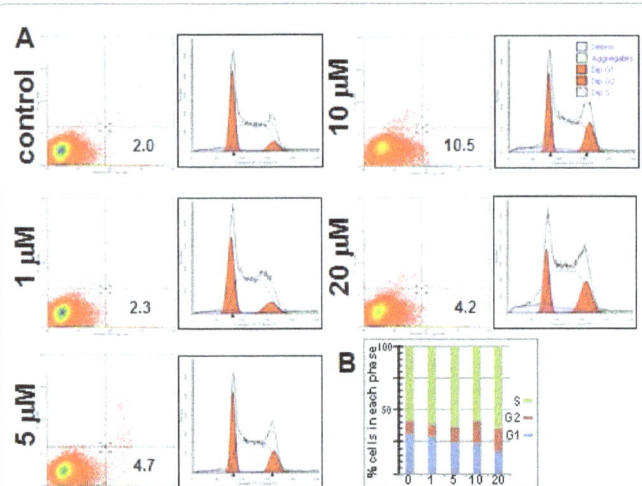

Figure 4: Effects of exogenous 4HNE addition on apoptosis and cell cycle by flow-cytometry For flow-cytometric assays, cell-cycle analyses were performed at 24 h after treating K562 cells with 1 to 20 μM 4-HNE and staining with Annexin V and propidium iodide (A) as described in Materials and Methods. Quantified cell-cycle phases are also presented (B).

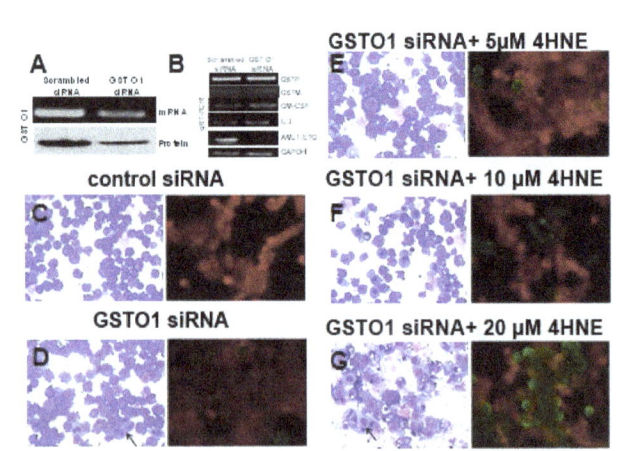

Figure 5: Effects of GSTO1 siRNA on GSTO1 depletion, cell morphology and apoptosis by TUNEL K562 cells were treated with GSTO1 siRNA or scrambled siRNA for 24 h prior to Western-blot (A) or RT-PCR assays (B). Commercially available specific anti-GSTO1 antibodies and secondary HRP-labeled antibodies were used for Western-blotting. RT-PCR analyses to quantify GSTO1, GSTM, GSTP, GM-CSG, IL3 and the AML1-ETO fusion gene mRNA were performed using specific primers. Wright-Giemsa stains and TUNEL assays were performed as described in Materials and Methods. Results for scrambled siRNA (C), GSTO1 siRNA (D) and GSTO1 siRNA without or with 5 μM (E), 10 μM (F), and 20 μM 4HNE (G) are presented. 4-HNE was added 24 h after siRNA and slides were prepared 24 h after addition of 4-HNE. All results presented are representative of three separate determinations.

supply of 4HNE resulting in greater overall exposure that can cause extensive protein and DNA cross-linking. In addition, the sub-cellular distribution of endogenously generated 4-HNE is dependent on differential production and metabolism of 4HNE in sub-cellular compartments; this cannot be replicated by exogenous 4-HNE inherently different biological effects are expected as seen in previous studies by others [37,38].

We considered the possibility that off-target effects of GSTO1

depletion by siRNA were responsible for the observed effects. Potential indirect effects unrelated to its GST activity, such as perhaps signaling or transcriptional changes that increase the oxidation of polyunsaturated fatty acids cannot be completely ruled out. A non-specific effect of siRNA is unlikely since the scrambled siRNA did not affect cellular 4-HNE, differentiation or apoptosis. Off target effects related to depletion of other GST isoenzymes are also unlikely because GSTO1 siRNA did not deplete GSTP or GSTM. Because there is no significant structural or sequence homology of GSTO1 with the only other 4-HNE metabolizing enzymes (cytochromes p450, aldehyde /aldose reductases or aldehyde dehydrogenases), it is very unlikely that increased cellular 4-HNE was due to a direct effect of the siRNA on these enzymes. The high catalytic efficiency of GSTO1 towards 4-HNE, the rise in cellular 4-HNE upon GSTO1 depletion, and the synergy between GSTO1 and exogenous 4-HNE also argue against the possibility that off-target effects are responsible for the observed apoptosis or differentiation.

4-HNE induces granulocytic maturation in the HL60 AML cell line known to express AML1. 4-HNE causes growth inhibition, apoptosis and necrosis in the CML-origin K562 erythroleukemia and increases surrogate markers of erythroid differentiation [20], but convincing morphological evidence for hematopoietic differentiation of K562 cells has not previously been presented. Unlike the differentiating effect in K562 cells, 4-HNE inhibits erythroid differentiation in non-malignant hematopoietic cells [39]. This indicates cell-dependent differential effect of 4-HNE and suggest a fundamentally opposite effect between normal and malignant erythroid cells, and could translate into a greater therapeutic index.

Because 4-HNE is not sufficiently reactive to directly initiate lipid-peroxidation, its actions are likely mediated through its alkylating activity towards signaling proteins and DNA. α,β-alkenal compounds such as 4-HNE directly bind DNA and modulate AP-1 [40,41], which in turn regulates the expression of GST, AML-1, IL-3, GM-CSF and β-hemoglobin. AP-1 and AML1 cooperate in hematopoietic differentiation by regulating the expression GM-CSF [24,41-46]. Our results indicated that 4-HNE regulates the expression of GM-CSF and IL3, associated with a remarkable down-regulation of the AML1-ETO fusion protein, through unknown mechanisms that require further investigation. Translocation involving AML1 are frequently seen in AML, a leukemia in which 4-HNE analogs have anticancer activity [47-49]. Though AML1 translocations are not seen in de-novo CML they are observed in drug-resistant CML during blast crisis. Thus GSTO1 targeting may be clinically applicable in drug-resistant CML for which there are few good options of therapy. Indeed, given the recently described role of GSTO1 in other malignancies, exploration of the implications of our findings in other cancer would also be of interest [48,49].

The potential therapeutic implications of our findings need to be considered in the wider context of targeting the mercapturic acid pathway for therapy of drug-resistant malignancy. The activity of the mercapturic acid pathway is frequently increased in treatment-resistant malignancy and this pathway plays a key role in the metabolism and excretion of 4-HNE and other pro-apoptotic electrophilic metabolites of lipid peroxidation. GST enzymes, the first committed step in the mercapturic acid pathway, catalyze the formation of thioether adducts of GSH with electrophiles such as 4-HNE. These GSH-electrophile adducts are removed from cells through energy dependent transport by membrane transporters such as RLIP76/RALBP1 prior to further metabolism to mercapturic acids by the kidney. A central role of RLIP76 in regulating cellular 4-HNE is clearly evident form studies that show marked increase in 4-HNE levels in tissues of RLIP76 knockout mice. Regression of multiple types of cancer with accompanying increase in cellular 4-HNE and lack of significant normal cell toxicity upon blocking RLIP76 strongly supports a key anti-apoptotic role of the mercapturic acid pathway in malignant cells and indicates that cancer cell-specific apoptosis is an inherent property of 4-HNE [50,51]. Its relevance in CML has also been demonstrated in studies showing apoptosis of K562 cells upon its blockade [52]. It is thus possible that combined targeting of GSTO1 and RLIP76 could be an even more effective therapy. Further investigations are needed to directly test this speculation.

In summary, our studies have demonstrated the expression of GSTO1 in a CML-derived cell line. Targeted depletion of GSTO1 increases cellular 4-HNE levels and causes differentiation, apoptosis and necrosis of K562 cells in a manner similar to that observed with exogenous treatment with 4-HNE. Modulation of intracellular 4-HNE by specific depletion of 4-HNE could be of clinical relevance in treatment of drug-resistant CML.

Acknowledgements

These studies were supported by NIH grant CA77495 to SA. The authors wish to thank Dr. Xiangle Sun (University of North Texas Health Science Center, Fort Worth, TX, Microscopy Facility) as well as Dr. Brian Armstrong, Ms. Mariko Lee, and Professor Ivan Todorov for help in microscopy (City of Hope). The authors also wish to thank the City of Hope Cytogenetics Core for karyotype assistance and the Analytical Cytometry Core for help in performing flow-cytometry and the Mass Spectrometry Facility at University of North Texas Health Science Center, Fort Worth, TX. KL also wishes to acknowledge her parents Beverly and James Leake, who courageously battled cancer and inspired her, and especially her husband Mr. Robert Bair, Jr., who has always been supportive.

Author Contributions

KL was the principal contributor in formulating the hypothesis, search and interpretation of literature, experimental protocol design and execution, and manuscript preparation. She was aided in performance of experiments by JS and SSS. SA is the senior author who personally supervised and advised KL in design and conduct of experiments, data analysis and manuscript preparation. KL and SA were aided by SSS in data collection, analysis, and manuscript preparation.

References

1. Druker BJ, Talpaz M, Resta DJ, Peng B, Buchdunger E, et al. (2001) Efficacy and safety of a specific inhibitor of the BCR-ABL tyrosine kinase in chronic myeloid leukemia. N Engl J Med 344: 1031-1037.

2. Gibbons DL, Pricl S, Posocco P, Laurini E, Fermeglia M, et al. (2014) Molecular dynamics reveal BCR-ABL1 polymutants as a unique mechanism of resistance to PAN-BCR-ABL1 kinase inhibitor therapy. Proc Natl Acad Sci USA 111: 3550-3555.

3. Brehme M, Hantschel O, Colinge J, Kaupe I, Planyavsky M, et al. (2009) Charting the molecular network of the drug target Bcr-Abl. Proc Natl Acad Sci USA 106: 7414-7419.

4. Rowley PT, Ohlsson-Wilhelm BM, Farley BA, LaBella S (1981) Inducers of erythroid differentiation in K562 human leukemia cells. Exp Hematol 9: 32-37.

5. Esterbauer H, Schaur RJ, Zollner H (1991) Chemistry and biochemistry of 4-hydroxynonenal, malonaldehyde and related aldehydes. Free Radic Biol Med 11: 81-128.

6. Petras T, Siems WG, Grune T (1995) 4-hydroxynonenal is degraded to mercapturic acid conjugate in rat kidney. Free Radic Biol Med 19: 685-688.

7. Guéraud F, Alary J, Costet P, Debrauwer L, Dolo L, et al. (1999) In vivo involvement of cytochrome P450 4A family in the oxidative metabolism of the lipid peroxidation product trans-4-hydroxy-2-nonenal, using PPARalpha-deficient mice. J Lipid Res 40: 152-159.

8. Habig WH, Pabst MJ, Jakoby WB (1974) Glutathione S-transferases. The first enzymatic step in mercapturic acid formation. J Biol Chem 249: 7130-7139.

9. Awasthi YC, Sharma R, Singhal SS (1994) Human glutathione S-transferases. Int J Biochem 26: 295-308.

10. Sharma R, Yang Y, Sharma A, Awasthi S, Awasthi YC (2004) Antioxidant role of glutathione S-transferases: protection against oxidant toxicity and regulation of stress-mediated apoptosis. Antioxid Redox Signal 6: 289-300.

11. Cheng JZ, Singhal SS, Saini M, Singhal J, Piper JT, et al. (1999) Effects of mGST A4 transfection on 4-hydroxynonenal-mediated apoptosis and differentiation of K562 human erythroleukemia cells. Arch Biochem Biophys 372: 29-36.

12. Jakoby WB (1978) The glutathione S-transferases: a group of multifunctional detoxification proteins. Adv Enzymol Relat Areas Mol Biol 46: 383-414.

13. Ruzza P, Rosato A, Rossi CR, Floreani M, Quintieri L (2009) Glutathione transferases as targets for cancer therapy. Anticancer Agents Med Chem 9: 763-777.

14. Di Pietro G, Magno LA, Rios-Santos F (2010) Glutathione S-transferases: an overview in cancer research. Expert Opin Drug Metab Toxicol 6: 153-170.

15. Tew KD, Townsend DM (2012) Glutathione-s-transferases as determinants of cell survival and death. Antioxid Redox Signal 17: 1728-1737.

16. He HR, Zhang XX, Sun JY, Hu SS, Ma Y, et al. (2014) Glutathione S-transferase gene polymorphisms and susceptibility to chronic myeloid leukemia. Tumour Biol 35: 6119-6125.

17. Kassogue Y, Quachouh M, Dehbi H, Quessar A, Benchekroun S, et al. (2014) Effect of interaction of glutathione S-transferases (T1 and M1) on the hematologic and cytogenetic responses in chronic myeloid leukemia patients treated with imatinib. Med Oncol 31: 47.

18. Schnekenburger M, Morceau F, Duvoix A, Delhalle S, Trentesaux C, et al. (2003) Expression of glutathione S-transferase P1-1 in differentiating K562: role of GATA-1. Biochem Biophys Res Commun 311: 815-821.

19. Singhal SS, Piper TT, Saini MK, Awasthi YC, Awasthi S (1999) Comparison of glutathione S-transferase isoenzymes in human leukemia K562, HL60 and U-937 cells. Biochem Arch. 15: 163-176.

20. Barrera G, Pizzimenti S, Dianzani MU (2004) 4-hydroxynonenal and regulation of cell cycle: effects on the pRb/E2F pathway. Free Radic Biol Med 37: 597-606.

21. Fazio VM, Barrera G, Martinotti S, Farace MG, Giglioni B, et al. (1992) 4-Hydroxynonenal, a product of cellular lipid peroxidation, which modulates c-myc and globin gene expression in K562 erythroleukemic cells. Cancer Res 52: 4866-4871.

22. Pizzimenti S, Barrera G, Calzavara E, Mirandola L, Toaldo C, et al. (2008) Down-regulation of Notch1 expression is involved in HL-60 cell growth inhibition induced by 4-hydroxynonenal, a product of lipid peroxidation. Med Chem 4: 551-557.

23. Pizzimenti S, Menegatti E, Berardi D, Toaldo C, Pettazzoni P, et al. (2010) 4-hydroxynonenal, a lipid peroxidation product of dietary polyunsaturated fatty acids, has anticarcinogenic properties in colon carcinoma cell lines through the inhibition of telomerase activity. J Nutr Biochem 21: 818-826.

24. Kutuk O, Basaga H (2007) Apoptosis signalling by 4-hydroxynonenal: a role for JNK-c-Jun/AP-1 pathway. Redox Rep 12: 30-34.

25. Lin MH, Yen JH, Weng CY, Wang L, Ha CL, et al. (2014) Lipid peroxidation end product 4-hydroxy-trans-2-nonenal triggers unfolded protein response and heme oxygenase-1 expression in PC12 cells: Roles of ROS and MAPK pathways. Toxicology 315: 24-37.

26. Ji GR, Yu NC, Xue X, Li ZG (2014) 4-Hydroxy-2-nonenal induces apoptosis by inhibiting AKT signaling in human osteosarcoma cells. ScientificWorldJournal 2014: 873525.

27. Sharma R, Sharma A, Chaudhary P, Pearce V, Vatsyayan R, et al. (2010) Role of lipid peroxidation in cellular responses to D,L-sulforaphane, a promising cancer chemopreventive agent. Biochemistry 49: 3191-3202.

28. Singhal SS, Saxena M, Ahmad H, Awasthi S, Haque AK, et al. (1992) Glutathione S-transferases of human lung: characterization and evaluation of the protective role of the alpha-class isozymes against lipid peroxidation. Arch Biochem Biophys 299: 232-241.

29. Prokai L, Stevens SM Jr, Rauniyar N, Nguyen V (2009) Rapid label-free identification of estrogen-induced differential protein expression in vivo from mouse brain and uterine tissue. J Proteome Res 8: 3862-3871.

30. Naumann S, Reutzel D, Speicher M, Decker HJ (2001) Complete karyotype characterization of the K562 cell line by combined application of G-banding, multiplex-fluorescence in situ hybridization, fluorescence in situ hybridization, and comparative genomic hybridization. Leuk Res 25: 313-322.

31. Schafhausen P, Dierlamm J, Bokemeyer C, Bruemmendorf TH, Bacher U, et al. (2009) Development of AML with t(8;21)(q22;q22) and RUNX1-RUNX1T1 fusion following Philadelphia-negative clonal evolution during treatment of CML with Imatinib. Cancer genetics cytogenetics. 189:63-67.

32. Bakshi R, Hassan MQ, Pratap J, Lian JB, Montecino MA, et al. (2010) The human SWI/SNF complex associates with RUNX1 to control transcription of hematopoietic target genes. J Cell Physiol 225: 569-576.

33. Jacobs AT, Marnett LJ (2009) HSF1-mediated BAG3 expression attenuates apoptosis in 4-hydroxynonenal-treated colon cancer cells via stabilization of anti-apoptotic Bcl-2 proteins. J Biol Chem 284: 9176-9183.

34. Walker JA, Quirke P (2001) Viewing apoptosis through a 'TUNEL'. J Pathol 195: 275-276.

35. Taatjes DJ, Sobel BE, Budd RC (2008) Morphological and cytochemical determination of cell death by apoptosis. Histochem Cell Biol 129: 33-43.

36. O'Brien V, Brown R (2006) Signalling cell cycle arrest and cell death through the MMR System. Carcinogenesis 27: 682-692.

37. Esterbauer H, Zollner H, Lang J (1985) Metabolism of the lipid peroxidation product 4-hydroxynonenal by isolated hepatocytes and by liver cytosolic fractions. Biochem J 228: 363-373.

38. Koster JF, Slee RG, Montfoort A, Lang J, Esterbauer H (1986) Comparison of the inactivation of microsomal glucose-6-phosphatase by in situ lipid peroxidation-derived 4-hydroxynonenal and exogenous 4-hydroxynonenal. Free Radic Res Commun 1: 273-287.

39. Skorokhod OA, Caione L, Marrocco T, Migliardi G, Barrera V, et al. (2010) Inhibition of erythropoiesis in malaria anemia: role of hemozoin and hemozoin-generated 4-hydroxynonenal. Blood 116: 4328-4337.

40. Minko IG, Kozekov ID, Harris TM, Rizzo CJ, Lloyd RS, Stone MP (2009) Chemistry and biology of DNA containing 1,N(2)-deoxyguanosine adducts of the alpha,beta-unsaturated aldehydes acrolein, crotonaldehyde, and 4-hydroxynonenal. Chem Res Toxicol. 22:759-758.

41. Camandola S, Scavazza A, Leonarduzzi G, Biasi F, Chiarpotto E, et al. (1997) Biogenic 4-hydroxy-2-nonenal activates transcription factor AP-1 but not NF-kappa B in cells of the macrophage lineage. Biofactors 6: 173-179.

42. Adunyah SE, Unlap TM, Wagner F, Kraft AS (1991) Regulation of c-jun expression and AP-1 enhancer activity by granulocyte-macrophage colony-stimulating factor. J Biol Chem 266: 5670-5675.

43. Park JH, Kaushansky K, Levitt L (1993) Transcriptional regulation of interleukin 3 (IL3) in primary human T lymphocytes. Role of AP-1- and octamer-binding proteins in control of IL3 gene expression. J Biol Chem 268: 6299-6308.

44. Duvoix A, Schnekenburger M, Delhalle S, Blasius R, Borde-Chiché P, et al. (2004) Expression of glutathione S-transferase P1-1 in leukemic cells is regulated by inducible AP-1 binding. Cancer Lett 216: 207-219.

45. Wang CY, Bassuk AG, Boise LH, Thompson CB, Bravo R, Leiden JM (1994) Activation of the granulocyte-macrophage colony-stimulating factor promoter in T cells requires cooperative binding of Elf-1 and AP-1 transcription factors. Mol Cell Biol. 14:1153-1159.

46. Quash G, Fournet G (2009) Methionine-derived metabolites in apoptosis: therapeutic opportunities for inhibitors of their metabolism in chemoresistant cancer cells. Curr Med Chem 16: 3686-3700.

47. Hassane DC, Guzman ML, Corbett C, Li X, Abboud R, et al. (2008) Discovery of agents that eradicate leukemia stem cells using an in silico screen of public gene expression data. Blood 111: 5654-5662.

48. Masoudi M, Saadat I, Omidvari S, Saadat M (2009) Genetic polymorphisms of GSTO2, GSTM1, and GSTT1 and risk of gastric cancer. Mol Biol Rep 36: 781-784.

49. Chung CJ, Pu YS, Su CT, Huang CY, Hsueh YM (2011) Gene polymorphisms of glutathione S-transferase omega 1 and 2, urinary arsenic methylation profile and urothelial carcinoma. Sci Total Environ 409: 465-470.

50. Awasthi S, Singhal SS, Yadav S, Singhal J, Drake K, et al. (2005) RLIP76 is a major determinant of radiation sensitivity. Cancer Res 65: 6022-6028.

51. Singhal SS, Wickramarachchi D, Yadav S, Singhal J, Leake K, et al. (2011) Glutathione-conjugate transport by RLIP76 is required for clathrin-dependent endocytosis and chemical carcinogenesis. Mol Cancer Ther 10: 16-28.

52. Yang Y, Cheng J, Singhal SS, Sharma A, Saini M, et al. (2001) Role of glutathione S-transferases in protection against lipid peroxidation: I. Overexpression of hGSTA2-2 in K562 cells protects against hydrogen peroxide induced apoptosis and inhibits JNK and caspase-3 activation. J Biol Chem. 276:19220-19230.

3

A Simplified Method for Measuring Secreted Invertase Activity in *Saccharomyces cerevisiae*

Harkness Troy AA* and Arnason Terra G#

*Departments of Anatomy and Cell Biology, and #College of Medicine, University of Saskatchewan, Saskatoon, Canada

Abstract

The measurement of sucrose hydrolysis to glucose and fructose in yeast is valuable for many aspects of yeast cell biology and metabolic analysis, and has been used extensively to understand the genetics of the SNF1 kinase. However, a simple and rapid method describing how to perform this assay for new users is lacking. Here, we review various methods used to measure invertase activity. We focus on a method based on a colorimetric assay that was first described by Goldstein and Lampen in 1975. Our report not only describes a simple and rapid application of this method to measure secreted invertase enzymatic activity from yeast whole cells for new users, but also establishes optimized times for assay conditions. The method utilizes a small volume of yeast culture in which the entire procedure can be performed in less than an hour. Very few reports offer a step-by-step method that can be readily used without prior knowledge of the procedure, providing the impetus for this report. The optimizations described in this report allow increased sensitivity when comparing subtle changes.

Keywords: Yeast; *SUC2*, Invertase; SNF1 kinase; Assay method

Introduction

The yeast external invertase enzyme exists as a dimer that can associate to form octamers [1]. Invertase converts the disaccharide sucrose into glucose and fructose [2]. Under conditions of low glucose, yeast cells express invertase as an attempt to use alternative carbon sources. The invertase enzyme is encoded by the *SUC2* gene, which produces two types of invertase enzymes, one that is glycosylated and secreted into the periplasmic space, and one that in not glycosylated and maintained within the cytosol [3,4]. The cytosolic form is expressed at low constitutive levels, whereas the periplasmic invertase is strictly regulated by glucose repression. The periplasmic localized invertase requires up to 3 hours for maximum activity when depressed, which then decreases slowly and is associated with a gradual release of invertase into the growth medium [5].

Under normal laboratory conditions yeast are grown in 2% glucose-supplemented media, where *SUC2* expression is actively repressed by the glucose activated transcriptional repressor Mig1 [6]. Low levels of glucose (0.014-0.067%), but not alternative carbon sources (such as galactose and glycerol), specifically activate *SUC2* expression [7]. Under these conditions, Mig1 repression is lifted by SNF1 kinase phosphorylation [8,9]. When glucose concentrations are high (2% for example) the SNF1 kinase is inactive and maintained in the cytosol, but under low glucose conditions becomes phosphorylated and transported into the nucleus, and other cellular compartments. Once active, SNF1 kinase phosphorylates a host of cellular factors that work to resist stress, and leads to the use of alternative carbon sources. The most studied of these targets is Mig1. Phosphorylation of Mig1 by SNF1 kinase leads to export of Mig1 from the nucleus, activation of *SUC2*, and expression of invertase. Sucrose in the media can then be converted to glucose and fructose. In fact, the SNF1 kinase complex was first identified as a sucrose non-fermentable mutant [10].

The study of invertase activity has been extensively used over the past 90 years to measure glucose in foods and various organisms, and more recently to assess SNF1 kinase activity. The invertase assay measures the amount of glucose converted from sucrose from yeast cells grown under activating (low glucose) or repressing (high glucose). This has been a powerful assay that has yielded valuable information about the genetics of SNF1 kinase function. Methods used to measure invertase activity have relied on the analysis of reducing sugars by spectrophotometry of colored reactions using dinitrosalicylic acid [11-14], or o-dianisidine [15], enzyme assay kits [16], polarimetry [17] (discussed in 13), HPLC [18], in-gel assays [10,19] and ultrasonic techniques [2]. Many recent reports that utilize the invertase assay refer to work based on spectrophotometric measurement of colored reactions using o-dianisidine at OD_{540} [20]. A recent report described measuring invertase activity [20] from invertase fused to the C-terminal 21 amino acids of the GPI (glycosylphosphatidylinositol) transamidase (GPI-T), which anchored the invertase enzyme to the plasma membrane [21]. Cells from this study were grown in media supplemented with 1% fructose (depressing conditions) for 36 hours. Methods have also been described where invertase activity is measured via preparation of cell lysates using glass beads [22]. However, a detailed simple and rapid protocol for performing the yeast invertase assay for new users is lacking. The purpose of this report is to provide a detailed and simple protocol for conducting the yeast invertase assay using whole cells and spectrophotometric measurement of product.

Materials and Methods

Strains, media, reagents and general methods

Strains used in this study were based on the S288c genetic background. The *mig1Δ* and *snf1Δ* mutants were described previously [23]. Cells were grown in YP media (1% yeast extract; 2% peptone) supplemented with 2% glucose for repressing conditions, or 0.05%

*Corresponding author: Harkness Troy AA, Department of Anatomy and Cell Biology, University of Saskatchewan, B313 Health Sciences Building, 107 Wiggins Road, Saskatoon, SK S7N 5E5, Canada
E-mail: troy.harkness@usask.ca

glucose for activating conditions. Glucose oxidase was purchased from Calbiochem, peroxidase, type I, from horseradish, was purchased from SIGMA, and o-dianisidine was obtained from Alfa Aesar. Westerns were performed according to our standard protocols [24].

Cell Preparation

Cells from a single yeast colony were used to inoculate 15 ml overnight YPD (2%) cultures (see Supplementary Materials for protocol). Plates were generally 2% YPD containing 2% agar. Typically, after 16 hours of growth at 30°C, the cells were at an optical density (OD) of 0.1 - 0.3, read at a wavelength of 600 nm (OD_{600}). It is important to start the experiment when the cells are in the early phase of log growth, as the *SUC2* gene is induced as glucose is depleted within the culture. Once the cells are at the appropriate OD, 1×10^6 cells are removed to assess invertase activity under repressed conditions. Cell concentrations were calculated using an OD_{600} of 1.0, which is roughly equivalent to 2×10^7 cells/ml. The remaining cells were then harvested and resuspended at an OD_{600} of 0.2 - 0.3 in YPD (0.05%). This condition is considered activating for *SUC2* expression and invertase activity. However, others have used 0.1% glucose for activating conditions, as well as 5% glucose for repressing conditions [22]. The cells were then incubated at 30°C for 2 hours. For 37°C experiments, the cells were incubated in 2% YPD at 37°C for 2 hours prior to addition of prewarmed 0.05% YPD. Cells were then harvested, resuspended in 0.05% YPD and incubated at 37°C for 2 hours. Following growth in activating conditions, 1×10^6 cells were removed to assess invertase activity. For time course studies, once the cells were resuspended in 0.05% YPD, 1×10^6 cells were removed every 20 minutes for 2 hours to assess invertase activity. Invertase activity in 2% glucose cultures prior to harvesting is considered time zero. Each aliquot of 1×10^6 cells was centrifuged washed 2 times with 200 µl sterile H_2O, then kept on ice until all samples were prepared. The pellets from 1×10^6 cells are small, so care must be taken to ensure the cell pellet is not pipetted away. Washing the cells in 10 mM Na Azide has been described [25], and this seems to result in a tighter cell pellet, which is easier to work with. When performing protein analyses in parallel with the invertase assay (such as for Western analysis), cultures were used that accommodated 5 - 10 ml of culture/protein lysate. We used the following formula to determine the amount of 2×SDS buffer (20% glycerol; 2% β-mercaptoethanol; 4% SDS; 0.13 M Tris pH 6.8; and 6.65 mg/100 ml Bromophenol Blue) to use when resuspending cell pellets, when preparing protein lysates: 2X SDS (µl) = OD_{600} × volume of cells used × 10. Once the cells were resuspended in 2×SDS buffer, the cells were boiled for 5 minutes, centrifuged and kept frozen at –20°C until needed.

Invertase Assay

Once the cells were washed 2 times with either sterile water or 10 mM Na Azide, the cell pellets were left on ice until needed. It is easiest to wash the cells directly after harvesting rather than at the end when many samples have accumulated. It is also more manageable to wash less than 10 samples at a time, as cell pellets loosen while awaiting pipeting. To start the reaction, all samples were resuspended in 50 µL 50 mM Na Acetate pH 5.1. Controls prepared for every assay were: a) cells without sucrose, b) no cells plus sucrose, and tubes containing c) 250 and d) 500 µM glucose (prepared from a 1 mM stock solution). Each control was brought to 50 µl with H_2O (c and d) or 50 mM NaAc (a and b). The controls were carried through the remainder of the assay. Next, 12.5 µl 0.5 M sucrose was added to all samples, except controls a, c and d, where 12.5 µl H2O was added. To ensure consistent start times, sucrose was added to the side of the eppendorf and then mixed when

ready to start the assay. Immediately following addition of sucrose, the tubes were incubated at 37°C. The reaction becomes saturated after 10 minutes of incubation, so incubation times longer than 10 minutes will not accurately reflect the µM Glucose converted/min in this reaction. Therefore, after 10 minutes at 37°C, stop the reaction by adding 75 µl of 0.2 M K_2HPO_4. The samples were then put on ice for 1 minute, boiled for 3 minutes and placed on ice again for 1 minute. Samples remained on ice at this point while additional samples were being treated. To begin the color reaction, 500 µl of the assay mix was added. The assay mix is made fresh by adding 50 µl of 5000 U/ml glucose oxidase, 62.5 µl 1 mg/ml peroxidase and 375 µl 10 mg/ml o-dianiside (suspend o-dianiside in 95% ethanol in a fume hood, as this is a toxic substance, and wrap in tin foil when stored at 4°C) into 25 ml 0.1 M potassium phosphate buffered to pH 7.0. The assay mix is wrapped in tin foil, stored at 4°C, and made fresh every week. The samples are then incubated at 37°C for 20 to 30 minutes. However, we find that this reaction is saturated after 10 minutes. In our hands, the invertase reaction is most sensitive when the sucrose to glucose conversion occurs for 10 minutes, followed by a 10-15 minute color reaction. Following the color conversion incubation, 500 µl 6 N HCl was added to develop the color. At this point, the reaction is complete and stable for a number of days at room temperature. The amount of sucrose converted to glucose is measured at OD_{540} after cellular debris has been pelleted. Control a (containing cells without sucrose; see above for control description) is used to zero the measurements. We find that the reading is saturated by anything greater than 500 µM glucose. Diluting the samples 20 fold (50 µl into 1 ml) into a 1:1 mixture of assay buffer:6 N HCl allows a more accurate measurement of the developed pink color. The amount of glucose converted is calculated by dividing the OD_{540} reading of the sample by the OD_{540} reading for 250 µM glucose (control c). This number is multiplied by 250 to give the total µM glucose converted and then divided by the time of the reactions (10 minutes in our hands). Invertase activity is given as µM glucose converted/minute/106 cells, as the number of cells assayed is 1×10^6. The formula is: (OD_{540} sample/ OD_{540} control c) ×(250/reaction time).

Results and Discussion

The invertase activity measured in this assay is predominantly the activity of the inducible enzyme that is secreted into the periplasmic space [4]. The invertase assay reported here is based on a protocol first described in 1975 [20] and used by many labs, but adequate description of the method for first time users is lacking. The assay essentially contains 3 keys steps: 1) cell preparation, 2) conversion of sucrose to glucose and fructose by the secreted invertase enzyme, and 3) quantitative measurement of the glucose produced. The number of cells used in the assay, the time required for the conversion of sucrose to glucose, and time for glucose measurement were optimized in this report for use in our laboratory. We found that measurement of 1×10^6 cells (100 µl of a culture at OD_{600} 0.5 will yield approximately 1×10^6 cells) produced values that approached the limit of the linear range of the experiment (Figure 1). Increasing the cell number to 1.5×10^6 or higher do not increase the amount of glucose measured. Using this assay to measure glucose production in repressed and depressed *mig1Δ* and *snf1Δ* mutants confirmed that the assay is correctly measuring Snf1 kinase activity at the *SUC2* promoter (Figure 2). The experiments in Figures 1 and 2 were performed with sucrose to glucose conversion time of 15 minutes and color development time of 30 minutes. When we optimized these conditions, we found that a sucrose to glucose conversion time of 10 minutes (Figure 3), and a color development time of 10-15 minutes was optimum (Figure 4), which differs from

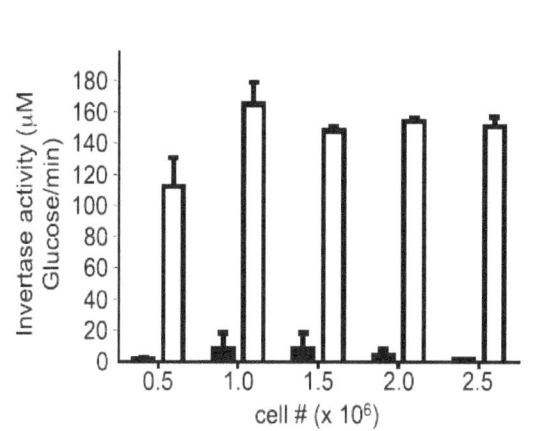

Figure 1: Invertase activity requires a maximum of 1 x 10⁶ cells for optimum measurements. WT yeast cells were grown overnight at 30°C to early log phase in 2% glucose. For the 2% glucose measurements, the number of cells indicated, based on OD_{600} readings, where an OD_{600} of 1 approximately equals 2 x 10⁷ cells/ml, were removed for invertase activity measurements. To measure invertase activity in 0.05% glucose (derepressed conditions), the cells were then centrifuged and resuspended in 0.05% glucose supplemented media. After 2 hours, the indicated cells were removed and again tested for invertase activity. The average of 2 experiments, with standard error is shown. The graphing and statistical program Prism 6.0 was used to analyze all data.

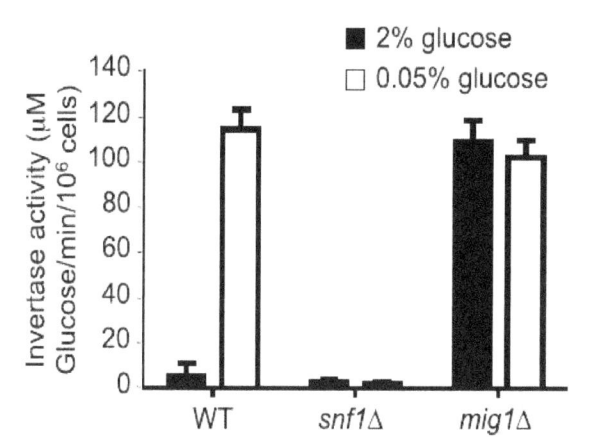

Figure 2: Cells deleted for SNF1 exhibit background invertase activity, whereas cells lacking *MIG1* are constitutively active. The invertase assay was conducted on the cells shown (WT, n=11; *snf1Δ*, n=5; *mig1Δ*, n=4), as described in Figure 1, with 1 x 10⁶ cells measured. The conversion of sucrose to glucose and fructose was stopped after 15 minutes and the color reaction proceeded for 30 minutes. Prism 6.0 was used for the analysis.

the reaction times commonly described in the literature (15 minutes for the sucrose to glucose conversion and 30 minutes for the color development). Furthermore, we found that the conversion of sucrose to glucose is most rapid at the beginning of the reaction and slows down over time (Figure 3B). It is therefore important to be accurate and consistent when performing the sucrose to glucose conversion reaction. We find that our reported incubation times provide the most sensitive results.

We tested invertase activity in wild type cells expressing endogenously TAP-tagged *MIG1* grown at 30°C and 37°C. The cells were grown overnight in YPD 2% glucose at 30°C. The next morning, when 20 ml cell cultures were in early log phase, the cells were split and

incubated at 30°C and 37°C in YPD 2%. After 2 hours, samples were taken for invertase activity measurement (1×10⁶ cells). Samples were also removed for protein lysate preparation (5 ml). The remaining cells were washed and resuspended in 0.05% glucose, and again incubated at 30°C and 37°C. After 2 hours, samples were removed for invertase activity determination and protein lysate preparation. Figure 5A shows that temperature has little effect on invertase activity after 2 hours in derepressing conditions. Western analyses using antibodies against phosphorylated mammalian AMPK, which recognizes phosphorylated yeast Snf1, shows that Snf1 is activated after growth in 0.05% glucose at both 30°C and 37°C. Likewise, antibodies that recognize the TAP epitope show that Mig1-TAP is also phosphorylated when grown in 0.05% glucose irrespective of temperature. In *snf1Δ* cells, as expected, there was no detectable signal from the phospho AMPK α antibody, no Mig1 phosphorylation and no invertase activity (Figure 5A). To take a more defined view of invertase activity at elevated temperatures, we conducted a time course, as previously described (Figure 5B) [22]. Our results demonstrate that shifting the temperature of the experiment to 37°C does not impact the assay. Although many studies have shown that yeast cells have a faster growth rate and a higher rate of glucose consumption when shifted from 28°C to 37°C [26-28], this does not influence the activation of the invertase enzyme. Nonetheless, the time course approach to analyzing invertase activity provides greater detail than the single time point approach demonstrated in Figures 4 and 5A.

Several other parameters should also be considered when measuring invertase activation. For example, while using cells in early logarithmic growth ensures higher glucose concentrations for repressed conditions, cells in later stages of growth, such as stationary phase, have thicker cell walls which may retain the invertase enzyme and block access to its substrate [29]. It also appears that sugars that derepress *SUC2* expression, such as inositol, may continue to do so even in the presence of concentrations of glucose (0.2%) that would normally repress its expression [30]. It was suggested that phosphatidylinositol (PI) may be involved in glucose derepression of secreted invertase activity. Furthermore, while it has been shown that deletion of *MIG1* allows expression of *SUC2* even in the presence of glucose, deletion of a gene encoding another transcription factor, *GCR1* (Glycolysis Regulation), which binds to the *SUC2* promoter, also renders *SUC2* transcription unresponsive to glucose [31]. Thus, expression of *SUC2* is regulated by

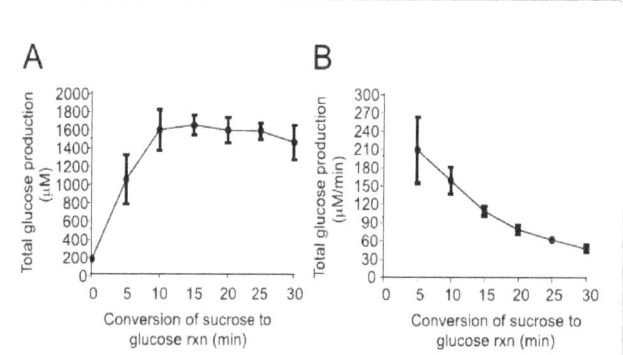

Figure 3: Optimization of the sucrose to glucose conversion reaction. A. The conversion of sucrose to glucose and fructose is saturated after 10 minutes. Wild type cells were treated as in Figure 1, except multiple samples of 1 x 10⁶ cells were evaluated for invertase activity after increasing sucrose to glucose and fructose conversion times. The experiment was repeated 3 times. Standard error of the mean is shown. B. The total glucose produced for each reaction was divided by the time of the reaction to provide glucose production/min. The conversion rate slows over time.

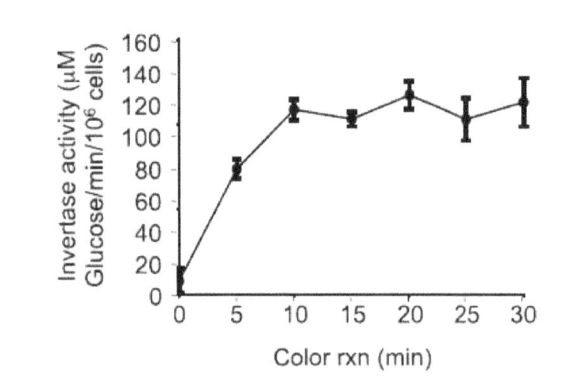

Figure 4: Optimization of the color development reaction. The color reaction is saturated after 10 minutes. Wild type cells were treated as in Figure 3, except multiple samples of 1 x 10⁶ cells were evaluated for invertase activity after increasing color development times. The experiment was repeated 3 separate times and analyzed using Prism 6.0.

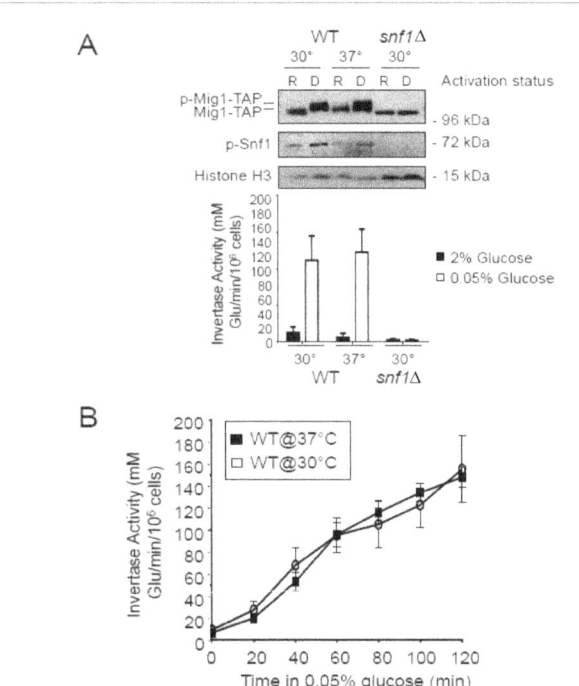

Figure 5: The influence of temperature shifts on the invertase reaction. A. Wild type and snf1Δ cells expressing an endogenously TAP-tagged *MIG1* allele were grown overnight to early log phase, at which time they were split with continued incubation at 30°C and 37°C. Samples were recovered for invertase measurements under repressed conditions. 10 ml samples were grown in order to isolate proteins (5 ml/sample) from cells under repressed and derepressed conditions. After 2 hours in repressing conditions, the cells were centrifuged and resuspended in 0.05% glucose media to activate the secreted invertase enzyme. After 2 hours, samples were removed for invertase measurements and protein purification (5 ml). For the inveratse experiments, WT at 30°C was performed 11 times, WT at 37°C was performed 7 times, and the snf1Δ experiment was repeated 5 times. Protein samples were analyzed by Western blotting with antibodies against TAP, phosphorylated Snf1 (mammalian phosphoAMPKα) and histone H3 as a load control. R represents repressed, while D represents derepressed samples. B. An invertase activity timecourse was conducted by removing 1 x 10⁶ cells every 20 minutes for 2 hours once the WT cells were switched to derepressing conditions at 30°C and 37°C. The 30°C timecourse was performed 6 times and the 37°C timecourse was repeated 5 times. As above, all data was analyzed using Prism 6.0.

a complex network of glucose responsive pathways.

This report describes a thorough step-by-step approach for determining activity of the invertase enzyme encoded by *SUC2* within the yeast genome. There are few such reports available in the literature, thereby allowing a researcher new to the field to rapidly conduct this experiment and obtain reproducible values.

Acknowledgements

This work was supported by Natural Science and Engineering Research Council (NSERC) grants to TAAH and TGA, and a New Investigator infrastructure grant from the Canadian Foundation for Innovation (CFI) to TAAH. Liubov Lobanova is acknowledged for assistance with statistical analyses. The authors declare no conflicts of interest.

References

1. Chu FK, Watorek W, Maley F (1983) Factors affecting the oligomeric structure of yeast external invertase. Arch Biochem Biophys 223: 543-555.

2. Resa P, Elvira L, Sierra C, Espinosa FM (2009) Ultrasonic velocity assay of extracellular invertase in living yeasts. Anal Biochem 384: 68-73.

3. Perlman D, Halvorson HO (1981) Distinct repressible mRNAs for cytoplasmic and secreted yeast invertase are encoded by a single gene. Cell 25: 525-536.

4. Carlson M, Botstein D (1982) Two differentially regulated mRNAs with different 5' ends encode secreted with intracellular forms of yeast invertase. Cell 28: 145-154.

5. Marten MR, Seo JH (1989) Localization of cloned invertase in Saccharomyces cerevisiae directed by the SUC2 and MFalpha1 signal sequences. Biotechnol Bioeng 34: 1133-1139.

6. Nehlin JO, Ronne H (1990) Yeast MIG1 repressor is related to the mammalian early growth response and Wilms' tumour finger proteins. EMBO J 9: 2891-2898.

7. Ozcan S, Vallier LG, Flick JS, Carlson M, Johnston M (1997) Expression of the SUC2 gene of Saccharomyces cerevisiae is induced by low levels of glucose. Yeast 13: 127-137.

8. Hedbacker K, Carlson M (2008) SNF1/AMPK pathways in yeast. Front Biosci 13: 2408-2420.

9. Zaman S, Lippman SI, Zhao X, Broach JR (2008) How Saccharomyces responds to nutrients. Annu Rev Genet 42: 27-81.

10. Carlson M, Osmond BC, Botstein D (1981) Mutants of yeast defective in sucrose utilization. Genetics 98: 25-40.

11. Sumner JB (1921) Dinitrosalicylic acid: a reagent for the estimation of sugar in normal and diabetic urine. J Biol Chem 47: 5-9.

12. Sumner JB (1925) More specific reagent for the determination of sugar in urine. J Biol Chem 65: 393-395.

13. Sumner JB, Howell SF (1935) A Method for determination of saccharase activity. J Biol Chem 108: 51-54.

14. Lee J (1954) A quick and simple method for blood-sugar estimation. Br Med J 2: 1087-1088.

15. Huggett AS, Nixon DA (1957) Use of glucose oxidase, peroxidase, and O-dianisidine in determination of blood and urinary glucose. Lancet 273: 368-370.

16. Bergmeyer H (1974) Abbreviations for Chemical and Biochemical Compounds. Methods of Enzymatic Analysis. Academic Press, New York 450-451.

17. Vosburgh WC (1921) The optical rotation of mixtures of sucrose, glucose and fructose. J Am Chem Soc 43: 219–232.

18. Tammi M, Ballou L, Taylor A, Ballou CE (1987) Effect of glycosylation on yeast invertase oligomer stability. J Biol Chem 262: 4395-4401.

19. Gabriel O, Wang SF (1969) Determination of enzymatic activity in polyacrylamide gels. I. Enzymes catalyzing the conversion of nonreducing substrates to reducing products. Anal Biochem 27: 545-554.

20. Goldstein A, Lampen JO (1975) Beta-D-fructofuranoside fructohydrolase from yeast. Methods Enzymol 42: 504-511.

21. Morissette R, Varma Y, Hendrickson TL (2012) Defining the boundaries of species specificity for the Saccharomyces cerevisiae glycosylphosphatidylinositol transamidase using a quantitative in vivo assay. Biosci Rep 32: 577-586.

22. Weiss P, Huppert S, Kölling R (2008) ESCRT-III protein Snf7 mediates high-level expression of the SUC2 gene via the Rim101 pathway. Eukaryot Cell 7: 1888-1894.

23. Harkness TA, Shea KA, Legrand C, Brahmania M, Davies GF (2004) A functional analysis reveals dependence on the anaphase-promoting complex for prolonged life span in yeast. Genetics 168: 759-774.

24. Postnikoff SD, Malo ME, Wong B, Harkness TA (2012) The yeast forkhead transcription factors fkh1 and fkh2 regulate lifespan and stress response together with the anaphase-promoting complex. PLoS Genet 8: e1002583.

25. Celenza JL, Carlson M (1984) Cloning and genetic mapping of SNF1, a gene required for expression of glucose-repressible genes in Saccharomyces cerevisiae. Mol Cell Biol 4: 49-53.

26. Jones RC, Hough JS (1970) The effect of temperature on the metabolism of baker's yeast growing on continuous culture. J Gen Microbiol 60: 107-116.

27. Postmus J, Canelas AB, Bouwman J, Bakker BM, van Gulik W, et al. (2008) Quantitative analysis of the high temperature-induced glycolytic flux increase in Saccharomyces cerevisiae reveals dominant metabolic regulation. J Biol Chem 283: 23524-23532.

28. Mensonides F, Brul S, Hellingwerf KJ, Bakker BM, Teixeira de Mattos MJ (2014) A kinetic model of catabolic adaptation and protein reprofiling in Saccharomyces cerevisiae during temperature shifts. FEBS J 281: 825-841.

29. Shi L, Li Z, Tachikawa H, Gao XD, Nakanishi H (2014) Use of yeast spores for microencapsulation of enzymes. Appl Environ Microbiol 80: 4502-4510.

30. Chi Z, Ma L, Gao L, Duan X (2007) Added inositol regulates invertase secretion and glucose-repressed SUC2 gene expression in Saccharomyces sp. W4. Indian J Biochem Biophys 44: 152-156.

31. Türkel S, Turgut T, López MC, Uemura H, Baker HV (2003) Mutations in GCR1 affect SUC2 gene expression in Saccharomyces cerevisiae. Mol Genet Genomics 268: 825-831.

4

Assessment of the Breast Milk Triglyceride, Protein and its Influencing Factors in Tehran, Iran

Hoda Boushehri[1], Shahnaz Khaghani[1*], Hossein Mirmiranpour[1], Sedigheh Shams[2] and Mohammad Zangooei[3]

[1]Department of Biochemistry, Tehran University of Medical Sciences, Tehran, Iran
[2]Medicine Department, Pathology division, Tehran University of Medical Sciences, Tehran, Iran
[3]Department of Biochemistry, Tehran University of Medical Sciences, Tehran, Iran

Abstract

Introduction: The composition of human milk is the biologic norm for infant nutrition. Human milk also contains many hundreds to thousands of distinct bioactive molecules that protect against infection and inflammation and contribute to immune maturation, organ development, and healthy microbial colonization.

Methods: 433 and 216 mothers were selected from Tehran southern and northern health care centers. The mother's diet was measured by a 24 hour diet history questionnaire for the past 3 days. All breast milk samples were frozen in plastic containers and stored immediately at −20°C until analysis. The samples were centrifuged at 3000 g for 15 minutes and the superficial fat layer was separated. Breast milk protein was measured by the Lowry method. Breast milk Triglyceride was measured by the triglyceride colorimetric assay kit.

Results: The breast milk triglyceride and protein by mother's age by age, mother's occupation and mother's diet were mentioned in the tables.

Discussion: These findings suggest that milk composition is more sensitive to maternal factors such as age, weight, height, occupation, education and mother's diet. The assessment between mother's diet carbohydrate and protein between two groups showed a significant difference, statistically (P = 0.001 and P = 0.000) and also between the breast milk protein between two groups showed a significant difference, statistically (P = 0.028). The assessment between the mother's diet fat in two groups was not significant (P = 0.069) and also the assessment of the breast milk triglyceride between the two groups did not show a significant difference (P = 0.258).

Conclusion: There was a significant difference between the mother's diet in the two groups and help us to change breast feeding malnourished mother's diet and convert it into a normal diet.

Keywords: Breast milk; Macronutrient; Protein; Triglyceride

Introduction

The composition of human milk is the biologic norm for infant nutrition. Human milk also contains many hundreds to thousands of distinct bioactive molecules that protect against infection and inflammation and contribute to immune maturation, organ development, and healthy microbial colonization. The phenomenon of nutrition in early life having lifetime effects on growth, metabolism and health has been termed "nutritional programming" and has been defined as a long-term change in the structure or function of an organism resulting from a stimulus acting at a critical period of development in early life [1]. International agencies and various US health organizations uniformly recommend breastfeeding as the preferred method of infant feeding for the entire first year of life and thereafter as long as is beneficial to the mother and infant. The effect of nutritional status of mothers on the quality and quantity of their milk is a frequent topic of discussion. The composition of human milk can be affected by the diet consumed by the lactating woman. The influence of the maternal diet on milk composition varies in magnitude between nutrients; for some nutrients no effect at all has yet been documented [2,3]. It has been proposed that poor intrauterine growth not only contributes to increased morbidity and mortality during infancy, but also that it has the potential to compromise adult health and well-being. These recommendations are based on knowledge that term infants nursed by nutritionally adequate mothers are provided with sufficient energy and the proper profile of nutrients to support normal growth and development without any additional foods through the first 4 to 6 months of life. After 6 months, complimentary foods are needed to furnish nutrients likely to become limiting. Also human milk furnishes an array of non-nutrient growth factors, immune factors, hormones and other bioactive components that can act as biological signals and confer protection against illness in infancy and later in life.

This phenomenon occurs when immaturity in tissues and organs involved in nutrient metabolism (i.e., the gastrointestinal tract, liver, and kidneys) limits the ability of an infant to respond to excesses or deficiencies in nutrient intakes. Human milk is species specific, and many of the nutrients it contains are secreted as bound components that can offer protection from digestion and facilitate absorption and utilization. The macronutrient composition of human milk varies within mothers and across lactation but is remarkably conserved across populations despite variations in maternal nutritional status. Lipids in comparison with the other nutrients of human milk have the greatest within and between sample variability. Studies on humans have shown the effect of maternal diet and anthropometric status on total milk fat content. The objectives of this study were to determine the possible relationship of breast milk fat content with maternal nutritional status.

*****Corresponding author:** Shahnaz Khaghani, Associate Professor of Biochemistry, Department of Biochemistry, Tehran University of Medical Sciences, Tehran, Iran, Poursina St, PO Box - 14155-6447, Tehran, Iran, E-mail: shahnaz_khaghani@yahoo.com

The mean macronutrient composition of mature, term milk is estimated to be approximately 0.9 to 1.2 g/dL for protein, 3.2 to 3.6 g/dL for fat, and 6.7 to 7.8 g/dL for lactose, 6.5-8% carbohydrates, 0.1-0.2% of electrolytes and the rest is water. Energy estimates range from 65 to 70 kcal/dL and are highly correlated with the fat content of human milk. A study examined the association between maternal characteristics and the composition of human milk macronutrient and found that after 4 months postpartum, the macronutrient concentrations of human milk are associated with one or more of the following factors: Maternal body weight for height, protein intake, parity, return of menstruation and nursing frequency [4].

Women who receive even a minimal basic education are generally more aware than those who are illiterate of the need to utilize available resources for the improvement of the health (particularly the nutritional status) of themselves and their families. In areas where cultural and religious beliefs seriously affect the mother's intake of food and or nutrients, every educational effort should be made to overcome these adverse practices. Special consideration must be given to ensure that intra-familial food distribution safeguards the mother's nutritional status.

Although maternal factors such as diet and body composition are plausible influences on this variation, most studies find weak or modest associations between maternal characteristics and the nutrient composition of the mother's milk. For instance, milk macronutrient composition appears to be largely independent of maternal diet and anthropometric measures of maternal body composition have inconsistent associations with milk composition. Milk protein is usually independent of body composition while the majority of studies report a modest association between body composition and milk fat, sugar, and total energy.

Associations between body fat and milk fat, if present, are usually positive, whereas milk sugar and maternal adiposity typically show an inverse relationship. Milk composition has also been shown to change over the course of lactation.

For the hypothesis, considering the significance of breast feeding, recognition of breast milk biochemical composition and their influencing factors is very important [5].

Information from such research will suggest strategies for nutrition intervention in areas of poor nutrition and provide dietary guidelines for lactating women [6-10].

The present study was performed to determine how and to what extent maternal nutritional status can be related to the breast milk amount and concentration of breast milk triglyceride and protein and produced by mothers of moderate to low socio-economic class and the changes in milk production.

The purpose of this article is to provide information for health care to guide the mothers.

The study protocol was approved by the Ethics Committee of Tehran University of Medical Science. All subjects were made aware of the content of the study and on agreeing to participate; a written informed consent document was obtained.

Materials and Methods

Subjects

The randomized sampling is easy and available. As shown in previous studies, the mean of protein in breast milk was 3.7 ± 1.3 g / 100 ml. 650 samples are sufficient for predicting of mean of protein in breast milk, confident interval %95 and accuracy 0.1, as done by the following formula:

$$N = (\delta^2 Z_{\alpha/2}^2)/d^2$$

(δ = 1, d = %1.5 = α, as the proportion of the population in the south to the north is about 2/1, so 433 and 216 mothers were selected from Tehran southern and northern health care centers, respectively.

Milk collection and analysis

Socio-economic data (working status), demographic data and clinical data (health status) were obtained through an interview. All breast milk samples were frozen in plastic containers and stored immediately at –20°C until analysis [11-15]. The samples were centrifuged at 3000 g for 15 minutes and the superficial fat layer was separated because high level of fat is an obstacle in accurate measurement [16,17]. Breast milk protein was measured by the Lowry method [13]. Breast milk triglyceride was measured by the triglyceride colorimetric assay kit. The assay is initiated with the enzymatic hydrolysis of the triglycerides by lipase to produce glycerol and free fatty acids. The glycerol released is subsequently measured by a coupled enzymatic reaction system with a colorimetric readout at 540 nm [14]. Information on mother's diet was collected by using a 24-hour recall method for 3 days (one week-end day included). Dietary intake of subjects was analyzed by Nutritionist III software programmer [18,19].

Statistical analysis

Data for the human milk are presented as mean and standard deviation. One way ANOVA was applied to find differences between triglyceride and protein concentrations in two groups. The correlation between other factors (Mother's age, mother's occupation and mother's diet) and triglyceride and protein concentrations in human milk was shown as Pearson's correlation coefficient. All statistical analyses were done using STATISTICA 10.0.

Results

Table 1 showed the breast milk triglyceride and protein in Tehran northern and southern health care centers. The breast milk triglyceride in northern was higher (499.68 ± 251.07 mg / 100 ml vs. 466.77 ± 205.33 mg / 100 ml) than southern but the assessment of the breast milk triglyceride did not show a significant difference between the two groups (P = 0.258).

The breast milk protein in southern was higher (0.99 ± 0.45 g / 100 ml vs. 0.87 ± 0.41 g / 100 ml) than northern and there was a significant difference between the two groups, statistically (P = 0.028). The breast milk protein in northern was less than RDA recommendations (0.9 to 1.2 g/dL).

Tables 2-4 showed the breast milk triglyceride and protein by age, occupation and mother's diet in Tehran northern and southern health care centers.

Discussion

These findings suggest that milk composition is more sensitive to maternal factors diet in the first few months. Assessment of the breast milk biochemical compositions and its influencing factors such as age, weight, height, occupation, education and mother's diet between two Tehran northern and southern health care centers showed that the greatest part of mothers in northern (42.5%) and southern (38.2%) health care centers were 20-24 year old and there was not a significant

Breast milk	Northern (N = 216) Mean ± SD	Southern (N = 433) Mean ± SD	P-value
Triglyceride (mg/100 ml)	499.68 ± 251.07	466.77 ± 205.33	0.258
Protein (g/100 ml)	0.87 ± 0.41	0.99 ± 0.45	0.028

Significant (P < 0.05)

Table1: Breast milk triglyceride and protein in Tehran northern and southern health care centers.

Breast milk / Age (year)	Northern (N = 216) Triglyceride (mg/100 ml) Mean ± SD	Northern (N = 216) Protein (gr/100 ml) Mean ± SD	Southern (N = 433) Triglyceride (mg/100 ml) Mean ± SD	Southern (N = 433) Protein (gr/100 ml) Mean ± SD
<20	538 ± 567.10	0.78 ± 0.48	509.06 ± 212.27	0.89 ± 0.32
21-25	483.75 ± 250.90	0.98 ± 0.43	477.07 ± 223.09	0.92 ± 0.37
26-30	482.63 ± 258.70	0.74 ± 0.36	457.52 ± 196.94	1.11 ± 0.61
31-35	620.94 ± 202.34	0.92 ± 0.42	419.47 ± 163.34	0.94 ± 0.32
>35	417.71 ± 208.87	0.79 ± 0.30	464.57 ± 227.60	1.39 ± 0.33
P-value	0.35	0.12	0.50	0.01

Significant (P < 0.05)

Table2: Breast milk triglyceride and protein by mothers age in Tehran northern and southern health care centers.

Breast milk / Occupation		Triglyceride (mg/100 ml) Mean ± SD	Protein (gr/100 ml) Mean ± SD
Groups: Northern (N=216)	Employed	517.20 ± 21	0.65 ± 0.40
	Housekeeper	498.74 ± 253.81	0.89 ± 0.41
	P-value	0.8	0.20
Southern (N = 433)	Employed	531.27 ± 198.55	1.14 ± 0.37
	Housekeeper	463.11 ± 205.60	0.98 ± 0.45
	P-value	0.29	0.26

Significant (P < 0.05)

Table3: Breast milk triglyceride and protein by mother's occupation in Tehran northern and southern health care centers.

Groups / Mothers` diet	Northern (N = 216) Mean ± SD	Southern (N = 433) Mean ± SD	P-value
Carbohydrate (g/d)	329.48 ± 156.35	372.88 ± 182.10	0.001
Fat (g/d)	87.01 ± 50.92	94.10 ± 42.86	0.069
Protein (g/d)	73.13 ± 2.98	86.29 ± 49.10	0.000

Significant (P < 0.05).

Table4: The mothers diet in Tehran northern and southern health care centers.

difference between the two groups, statistically (P = 0.31).Assessment of mother's weight in the two groups showed that their weigh were 55-64 kg in northern (30.8%) and southern (29.7%) groups and there was not a significant difference between the two groups, statistically (P = 0.13). Assessment of mother's height in the two groups showed that they were 155-159 cm in northern groups (34.7%) and 160-164 cm in southern groups (34%) and there was not a significant difference between the two groups, statistically (P = 0.5). Assessment of education in the two groups showed that they have degree in northern (54.7%) and southern (44.6%) groups. The statistical tests did not show a significant difference between the two groups by education (P = 0.37) because they were illiterate of the need to utilize available resources for the improvement

of the health (particularly the nutritional status) of themselves and their families. In areas where cultural and religious beliefs seriously affect the mother's intake of food and or nutrients, every educational effort should be made to overcome these adverse practices. Assessment of mother's occupation in two northern and southern groups showed that most of them in northern (96.6%) and southern (94.1%) groups were housekeepers and there was not a significant difference between the two groups by occupation (P = 0.17). Assessment of the breast milk triglyceride and protein by mother's occupation in the two groups did not show a significant difference, statistically (P = 0.11). Assessment of mother's diet showed that the mother's diet carbohydrate, protein in southern was higher than northern and also the breast milk protein in southern was higher than northern. Mother's diet fat were higher in southern than northern but the breast milk triglyceride in northern was higher than southern while Mother's diet triglyceride was significantly inversely associated with breast milk triglyceride. Current maternal diet was not associated with milk composition.

The mother's diet carbohydrate in northern was less than southern (329.48 ± 156.35 g/d vs. 372.88 ± 182.10) and there was a significant difference between the two groups, statistically (P = 0.001). The assessment of the mother's diet protein between two groups showed a significant difference, statistically (P = 0.001 and P = 0.000) and also the assessment of the breast milk protein between two groups showed a significant difference, statistically (P = 0.028).

The assessment between the mother's diet fat in two groups was not significant (P = 0.069) and also the assessment of the breast milk triglyceride between the two groups did not show a significant difference (P = 0.258).

Therefore recognition of breast milk biochemical composition and their influencing factors can help us to change breast feeding malnourished mother's diet and convert it into a normal diet.

Human milk is a dynamic, multi-faceted fluid containing nutrients and bioactive factors needed for infant health and development. While many studies of human milk composition have been conducted, components of human milk are still being identified. Standardized, multi-population studies of the breast milk triglyceride and protein are sorely needed to create a rigorous, comprehensive reference inclusive of nutrients and bioactive factors.

In sum, we document considerable individual variation in human milk composition in these two group's mothers. Consistent with prior research, we find evidence that composition changes with the age of the mother and that this is likely partially reflecting changes in nursing frequency. Similar to past studies that report minimal evidence for associations between the milk nutritional variation and maternal diet or nutritional status as measured during lactation.

Conclusion

There was a significant difference between the mean of mother's diet carbohydrate and mother's diet protein in the two groups and help us to change breast feeding malnourished mother's diet and convert it into a normal diet.

Acknowledgment

The authors wish to thank the Vice Chancellor of Tehran University of Medical Sciences for the research grant and for permission this study that was conducted following the approval of our institutional review board.

References

1. Picciano MF (1998) Human milk: Nutritional aspects of a dynamic food. Biol Neonate 74: 84-93.

2. Raiten DJ, Raghavan R, Porter A, Obbagy JE, Spahn JM, et al. (2014) Executive summary: Evaluating the evidence base to support the inclusion of infants and children from birth to 24 months of age in the Dietary Guidelines for Americans — "the B-24 Project". The American journal of clinical nutrition 99: 663S-691S.

3. Junqueira LCU, Mescher AL (2010) Junqueira's basic histology: Text and atlas. New York: McGraw-Hill Medical.

4. Beal VA (1980) Nutrition in the life span. New York: Wiley.

5. Hofvander Y (1983) Maternal and young child nutrition: Excerpts from a United Nations expert group: UNESCO, Division of Sciences, Technical and Vocational Education.

6. Goldman A, Goldblum R, Jensen R (1995) Defense agents in milk. A defense agent in human milk. Handbook of milk composition Academic Press, San Diego 727-745.

7. Mandel D, Lubetzky R, Dollberg S, Barak S, Mimouni FB (2005) Fat and energy contents of expressed human breast milk in prolonged lactation. Pediatrics 116: e432-435.

8. Behrman RE, Kliegman R, Jenson HB (2000) Nelson textbook of pediatrics. Philadelphia: WB Saunders Co.

9. Worthington Roberts BS, Williams SR (1989) Nutrition in pregnancy and lactation. St. Louis: Times Mirror/Mosby College Pub.

10. Hadders-Algra M, Bouwstra H, van Goor SA, Dijck-Brouwer DA, Muskiet FA (2007) Prenatal and early postnatal fatty acid status and neurodevelopmental outcome. J Perinat Med 35 Suppl 1: S28-34.

11. Lönnerdal B (1985) Biochemistry and physiological function of human milk proteins. Am J Clin Nutr 42: 1299-1317.

12. Hill RM, American Academy of P (1981) Breast feeding. Evanston, Ill.: American Academy of Pediatrics.

13. Anderson NG, Powers MT, Tollaksen SL (1982) Proteins of human milk. I. Identification of major components. Clin Chem 28: 1045-1055.

14. Bucolo G, David H (1973) Quantitative determination of serum triglycerides by the use of enzymes. Clin Chem 19: 476-482.

15. Fossati P, Prencipe L (1982) Serum triglycerides determined colorimetrically with an enzyme that produces hydrogen peroxide. Clinical chemistry 28: 2077-2080.

16. Burtis CA, Ashwood ER, Bruns DE (2012) Tietz textbook of clinical chemistry and molecular diagnostics. Philadelphia, Pa.; London: Saunders.

17. Wachtel MS, Dahm PF (2003) The ASCUS: SIL ratio and the reference laboratory pathologist. Cytopathology 14: 249-256.

18. Arslanoglu S, Moro GE, Ziegler EE (2006) Adjustable fortification of human milk fed to preterm infants: Does it make a difference? J Perinatol 26: 614-621.

19. National Research C (1980) Committee on Dietary A. Recommended dietary allowances. Washington, D.C.: National Academy of Sciences.

5

Biological Activities of Compounds Isolated from *Loxostylis alata* (Anacardiaceae) Leaf Extract

Mohammed M Suleiman[1,2*], Esameldin E Elgorashi[1], Babatunde B Samuel[1], Vinasan Naidoo[1] and Jacobus N Eloff[1]

[1]Phytomedicine Programme, Department of Paraclinical Sciences, Faculty of Veterinary Science, University of Pretoria, Private Bag X04, Onderstepoort, 0110, South Africa

[2]Department of Pharmacology and Toxicology, Faculty of Veterinary Medicine, Ahmadu Bello University, Zaria, Nigeria

Abstract

In a random screening of antimicrobial activity of tree leaves, *Loxostylis alata* (Spreng.) f. ex Reichb had shown activity against the pathogenic fungi; *Cryptococcus neoformans*. This stimulated further interest to investigate its antimicrobial activity. Extracts and compounds isolated from leaves of *Loxostylis alata* by bioassay-guided fractionation were evaluated for their *in vitro* antimicrobial, anti-inflammatory (Cyclooxygenase-1 and -2) activities and for their potential toxic effects using 3-(4,5-dimethylthiazolyl-2)-2,5-diphenyltetrazolium bromide (MTT) and *Salmonella typhimurium* tester strains TA98 and TA100. Antimicrobial activity was evaluated using a serial dilution microplate assay. The bacterial strains used were *Staphylococcus aureus* (ATCC29213), *Enterococcus faecalis* (ATCC 29212), *Pseudomonas aeruginosa* (ATCC 27853) and *Escherichia coli* (ATCC 25922). While the fungal strains used were isolates of *Cryptococcus neoformans*, *Sporothrix schenckii*, *Aspergillus fumigatus*, *Microsporum canis* and *Candida albicans*. A bioassay guided fractionation of the crude extract yielded two antimicrobial compounds namely, Lupeol 1 and β-sitosterol 2. In addition β-sitosterol exhibited selective inhibition of COX-1 (IC_{50} = 55.3 ± 2) None of the compounds isolated were toxic in the *Salmonella typhimurium*/microsome assay and MTT cytotoxicity test. The isolation of these two compounds is reported for the first time from *Loxostylis alata*.

Keywords: *Loxostylis alata*; Antimicrobial activity; Anti-inflammatory activity; Cytotoxicity; Genotoxicity

Introduction

About 60% of the world's population relies almost entirely on herbal remedies to treat different ailments [1]. Plant derived drugs have for ages been regarded as an essential source of therapeutically effective medicines and still remain important with about 25% of the drugs prescribed worldwide being herbal formulations [1]. Of the 252 drugs considered as basic and essential by the WHO, 11% are exclusively of plant origin and a significant number are synthetic drugs obtained from natural precursors [1]. In 1997, the world market for phytomedicine products was estimated at US$10 billion [2]. Recent development of natural products into chemotherapeutic armamentarium include the antimalarial drug artemisinin and the anticancer agents taxol, docetaxel and camptothecin Therefore, the use of natural products is one of the most successful strategies for the discovery of new medicines [3]. Where natural compounds failed to show sufficient activity or were too toxic, they may serve as lead compounds, allowing the design and rational planning of new drugs that could be more effective [4].

As plants produce an array of diverse chemical compounds, the separation and determination of their active compounds will provide an insight into their pharmacological, pharmacokinetic and toxicological properties [5].

Loxostylis alata is a member of the family Anacardiaceae [6]. The bark and leaves of *Loxostylis alata* are used in South African traditional medicine during childbirth to relieve pain [7] and also to stimulate the immune system [8] but no indication of its use in combating microbial infections could be found. Ginkcol (3-(8Z-pentadecenyl) phenol) and ginkgolic acid (6-(8Z-pentadecenyl) salicylic acid) were previously isolated from the leaves of *L. alata* [9]. To date no studies have been carried out on the plant to determine its pharmacologically active constituents.

In a screening study of seven South African plant species active against *Cryptococcus neoformans*, *Loxostylis alata* had the highest activity [10]. The primary objective of this study was to isolate the antimicrobial compound(s) from the crude extracts of *Loxostylis alata* based on bioautography assays. The isolated compounds were investigated further for their anti-inflammatory (cyclooxygenase-1 and -2), mutagenic (*Salmonella*/microsome assay) and cytotoxic (MTT assay) effects in order to find a safer, efficacious and cheap chemical compounds that could be used to treat microbial infections and other related diseases.

The plant extract had activity against experimental infection with *Aspergillus fumigatus* in chickens [11]. It will be worthwhile to identify and isolate compound(s) that are responsible for the antifungal effect of the plant. Therefore, the study was aim at identifying and isolating the biologically active compounds in the crude extract of *L. alata*.

Materials and methods

Plant collection

Leaves of *Loxostylis alata* (Spreng.) f. ex Reichb were collected at the Botanical Garden of the University of Pretoria, South Africa. Samples of the plant were identified and authenticated by Lorraine Middleton and Magda Nel of the Botanical Garden of the University of Pretoria. Voucher specimen of the plant (number; PRU PRU96508)

*Corresponding author: Mohammed M Suleiman, Department of Pharmacology and Toxicology, Faculty of Veterinary Medicine, Ahmadu Bello University, Zaria, Nigeria, E-mail: mohsulai@yahoo.com

was deposited at the Schweikert Herbarium of the Department of Plant Science, University of Pretoria, South Africa.

Extraction, isolation and identification of constituents

Leaves of *Loxostylis alata* were dried at room temperature, milled to a fine powder and stored at room temperature in closed containers in the dark until used. The ground plant material (500 g) was extracted with acetone (5 litres × 3). The solvent of the combined extracts was removed *in vacuo*.

The acetone extract (70 g) was subjected to solvent-solvent fractionation using carbon tetrachloride, hexane, chloroform, aqueous methanol, butanol and water [12]. The carbon tetrachloride (CCl_4) fraction had the highest antimicrobial activity and were therefore, chosen for further isolation of active compounds. Column chromatography (37×5 cm, silica gel 60) of the CCl_4 fraction (10 g) using a hexane: ethyl acetate step gradient followed by ethyl acetate: methanol step gradient was performed. Initially, 100% hexane was used, and then reduced to 0% hexane by the addition of 10% ethyl acetate in successive steps. This was followed by an ethyl acetate: methanol gradient where ethyl acetate was reduced to 0% by the addition of 10% methanol in successive increments. Thirteen fractions were collected and each tested for activity against *S. aureus* using the bioautographic method [13]. Based on the bioautography profile, fractions containing active compounds with the same R_f value (F3-F8, F9-F13) were combined and referred to as F2-1 and F2-2 respectively. Fractions F2-1 (3 g) and F2-2 (2 g) were further fractionated by column chromatography eluted isocratically with hexane: ethylacetate (7:3) to give lupeol as a white amorphous powder and β-sitosterol as white-yellowish amorphous powder respectively.

Antimicrobial activity

Fungal and bacterial cultures: Bacterial strains used for antibacterial testing were the Gram-positive *Staphylococcus aureus* (ATCC29213), *Enterococcus faecalis* (ATCC 29212), and the Gram-negative *Pseudomonas aeruginosa* (ATCC 27853) and *Escherichia coli* (ATCC 25922). Pathogenic fungal isolates used were *Cryptococcus neoformans*, *Sporothrix schenckii*, *Aspergillus fumigatus*, *Microsporum canis* and *Candida albicans* (obtained from the Microbiology Unit, Department of Veterinary Tropical Diseases, University of Pretoria). Bacterial cells were inoculated into fresh Müller-Hinton (MH) broth (Fluka, Switzerland) and incubated at 37°C for 14 h prior to the screening procedures. Fungal cultures were grown in Sabouraud dextrose (SD) broth at 37°C and maintained on SD agar at 4°C.

Bioautography

The antibacterial and antifungal bioautographic assays were carried out according to the method described by Begue and Kline [13] with slight modification for fungi by Masoko et al. [14]. Briefly, Thin Layer Chromatography (TLC) plates were loaded with 100 µg of each fraction or 10 µg of pure compound, and dried before developing in Chloroform/Ethyl acetate/Formic acid (5:4:1): [CEF] and Hexane/Ethyl acetate (7:3) [HE] mobile phases for the fractions and the pure compounds, respectively. The solvent was allowed to evaporate from the plates under a stream of fast moving cold air for 2-5 days. Plates were then sprayed with concentrated cultures of bacteria or fungal species until completely moist. The moist plates were incubated at 37°C for 24 h. Thereafter, the plates were sprayed with 2 mg/ml of p-iodonitrotetrazolium violet (INT) and incubated for a further 1 h in case of bacteria and 24 h for fungi [11]. White areas over a purple background on the TLC plate indicate the non-reduction of INT to

coloured formazan and therefore an indication of microbial inhibition by the compounds present.

Minimum Inhibitory concentration (MIC)

Minimum inhibitory concentrations of extracts, column fractions and isolated compounds against bacteria and fungi were determined using the serial microdilution assays [14,15]. In brief, two-fold serial dilutions of the samples were prepared in wells of 96-well microtitre plates. Bacterial or fungal culture (100µl of an overnight culture) was then added to each well before incubation for 24 h for bacteria or 48 h in case of fungi at 37°C. p-Iodo Nitro Tetrazolium chloride (INT, Sigma) was added to each well as indicator of bacterial or fungal growth. The minimum inhibitory concentration (MIC) was read as the concentration of sample that inhibited microbial growth, as indicated by a visible reduction in the red colour of the INT formazan. In each assay, negative solvent controls, growth controls and a positive control were included. Gentamicin and amphotericin B (Sigma) were used as the antibacterial and antifungal positive controls, respectively with the solvents as negative controls. The samples were tested in triplicate and the assays were repeated twice to confirm results.

Cytotoxicity assay

The isolated compounds were tested for cytotoxicity against the Vero monkey kidney cell line. The cells were maintained in minimal essential medium (MEM, Highveld Biological, Johannesburg, South Africa) supplemented with 0.1% Gentamicin (Virbac) and 5% foetal calf serum (Adcock-Ingram). Cell suspensions were prepared from confluent monolayer cultures and plated at a density of $0.5×10^3$ cells into each well of a 96-well microtitre plate. After overnight incubation at 37°C in a 5% CO2 incubator, the subconfluent cells in the microtitre plate were used in the cytotoxicity assay. Stock solutions of the compounds were prepared by reconstitution to a concentration of 10 mg/ml in dimethylsulphoxide (DMSO). Serial 10-fold dilutions of each extract were prepared in growth medium (1-1000 µg /ml). The method described by Mosmann [16] was used to determine the viability of cell growth after 5 days incubation with the compounds. MTT was used as an indicator for cell growth. The absorbance was measured at 570 nm. Berberine chloride (Sigma) and DMSO were used as positive and negative controls, respectively. Tests were carried out in quadruplicate and each experiment was done in triplicate. Furthermore, the selectivity index of each fraction was calculated as shown by Shai et al. [17]

Selectivity index (SI) = Lethal concentration 50 (LC50)/Minimum inhibitory concentration (MIC)

This ratio gives the relative safety of each fraction.

Genotoxicity test

The potential mutagenic effects of the investigated plant compounds were detected using the Ames test. The Ames assay was performed with *Salmonella typhimurium* (TA98 and TA100) strains. One hundred microliters of bacterial stock was incubated in 20 ml of Oxoid Nutrient for 16 h at 37°C on an orbital shaker. The overnight culture (0.1 ml) was added to 2 ml top agar (containing traces of biotin and histidine) together with 0.1 ml test solution (plant extract, solvent control or positive control) and 0.5 ml phosphate buffer (for exposure without metabolic activation). The top agar mixture was poured over the surface of the agar plate and incubated for 48 h at 37°C. After incubation, the number of revertant colonies (mutants) was counted [18]. All cultures were made in triplicate (except the solvent control where five replicates were made) for each assay. The assays were repeated twice. The positive control used was 4-NitroQuinoline-1-Oxide (4-NQO) at a concentration of 2 μg/ml.

Anti-inflammatory assay

Inhibition of prostaglandin biosynthesis by the plant extract and isolated compounds was investigated using both the COX-1 and COX-2 assays [19,20]. The COX-1 enzyme (from ram seminal vesicles, Sigma Aldrich) and COX-2 (human recombinant, Sigma-Aldrich) were activated with co-factor solution and pre-incubated on ice for 5 min. Sixty microliters of this enzyme/co-factor solution was added to 20 μl of crude extract of *Loxostylis alata* extract (20 μl of extract solution) or 20 μl of compound and pre-incubated for 5 min at room temperature. Twenty microliters of [^{14}C] arachidonic acid was added to the tested samples and incubated at 37°C for 10 min. After incubation, the reaction was terminated by adding 10 μl of 2 N HCl. Four microliters of a 0.2 mg/ml carrier solution of unlabelled prostaglandins was added. In each assay, four controls were run. Two were background in which the enzyme was inactivated with HCl before the addition of [^{14}C] arachidonic acid, and two were solvent blanks. Indomethacin was included in each test assay as a standard. Percentage inhibition of plant extracts was calculated by comparing the amount of radioactivity present in the sample to that in the solvent blank. IC^{50} was calculated from at least 5 concentrations. Results are presented as mean ± SEM. of two experiments carried out in duplicate.

Results and Discussion

Biological activity of the extract

In a preliminary random screening of antimicrobial activity of acetone extracts of tree leaves, *Loxostylis alata* had promising activity against Cryptococcus neoformans. In this study, an investigation on the antifungal effect of the acetone extracts of *Loxostylis alata* against *Aspergillus fumigatus* confirmed earlier findings. The yield, MIC value together with the total activity of the crude extract and the different fractions resulted from solvent - solvent fractionation of the acetone extract (70 g) are presented in Table 1. Total Activity (TA) is calculated by dividing the quantity extracted by each solvent in mg with the MIC value in mg/ml. This value indicates the volume to which the active constituent present in one gram of the fraction can be diluted and still inhibit the growth of the test organism [21]. A higher value of total activity indicates increased usefulness and economic value of the plant species and is of benefit in enabling rural use of extracts of the species. The CC$_{14}$ fraction was the most active fraction with MIC and TA value of 0.08 mg/ml and 3201.79 ml/g, respectively. It therefore means that 1 gram of CCl4 fraction can be diluted in 3201.79 ml of the solvent used and still inhibit the growth of *A. fumigatus*. Similarly, the CC$_{14}$ fraction had a greater area of inhibition against all the tested pathogens. Hexane and aqueous methanol fractions had a low area of inhibition, while

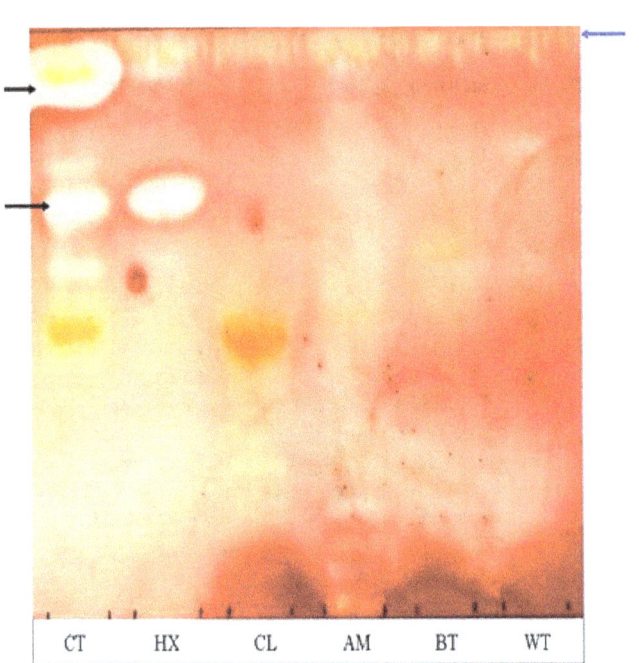

Figure 1: Carbon Tetrachloride (CT), Hexane (HX), Chloroform (CL), Aqueous Methanol (AM), Butanol (BT) and Water (WT) fractions of *Loxostylis alata* separated on TLC plates using CEF and sprayed with S. aureus and 24 h later by INT. White areas indicate inhibition of microbial growth (black arrow) after 60 minutes of incubation at 37oC. The blue arrow (right) indicates solvent front.

butanol and water fractions did not have any areas of inhibition when the TLC bioautographic method was used (Figure 1).

Bioactivity guided fractionation of the CC$_{14}$ fraction led to the isolation of two compounds 1 and 2. These compounds were identified, based on comparison of ^{1}H NMR, ^{13}C NMR and mass spectroscopic (MS) data with literature values, as lupeol and β-sitosterol, respectively.

The ^{1}H NMR and ^{13}C NMR spectral data of compound 1 exhibited characteristics spectra features of pentacyclic triterpene. The presence of olefinic protons (4.68 broad signal at H-29a, 4.56 broad signal at H-29b), 3.18 dd, with seven methyl signals are due to lupeol type triterpene. Signals were readily characterised by comparison with signals of lupeol from previous reports [22-25]. Mass spectrum of the compound with M+426, and prominent signals at 218 and 207 confirmed that the compound is lupeol [24]. Analysis and interpretation of the spectroscopic data

obtained with previously reported data led to the proposed structure for the compound as lupeol (Figure 2a) with a molecular formula C$_{30}$H$_{50}$O. Lupeol, although a compound commonly found in higher plants, is been reported for the first time in *L. alata*.

The characteristic signal of compound 2 is the chemical shift of the 4-6 olefinic signal (5.35) and multiplet at 3.55 due to H-3. This confirmed the isolated compound to be a 24-steroid derivative. Comparison of the carbon spectral data for compound 2 with previously compiled data [26-28] led to the proposed structure of the compound to be β-sitosterol (Figure 2b). Mass spectroscopy with molecular ion of 414 and prominent peaks at 396 and 105 served to confirmed the compound to be β-sitosterol with a molecular formula C$_{30}$H$_{50}$O [26-28].

Fraction	Fraction yield (%)	MIC (mg/ml)	Total activity (ml/fraction)	Cytotoxicity (LC50 ± SEM in mg/ml)	Selectivity index
Hexane	3.33	0.24	138.69	0.41 ± 0.003	
Carbon tetrachloride	25.61	0.08	3201.79	0.23 ±0.001	1.71
Chloroform	1.86	0.94	19.76	0.67 ±0.002	2.88
Aqueous methanol	3.50	1.88	18.62	NT	0.71
Butanol	38.64	2.5	15.46	NT	NA
Water	11.91	2.5	47.66	NT	NA
Amphotericin B	-	0.091	NA	NT	NA
DMSO	-	NT	NA	NDT	NA

NT = not tested; NA= not available; NDT= no detectable toxicity

Table 1: Minimal inhibitory concentrations and safety evaluation of various fractions of Loxostylis alata against Aspergillus fumigatus.

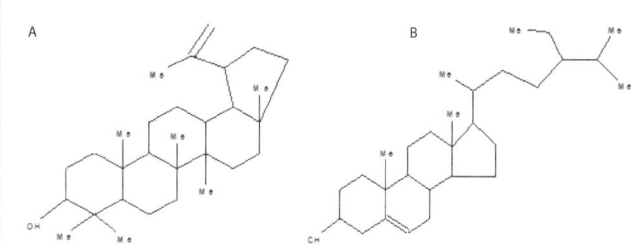

Figure 2: Structure of lupeol (a) and β-sitosterol (b) isolated from *Loxostylis alata* leaves.

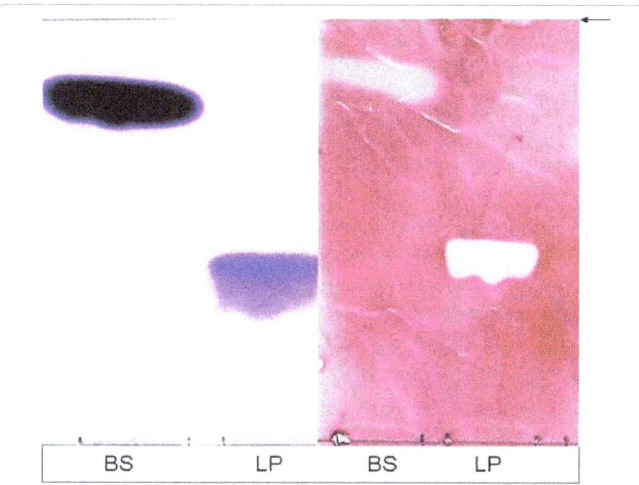

Figure 3: TLC plates indicating activity of *Loxostylis alata* isolated compounds. The compounds (spotted left to right) 10 µg β-sitosterol (BS) and 10 µg lupeol (LP) and eluted using hexane:ethyl acetate (7:3). The plates were sprayed with acidified vanillin (A) or *Staphylococcus aureus* culture (B). White areas on plate B indicate inhibition of microbial growth after 60 minutes of incubation at 37°C.

Antimicrobial activity of isolated compounds

The two compounds isolated from CCl_4 fraction of *Loxostylis alata* were active against *S. aureus* and *E. coli* with R_f values in hexane: ethyl acetate (7:3) solvent system of 0.47 for lupeol and 0.81 for β-sitosterol (Figure 3). Lupeol showed the most pronounced zone of inhibition against *S. aureus*. Only lupeol was active when tested against the five fungal pathogens using bioautographic means (results not shown). Similarly, when MICs of the 2 compounds were determined, only lupeol had activity against the fungal pathogens. However, β-sitosterol showed some activity against *S. aureus* and *E. coli* (Table 2). In a similar study, lupeol had low activity against *Candida albicans* with MIC values of more than 250 µg/ml but showed high activity against *Sporothrix schenckii* and *Microsporum canis* (MIC values of 12 and 16 µg/ml,

respectively), this is in agreement with what Shai et al. [17], reported. Lupeol and β-sitosterol, previously isolated from the stem bark of *Buchholzia coriacea*, have been shown to have activity against some species of pathogenic bacteria and fungi [29]. Similarly, β-sitosterol was found to have good inhibitory activity against the fungi *Aspergillus niger, C. cladosporioides, and Phytophthora sp.* [30].

Anti-inflammatory assay

The results from screening against cyclooxygenase enzymes -1 and -2 (COX-1 and -2) showed that the crude extract of *Loxostylis alata* and lupeol inhibited COX-1 in a concentration dependent manner (IC50=92.5 ± 1.6 and 134.0 ± 5.1 µM, respectively). Indomethacin had an IC_{50} of 3.30 ± 0.006 and 122.5 µM against COX-1 and COX-2, respectively. Neither the crude extract nor lupeol or 2 inhibited the activity of COX-2. Although lupeol was not active against COX-2, it did produce a dose-dependent inhibition of carrageenan induced paw oedema in rats [31]. The *in vivo* action exhibited by lupeol may probably be ascribed to the fact that when administered into the body, it undergoes biotransformation to an active moiety that confers its anti-inflammatory action. In some cases a drug becomes pharmacologically active only after it has been metabolized in the body [32]. Both COX -1 and -2 regulate the biosynthesis of prostaglandins from arachidonic acid. COX-1 is a constitutive form and has a clear physiological function while COX-2 is mainly induced by inflammatory mediators. It is the inhibition of prostaglandin synthesis by COX-1 and -2 that is believed to be behind the anti-inflammatory mechanism of action of NSAIDs [32]. However, prolonged use of both enzymes inhibitors may cause detrimental myocardial infarction (COX-2) [33], gastrointestinal damage and nephrotoxicity (COX-1) [32]. In addition, COX-1 selective inhibitors have beneficial anti-thrombotic effect. Inhibition of COX-1 by both the crude extract and lupeol may exert beneficial anti-thrombotic effect and protect from heart diseases. Further supporting evidence is that the crude extract inhibited equine platelet aggregation [34]. Moreover, lupeol could form a base for the development of new semi-synthetic drugs for the management of thrombolic disorders.

In vitro safety test

Compounds 1 and 2 were relatively non toxic with LC_{50} of 76.66 ± 4.13 and 136.60 ± 7.20 µg/ml, respectively compared to the reference compound berberine with LC_{50} of 6.36 ± 0.81 µg/ml (Table 2). β-sitosterol which occurs as an sterol in many plants has activities potentially useful in improving human health such as anti-inflammatory, antipyretic, immunomodulating, and antineoplastic [35,36].

Results obtained from the mutagenicity test of the 2 compounds using *Salmonella* TA98 and TA100 strains are expressed as mean ± SEM (Table 3) and are based on number of induced revertant colonies. Substances are considered active if the number of induced revertant colonies is twice the revertant colonies of the negative control (blank) [18]. The two compounds were not mutagenic in the Salmonella/

Compound	MIC values against the tested pathogens (µg/ml)									Cytotoxicity (LC50 ± SEM in µg/ml)
	SA	EF	EC	PA	AF	CA	CN	MC	SS	
Lupeol	29	67	83	150	92	120	47	63	57	76.66 ± 4.1
β-sitosterol	90	>250	110	>250	>250	>250	>250	>250	>250	136.60 ± 7.2
Gentamicin	6.7	4.2	15.2	12.67	NA	NA	NA	NA	NA	NA
Amphotericin B	NA	NA	NA	NA	6.4	0.81	0.32	0.41	0.45	NA
Berberine	NA	NA	NA	NA	NA	NA	NA	NA	NA	6.36 ± 0.8

Staphylococcus aureus (SA), Enterococcus faecalis (EF), Escherichia coli (EC), Pseudomonas aeruginosa (PA), Aspergillus fumigatus (AF), Candida albicans (CA), Cryptococcus neoformans (CN), Microsporum canis (MC), Sporothrix schenckii (SS)
NA = not available

Table 2: Minimal inhibitory concentrations and safety evaluation of compounds isolated from Loxostylis alata.

Treatment	Revertant/plate in Salmonella typhimurium strains					
	TA98 (µg/plate ± SEM)			TA100 (µg/plate ± SEM)		
	2000	200	20	200	20	2
Lupeol	29.30 ± 1.5	29.67 ± 3.6	27.33 ± 1.8	161.33 ± 7.9	167.00 ± 20.1	158.50 ± 8.5
β-sitosterol	22.30 ± 2.2	28.00 ± 2.0	26.67 ± 2.7	179.00 ± 5.9	170.70 ± 1.1	163.30 ± 1.1
Crude extract	NT	NT	NT	NT	NT	NT

Negative control for the *Salmonella typhimurium test* is DMSO (100 µl/plate; TA98: 19.30 ± 2.89; TA100: 152.60 ± 7.07), while the positive control is 4-nitroquinoline 1-oxide (4-NQO) (10 µg/plate; TA98: 170.33 ± 14.14; TA100: 960 ± 24.89). All values quoted are mean ± SEM

Table 3: Mutagenic activity expressed as the mean and standard error of mean of the number of revertants/plate in Salmonella typhimurium strains TA98 and TA100 exposed to extract and compounds of *Loxostylis alata,* at different concentration.

microsome tester strains TA98 and TA 100. The lack of cytotoxic or mutagenic effects of these compounds does not guarantee their safe use as traditional medicines. Detailed laboratory and clinical evaluations are needed to justify their use as medicines [37].

Conclusion

The compounds isolated from the leaf extract of *Loxostylis alata* had varying degrees of antimicrobial and cyclooxygenase inhibitory activities. However, detailed toxicity and efficacy studies of the extracts or isolated compounds in both laboratory and target animal species are required to justify its use in clinical practice. If these are effective, there is also need for investigating the mechanism underlying the antimicrobial actions of these compounds from *Loxostylis alata*.

Acknowledgements

The authors thank the South African National Research Foundation (SA-NRF) and the University of Pretoria Research Fund for financial support. MM Suleiman is grateful to authorities of Ahmadu Bello University, Zaria, Nigeria for the award of PhD study Fellowship at the University of Pretoria, South Africa.

References

1. Rates SM (2001) Plants as source of drugs. Toxicon 39: 603-613.

2. Soldati F (1997) The registration of medicinal plant products, what quality of documentation should be required? The industrial point of view. World congress on medicinal and aromatic plants for Human welfare 2, abstracts. Mendoza: ICMPA/ ISHS/ SAIPOA, P.L-48.

3. Harvey AL, Waterman PG (1998) The continuing contribution of biodiversity to drug discovery. Curr Opin Drug Discov Devel 1: 71-76.

4. Hamburger M, Hostettmann K (1991) Bioactivity in plants: the link between phytochemistry and medicine. Phytochem 30: 3864-3874.

5. Sun JW, Sheng JF (1998) A Handbook of bioactive compounds from plants. China medical-pharmacological science and Technology Publishing House, Beijing, China.

6. Coates-Palgrave M (2002) Keith Coates-Palgrave Trees of Southern Africa: 3rd edition, Struik Publishers, Cape Town, South Africa, pp. 1212.

7. Pooley E (1993) The Complete Field Guide to Trees of Natal, Zululand and Transkei. Natal Flora Publications Trust, South Africa.

8. Pell SK (2004) Molecular systematics of the cashew family (Anacardiaceae).

9. Drewes SE, Horn MM, Mabaso NJ (1998) *Loxostylis alata* and Smodingium argutum- a case of phytochemical bedfellows. S Afr J Bot 64: 128-129.

10. Suleiman MM, McGaw LJ, Naidoo V, Eloff JN (2010) Evaluation of several tree species for activity against the animal fungal pathogen Aspergillus fumigatus. S Afr J Bot 76: 64-71.

11. Suleiman MM (2009) The *in vitro* and in vivo biological activities of antifungal compounds isolated from *Loxostylis alata* A. Spreng. ex Rchb. PhD Thesis, Phytomedicine Programme, Paraclinical Sciences, Faculty of Veterinary Science, University of Pretoria.

12. Suffness M, Douros J (1979) Drugs of plant origin. Method Cancer Res 26: 73-126.

13. Begue WJ, Kline RM (1972) The use of tetrazolium salts in bioautographic procedures. J Chromatogr 64: 182-184.

14. Masoko P, Picard J, Eloff JN (2005) Antifungal activities of six South African Terminalia species (Combretaceae). J Ethnopharmacol 99: 301-308.

15. Eloff JN (1998) A sensitive and quick microplate method to determine the minimal inhibitory concentration of plant extracts for bacteria. Planta Med 64: 711-713.

16. Mosmann T (1983) Rapid colorimetric assay for cellular growth and survival: application to proliferation and cytotoxicity assays. J Immunol Methods 65: 55-63.

17. Shai LJ, McGaw LJ, Aderogba MA, Mdee LK, Eloff JN (2008) Four pentacyclic triterpenoids with antifungal and antibacterial activity from Curtisia dentata (Burm.f) C.A. Sm. leaves. J Ethnopharmacol 119: 238-244.

18. Maron DM, Ames BN (1983) Revised methods for the Salmonella mutagenicity test. Mutat Res 113: 173-215.

19. Jäger AK, Hutchings A, van Staden J (1996) Screening of Zulu medicinal plants for prostaglandin-synthesis inhibitors. J Ethnopharmacol 52: 95-100.

20. Noreen Y, Ringbom T, Perera P, Danielson H, Bohlin L (1998) Development of a radiochemical cyclooxygenase-1 and -2 in vitro assay for identification of natural products as inhibitors of prostaglandin biosynthesis. J Nat Prod 61: 2-7.

21. Eloff JN (2004) Quantification the bioactivity of plant extracts during screening and bioassay guided fractionation. Phytomedicine 11: 370-371.

22. Sholichin M, Yamasaki K, Kasai R, Tanaka C (1980) 13C Nuclear magnetic resonance of lupane-type triterpenes, lupeol, betulin and betulinic acid. Chemical and Pharm Bull 28: 1006-1008.

23. Mahato SB, Kundu AP (1994) 13C NMR spectra of pentacyclic triterpenoids-A compilation and some salient features. Phytochem 37: 1517-1575.

24. Tomosaka H, Koshino H, Tajika T, Omata S (2001) Lupeol esters from the twig bark of Japanese pear (Pyrus serotina Rehd.) cv. Shinko. Biosci Biotechnol Biochem 65: 1198-1201.

25. Imam S, Azhar I, Hasan MM, Ali MS, Ahmed SW (2007) Two triterpenes lupanone and lupeol isolated and identified from Tamarindus indica linn. Pak J Pharm Sci 20: 125-127.

26. Rubinstein I, Goad LJ, Clague ADH, Mulheirn LJ (1976) The 220 MHz NMR spectra of phytosterols. Phytochem 15: 195-200.

27. Chaurasia N, Wichtl M (1987) Sterols and steryl glycosides from Urtica dioica. Journal of Natural Product 50: 881-885.

28. Lopes MN, Mazza FC, Young MCM, Bolzani VS (1999) Complete assignments of 1H and 13C-NMR spectra of the 3,4-seco-triterpene canaric acid isolated from Rudgea jasminoides. J Brazilian Chem Soc 10: 237.

29. Ajaiyeoba EO, Onocha PA, Nwozo SO, Sama W (2003) Antimicrobial and cytotoxicity evaluation of *Buchholzia coriacea* stem bark. Fitoterapia 74: 706-709.

30. Lall N, Weiganand O, Hussein AA, Meyer JJM (2006) Antifungal activity of naphthoquinones and triterpenes isolated from the root bark of Euclea natalensis. S Afr J Bot 72: 579-583.

31. Agarwal RB, Rangari VD (2003) Anti-inflammatory and antiarthritic activities of lupeol and 19a-H lupeol isolated from Strobilanthus callosus and Strobilanthus ixiocephala roots. Indian J Pharmacol 35: 384-387.

32. Rang HP, Dale MM, Ritter JM, Moore PK (2003) Pharmacology. Fifth edition, Churchill, Livingstones, Edinburgh, UK, 797 pages.

33. Boers M (2001) NSAIDS and selective COX-2 inhibitors: competition between gastroprotection and cardioprotection. Lancet 357: 1222-1223.

34. Suleiman MM, Bagla V, Naidoo V, Eloff JN (2010) Evaluation of selected South African plant species for antioxidant, antiplatelet, and cytotoxic activity. Pharm Biol 48: 643-650.

35. Gupta MB, Nath R, Srivastava N, Shanker K, Kishor K, et al. (1980) Anti-inflammatory and antipyretic activities of beta-sitosterol. Planta Med 39: 157-163.

36. Bouic PJ (2001) The role of phytosterols and phytosterolins in immune modulation: a review of the past 10 years. Curr Opin Clin Nutr Metab Care 4: 471-475.

37. Debnath AK, Lopez de Compadre RL, Debnath G, Shusterman AJ, Hansch C (1991) Structure-activity relationship of mutagenic aromatic and heteroaromatic nitro compounds. Correlation with molecular orbital energies and hydrophobicity. J Med Chem 34: 786-797.

6

Design Self-Assembling Peptide DSAP-2 for 3d Cell Culture and Rapid Hemostasis

Mengmeng Li[1,8,†], Xiaofan Xu[1,8,†], Ran Wang[2,†], Duanhua Li[3,†], Yuelin Sun[4], Nan Liu[5], Yuanyuan Yue[1,8], Tianxin Zhao[4], Jianping Gong[6], Kanran Wang[3], Xinyuan Li[3], Mao Tan[3], Shanshan Zhang[3], Kunyue Tan[7], Zhenyin Chen[1,8], Huinan Zhang[1,8], Feng Li[2], Lifeng Jin[2], Zhongli Luo[1,8*]

[1]The College of Basic Medical Sciences, Chongqing Medical University, Chongqing 400016, China
[2]China Tobacco Gene Research Center, Zhengzhou Tobacco Research Institute, Zhengzhou, 450001, China
[3]Sichuan Industrial Institute of Antibiotics, Chengdu University, Chengdu, 610051, China
[4]The College of Clinical Pediatrics, Chongqing Medical University, Chongqing 400016, China
[5]China National Tobacco Quality Supervision& Test Centre, Zhengzhou, 450001, China
[6]The College of Clinical Medicine, The First Affiliated hospital of Chongqing Medical university, Chongqing Medical University, Chongqing 400016, China
[7]The College of Clinical Medicine, The Second Affiliated hospital of Chongqing Medical university, Chongqing Medical University, Chongqing 400016, China
[8]Molecular Medicine and Cancer Research Center, Chongqing Medical University, Chongqing 400016, China
†: These authors contributed equally to this work, and they are first authors to this work.

Abstract

Traditional self-assembling peptide can form nanofiber scaffolds to meet the challenges of advance biomaterial, cell culture, tissue engineering and regeneration. L-amino acids have been widely used instead of D-amino acids to design nanomaterial since some D-amino acids have toxicity of cells. Here we report that using D-amino acids to design a new D-form self-assembling peptide DSAP-2 and the circular dichroism, atomic force microscopy and scanning electron microscopy show that the peptide can form nanofiber scaffold as well. Furthermore, cell inhibition assay confirmed this D-form peptide show no toxicity of cells that can support cell growth. Fluorescence microscopy results show that cells had less cell apoptosis in the 3D environment and displayed a fast proliferation after cultured for 7days. Peptide's hydrogel not only formed nano-scaffolds surrounded by cells in a 3-D cell culture, but achieved rapid hemostasis in a rabbit liver wound model. Our study suggests this peptide could be used in the wound and beyond in the future. This work could also inspire us to design more novel D-form self-assembling peptide in biomaterials and biomedical areas.

Keywords: Self-assembling peptide; D-Amino acid; Nanofiber; 3D Cell culture; Rapid hemostasis

Introduction

At present, self-assembling peptides have been extensively studied in biomaterials and biomedical areas. More and more recent designs have shown their surprising results in structures, properties, functions and even in applications [1]. They can form well-ordered nanostructures such as nanofiber, nanotube and nanovesicle. They have multiple advantages, including stability, safety, efficiency, non-biological, biocompatibility, biodegradability and non-immunogenicity [2]. And they are widely applied to 3D cell culture [3-5], rapid hemostasis [6,7], wound-healing [8,9], drug control release [9-11], membrane proteins stabilization [12-16] and solar cell devices [17-21]. Compared with the topical cell culture media such as engineered substrates, animal-derived extracellular matrix or synthetic mimics, self-assembling peptides are competitive for helping the understanding and manipulation of 3-dimensional (3D) microenvironment cellular processes to proliferation, differentiation, migration, cell-cell contact interactions and apoptosis in tissue engineering and regenerative medicine [1]. Partially to 3D print bioink for soft-tissue, it is necessary to develop a kind of biomaterials which prevents body enzymes from quick degradation, where every single ingredient is known to achieve the fine-tuning and control, or suit for basic individual needs of studies and applications [22]. Peptides and proteins made of D-amino acids are more stable in the body environment since proteases can readily degrade L-form peptide bonds, but difficult to degrade D-form peptide bonds [23-26]. Proteins of animals are all synthesized by L-amino acids and some D-amino acid like D-Ala and D-Asp have toxicity of cells [23,26-29]. Therefore, most of them were designed by L-amino acid and a few by D-amino acids [1,2]. Up till now, there have been a few reports that D-form self-assembling peptide did not obtain toxicity to cell stains and was also resistant to protease digestion, as a 3D biological matrix for cell culture [6,30-32]. Amino acids and theirs isomers are a

good option of nano-biomaterials for biotechnology and biomedical areas [33-36]. Here we utilized two D-amino acids, D-Ala and D-Asp, which were reported to have toxicity of cells, and designed a new chiral self-assembly peptide DSAP-2. We got D-form self-assembling peptide hydrogel, investigated its physicochemical properties by circular dichroism spectroscopy, and examined microstructures by AFM and SEM. We also assessed the situations of cell behaviors in 3D cell culture, and some of its simple applications. Our study could prompt more designers working in basic medical and clinical studies to find more similar peptides.

Materials and Method

Peptides synthesis and purification

The sequence of peptide DSAP-2 is Ac-(^{D}Arg-^{D}Ala-^{D}Asp-^{D}Ala)$_4$-CONH$_2$, and the peptide was commercially custom-synthesized by solid-phase peptide synthesis (Chengdu CP Biochem Co., Ltd., Chengdu, China). The peptide was purified to 95.27% by HPLC and characterized by mass spectroscopy. The lyophilized white powder was stored at 4°C. Solutions of the peptides were prepared at mass concentration of 1.0% in water (18.2 KΩ/cm², Millipore Milli-Q system) and stored at 4°C before use.

*Corresponding author: Zhongli Luo, The College of Basic Medical Sciences and Molecular Medicine and Cancer Research Center, Chongqing Medical University, Chongqing 400016, China, E-mail: Zhongliluo@163.com

Molecular modeling

Design of molecular models of these peptides was based on the principle of minimum energy and models were constructed using free modeling software from China (Hyperchem professional version 7.5, http://www.hyper.com). The software package was run on a PC machine.

DSAP-2 hydrogel

1.0 ml of the stock solution of DSAP-2 peptide (10 mg/ml) was added to 1.0 ml of phosphate-buffered saline (0.058 M Na_2HPO_4, 0.017 M NaH_2PO_4, 0.069 M NaCl, 0.002 M Mg^{2+}, pH=7.2) which induced DSAP-2 self-assembling to form hydrogel, then the secondary structure of DSAP-2 was test by CD spectroscopy and the stable hydrogel was stained with Congo red at a glass slide after cultured for 24 h in room temperature. In vitro physiological environment: d-DARA16 solution (1%) was mixed with culture medium (DMEM or MEM or RPMI-1640) (Gibco) which include 8-10% fetal calf serums, added the same volume (100 μl) solution into 96 well-plates, cultured it for 24 h in the incubator (37°C, 5% CO_2), and dyed by Congo red in a glass slide.

Atomic force microscopy

500-1000 mmol/l peptide solution was prepared and cultured in different pH regulated by HCl, PBS and NaOH over 12 h. Then 5-10 μl peptide solution was applied onto a freshly cleaved mica surface. Each aliquot was left on mica for 30-60 s, washed with 1000 ml deionized water at least three times, dried in the air and imaged immediately. The images were obtained to scan the mica surface in the air in the Tapping Mode of AFM (Hitachi SPM400, Japan). It was important to minimize the tip tapping force to image soft biopolymer with AFM at resolution. AFM images were taken at 512 × 512 pixels resolution and displayed topographic images of the samples, in which the brightness of features increases as a function of height.

Cell cultures preparation

Human hepatoma cells SMMC-7721 and normal human hepatocyte cell L-02 (Transplantation engineering and transplantation immunity laboratory, Sichuan University) were dissolved rapidly in 37°C water bath, suspended in RPMI-1640 (Gibco Corp), added into 25 cm^2 culture vessels and cultured in the incubator (37°C, 5% CO_2). RPMI-1640 (Gibco Corp) medium contained 1% double-antibody solution (mycillin) and 8-10% (volume concentration) fetal bovine serum (Gibco Corp).

Cell inhibition assay

Two liver cell strains, normal cell line L-02 cells and cancer cell line SMMC-7721 cells, were seeded into 96 well plates with 10% FBS RPMI-1640 medium at a certain concentration of 1.2×10^4 cells/well (L-02 cells) and 1.5×10^4 cells/well (SMMC-7721 cells) respectively and incubated for overnight in 5% CO_2 at 37°C. Here we set four control groups: blank control (C); before Medication control (T0); experimental groups (Te(1-5)) and positive control groups(Tp(1-5)). Cell growth rate=(T-T0/(C-T0) × 100, the relative Growth Rate (GR) was calculated by OD value as follows: GR=(T-T0)/(C-T0) × 100 if T ≥ T0, GR=(T-T0)/T0 × 100 if T<T0, here T is Te(1-5) or Tp(1-5). When the GR is less than 50%, calculate the GI_{50} with Xlfit software in 4 Parameter Logistic Model. Samples of experimental group were DSAP-2 with different concentrations (0.025, 0.074, 0.22, 0.67 and 2.0 mg/ml) and the positive control groups were paclitaxel [37] (0.001, 0.01, 0.1, 1 and 10 mg/ml). 20 μl samples were added into each hole of Te, Tp groups (added PBS into blank control) and cultured for 48 h. Cells

of these groups were immobilized by TCA (30 μl, 50%) for 1 h in 4°C, free from the stationary liquid, washed five times with distilled water and dried in the air. Fixed cells were stained for 20 min by 0.4% SRB (Sulforhodamine B) at room temperature, washed by 1% acetum and dried in the air. Mixed Tris buffer solution into cells (10 mM, 200 μl/hole), and tested the optical density (OD) value at 490 nm.

Morphology of cells in 3D cell culture

Here L-02 cells were cultured as a model for 3D cell culture. When cells spread over the whole bottom of culture bottle, removed medium and trypsinized by 1 ml 0.25% trypsin to dissociate adherent cells. 1-2 ml RPMI-1640 is added into culture bottle to terminate trypsin action. Centrifuged cells for 8 min in 1000 turn/min, discarded supernatant, resuspended culture cell by RPMI-1640 and subcultured in culture bottles, mixed the cells with peptide solution for 3D culture. More detail processes can be seen in the reference [32]. The procedures of L-02 cell 3D culture in copper wire were mentioned above, and the ingrowth of cells in the pore of copper wire mesh can be clearly observed by phase contrast microscope.

Scanning electron microscopy

L-02 cells overlap on copper wire mesh and was detected by scanning electron microscope after being cultivated for 2-3 days. At the temperature of 4°C, used 5% (volume ratio) glutaraldehyde and fixed the hydrogel and the cells for 30-60 min. The cells were dehydrated with 20%, 50%, 70%, 90% and 100% ethanol gradient and dried for 2-4 hours in critical CO_2 liquid services. Metal spraying the sample after vacuum drying, then observed it by scanning electron microscope(JSM-5900, JEOL, Japan).

Fluorescence microscopy

L-20 cells were 3D cultured in 96 well plates, the positive control was added cis-platin (2.5 mg/kg) and the negative control is 3D culture system. Cells were washed twice by PBS, mixed with 500 μl binding buffer which included 2 μl Annexin V-FITC and 5 μl Propidium Iodide and shielded from light, reacted for 5 min at room temperature. When Annexin V was used in combination with PI, PI were excluded from living cells (Annexin V- / PI-) and early apoptotic cells (Annexin V+ / PI-), while late apoptotic cells and necrotic cells are simultaneously FITC and PI staining combined showed double positive (Annexin V+ / PI+). Cell apoptosis observed by using inverted Fluorescence Microscopy with double color filter (FITC and rhodamine).

The hemostasis of rabbit liver mode

In the rabbit liver transverse hemostasis experiments, 10 white New Zealand rabbits (1-3 kg, random distribution of male and female) (animal experimental center, West China hospital, Sichuan university) were chosen. The animals were anesthetized with an intraperitoneal injection of sodium pentobarbital (50 mg/kg), and then chose 3 bigger livers in each rabbit and made a sagittal liver cut about 1.5 cm long, 0.1-0.2 cm wide and 0.2-0.4 cm deep. Applied 200 μl of 10 mg/ml DSAP-2 peptide solution into the wound and recorded the hemostasis time. In addition, we chose two rabbits as a negative control that treated with saline, and found the hemostasis time were 90-120 s. Experiment was repeated at least 10 times on different rabbits and the average time for hemostasis was recorded. Here we focus on the chiral peptide as a catalyst to hemostasis and do not estimate the clinical relevance of our findings, so some positive controls (current treatment protocol, other hydrogels) are not taken into consideration here. All our studies followed the rule of animal ethics and were approved by the Animal

Ethics Committee of the Sichuan University or Chongqing Medical University.

Results

The structure of DSAP-2

We present the molecular model of DSAP-2 (Figure 1A), and we had an interest in what structure this peptide would adopt. CD spectroscopy revealed it indeed has an inverted spectrum with an ellipticity at 222 nm and a minimum ellipticity at 208 nm (Figure 1B). The CD profile suggests the secondary structure of this D-form peptide is dominated, none-typical β-sheet, but the α-helix in aqueous solution.

The nanostructure of DSAP-2 cultured in various pH value solution

The nanostructures of chiral peptide were obtained by AFM. Cultured in acidic solution (pH=3), DSAP-2 can form some nanofibers and nanoparticles (Figure 2A). In the neutral environment (pH=7), it can self-assembly to a large number of well-ordered nanofibers, with a diameter between 10-20 nm and a length of 1000 to 5000 nm and more (Figure 2B). In the alkaline solution (pH=10), only nanoparticles were obtained (Figure 2C). The results in the process of D-form peptide forming nanostructures were significantly affected by the pH environment. Furthermore, the self-assembly processes of this peptide were much sensitive to pH change. The results suggested that we can easily control the pH value and get the target nanostructure in our study.

Cell Inhibition and cell apoptosis in DSAP-2 solution

Some D-amino acids like D-Ala and D-Asp have toxicity of cells, but it is not clear whether the D-form peptide is toxic for cell strains or not [32,38]. We added peptide solutions with different concentrations into cell culture medium and tested OD value in each group compared with positive control. The data showed that, in different concentration peptide solutions, there was no significant difference in relative growth rate between normal cell line L-02 and cancer cell line SMMC-7721, and all of the growth rates were higher than 90% (Figure 3B and 3D). In the positive control drug paclitaxel group, cell inhibition increased significantly in both cell lines when the concentration was greater than 0.1 mg/ml (Figure 3A and 3C). The results confirmed DSAP-2 had no inhibited cells growth, and it was not proved this D-form peptide had toxicity of cell strains. Furthermore, Annexin V-FITC and Propidium Iodide were used to evaluate the cell apoptosis of DSAP-2 by fluorescence microscope. We found that L02 in DSAP-2 grew well and few cell apoptosis (Figure 4A-4C), and some cell apoptosis in positive control (Figure 4D-4F). When cultured for 7 days, cell proliferation is very fast, forming cell mass (Figure 5A-5D). The results confirmed that this D-form peptide can support cell growth and do not induce cell apoptosis or death.

Hydrogel of DSAP-2

Stable hydrogel can be formed by DSAP-2, with >99% water content, not only in solution with ions but also in vitro physiological environment (RPMI-1640, Gibco) and the hydrogel was transparent in the naked eye. We can observe the morphology of the hydrogel by the light microscope after stained by Congo red (Figure 6A). The picture suggested that the hydrogel had a capability of moisture-keeping, providing the environment for cells growth. DSAP-2 peptides can self-assemble to ordered-nanofibers scaffolds, form the stable hydrogel scaffold in physiological environment, support cell growth without cell

inhabitation or cell apoptosis, which suggests it, could be used as nano-biomaterial for three-dimensional (3D) cell culture.

Three-dimensional cell culture microenvironment of DSAP-2

Having learned about the self-assembly property of DSAP-2, we obtained different morphology of cells (L-02 and SMMC-7721) in the two-dimensional (2D) and 3D cultured in DSAP-2 peptide solution (Figure 5A-5D). To check the 3D morphology of cells microenvironment, we cultured cells in copper wire meshes and confirmed by SEM. The nanofibers diameter was ~ 10-30 nm, and the pores between nanofibers were about 10-100nm. L-02 cells can adhere, grow and proliferate in the scaffolds interspace. The cell surface was covered with piled-nanofibers which provided 3D scaffolds support like extracellular matrix (Figure 6B). The interspaces of peptide scaffolds retained a little water and the small molecular bioactive substances can be interchanged through these interspaces. The truly nano-scaffolds microenvironment proved this D-form self-assembling peptide DSAP-2 can be applied to 3D cell culture as the matrix material, and support cell growth, proliferation and beyond.

The rapid hemostasis function of DSAP-2

In our previous report, we found the chiral peptide d-EAK16 had an amazingly rapid hemostasis effect [6]. Here is the transverse wound model of rabbit liver. We wiped oozing bleeding 2-4 times with clean gauze on the liver surface of rabbit before adding DSAP-2 solution (Figure 7A). The weight of bleeding was 448mg on average (Figure 7C). After applying 200 μl 10 mg/ml peptide solution to the wound of rabbit liver (Figure 7B), we found that a layer of hydrogel was formed rapidly on the wound and bleeding was stopped. Hemostatic time was 18.3 ± 5.1 s (Figure 7D) compared with 106.1 ± 10.4 s (P<0.05) when treated with saline. The results confirmed that DSAP-2 has a satisfying hemostatic effect. DSAP-2 can not only support cell growth but also achieve rapid hemostasis.

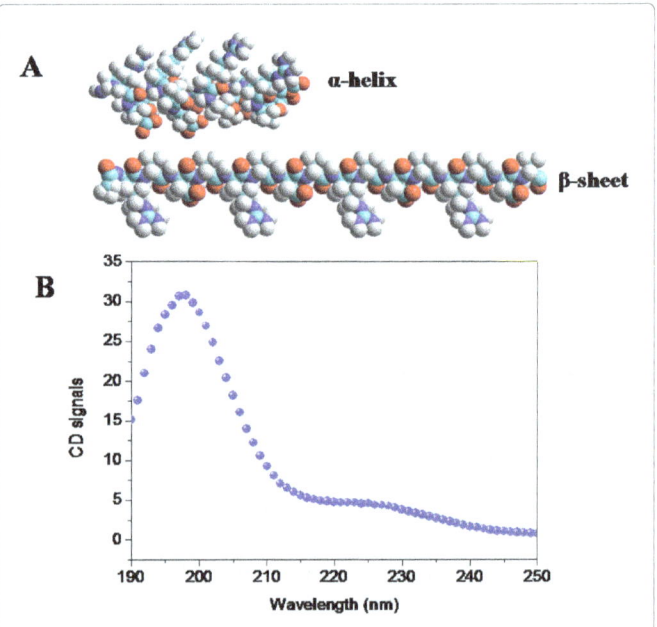

Figure 1: (A) Molecular model of the DSAP-2. The peptide is modeled with α-helix and β-sheet in the extended (N–>C). Color code: hydrogen=white, carbon=cyan, oxygen=red and nitrogen=blue; (B) CD spectrum of DSAP-2 at room temperature. Peptide (10 mg/ml) was incubated in 1.0 ml of phosphate-buffered saline (0.058 M Na₂HPO₄, 0.017 M NaH₂PO₄, 0.069 M NaCl, 0.002 M Mg²⁺, pH=7.2) after 24 h.

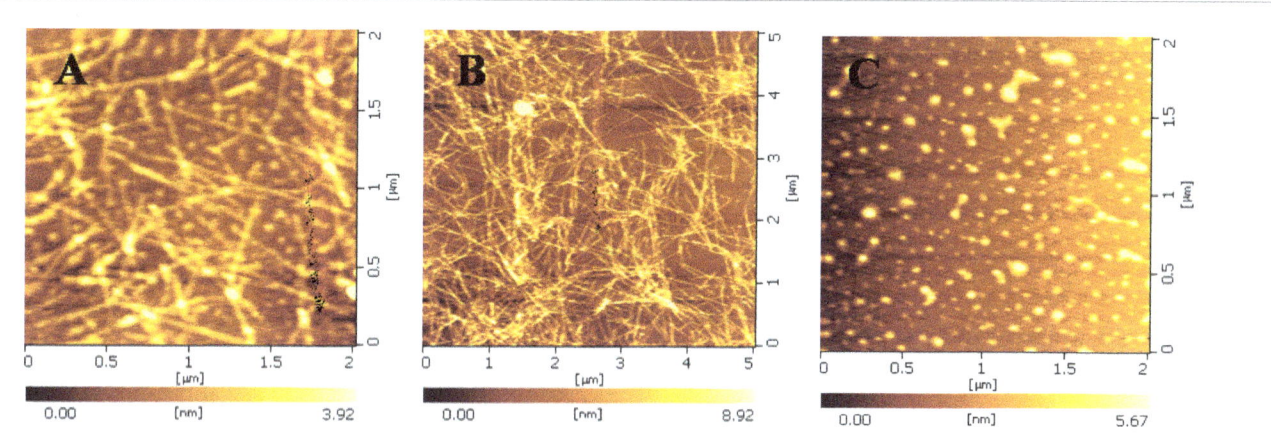

(A) DSAP-2 is self-assembled to nanofibers and nanoparticles when pH=3 (Regulated by HCl); (B) DSAP-2 is self-assembled to nanofibers completely when pH=7 (PBS); (C) While under the condition of pH=10 (Regulated by NaOH), few nanofibers obtained, most of them are nanoparticles.

Figure 2: AFM images with DSAP-2 cultured in various pH solution.

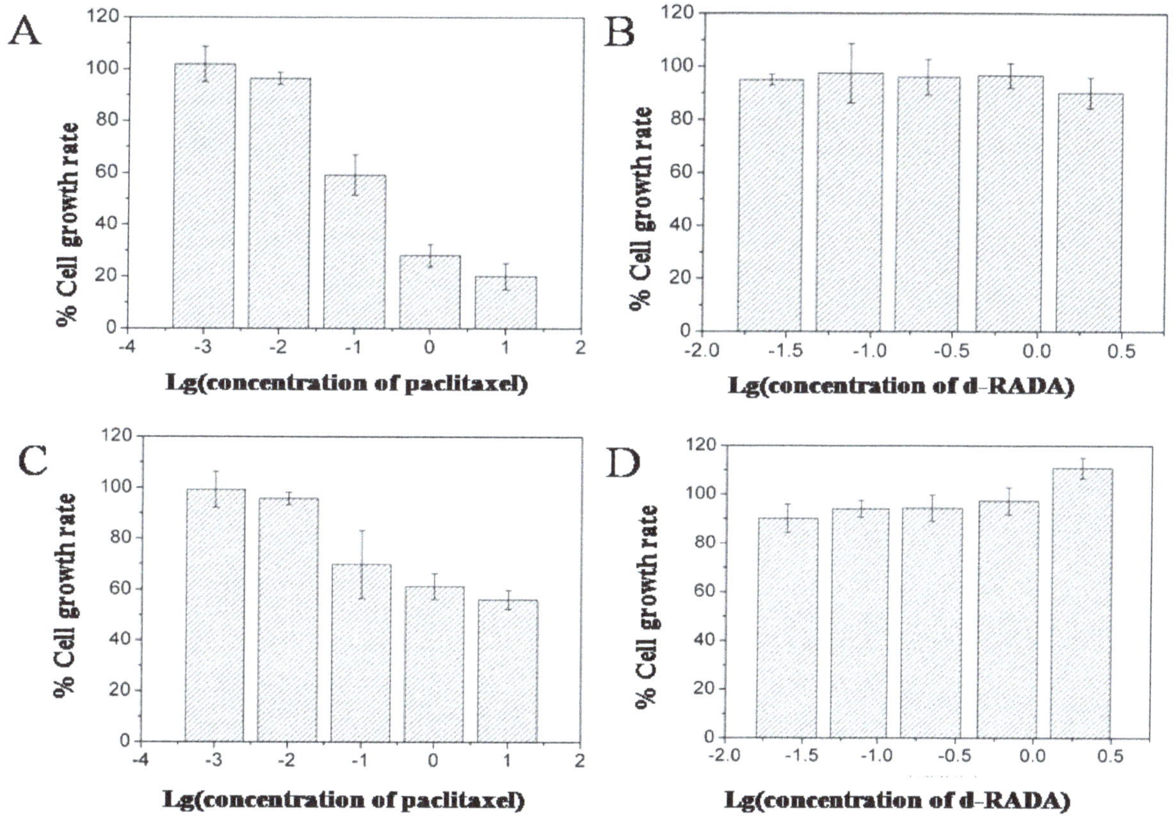

(A) Paclitaxel on Hepatocyte L02; (B) DSAP-2 on L02; (C) Paclitaxel on Hepatic cancer cell SMMC7721; (D) DSAP-2 on SMMC7721. Cells cultured in the 2D plate for 48 hours. The X-axe means lg (concentration of DSAP-2 or Paclitaxel), and the Y-axe means the cell growth rate. The concentration of DSAP-2 is 0.025, 0.074, 0.22, 0.67 and 2.0 mg/ml, and the Paclitaxel is 0.001, 0.01, 0.1, 1.0 and 10.0 mg/ml respectively.

Figure 3: Compare DSAP-2 and Paclitaxel solution with the cell growth rate.

Discussion

The advantage of DSAP-2 for 3D cell culture

The self-assembling processes also require some induced factors such as peptide concentration, pH, ions and temperature. They can easily meet these factors in the body physiological condition, and be widely used in the biomaterial area and medical areas. In general, cell cycle, cell differentiation and cell communication are determined by molecular gradient [39,40]. The interactions of protein-protein or protein-receptor, the cellular membrane structure, the extracellular matrix (ECM) and ligand play a vital role in cellular activities and

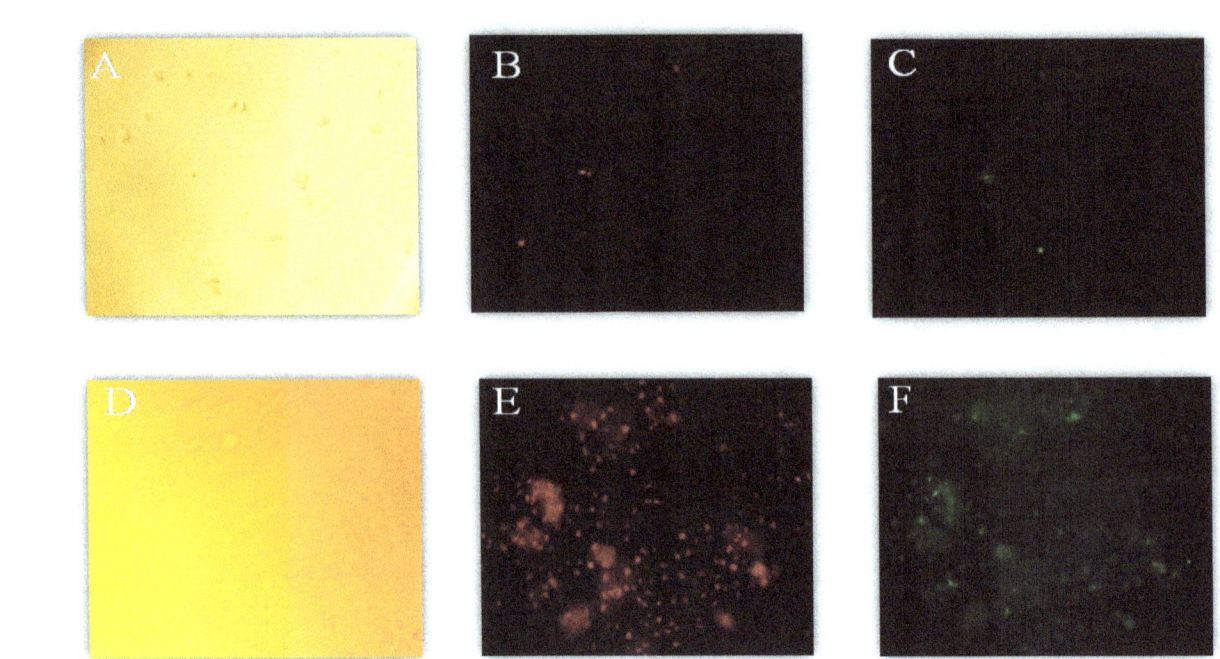

Figure 4: The apoptosis of cells cultured in DSAP-2 and cisplatin solution in first three days. (A) The bright field image of DSAP-2 cell culture;(B) The PI image of DSAP-2 cell culture;(C) The Annexin V-FITC image of DSAP-2 cell culture; (D) The bright field image of cell culture in cisplatin; (E) The PI image of cell culture in cisplatin; (F) The Annexin V-FITC image of cell culture in cisplatin. We did not obtain significantly the apoptosis of L02 in DSAP-216.

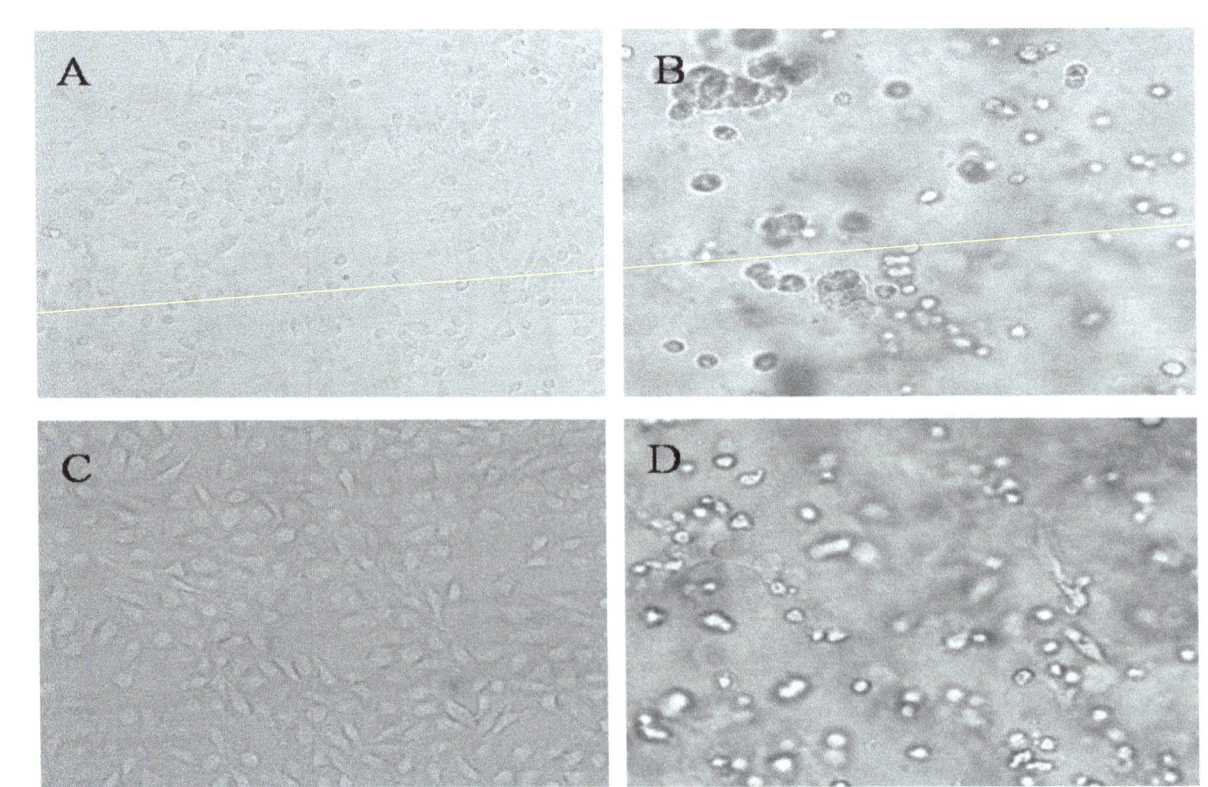

Figure 5: Morphology of cell growth in 7 days. (A) L02 cultured in 2D plate. (B) L02 cultured in 3D environment of DSAP-2 hydrogel. (C) SMMC7721 cultured in 2D plate. (D) SMMC7721 cultured 3D micro-environment of DSAP-2 hydrogel as well.

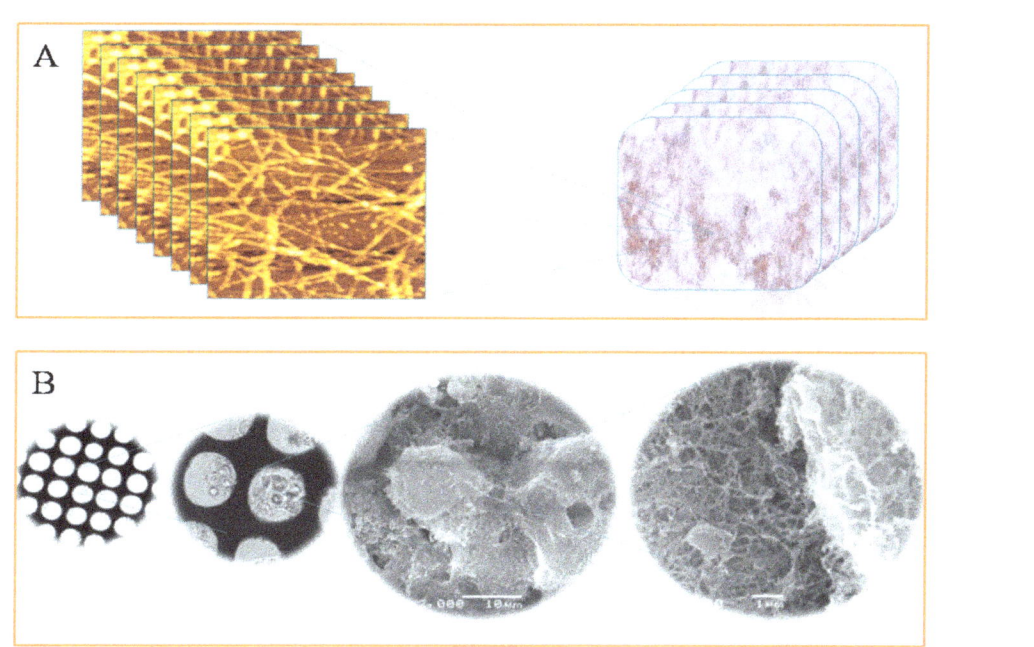

Figure 6: The cell covered with nanofibers by 3D cell cultured model. (A) AFM images of the DSAP-2 in Na⁺ solution. DSAP-2 hydrogel of Congo red stain (10 × 40). Specially to copy the same AFM images to pile together with one picture, which could show mimicking at the truly station of hydrogel and its nanofiber scaffolds; (B) 3D cell culture to copper wire meshes. The ingrowth of cells in the pore of copper wire mesh can be clearly observed by phase contrast microscope. SEM confirmed cell surface covered with nanofibers in 3D cell culture model (2000X), and the other one is zoomed to 10000X.

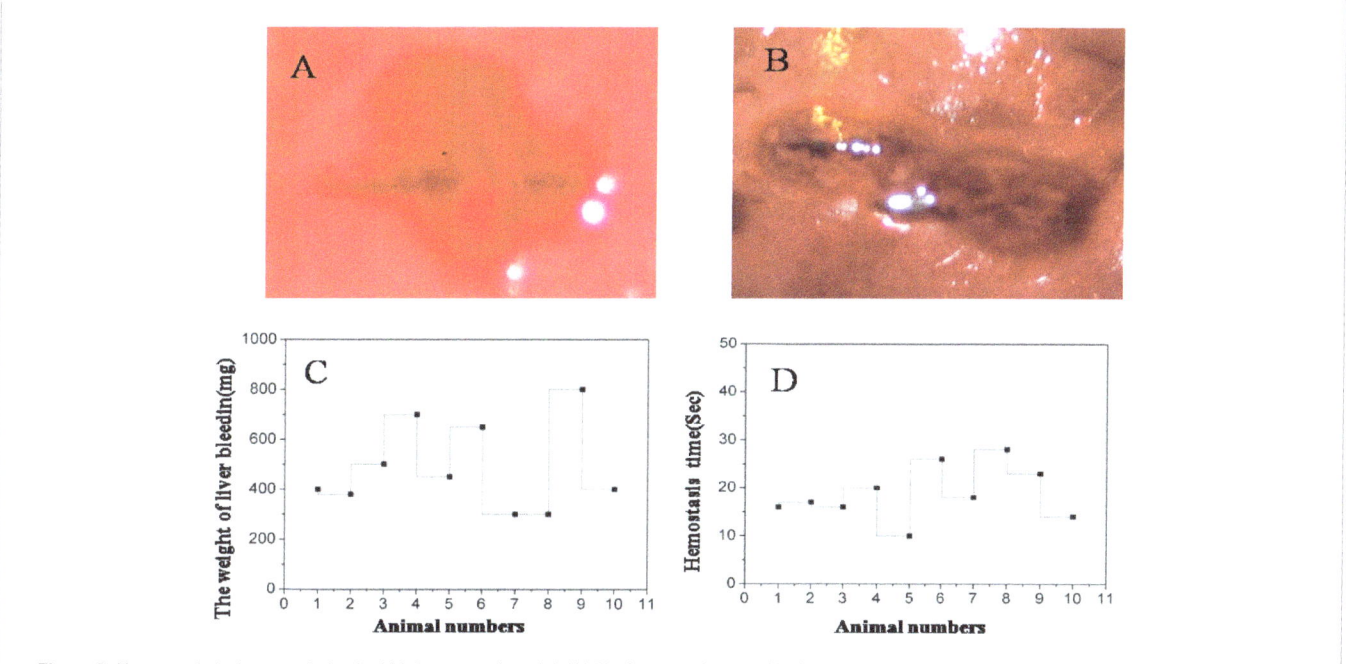

Figure 7: Hemostasis in the vascularized rabbit liver wound model. (A) The hemostatic wound in the rabbit liver. (B) After adding the peptide DSAP-2 solution, the bleeding stopped quickly. Complete hemostasis was achieved in 18.3 ± 5.1 seconds, statistically significant compared with 106.1 ± 10.4 seconds when irrigated with saline. (C) The weight of liver bleeding of the ten respective rabbits. (D) The separate hemostasis time of the ten rabbits treated with DSAP-2.

metabolism in cell culture. 2D cell culture system can't establish a dedicated 3D molecular gradient and thus alter these cells' metabolism or gene expression [4,41]. DSAP-2 can self-assemble to well-ordered nanofibers then aggregate to 3D scaffolds under a certain condition like other self-assembly peptides. It has no cell growth inhibition and no cell apoptosis (Figure 5 and 6), and its nanofiber scaffolds are similar to extracellular matrix surrounded the cells (Figure 2B). These kinds of 3D tissue cell cultures systems could provide a more realistic biophysical microenvironment that can enhance cell proliferation, migration, differentiation and performing their biological function [42-44], and suggest this peptide has a potential extracellular matrix to be used in 3D tissue culture system or 3D print soft-ink.

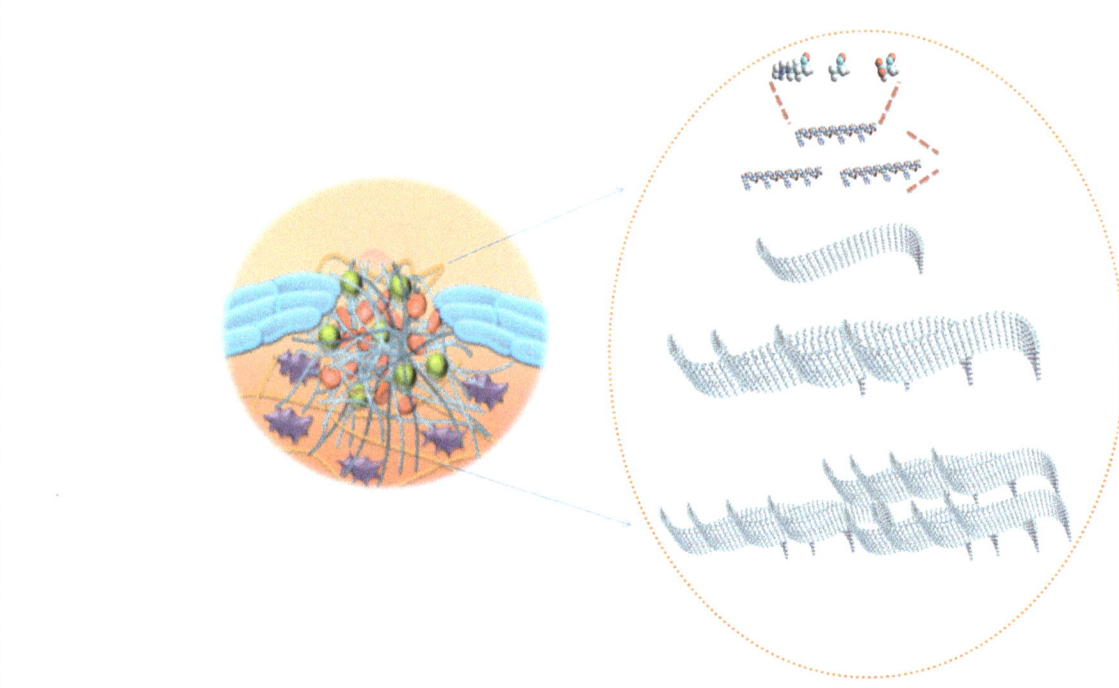

Figure 8: A plausible model of DSAP-2 worked on hemostasis. The DSAP-2 composed of 16 d-amino acid, and this peptide can self-assemble into ordered-nanofibers from molecules bottom up to these piled-nanofibers, and to scaffold, then associated with hydrogen bond of water to hydrogel. Covered this hydrogel to wound healing, these nanofibers could not only allow attachments of cells but also allow access to oxygen, hormones, nutrients and remove of waste products. The nanofiber scaffolds could prevent the escape of cells and fluid like multi-layered fish-net, which could also absorb coagulation factors as a medium to accelerate the process of hemostasis. (Blue cells: the vessel endotheliocyte, blue fibers: chiral peptide nanofibers, brown fibers: fibrin, purple cell: platelet, green cells: regenerated cells.

Rapid hemostasis of DSAP-2 and its proposed plausible model

We had reported the nanofiber scaffold can stop bleeding quickly, which is associated with the nano-mechanically force [32]. Here DSAP-2 can stop bleeding quickly as well. A plausible hypothesis of rapid hemostasis of DSAP-2 is the ions induced peptide molecules self-assembling to nanofibers, and these nanofibers by forming tight nano-seals to prevent leakage of liquid and cells (Figure 8). The mechanism of hemostasis could be a complicated process like promoting/resisting platelet activation, coagulation, fibrinolysis, cell interaction and so on [45,46]. When wound bleeds without this peptide hydrogel solution, coagulation factors normally distribute in decentralized spaces and simultaneously cascade reaction center was not centralized, generating longer coagulation time. Covered the hydrogel to the wound bleeding, diversified factors could be captured in nanofibers web to fleetly form a relatively stable central bed of coagulation activation which may accelerate the hemostasis process [45,47]. More detailed evidence still needs to be found in the future.

Conclusion

Here we designed a D form self-assembling peptide DSAP-2, obtained its nanostructure, which can be affected by pH value, and got its nanofiber hygrogel in vitro physiological environment. We also confirmed this D-form peptide can support cell growth, and nano-scaffolds surrounded by cells can use it as a 3D cell culture matrix material to support cell growth, proliferation and beyond. DSAP-2 can also achieve rapid hemostasis as well. Our study suggests this peptide could work in the wound healing in the future.

Contributors

Z.L. and M.M. designed research; all members of the team contributed new reagents, analytic tools and finished the experiment; Z.L., M.M., X.F., W.R. and L.L. analyzed data; Z.L., M.M., X.F. and L.L. wrote the paper.

Funding Acknowledgement

ZL was supported by Nature Science Foundation Project of CQ (CSTC) (cstc2015jcy jB X0072), and the grant from the National Nature Science Foundation of China (NSFC 31540019), Antibiotic Research and Re-evaluation of Sichuan Provincial Key Laboratory Topics (ARRLKF14-01), Chongqing Medical University Basic Medical Science Support Foundation (JC201514), and Chongqing Medical University Research Cultivate Foundation (Natural Science) (201417).

References

1. Luo Z, Zhang S (2012) Designer nanomaterials using chiral self-assembling peptide systems and their emerging benefit for society. Chem Soc Rev 21: 4736-4754.

2. Hauser CA, Zhang S (2010) Designer self-assembling peptide nanofiber biological materials. Chem Soc Rev 39: 2780-2790.

3. Zhang S, Holmes TC, DiPersio CM, Hynes RO, Su X, et al. (1995) Self-complementary oligopeptide matrices support mammalian cell attachment. Biomaterials 16: 1385-1393.

4. Zhang S, Gelain F, Zhao X (2005) Designer self-assembling peptide nanofiber scaffolds for 3D tissue cell cultures. Semin Cancer Biol 15: 413-420.

5. Hao Y, Shih H, Munoz Z, Kemp A, Lin CC (2014) Visible light cured thiol-vinyl hydrogels with tunable degradation for 3D cell culture. Acta Biomater 10: 104-114.

6. Luo Z, Wang S, Zhang S (2011) Fabrication of self-assembling D-form peptide nanofiber scaffold d-EAK16 for rapid hemostasis. Biomaterials 32: 2013-2020.

7. Liu X, Wang X, Ren H, He J, Qiao L, et al. (2013) Functionalized self-assembling peptide nanofiber hydrogels mimic stem cell niche to control human adipose stem cell behavior in vitro. Acta Biomater 9: 6798-6805.

8. Kandyba EE, Hodgins MB, Martin PE (2008) A murine living skin equivalent amenable to live-cell imaging: analysis of the roles of connexins in the epidermis. J Invest Dermatol 128: 1039-1049.

9. Gelain F, Unsworth LD, Zhang S (2010) Slow and sustained release of active cytokines from self-assembling peptide scaffolds. J Control Release 145: 231-239.

10. Nagai Y, Unsworth LD, Koutsopoulos S, Zhang S (2006) Slow release of molecules in self-assembling peptide nanofiber scaffold. J Control Release 115: 18-25.

11. Zhao Y, Ji T, Wang H, Li S, Nie G (2014) Self-assembled peptide nanoparticles as tumor microenvironment activatable probes for tumor targeting and imaging. J Control Release 177: 11-19.

12. Keyes-Baig C, Duhamel J, Fung SY, Bezaire J, Chen P (2004) Self-assembling peptide as a potential carrier of hydrophobic compounds. J Am Chem Soc 126: 7522-7532.

13. Ho DN, Pomroy NC, Cuesta-Seijo JA, Prive GG (2008) Crystal structure of a self-assembling lipopeptide detergent at 1.20 A. Proc Natl Acad Sci U S A 105: 12861-12866.

14. Matson JB, Zha RH, Stupp SI (2011) Peptide Self-Assembly for Crafting Functional Biological Materials. Curr Opin Solid State Mater Sci 15: 225-235.

15. Zhuang F, Oglecka K, Hauser CA (2011) Self-Assembling Peptide Surfactants A6K and A6D Adopt a-Helical Structures Useful for Membrane Protein Stabilization. Membranes (Basel) 1: 314-326.

16. Midtgaard SR, Pedersen MC, Kirkensgaard JJ, Sorensen KK, Mortensen K, et al. (2014) Self-assembling peptides form nanodiscs that stabilize membrane proteins. Soft Matter 10: 738-752.

17. Kiley P, Zhao X, Vaughn M, Baldo MA, Bruce BD, et al. (2005) Self-assembling peptide detergents stabilize isolated photosystem I on a dry surface for an extended time. PLoS Biol 3: e230.

18. Mukherjee D, May M, Vaughn M, Bruce BD, Khomami B (2010) Controlling the morphology of Photosystem I assembly on thiol-activated Au substrates. Langmuir 26: 16048-16054.

19. Mukherjee D, Vaughn M, Khomami B, Bruce BD (2011) Modulation of cyanobacterial photosystem I deposition properties on alkanethiolate Au substrate by various experimental conditions. Colloids Surf B Biointerfaces 88: 181-190.

20. Kim JH, Lee M, Lee JS, Park CB (2012) Self-assembled light-harvesting peptide nanotubes for mimicking natural photosynthesis. Angew Chem Int Ed Engl 51: 517-520.

21. Mershin A, Matsumoto K, Kaiser L, Yu D, Vaughn M, et al. (2012) Self-assembled photosystem-I biophotovoltaics on nanostructured TiO(2)and ZnO. Sci Rep 2: 234.

22. Ozbolat IT, Yu Y (2013) Bioprinting toward organ fabrication: challenges and future trends. IEEE Trans Biomed Eng 60: 691-699.

23. Kaneda Y, Yamamoto Y, Okada N, Tsutsuml Y, Nakagawa S, et al. (1997) Antimetastatic effect of synthetic Glu-Ile-Leu-Asp-Val peptide derivatives containing D-amino acids. Anticancer Drugs 8: 702-707.

24. Jorgensen NO, Stepanaukas R, Pedersen AG, Hansen M, Nybroe O (2003) Occurrence and degradation of peptidoglycan in aquatic environments. FEMS Microbiol Ecol 46: 269-280.

25. Martinez-Rodriguez S, Martinez-Gomez AI, Rodriguez-Vico F, Clemente-Jimenez JM, Las Heras-Vazquez FJ (2010) Natural occurrence and industrial applications of D-amino acids: an overview. Chem Biodivers 7: 1531-1548.

26. Sugiki T, Utsunomiya-Tate N (2013) Site-specific aspartic acid isomerization regulates self-assembly and neurotoxicity of amyloid-beta. Biochem Biophys Res Commun 441: 493-498.

27. Schieber A, Bruckner H, Rupp-Classen M, Specht W, Nowitzki-Grimm S, et al. (1997) Evaluation of D-amino acid levels in rat by gas chromatography-selected ion monitoring mass spectrometry: no evidence for subacute toxicity of orally fed D-proline and D-aspartic acid. J Chromatogr B Biomed Sci Appl 691: 1-12.

28. Stegman LD, Zheng H, Neal ER, Ben-Yoseph O, Pollegioni L, et al. (1998) Induction of cytotoxic oxidative stress by D-alanine in brain tumor cells expressing *Rhodotorula gracilis* D-amino acid oxidase: a cancer gene therapy strategy. Hum Gene Ther 9: 185-193.

29. Zhang G, Sun HJ (2014) Racemization in reverse: evidence that D-amino acid toxicity on Earth is controlled by bacteria with racemases. PLoS One 9: e92101.

30. Luo Z, Zhao X, Zhang S (2008) Self-Organization of a Chiral D-EAK16 Designer Peptide into a 3D Nanofiber Scaffold. Macromole Biosci 8: 785-791.

31. Luo Z, Zhao X, Zhang S (2008) Structural Dynamic Behaviors of a Self-Assembling Peptide EAK16 Made of Only D-amino acids. PLoS One 3: e2364.

32. Luo Z, Yue Y, Zhang Y, Yuan X, Gong J, et al. (2013) Designer D-form self-assembling peptide nanofiber scaffolds for 3-dimensional cell cultures. Biomaterials 34: 4902-4913.

33. Aggeli A, Nyrkova IA, Bell M, Harding R, Carrick L, et al. (2001) Hierarchical self-assembly of chiral rod-like molecules as a model for peptide beta -sheet tapes, ribbons, fibrils, and fibers. Proc Natl Acad Sci U S A 98: 11857-11862.

34. Zhao Y, Tanaka M, Kinoshita T, Higuchi M, Tan T (2009) Controlled release and entrapment of enantiomers in self-assembling scaffolds composed of beta-sheet peptides. Biomacromolecules 10: 3266-3272.

35. Belanger D, Tong X, Soumare S, Dory YL, Zhao Y (2009) Cyclic peptide-polymer complexes and their self-assembly. Chemistry 15: 4428-4436.

36. Chronopoulou L, Sennato S, Bordi F, Giannella D, Di Nitto A, et al. (2014) Designing unconventional Fmoc-peptide-based biomaterials: structure and related properties. Soft Matter 10: 1944-1952.

37. Liebmann J, Cook JA, Fisher J, Teague D, Mitchell JB (1994) In Vitro Studies of Taxol as a Radiation Sensitizer in Human Tumor Cells. J Natl Cancer Inst 86: 441-446.

38. Kamei N, Morishita M, Eda Y, Ida N, Nishio R, et al. (2008) Usefulness of cell-penetrating peptides to improve intestinal insulin absorption. J Control Release 132: 21-25.

39. Wilson PA, Melton DA (1994) Mesodermal patterning by an inducer gradient depends on secondary cell-cell communication. Curr Biol 4: 676-686.

40. Bosch TC, Fujisawa T (2001) Polyps, peptides and patterning. Bioessays 23: 420-427.

41. Cimetta E, Sirabella D, Yeager K, Davidson K, Simon J, et al. (2013) Microfluidic bioreactor for dynamic regulation of early mesodermal commitment in human pluripotent stem cells. Lab Chip 13: 355-364.

42. Driskell RR, Lichtenberger BM, Hoste E, Kretzschmar K, Simons BD, et al. (2013) Distinct fibroblast lineages determine dermal architecture in skin development and repair. Nature 504: 277-281.

43. Swift J, Ivanovska IL, Buxboim A, Harada T, Dingal PC, et al. (2013) Nuclear lamin-A scales with tissue stiffness and enhances matrix-directed differentiation. Science 341: 12401-12404.

44. Discher DE, Mooney DJ, Zandstra PW (2009) Growth factors, matrices, and forces combine and control stem cells. Science 324: 1673-1677.

45. Mankad PS, Codispoti M (2001) The role of fibrin sealants in hemostasis. Am J Surg 182: 21S-28S.

46. Kumar V, Chapman JR (2007) Whole blood thrombin: development of a process for intra-operative production of human thrombin. J Extra Corpor Technol 39: 18-23.

47. Shah SK, Fogle LN, Aroom KR, Gill BS, Moore-Olufemi SD, et al. (2010) Hydrostatic intestinal edema induced signaling pathways: potential role of mechanical forces. Surgery 147: 772-779.

7

Determination of Kanamycin Plasma Levels using LC-MS and its Pharmacokinetics in Patients with Multidrug-Resistant Tuberculosis with and without HIV-Infection

Pierre Mugabo[1]*, Mercy I Abaniwonda[1], Danie Theron[2], Leonie Van Zyl [2], Shafick M Hassan[3], Marietjie Stander[4], Helen McIlleron[5] and Richard Madsen[6]

[1]School of Pharmacy, University of the Western Cape, Private Bag X17, 7535. Bellville, South Africa
[2]Brewelskloof Hospital, Department of Health, Province of Western Cape, South Africa
[3]Department of Nursing and Radiology, Cape Peninsula University of Technology, Bellville, South Africa
[4]Department of Biochemistry, University of Stellenbosch, South Africa
[5]Department of Medicine, Division of Clinical Pharmacology, University of Cape Town, South Africa
[6]Department of Statistics, University of Missouri, USA

Abstract

Purpose: The objectives of the study were: (1) to determine kanamycin plasma concentrations using liquid chromatography coupled with mass spectrometry (LC-MS), (2) to investigate kanamycin pharmacokinetics (PK) in patients with multi-drug resistant tuberculosis (MDR-TB), (3) to find out whether HIV infection, kidney dysfunction and antiretroviral drugs influence kanamycin PK.

Methods: The study was designed as a non-randomized study involving male and female HIV- positive and HIV-negative patients admitted for MDR-TB treatment. Blood samples were collected before (baseline) and ½, 1, 2, 4, 8 and 24 hours after intramuscular injection of kanamycin. LC-MS was used to quantify kanamycin plasma concentrations.

Results: Thirty one patients including 13 HIV (+) participated in the study. The lower limit of detection and lower limit of quantification of kanamycin were 0.06 µg/ml and 0.15 µg/ml respectively. Kanamycin PK parameters were described and there was no significant difference between HIV-positive and HIV-negative patients. A statistical significant difference (p=0.0126) was found in the renal function in HIV - positive and HIV - negative patients. However, this difference did not affect kanamycin elimination. No interactions have been identified between antiretroviral drugs and kanamycin. Conclusion: LC-MS analysis method is highly specific and highly sensitive in the detection and quantification of kanamycin plasma concentrations. Kanamycin PK in patients with MDR-TB was described. Due to a limited number of patients, we cannot rule out any influence of HIV - infection, renal impairment and antiretroviral drugs on kanamycin pharmacokinetics. The relationship between the area under the curve of kanamycin free plasma concentrations (fAUC) and its minimum inhibitory concentrations (MIC) on M.tuberculosis isolated from the sputum of each patient should be assessed. Therefore, kanamycin free plasma concentrations and MIC should be determined

Keywords: Multi-drug resistant tuberculosis; Human immunodeficiency virus; Liquid Chromatography-Mass Spectrometry; Plasma concentrations; Pharmacokinetics; Kanamycin

Introduction

The surge of multidrug- resistant tuberculosis (MDR-TB) is raising concerns globally and in sub-Saharan Africa [1-6]. Although the epidemiological relationship between HIV infection and MDR-TB has not been established in sub- Saharan Africa [7-10], clinical evidence has shown that there is a link between HIV infection and the development of MDR-TB [11-14].

Many studies have confirmed that HIV -positive patients do not adequately absorb anti-TB drugs resulting in sub-therapeutic outcomes of anti-TB therapy that may result in the development of resistance to anti-TB drugs [12,13,15]. This evidence has not yet been confirmed for many of the second-line anti-TB drugs.

Interactions between anti-retroviral drugs and anti-TB drugs alter the plasma concentrations of anti-TB drugs and these interactions could result in sub-therapeutic anti-TB drugs plasma concentrations. For first-line anti-TB drugs, major drug/drug interactions occur between rifampicin (RIF) and highly active anti-retroviral therapy (HAART) drugs, protease inhibitors (PIs) and non-nucleoside reverse transcriptase inhibitors (NNRTIs) [16, 17]. Furthermore, interaction between tenofovir and kanamycin as a result of reduced elimination by the kidney could result in an increase in the plasma concentration of kanamycin.

Consequently, a better understanding of the pharmacokinetics (PK) and pharmacodynamics (PD) of anti-TB drugs should improve treatment outcomes in patients with MDR-TB infection and in patients with MDR-TB co-infected with HIV [18].

Kanamycin is one of the drugs used in the intensive phase treatment of MDR-TB. The PK of kanamycin has been studied in healthy volunteers using microbiological assay methods and to a limited extent in patients with MDR-TB [19,20]. To the best of our knowledge, there is no recently published study on the analysis of kanamycin plasma concentrations using liquid chromatography coupled with mass spectrometry (LC-MS). In addition, little information exists on the PK of kanamycin in HIV -negative patients infected with MDR-

*Corresponding author: Pierre Mugabo, University of the Western Cape, Private Bag X17, 7535. Bellville, South Africa, E-mail: pmugabo@uwc.ac.za

TB [21], and currently there is no information on its PK in South African patients with MDR-TB infection and in patients with MDR-TB co-infected with HIV [22]. Therefore, information obtained from this study might help for future development of therapeutic drug monitoring (TDM) in order to improve patients' treatment outcome and optimise drug therapy.

Hence, we determined kanamycin plasma concentrations using LC-MS and evaluated the PK of kanamycin in patients with MDR-TB and in patients with MDR-TB co-infected with HIV during their course of treatment. We also examined the influence of HIV infection on kanamycin PK. We evaluated the effect of the kidney dysfunction on kanamycin PK and assessed the interaction between antiretroviral drugs and kanamycin.

Methods

Study site, design and subjects

The study was conducted at Brewelskloof Hospital (BKH), South Africa. BKH is one of the South African hospitals specialized in the treatment of MDR-TB. The study was designed as a prospective, non randomized pharmacokinetic study involving male and female HIV-positive and HIV-negative patients admitted for MDR-TB treatment.

Inclusion and exclusion criteria

A patient was included in the study if he/she complied with all of the following: (1) Signature of informed written consent; (2) Informed consent for HIV test; (3) On kanamycin treatment for at least 2 weeks; (4) Adult patients 18 - 65 years old; (5) MDR-TB sensitive to second -line anti-TB drugs.

Patients were excluded from the study in case any of the following criteria applied: (1) Patient request; (2) History of congestive cardiac failure; (3) Uncontrolled hypertension; (4) Ischemic heart disease; (5) Pregnancy or breast feeding; (6) Hypersensitivity to kanamycin; (7) Patients on drugs other than anti-retroviral drugs, known to interact with kanamycin; (8) Older than 65 years and younger than 18 years; (9) Haemoglobin less than 10g%, and (10) severe dehydration.

Kanamycin dose and blood sampling

Patients received kanamycin at a dose of 500, 600, 660, 750, 1000 mg daily based on their body weight. On the study day, after an 8-hour overnight fast, blood samples were collected in a heparinised tube via an intravenous catheter fixed on the forearm vein before (baseline) and ½, 1, 2, 4, 8 and 24 hours after intramuscular administration of kanamycin. Blood samples were immediately centrifuged at 5,250 rpm for 5 minutes. Then, plasma was separated and stored at -80°C until the day of analysis. Blood was also collected for renal and liver function tests, CD4 counts, viral load and haematology tests.

Determination of kanamycin plasma concentrations and chemicals used

Plasma levels of kanamycin were determined using LC-MS. The following chemicals were used in the study: analytical grade dimethyl sulfoxide (DMSO), acetonitrile (ACN), trichloroacetic acid (TCA), phosphoric acid and HPLC grade trifluroacetic acid (TFA). All of them were obtained from Sigma-Aldrich (Cape Town, Western Cape). Kanamycin was supplied by BKH and used as a working standard.

Liquid Chromatography-Mass Spectrometry

LC-MS was performed with Waters Acquity UPLC system connected to a Xevo triple quadrupole mass spectrometer (Waters, Milford, MA, USA). The Waters Atlantis is a reversed phase packing with a difunctional C_{18} ligand, designed to retain polar compounds better. The mobile phase used was 1 % formic acid in water (v/v) as solvent A, solvent B consisted of acetonitrile. A flow rate of 0.23 ml/min was applied and an injection volume of 5 µl. The gradient started at 98% solvent A for the first 2 minutes followed by a linear gradient over 8 minutes to 70 % solvent B. The column was washed for 1 minute at 100% solvent B and re-equilibrated for another 6 minutes at the starting conditions.

The MS conditions were as follows: electrospray ionization in the positive mode was applied, the ion source and desolvation temperature were held at 140 °C and 400 °C, respectively. The capillary voltage was 2.8 kV. The desolvation gas at 1000 L/h and the cone gas was 50 L/h. The instrument was operated at multiple reactions monitoring (MRM) mode. The MRM settings for kanamycin was 485 > 163 at collision energy 20 eV.and cone voltage of 20 V. Propanolol was used as internal standard and was monitored at an MRM of 260.3 >183 at a collision energy of 20eV and cone voltage of 18 V. Waters MassLynx™ software was used for the data collection and processing.

Preparation of standards

The stock solution of 1 mg/ml was serially diluted with acetonitrile to obtain working solutions with the concentrations 10, 5, 1, 0.5, 0.1, 0.05 and 0.01µg/ml. All these standards contained 10 ppm propanolol as internal standard.

Patient samples preparation

To prepare the patients' plasma samples for the LC-MS assay, trichloroacetic acid (30 µl) was added to 50 µl plasma followed by 170 µl internal standard solution (10 ppm propanolol in water). The mixture was vortexed for 1 minute, followed by centrifugation at 6000 g for 5 minutes. The supernatant was injected onto the LC-MS. Blank plasma was spiked with 1 and 5 ppm of kanamycin in triplicate to determine the recoveries and repeatability. The relative standard deviation was better than 12%. This relatively high standard deviation and relatively high limit of detection and quantification is due to the fact that kanamycin elutes just after the void volume of the column. The use of a C18 column with similar selectivity as the Waters Atlantis column used here is very important for this analysis.

Determination of pharmacokinetic parameters

The plasma concentration-time profile for each patient was plotted using a semi-log graph paper. Kanamycin PK parameters were calculated based on the non-compartmental analysis [22-24] and expressed as median and range (lowest to highest).

Statistical analysis

Patients' data were organised and coded onto data collection forms and captured into Microsoft Excel spreadsheets. Kanamycin concentrations and PK parameters were analysed using descriptive statistics. Analysis was done using SAS version 9.0 (SAS Institute Inc., Cary, NC, USA).

Since the data is highly skewed in many cases, the HIV+ and HIV- groups were compared using the Wilcoxon Rank Sum test rather than a t-test. PK parameters were reported as mean and standard deviation. The Kruskal-Wallis one-way analysis of variance was used in comparing more than two groups to see if they originate from the same population. Statistical significance was assumed at the $p < 0.01$ level to avoid a type 1 error (false positive).

The number of patients in HIV-positive and HIV-negative groups was sufficient to give a power of about 80% in detecting a statistical significant difference in the means of about 1.2 standard deviations based on our power calculations. Also, the number of patients who participated in previously published studies [21,25-28] was similar to the number of patients in our study.

Ethics consideration

The study was approved by the ethics committee of the University of the Western Cape and the University of Cape Town. Permission to conduct the study was granted by the Western Cape Department of Health. It was conducted according to the national and international ethics requirements. The information collected was kept confidential and saved in a safe file which can only be accessed by the researcher. Patient confidentiality and privacy was maintained at all times.

Results

Patients' demographic data

Thirty-one patients (17 males and 14 females) infected with MDR-TB participated in the study. Of these 31 patients, 13 (8 males and 5 females) were infected with HIV. The median (range) age and weight of patients were 32 (18–54) years and 53.0 (41.8–90.0) kg, respectively.

Renal and liver function profile

The renal function was normal in 5 HIV (+) and 15 HIV (-) patients, mildly impaired (60-89 GFR) in 6 HIV (+) and 3 HIV (-) patients, moderately impaired (40-59 GFR) in 2 HIV (+) patients. Liver function tests were normal in both HIV (+) and HIV (-) patients.

Virological profile

In HIV (+) patients the CD4 count (cells/mm^3) was <100 in 5 patients, 100-299 in 3 patients and > 300 in 5 patients. The viral load was less than 40 copies/ml in 10 patients and 5,000 to 1,000,000 copies/ml in 3 patients.

Validation of the method of kanamycin liquid chromatography-mass spectrometry analysis

Liquid chromatography coupled with mass spectrometry was used in the quantification of kanamycin plasma concentrations. This method was validated by determining linearity, recovery, precision and accuracy, low limit of detection, low limit of quantification, and specificity.

The overall precision expressed as relative standard deviation (RSD %), was less than 12%. The accuracy, expressed in terms of recovery was 74 ± 9.1% and 111 ± 6.2% for 1 µg/ml and 5 µg/ml, respectively.

The lower limit of detection of kanamycin was 0.06 µg/ml. The lower limit of quantification of kanamycin in the plasma was 0.15 µg/ml.

There were no interfering peaks from the plasma components with kanamycin peak in the blank plasma, which was detected at a retention time of 2.65 minutes. Figure 1 shows the chromatograms of kanamycin and internal standard of a patient's plasma. This relatively high standard deviation and relatively high limit of detection and quantitation is due to the fact that kanamycin elutes just after the void volume of the column. The use of a very polar C18 column is very important for this analysis as most other columns and solvent systems tested were unable to retain kanamycin.

Kanamycin pharmacokinetic parameters

Table 1 and Figure 2 present kanamycin mean plasma concentrations in HIV-negative and HIV-positive patients at different times of blood sampling as indicated in the methods. The standard deviations (STD) and P-values between HIV-negative and HIV–positive are also shown. Before kanamycin administration there were no detectable plasma concentrations from previous day kanamycin administration in both HIV - positive and HIV - negative patients. However, 24 hours after current study kanamycin dosing, the mean plasma concentrations we 1.27 ± 2.89 µg/ml in HIV (+) and 0.97 ± 2.54 µg/ml in HIV (-) patients.

Table 2 and Figures 3-5 present kanamycin pharmacokinetic parameters in HIV-negative and HIV-positive patients. The elimination rate constant (K_e), the elimination half-life ($T_{1/2}$), the area under the plasma concentration curve during 24 hours (AUC_{0-24}), the area under the plasma concentration curve from zero to infinity ($AUC_{0-\infty}$), the maximum plasma concentrations (C_{max}), the time to the maximum plasma concentrations (T_{max}), the absorption rate constant (k_a), the absorption half-life ($t_{1/2}$), the volume of distribution (V_d), the total clearance (Cl_{tot}), and the mean residence time (MRT) are given in Table 2 in the order at which they appear. Each parameter is shown as mean value plus STD. P-values between HIV (-) and HIV (+) patients are also indicated.

Discussion

Determination of kanamycin plasma concentrations using liquid chromatography-mass spectrometry

The LC-MS method is a proven method and has been widely used in the quantification of anti-TB drugs [22-24]. The plasma levels of kanamycin were determined using LC-MS method and analysis was conducted according to scientific standards. The linearity, lowest limit of detection, lowest limit of quantification, specificity, precision, recovery and accuracy were conducted to validate the assay. All chemicals used were prepared and standardised regularly. Chemicals were obtained from a reputable source (Sigma-Aldrich, Cape Town). Separation of kanamycin was achieved at a retention time of 1.50 minutes with a high recovery percentage of 92.5%.

Previously published studies have used microbiological and fluoroimmunoassay in the quantification of kanamycin [21,25-28]. This study results demonstrate that the LC-MS analysis method is highly successful and accurate in the detection and quantification of kanamycin concentrations in plasma.

At baseline kanamycin plasma concentrations were below detectable levels (0.05 µg/ml). This could be as a result of an insufficient amount of kanamycin remaining in the body 24hrs after previous dosing that could be detected at baseline.

Kanamycin pharmacokinetics

Kanamycin PK parameters have been described in 3 studies in healthy volunteers [25,26,28] and in one study involving HIV -negative patients infected with MDR-TB [21] using immunoassay methods. C_{max}, T_{max}, K_e, $T_{1/2}$, Cl_{tot} and V_d results of these studies range from 20 to 35 µg/ml, 1 to 2 hours, 0.29 to 0.30 hr^{-1}, 2 to 4 hours, 5 to 6 L/hr and 17–23 L respectively [21,25,26,28].

When comparing kanamycin PK parameters in previous studies to that of HIV -negative patients in the study, the mean C_{max} (18.39 µg/

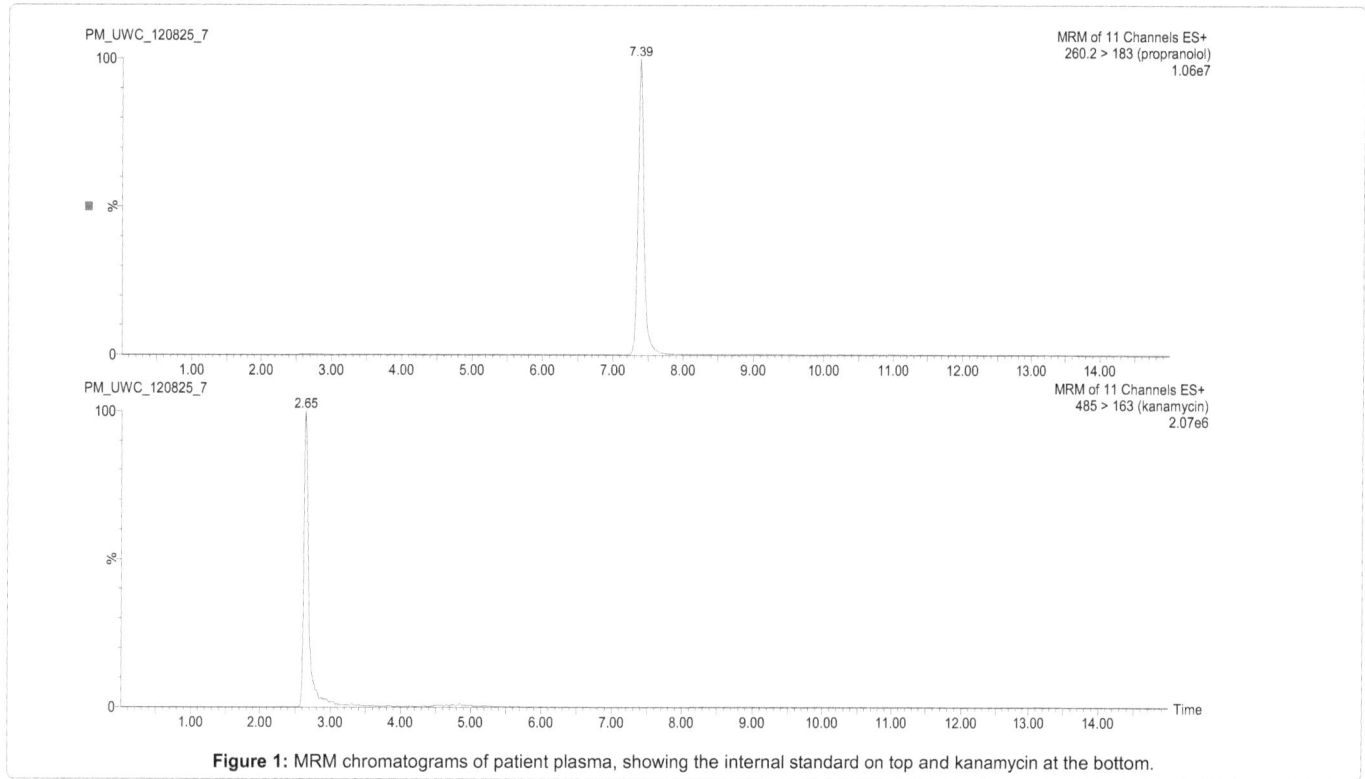

Figure 1: MRM chromatograms of patient plasma, showing the internal standard on top and kanamycin at the bottom.

Time	HIV - NEG	(N=18)	HIV - POS	(N=13)	P-value
(hr)	Mean (µg/ml)	STD	Mean (µg/ml)	STD	
t0	0.00	0	0.00	0	1
t0.5	1.94	3.83	3.83	5.27	0.3472
t1	16.43	5.63	15.94	7.47	0.9447
t2	14.33	5.92	14.46	4.78	0.9916
t4	9.06	3.79	9.83	3.18	0.7004
t8	4.96	4.13	5.64	4.14	0.4105
t24	0.97	2.54	1.27	2.89	0.5139

Table 1: Kanamycin plasma concentrations in HIV-negative and HIV-positive patients.

ml) was lower, T_{max} (1hr) was similar, K_e (0.13hr^{-1}) was lower, $T_{1/2}$ (5.37 hrs) was longer, Cl_{tot} (4.00L/hr) was higher and V_d (33.02L) was higher. The increased V_d kanamycin could be responsible for the long time kanamycin molecules resided in HIV-negative patients [20,25,26,28].

Influence of human immunodeficiency virus on the pharmacokinetics of kanamycin

The rate and extent of absorption of kanamycin as represented by the T_{max} and C_{max} were similar in both HIV -positive and HIV -negative patients. The AUC_{0-24}, which quantifies the extent of absorption of kanamycin was also similar in HIV -positive and HIV -negative patients. HIV -positive patients were not severely affected by HIV. Many HIV positive patients had good immunological and virological profile. Eight out of thirteen patients had a CD4 count within the ranges of (100-599) cells/mm^3 and ten had a viral load of less than 40 copies/ml.

When compared to other HIV -positive patients in the study, a reduction in the extent of distribution of kanamycin in two patients with CD4 count of 382 and 336 cells/mm^3 and represented by a V_d of 13.28 and 15.39 L, respectively, might be associated with the short elimination $T_{1/2}$ of 2.10 and 3.15 hours and MRT of 2.39 and 2.87 hrs,

respectively that was observed. The $T_{1/2}$ of a drug is a PK parameter dependent on both V_d and CL_{tot} and is a reflection of the extent of the distribution or elimination of a drug [29-32]. Similarly, an increase in the V_d (60.22, 51.92, 26.26 and 30.17 L) of kanamycin in some patients as compared to other HIV -positive patients resulted in the lengthening of the elimination $T_{1/2}$ of 6.30, 8.77, 11.00 and 5.33 hrs and MRT of 7.92, 8.80, 12.96 and 4.69 hrs, respectively.

There were no significant differences in the PK parameters of kanamycin in HIV -positive patients when compared to the mean PK parameters in HIV -negative patients. The smallest observed p-value is about 0.48 However, it should be remembered that the sample sizes are relatively small so that there is limited power to detect differences. Differences may in fact exist but could not be detected statistically.

Influence of renal dysfunction on the pharmacokinetics of kanamycin:

There was a significant difference (p=0.013) in the renal function between the HIV -positive and HIV -negative patients. However there was no significant difference (p=0.31) when we correlated the GFR values and the PK parameters in the two groups of patients to see if changes in the renal function affected the PK of kanamycin. HIV could be responsible for the significant difference in the renal function between HIV -positive and HIV -negative patients. A decline in renal function and low CD4 count are associated with HIV-related nephropathy, due to HIV infecting the renal cells directly [33-35]. Also, we had more patients with impaired renal function in the HIV -positive group than in the HIV -negative group and this could have contributed to the statistical difference. This result is consistent with a study done in South African patients, reporting that HIV-related nephropathy is exhibited in HIV positive patients at any stage of HIV infection and is characterised with varying degrees of GFR [33].

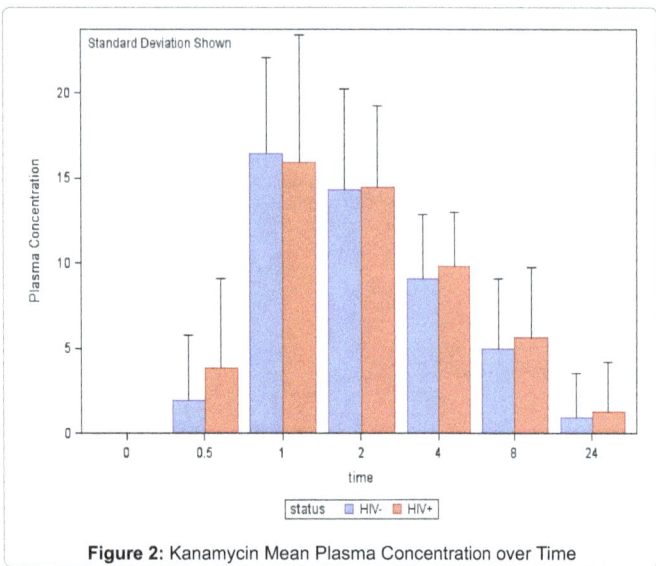

Figure 2: Kanamycin Mean Plasma Concentration over Time

PK	HIV - NEG (N=18)		HIV - POS (N=13)		P-value
Parameters	Mean (µg/ml)	STD	Mean (µg/ml)	STD	
K_e (hr^{-1})	0.20	0.11	0.19	0.08	0.8205
T_{max} (hr)	1.16	0.49	1.27	0.53	0.6159
K_a (hr^{-1})	1.29	1.32	1.05	0.88	0.8357
$t_{1/2}$ (hr)	1.67	1.86	1.29	1.59	0.9273
$T_{1/2}$ (hr)	4.45	2.25	4.62	2.66	0.8205
Cl_{tot} (L/hr)	7.72	5.49	9.13	8.93	0.7153
MRT (hr)	3.99	3.01	4.16	3.56	0.7674
C_{max} (µg/ml)	18	4.69	16.35	5.76	0.4892
V_d (L)	38.62	18.56	50.18	45.34	0.7078
AUC_{0-24} (µg/ml.hr)	122.53	58.58	122.89	77.94	0.6217
$AUC_{0-\infty}$ (µg/ml.hr)	170.26	91.37	169.08	115.32	0.5669

Table 2: Kanamycin PK parameters in HIV-negative andHIVpositive patients.

Influence of antiretroviral drugs on the pharmacokinetics of kanamycin?

Kanamycin was administered with other MDR-TB drugs to all patients. Some of the HIV positive patients were also given lamivudine, stavudine and efavirenz. None of these drugs affected the metabolism, distribution and renal elimination of kanamycin.

Therapeutic implications

The two common PK parameters associated with the clinical efficacy of aminoglycosides are C_{max} and AUC_{0-24} [36]. High peak plasma concentration of aminoglycosides is associated with increased rate of elimination of Mycobacterium tuberculosis (MTB) and better therapeutic response in patients [4,12]. However, due to the narrow therapeutic range (20-35) µg/ml of aminoglycosides [12], care must be taken when administering kanamycin in patients with renal impairment.

Kanamycin shows inhibitory activity against MTB at concentration of about 6 µg/ml in vitro and an intramuscular dose of 15 mg/kg produces a C_{max} of 35-45 µg/ml [4,12]. Most of our patients had a low peak plasma concentration of kanamycin when compared to the literature [25-28]. A median dose of 18.9 mg/kg of kanamycin in both HIV -positive and HIV –negative patients in the study resulted in a peak plasma level of 18.19 (8.40-27.63) µg/ml and 18.39 (13.32-25.26) µg/ml, respectively. The low C_{max} could result in poor response

to therapy and increased risk of selection of drug-resistant organisms. This is because kanamycin has a concentration-dependent bactericidal activity as the rate of bacterial killing increases as the concentration increases [37-40]. In addition, the C_{max}: MIC ratio correlates best with bacterial killing and it is important to have a high C_{max}: MIC ratio of at least 8–10 to prevent resistance for aminoglycosides [40,41]. Therefore, the ideal dosing regimen of kanamycin would maximise concentration, because the higher the concentration, the higher the extent of bacterial killing [40].

It has been suggested that clinicians should aim for a C_{max} of between 20 and 35 µg/ml to maximise the rate and extent of bacterial killing and a C_{trough} (trough level) of <10 µg/ml to prevent toxicity when kanamycin is given intramuscularly [12]. Based on our results, the mean C_{trough} of kanamycin in HIV -positive and in HIV -negative patients was 1.27 ± 2.89 µg/ml and 0.97 ± 2.54 µg/ml respectively. This explains that kanamycin plasma levels were not toxic in our patients.

Furthermore, a high C_{max}: MIC ratio suggests a persistent prolonged period of bacterial growth inhibition after exposure to aminoglycosides. Clinically, the post antibiotic effect (PAE) for aminoglycosides is usually between 2 and 4 hours [42]. The PAE of aminoglycosides suppresses bacterial regrowth when serum concentrations are below the MIC [42,43].

Limitations of the Study

We had an unequal distribution of patients in the HIV-positive and HIV-negative groups. Thirty-one patients volunteered to participate in the study, of which 13 were HIV-positive. Also, there were very few patients with kidney dysfunction and no drug–drug interaction was observed between kanamycin and co-administered medications.

There was no balance in the CD4 count and viral load in HIV-positive patients. Five patients had a CD4 count of <100 cells/mm³ and eight had a CD4 count of >100 cells/mm³. Some patients were in the early stage of the disease, while some had advanced HIV infection. In addition, studies on the PK of kanamycin are very scarce, especially in sub-Saharan Africa. Thus, comparison of our results with previously published studies for similarities or differences in the PK parameters was limited. Future studies involving more volunteers are needed.

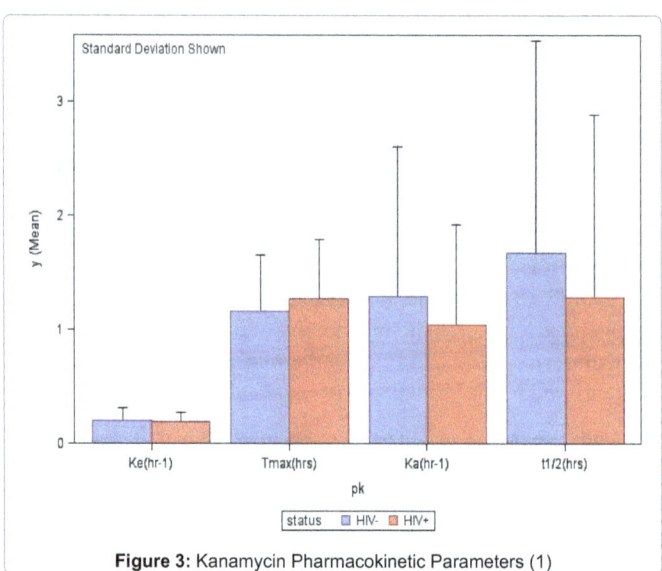

Figure 3: Kanamycin Pharmacokinetic Parameters (1)

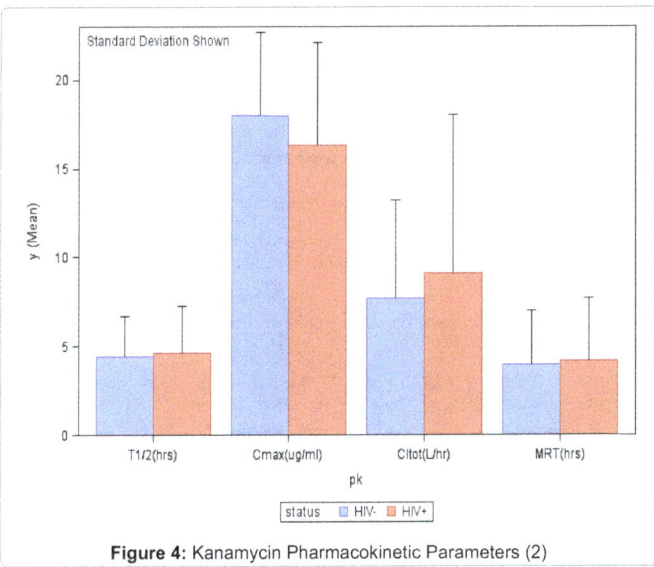

Figure 4: Kanamycin Pharmacokinetic Parameters (2)

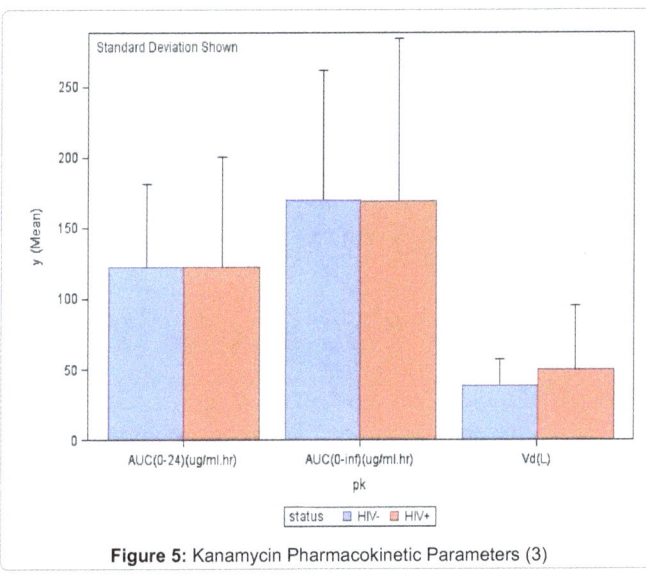

Figure 5: Kanamycin Pharmacokinetic Parameters (3)

Conclusion

Based on the results obtained, we can conclude that objectives of the present study were achieved.

The LC-MS analysis method is highly specific and highly sensitive in the detection and quantification of the plasma concentrations of kanamycin. The PK of kanamycin in patients with MDR-TB and in those with MDR-TB co-infected with HIV was described. Furthermore, HIV infection does not have any influence on the PK of kanamycin. Finally, changes in renal function do not influence the PK of kanamycin.

Recommendations

Based on the results of this study, the following should be considered for future studies.

Kanamycin-free plasma concentrations should be evaluated, in order to determine the AUC of the free plasma concentrations (fAUC) which, together with the MIC will be used to determine the relationship between fAUC and MIC of kanamycin.

Therefore, the MIC of kanamycin on *M.tuberculosis* isolated from the sputum of each patient should be determined.

PK/PD relationship of kanamycin should be determined, because it quantifies the activity of an antibiotic and describes the time course of action of the antibiotic.

Acknowledgement

The following people and departments are acknowledged:

The medical superintendent at Brewelskloof Hospital for permission to conduct the study.

Staff members at Brewelskloof Hospital for their support.

The Pharmaceutical Services, Provincial Administration of the Western Cape for supplying anti-tuberculosis tablets.

The Department of Health, Province of the Western Cape for the permission to conduct the study at Brewelskloof Hospital.

Patients who participated in the study.

The research department, University of the Western Cape for financial support of the study.

The Medical Research Council for financial support of the study.

References

1. Weyer K (2004) Dots-plus for standardized management of multidrug resistant tuberculosis in South Africa- Policy guidelines, Pretoria, South Africa: Medical Research Council of South Africa, Department of Health.

2. Andrews JR, Shah NS, Gandhi N, Moll T, Friedland G, et al. (2007) Multidrug-resistant and extensively drug-resistant tuberculosis: implications for the HIV epidemic and antiretroviral therapy rollout in South Africa. J Infect Dis 196 Suppl 3: S482-490.

3. Wells CD, Cegielski JP, Nelson LJ, Laserson KF, Holtz TH, et al. (2007) HIV infection and multidrug-resistant tuberculosis: the perfect storm. J Infect Dis 196 Suppl 1: S86-107.

4. Budha NR, Lee RE, Meibohm B (2008) Biopharmaceutics, pharmacokinetics and pharmacodynamics of antituberculosis drugs. Curr Med Chem 15: 809-825.

5. Mitnick CD, Appleton SC, Shin SS (2008) Epidemiology and treatment of multidrug resistant tuberculosis. Semin Respir Crit Care Med 29: 499-524.

6. World Health Organization (2009) Treatment of tuberculosis: Guidelines for national programmes. Fourth edition, World Health Organization: Geneva, Switzerland.

7. Wilkinson D, Pillay M, Davies GR, Sturm AW (1996) Resistance to antituberculosis drugs in rural South Africa: rates, patterns, risks, and transmission dynamics. T Roy Soc Trop Med, Vol.90, No.6, pp. 692-695.

8. Kenyon TA, Mwasekaga MJ, Huebner R, Rumisha D, Binkin N, et al. (1999) Low levels of drug resistance amidst rapidly increasing tuberculosis and human immunodeficiency virus co-epidemics in Botswana. Int J Tuberc Lung Dis 3: 4-11.

9. Churchyard GJ, Corbett EL, Kleinschmidt I, Mulder D, De Cock KM (2000) Drug-resistant tuberculosis in South African gold miners: incidence and associated factors. Int J Tuberc Lung Dis 4: 433-440.

10. World Health Organization (2004) Anti-tuberculosis drug resistance in the world: third global report. WHO/International Union against Tuberculosis and Lung Disease Global Project on Anti-tuberculosis Drug Resistance Surveillance, Geneva, Switzerland.

11. Patel KB, Belmonte R, Crowe HM (1995) Drug malabsorption and resistant tuberculosis in HIV-infected patients. N Engl J Med 332: 336-337.

12. Peloquin CA (2002) Therapeutic drug monitoring in the treatment of tuberculosis. Drugs 62: 2169-2183.

13. Gurumurthy P, Ramachandran G, Hemanth Kumar AK, Rajasekaran S, Padmapriyadarsini C, et al. (2004) Decreased bioavailability of rifampin and other antituberculosis drugs in patients with advanced human immunodeficiency virus disease. Antimicrob Agents Chemother 48: 4473-4475.

14. Tappero JW, Bradford WZ, Agerton TB, Hopewell P, Reingold AL, et al. (2005) Serum concentrations of antimycobacterial drugs in patients with pulmonary tuberculosis in Botswana. Clin Infect Dis 41: 461-469.

15. Choudhri SH, Hawken M, Gathua S, Minyiri GO, Watkins W, et al. (1997) Pharmacokinetics of antimycobacterial drugs in patients with tuberculosis, AIDS, and diarrhea. Clin Infect Dis 25: 104-111.

16. Burman WJ, Gallicano K, Peloquin C (1999) Therapeutic implications of drug interactions in the treatment of human immunodeficiency virus-related tuberculosis. Clin Infect Dis 28: 419-429.

17. Aaron L, Saadoun D, Calatroni I, Launay O, Mémain N, et al. (2004) Tuberculosis in HIV-infected patients: a comprehensive review. Clin Microbiol Infect 10: 388-398.

18. Derendorf H, Lesko LJ, Chaikin P, Colburn WA, Lee P, et al. (2000) Pharmacokinetic/pharmacodynamic modeling in drug research and development. J Clin Pharmacol 40: 1399-1418.

19. Kirby WM, Clarke JT, Libke RD, Regamey C (1976) Clinical pharmacology of amikacin and kanamycin. J Infect Dis 134 SUPPL: S312-315.

20. Coyne KM, Pozniak AL, Lamorde M, Boffito M (2009) Pharmacology of second-line antituberculosis drugs and potential for interactions with antiretroviral agents. AIDS 23: 437-446.

21. Yew WW, Cheung SW, Chau CH, Chan CY, Leung CK, et al. (1999) Serum pharmacokinetics of antimycobacterial drugs in patients with multidrug resistant tuberculosis during therapy. Int J Clin Pharm Res 19: 65-71.

22. Mugabo P, Taha E, Stander M, Hassan S, Moeti S, et al. (2009) Determination of plasma concentration using LC/MS and pharmacokinetics of ofloxacin in patients using multi-drug resistant tuberculosis and in patients co-infected with multi-drug resistant tuberculosis and HIV. 5th IAS Conference on HIV pathogenesis, Treatment and Prevention, Cape Town.

23. Niessen WM (1998) Analysis of antibiotics by liquid chromatography-mass spectrometry. J Chromatogr A 812: 53-75.

24. Peng GW, Gadalla MA, Peng A, Smith V, Chiou WL (1977) High-pressure liquid-chromatographic method for determination of gentamicin in plasma. Clin Chem 23: 1838-1844.

25. Doluiso JT, Dittert LW, LaPiana JC (1973) Pharmacokinetics of kanamycin following intramuscular administration. J Pharmacokinet Biop 1: 253-265.

26. Cronk GA, Naumann DE (1959) The absorption and excretion of kanamycin in human beings. J Lab Clin Med 53: 888-895.

27. Clark SJ, Creighton S, Portmann B, Taylor C, Wendon JA, et al. (2002) Acute liver failure associated with antiretroviral treatment for HIV: a report of six cases. J Hepatol 36: 295–301.

28. Cabana BE, Taggart JG (1973) Comparative pharmacokinetics of BB-K8 and kanamycin in dogs and humans. Antimicrob Agents Chemother 3: 478-483.

29. Peloquin CA, Nitta AT, Burman WJ, Brudney KF, Miranda-Massari JR, et al. (1996) Low antituberculosis drug concentrations in patients with AIDS. Ann Pharmacother 30: 919-925.

30. Weyer K (2005) Multidrug-resistant tuberculosis. Continuing Medical Education Journal 23: 75–84.

31. Gurumurthy P, Ramachandran G, Hemanth Kumar AK, Rajasekaran S, Padmapriyadarsini C, et al. (2004) Malabsorption of rifampin and isoniazid in HIV-infected patients with and without tuberculosis. Clin Infect Dis 38: 280-283.

32. Mehvar R (2004) The relationship among pharmacokinetic parameters: effect of altered kinetics on the drug plasma concentration-time profiles. Am J Pharm Educ 8: 1–9.

33. Gerntholtz TE, Goetsch SJ, Katz I (2006) HIV-related nephropathy: a South African perspective. Kidney Int 69: 1885-1891.

34. Roe J, Campbell LJ, Ibrahim F, Hendry BM, Post FA (2008) HIV care and the incidence of acute renal failure. Clin Infect Dis 47: 242-249.

35. Leventhal JS, Ross MJ (2008) Pathogenesis of HIV-associated nephropathy. Semin Nephrol 28: 523-534.

36. Yew WW (2001) Therapeutic drug monitoring in antituberculosis chemotherapy: clinical perspectives. Clin Chim Acta 313: 31-36.

37. Burgess DS (1999) Pharmacodynamic principles of antimicrobial therapy in the prevention of resistance. Chest 115: 19S-23S.

38. Berning SE, Huitt GA, Iseman MD, Peloquin CA (1992) Malabsorption of antituberculosis medications by a patient with AIDS. N Engl J Med 327: 1817-1818.

39. Arbex MA, Varella Mde C, Siqueira HR, Mello FA (2010) Antituberculosis drugs: drug interactions, adverse effects, and use in special situations. Part 2: second line drugs. J Bras Pneumol 36: 641-656.

40. Nuermberger E, Grosset J (2004) Pharmacokinetic and pharmacodynamic issues in the treatment of mycobacterial infections. Eur J Clin Microbiol Infect Dis 23: 243-255.

41. Nicolau DP (2003) Optimizing outcomes with antimicrobial therapy through pharmacodynamic profiling. J Infect Chemother 9: 292-296.

42. Douglas JG, McLeod MJ (1999) Pharmacokinetic factors in the modern drug treatment of tuberculosis. Clin Pharmacokinet 37: 127-146.

43. Turnidge J (2003) Pharmacodynamics and dosing of aminoglycosides. Infect Dis Clin North Am 17: 503-528.

8

Effectiveness of the Androctonus Australis Hector Nanobody NbF12-10 Antivenom to Neutralize Significantly the Toxic Effect and Tissue Damage Provoked by Fraction of *Androctonus mauretanicus* (Morocco) Scorpion Venom

Chgoury F[1,4*], Benabderrazek R[2], Tounsi H[3], Oukkache N[1], Hmila I[2], Boubaker S[3], Ayeb ME[2], Saïle R[4] Ghalim N[1] and Bouhaouala-Zahar B[2,5*]

[1]Laboratory of Venoms and Toxins, Institut Pasteur du Maroc, 1- Place Louis Pasteur, Casablanca 20360, Morocco
[2]Laboratory of Venoms and Therapeutic Molecules, Pasteur Institute of Tunis/University of Tunis El Manar, 13 Place Pasteur, BP74, 1002 - Tunis, Tunisia
[3]Laboratory of Human and Experimental Pathology, Pasteur Institute of Tunis/University of Tunis El Manar, 13 Place Pasteur, BP74, 1002 - Tunis, Tunisia
[4]Laboratory of Biology and Health, URAC 34, Hassan II University Casablanca, Faculty of Science Ben M'sik, Morocco
[5]Medical School of Tunis, 15 Rue Djebel Lakhdhar, La Rabta 1007, Tunis-Tunisia-University of Tunis El Manar

Abstract

Scorpion stings are life threatening in large parts of the world. Toxins from scorpion venom are responsible for severe metabolic and tissue disruption and immunotherapy is the only specific treatment able to neutralize the toxic effects of scorpion venom. The *Androctonus mauretanicus* (Am) is the most dangerous scorpion in Morocco, whereas in Tunisia *Androctonus australis hector* (Aah) is causing most casualties. In this work, we investigated the potential of NbF12-10, a new immunotherapeutic concept based on anti-toxin Nanobodies (Nbs) to neutralize Am scorpion venom. We first explored the immune cross-reactivity between Am and Aah scorpions venoms using anti-AahI and anti-AahII polyclonal, NbAahI'F12 (anti-AahI'), monospecific NbAahII10 (anti-AahII) monospecific and bispecific NbF12-10 (anti-AahI'/anti-AahII) monoclonal antibodies and subsequently we study the histological damages observed after envenomation with the F3 toxic fraction of Am scorpion venom by intra-cerebroventricular (i.c.v) injection and the capacity of NbF12-10 to reduce tissue damage induced by F3 fraction after i.c.v administration of F3:NbF12-10 mixture, in mice. Results showed significant para-specific activity of anti-Aah polyclonal and monoclonal antibodies towards Am venom fractions. Histological investigations revealed severe tissue damage in brain, lung and liver after i.c.v. administration of F3 fraction. The NbF12-10 pre-mixed with F3 fraction showed an efficient neutralizing capacity against lethal effect of this toxic fraction. Moreover, *in vitro* pre-incubation of F3 with NbF12-10 at 8-fold molar excess led to significantly reduced tissue damage. Further, NbF12-10 displays a noteworthy potential to neutralize Am toxins and to rescue 50% of envenomed mice from dying. This study provides first evidence that NbF12-10 nano-therapeutic has promising prospective to treat scorpion envenoming in the Maghreb area.

Keywords: Scorpion venom; Damage tissue; Nanobody; Immune cross-reactivity

Abbreviations

Aah: *Androctonus australis hector*; AahI-AahI'-AahII: Toxins of Aah Venom; Am: *Androctonus mauretanicus*; BSA: Bovin Serum Albumin; ELISA: Enzyme-Linked Immuno Sorbent Assay; F3: Gel Filtration Toxic Fraction of Am Venom; HCAbs: Heavy-Chain Antibody; i.c.v: Intra-Cerebroventricular; MW: Molecular Weight; Nbs: Nanobody; PBS: Phosphate Buffer Saline; scFv: Single Chain Variable Fragment; SDS-PAGE: Sodium Dodecyl Sulfate Polyacrylamide Gel; VHH: variable domain of the heavy chain of a HCAb; ng: nanogram

Introduction

Envenoming by stings from dangerous scorpions constitute a frequent medical emergency and an important public health problem in many countries [1-8]. In Maghreb countries, this so-called scorpionism, is considered as a major public health problem (Direction du soin et de santé de base, DSSB, Ministère de la santé-Tunisie; Centre antipoison et de pharmacovigilance-Ministère de la santé-Morocco [9]). Various scorpion species are encountered in these regions. For the *Androctonus* genus, the *Androctonus mauretanicus mauretanicus* (Amm) renamed *Androctonus mauretanicus* (Am) is endemic exclusively in the arid region of Morocco (i.e. Marrakech-Tensit-Al Haouz) [6], whereas the natural biotope of *Androctonus australis hector* (Aah) is in south of Tunisia. The *Buthus* scorpion genus has the widest spreading throughout the Maghreb. Both Am and Aah sub-species are

responsible for the majority of stings, especially in children [4,10]. It is well established that the toxicity of scorpion venom is mainly due to the fast diffusion of toxins throughout the body [11,12]. These toxins affect ionic channels (i.e. Na^+, K^+ Ca^{2+} or Cl^- channels) and modulate the transmission of nervous impulses by increasing the discharge of mediators (catecholamines, cytokines, neuropeptide...) causing the release of metabolic serum biomarkers and tissue damages [13-17]. Sodium channel specific toxins are the most represented venom proteins that have been structurally defined and classified in different antigenic groups as identified by polyclonal antibodies. Among these toxins, Amm V is one of the most abundant (46% of the whole Amm venom) and active toxin displaying a 75% sequence identity with

*Corresponding authors: Fatima Chgoury, Laboratory of Venoms and Toxins, Institut Pasteur du Maroc, 1- Place Louis Pasteur, Casablanca 20360, Morocco Balkiss Bouhaouala-Zahar,Medical School of Tunis, 15 Rue Djebel Lakhdhar, La Rabta 1007, Tunis-Tunisia-University of Tunis El Manar
E-mail: fchgoury@ gmail.com, balkiss.bouhaouala@gmail.com

AahII [18,19]. However, mass spectrometry analysis of Amm and Aah scorpion venoms revealed other compounds with molecular weight of about 7 kDa. Experimental data has well established that polyclonal antibodies exhibit a cross reactivity to toxins with more than 40% amino acid sequence identity (i.e., AahII/AmmV/AmmVIII) [20]. However, the idea of the cross neutralizing capacity of polyclonal antibodies has been challenged [21].

To combat clinical symptoms of such hazardous disease, it is absolutely essential to administer the venom-specific antibody as soon as possible after an effective scorpion envenoming. In Tunisia, the use of F(ab)'2 polyclonal antibodies obtained from hyper-immunized horses (with Aah and Bot venoms) is currently recommended as therapy for severe cases, in hospitals. In Morocco, a similar treatment was applied till 2000. Indeed, Fab fragments were also used in some clinical studies [22]. However, the neutralizing potency as well as the specificity of F (ab)'2 or Fab against scorpion toxins were limited due to their polyclonal origin and bio-distribution properties [10,12], [23-25]. Hence, the treatment could fail to rescue patients that are severely envenomed because of the very fast diffusion of scorpion toxins reaching their targets and causing major complications (i.e., pulmonary edema, and respiratory disorder) [26-28] and heart failures [29,30].

In order to improve the immunotherapy against scorpion envenoming, we explored the performance of a novel small antibody fragment that diffuses more rapidly in tissues. This product is derived from the unique Heavy-chain only antibodies (HCAbs) occurring in Camelidae and comprises a single-domain, antigen-binding fragment known as VHH, also referred to as Nbs [31]. Interestingly, the Nbs share a high sequence identity with human VH of family III [32,33]. From VHH library screenings, several Nbs have been retrieved using phage display technology, from which we further selected NbAahI'F12 and NbAahII10 against AahI' and AahII toxins, respectively [34-36]. The corresponding bispecific NbF12-10 format of only 29 kDa yielded a therapeutic compound with a strong protective capacity against the whole Aah venom in mice [35].

However, the potential of NbF12-10 to neutralize venoms of other scorpions such as that from *Androctonus mauretanicus* scorpion, living in Morocco remains unexplored. Turning this challenge into practice, we first investigated the para-specificity by testing the capacity of polyclonal (anti-AahI and anti-AahII), monoclonal (NbAahI'F12 and NbAahII10) and bispecific antibodies (NbF12-10) to recognize and to bind Am venom compounds of black Morocco scorpion, using an ELISA assay. Thereafter, we assessed the potency of NbF12-10 to reduce histological lesions, observed in vital organs, after experimental pre-incubation with the most toxic fraction from Am venom. Our data demonstrate the capacity of NbF12-10 to reduce fatal disturbances provoked by a lethal dose of toxic fraction from Moroccan scorpion venom.

Materials and Methods

Animals

Male Swiss mice (20 ± 2 g) were housed under controlled temperature in the animal breeding unit at Pasteur Institute of Tunis. Animals used for toxicity assays and histological experiments were approved by the institution Research Board of the Pasteur Institute of Tunis and carried out according to the European Community Council Directive (86/609/EEC) for experimental animal care and procedures.

Scorpion venom

The venom of *Androctonus mauretanicus* individual scorpions was collected at the Pasteur institute of Morocco using electrical stimulation. The lyophilized venom was diluted in cold water (2 v/v) and centrifuged for 15 min at 4°C to remove lipid compounds and debris. The venom supernatant was stored at -20°C. The protein concentration was determined according to the Bradford method [37] using and BSA (Bovine serum albumin) as standard and the Bio-Rad reagent.

Production of polyclonal antibodies

Immune sera against AahII and AahI, the most active toxins from Aah scorpion venom, were expressed by immunizing New Zealand rabbits as described previously [38]. After collection of pre-immune sera, each animal was first injected intradermally at 10 µg of toxin (AahI or AahII) in Freund's Adjuvant complete (Sigma) and then, rabbit received two injections of 10 µg and two injections of 15 µg of toxins in Freund's Adjuvant incomplete (Sigma) through the subcutaneous route every 3 weeks.

Production of nanobodies

The production and purification of Nanobodies (i.e., NbAahI'F12, NbAahII10 and NbF12-10) was according to previously reported protocols [34,35]. Briefly, the clone harboring the gene for the AahI', the AahII or the bispecific NbF12-10 protein was cultured separately in shaker flasks with Terrific Broth supplemented with 100 µg ampicillin/ml and 0.1% glucose, until the absorbance at 600 nm reached a value between 0.6 and 0.9. At this time, the recombinant protein expression was induced with 1 mM isopropyl-thiogalactopyranoside and incubation for at least 16 h at 28°C. From the periplasmic compartment, proteins were extracted by osmotic shock [39] and loaded on a Ni-NTA super-flow Sepharose column (Qiagen). The purity of His-6 tagged NbF12-10 was checked by sodium dodecyl sulfate polyacrylamide gel electrophoresis (SDS-PAGE) and the final yield was monitored from the UV absorption at 280 nm and the theoretical extinction coefficient of the Nb, calculated from its amino acid content, as previously described [35].

Gel-filtration chromatography of venom

The supernatant of the Am venom was loaded on a Sephadex G50 column (2.6 × 100 cm) (Sigma) for size exclusion chromatography using 1.6 M acetic acid as equilibration and running solution (28 ml/h) according to Miranda et al. [40] with minor modifications [41]. Fractions (2.5 ml/tube) were collected in a fraction collector (Frac-920, GE). Absorbance was assessed at 280 nm using a spectrophotometer (Beckman DU 640-UV/Visible). Pooled fractions were stored at -20°C till used for toxicity and histological assays.

In vivo assay

The toxicity of scorpion venom Am and derived fractions was measured in mice by i.c.v injection. The LD_{50} represents as amount of venom or toxic fraction leading to 50 % of mice surviving the injection [34,36]. Survivors were counted after 24h.

Polyacrylamide gel electrophoresis

Determination of molecular weight (MW) of Am venom and its toxic fraction F3 were performed in sodium dodecyl sulfate-containing polyacrylamide gels [42]. SDS-PAGE was performed under reducing conditions. Proteins were stained with Coomassie brilliant blue.

Immunological tests: indirect ELISA

ELISA were carried out using anti-AahI, anti-AahII specific polyclonal antibodies, NbAahI'F12 and NbAahII10 monospecific and NbF12-10 bispecific nanobodies, following standard protocols to explore their antigenic cross-reactivity against Am scorpion whole venom as well as F2 and F3 toxic fractions of Am venom. Micro titer 96 wells plates (Nunc Maxisorp Plate) were coated overnight at 4°C with 100 µl of 1 µg/ml of Am venom, F2 or F3 fractions in PBS buffer (Phosphate-Buffered-Saline). After washing with 0.1% Tween-PBS, the residual protein binding sites were blocked with 3 % milk in PBS, for 1 hr at 37°C. Subsequently, after washing steps as before, 100 µl of primary antibody (i.e. mouse anti-AahI or anti-AahII polyclonal antibodies, kind gift from Dr Christiane Devaux) or NbAahI'F12, NbAahII10 and NbF12-10 monoclonal antibodies) (at appropriate dilution or concentration as indicated below) were added. After a washing step, secondary peroxidase conjugated antibody (i.e. rabbit anti-mouse IgG (Sigma) or mouse anti-his-6 clone BMG-His-1, Roche laboratory, as appropriate) were added, After washing, ortho-phenylenediamine dihydrochloride-H_2O_2 (Sigma) was added as substrate and the reaction was stopped using 2N sulfuric acid. Absorbance was measured with a spectrophotometer (Multiskan EX, Thermo Electron Corporation) at 492 nm. All samples were applied in duplicate and ELISA procedures were repeated three times. All polyclonal antibodies concentrations have been adjusted to give similar optical density readout in the ELISA.

Pathophysiological study of F3 fraction from Am scorpion venom in mice

To highlight the tissue damage induced by F3 fraction, three groups of 4 mice were used. The first group as control received physiological saline. Second and third groups were challenged with 30 and 35 ng of F3 toxic fraction, an amount corresponding to 2 and 2.3 LD_{50} respectively. All injections were carried out intra-cerebroventricularly. The levies of organs: brain, lungs and liver were performed in postmortem animals.

In vivo neutralizing of the F3 toxic fraction with NbF12-10

To investigate the *in vivo* neutralizing capacity of NbF12-10 against toxic effect of F3 fraction, five groups of mice were injected with two lethal doses of F3 fraction: 30 and 35 ng (corresponding to 2 and 2.3 LD_{50}) pre-incubated for 1 hour at 37°C with NbF12-10 at molar ratios in cascade from 1:1 to 1:8 molar excess of NbF12-10 dose (Table1).

Organs: brain, lungs and liver were conducted in postmortem animals or in survivors after 24 hours of experimentation.

Experimental conditions for histological analysis

To analyze the histopathological effect on tissues induced by the F3 fraction of Am scorpion venom and the effectiveness of the NbF12-10 to neutralize the F3 that we checked for possible reduced tissue damage after i.c.v. injection of F3 toxins pre-incubated with the bispecific Nb construct. Brain, lung and liver were extracted from control animals, envenomed mice or treated with F3:NbF12-10 mixture. The organs

were fixed in 10 % formalin solution, embedded in paraffin, sliced (2 to 4 µm) and stained with hematoxylin-eosin for microscopic analysis using a Carl Zeiss Axiskop 50 microscope (Germany).

Statistical analysis

Significance of the differences in the immune-reactivity towards Am venom and its fractions F2 and F3 of the polyclonal (anti-AahI, anti-AahII) and monoclonal antibodies (NbF12-10, NbAahI'F12 and NbAahII10) was assessed by Student's t-test (the level of significance was $p < 0.05$).

Results

Venom fractions

The fractionation of soluble Am venom by gel filtration on Sephadex G50 shows six distinct fractions: F1-F6 (Figure 1). Bradford protein quantification showed that F3 (15 µg/µl of protein) fraction represents 41.15% of the venom proteins (Figure 2).

In vivo toxicity assay

The toxicity of F1, F2 or F3 fractions was assessed in mice by i.c.v injection of different amounts (between 5 ng to 2 µg) into Swiss mice (weighting 18-20 g). The number of surviving mice was monitored at 24 hr after toxin injection. As negative control, mice received only

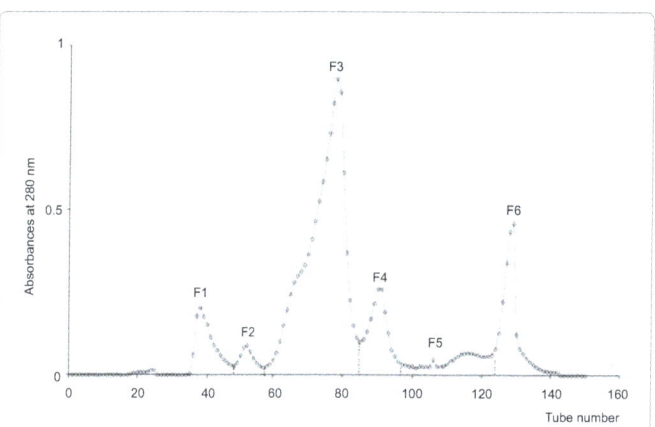

Figure 1: Size exclusion chromatography profile on Sephadex G50 of *Androctonus mauretanicus* scorpion venom. The soluble venom was fractionated using a 2.6 x 100 cm column and fractions were eluted with acetic acid 1.6 M.

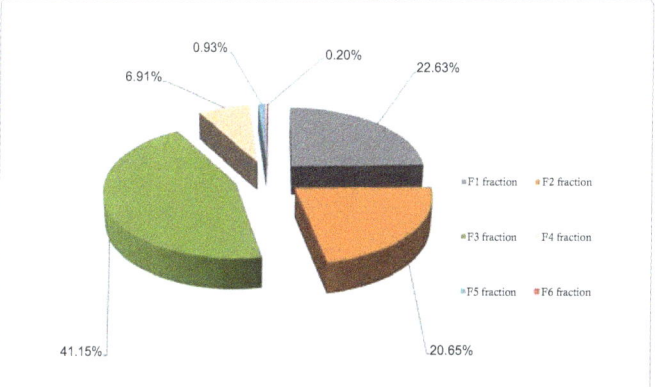

Figure 2: Representative yield of Am venom fractions acquired by gel filtration on SephadexG50 column, in percentages. F1 to F6 represent the eluted fractions from Am venom fractionation.

Group of four mice	LD_{50} (F3 fraction)	Molar ratio F3:NbF12-10
1	2	1:1
2	2	1:2
3	2	1:4
4	2.3	1:4
5	2.3	1:8

Table 1: Different molar ratios of F3 : NbF12-10 pre-incubated mixtures. Each mixture is administered by i.c.v route in mice

physiological solution (NaCl 0.9%). Results showed that F1 is not toxic below 2 µg injected per mouse while F2 causes envenoming symptoms, no mortality was recorded. In contrast, F3 is causing highly toxic symptoms and mortality. The LD_{50} of F3 fraction was estimated (using cohorts of 4 mice) to approximately 15 ng/mouse. F4 to F6 fractions showed small low molecular weight peptides displaying low toxicity. As expected, F3 fraction contains peptides with apparent molecular weight (MW) related to toxin's MW (Figure 3).

Immune cross-reactivity between Am and Aah using AahI and AahII-specific polyclonal: Indirect ELISA

The cross-reactivity of polyclonal antibodies directed against the major toxins from Aah venom: anti-AahI, anti-AahII, towards Am venom or fractions F2 and F3, showed successful recognition of the F3 Am fraction by both anti-AahI and anti-AahII polyclonal antibodies with a very high significant p value (p = 0.0008 and p = 0.001, respectively). Also, anti-AahI and anti-AahII reacted immunologically with Am venom (p = 0.02; p = 0.004 respectively) (Figure 4A,4B) whereas F2 fraction revealed low reactivity to anti-AahII (p = 0.035) (Figure 4B).

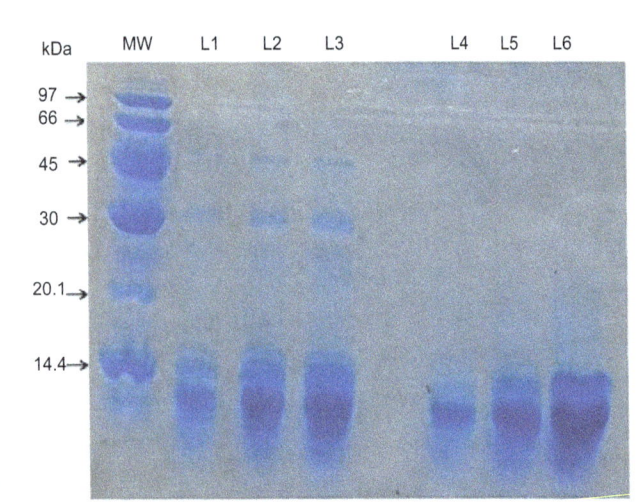

Figure 3: SDS-PAGE of *Androctonus mauretanicus* scorpion venom and its toxic fraction F3. After electrophoresis, 15 % polyacrylamide gel is stained with coomassie blue. Am venom displays several apparent molecular weights. The estimated mass for F3 fraction is below 14.4 kDa MW. L1-L3 Lanes: 5 µg, 10 µg and 20 µg of Am venom, respectively. L4-L6 Lanes:5 µg, 10 µg, 20 µg of F3 fraction respectively. MW: molecular weight markers.

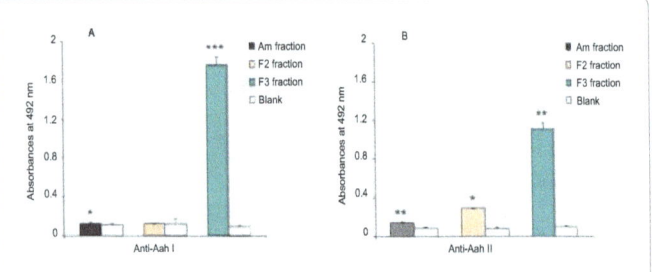

Figure 4: Antigenic cross-reactivity of polyclonal anti-AahI (Figure 4A) and anti-AahII (Figure 4B) antibodies on Am venom and F2 and F3 fractions. Highly significant recognition (***) (p < 0.001); Very significant recognition (**) (0.001 < p < 0.01); significant recognition (*) (0.01 < p < 0.05). p: probability value.

Immune cross-reactivity between Am and Aah scorpion venoms using NbF12-10, NbAahI'F12 and NbAahII10 specific monoclonal antibodies: Indirect ELISA

We evaluated immunological binding capacity of monoclonal Nbs: NbF12-10, NbAahI'F12 and NbAahII10 towards Am venom and its fractions F2 and F3. An antigenic cross-reactivity against F3 fraction is observed when NbF12-10 (Figure 5A) and NbAahI'F12 (Figure 5B) are used at concentration of 5µg/ml, and the p-values are highly significant (p = 0.0028 and 0.0022, respectively). A significant reactivity of NbAahI'F12 against Am venom is noted (p = 0.0025) (Figure 5B). Remarkably, only poor binding of NbAahII10 to Am venom as well as to F3 fraction is noticed (Figure 5C). No affinity has been noted between Nbs (NbF12-10, NbAah'F12 and NbAahII10) and F2 fraction.

Histology of brain, lung and liver tissues upon F3 injection with or without NbF12-10

Pathophysiological effects of F3 fraction have been investigated in mouse by i.c.v injection. Histological screening of organs sections from mice envenomed by F3 toxic fraction with two doses of 30 ng and 35 ng (corresponding to 2 LD_{50} and 2.3 LD_{50}, respectively), showed 100% mortality of mice poisoned and structural changes in brain, lung and liver tissues. Indeed, in brain tissue, a marked congestion, vasodilatation, hemorrhage, edema and neuronal constriction were observed (Figure 6: panels B-B1 and K). In lung parenchyma, we observed many edemas in intra-alveolar and bronchiolar levels, and half of the lung tissue was invaded by edema and congestion. Moreover, several hemorrhagic foci, large fibrin deposition, infiltration of inflammatory cells and loss of alveolar walls were observed (Figure 6: panels E and M-M1). In liver tissue, F3 fraction caused congestion, sinusoidal dilatation, hepatocyte turgescence, hepatocyte with nuclear hypertrophy or bi-nucleating (Figure 6: panels H and O). Histological slices of control animals showed normal architecture structural (Figure 6: panels A, D-D1 and G).

To evaluate the capacity of NbF12-10 to neutralize the toxicity caused by 30 or 35 ng (i.e. 2 LD_{50} and 2.3 LD_{50}) of the F3 toxins from Am scorpion venom per mice, we pre-incubated the toxins with NbF12-10 at various molar ratios before i.c.v. injection (Table 1). The

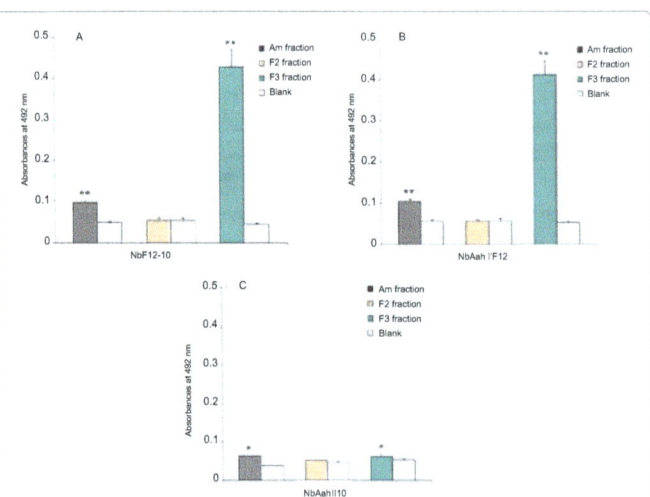

Figure 5: Antigenic cross-reactivity of Aah-specific NbF12-10 (Figure 5A), NbAahI'F12 (Figure 5B), NbAahII10 (Figure 5C) nanobodies towards Am venom, F2 and F3 fractions. Very significant recognition (**) (0.001 < p < 0.01); significant (*) (0.01 < p < 0.05). p: probability value.

Group of four mice	Molar ratio F3:NbF12-10	Survivors mice
1	1 : 1	0/4
2	1 : 2	0/4
3	1 : 4	0/4
4	1 : 4	0/4
5	1 : 8	2/4

Table 2: Efficiency of NbF12-10 against the toxic effects of F3 fraction. Results of mice groups challenged with molar ratios of F3: NbF12-10 by i.c.v injection.

NbF12-10 was added at an estimated 1 to 8 molar excess over the toxins in the F3 fraction, as indicated. The mice from the first, second and third group received 30 ng of F3 pre-incubated with either 120 ng, 240 ng or 480 ng of NbF12-10 (that correspond to a molar ratio of toxin: Nb of 1: 1, 1:2 and 1:4, respectively). The fourth and fifth groups of mice received 35 ng of F3 pre-incubated with 560 ng or 1120 ng of NbF12-10 (corresponding to 4 or 8-fold molar excess of Nb, respectively).

Our results revealed that NbF12-10 ensures the survival of 50 % of mice injected with 35 ng of the F3 fraction with an 8 fold molar excess of Nb (Table 2). Hence, a significant Am-neutralizing capacity of the NbF12-10 was noticed under these conditions whereas a reduced excess of NbF12-10 (i.e. equimolar to 1:4 ratio) in the mixtures failed to neutralize a 2 LD_{50} of F3-Am fraction as all mice died from F3 poisoning and important structural changes in tissues were observed experimentally.

Interestingly, the survivals didn't exhibit any severe symptoms of envenoming (e.g. neurological signs, agitation and lumps dorsal are missing) and damages were clearly less significant in the target

tissue of envenomed mice that survived following injection. Indeed, the detailed histological study of tissue structure demonstrates a significant reduced proportion of tissue damage within the organ sections. In particular, brain parenchyma was completely devoid of edema and nerve cells display their common feature (Figure 6: panel L). Regression of lung edema was evident. The number of hemorrhagic areas was less important nearby minor congestions and no deposited fibrin was noticed (Figure 6: panel N-N1). Moreover, liver tissue revealed a similar architecture to control tissue without dilatation of sinusoids, neither cell turgescence (Figure 6: panel P). However, a lower molar excess of NbF12-10 (30 ng of F3 fraction mixed to 4-fold molar excess of NbF12-10) resulted in a severely reduced experimental neutralizing efficacy and mice from this cohort failed to survive. Hence, histological analysis of post-mortem animals showed tissue damage as well. In cerebral cortex, we noted extravasation of blood (data not shown), edema, less regression of neurons and congestion of a large vessel (Figure 6: panel C). Pulmonary tissue was invaded by edema (Figure 6: panel F). Sinusoidal dilatation and a minority of hepatocyte turgescence were observed (Figure 6: panel I).

Discussion

In the present study, we have demonstrated that F3, a toxic fraction from Am scorpion venom has led to structural abnormalities. This fraction corresponds to most abundant toxic component, obtained after analytical filtration of Am venom (Figure 1). F3 fraction showed a similar retention time as that of AahG50 (derived from Aah venom) fraction whereas the eluted fractions on either side of this F3 peak display significant divergence in retention time [34,36]. The LD_{50} of F3 fraction, estimated as the amount of toxins whereby 50% of the mice (cohorts of 4 mice) survived the injection that corresponds to

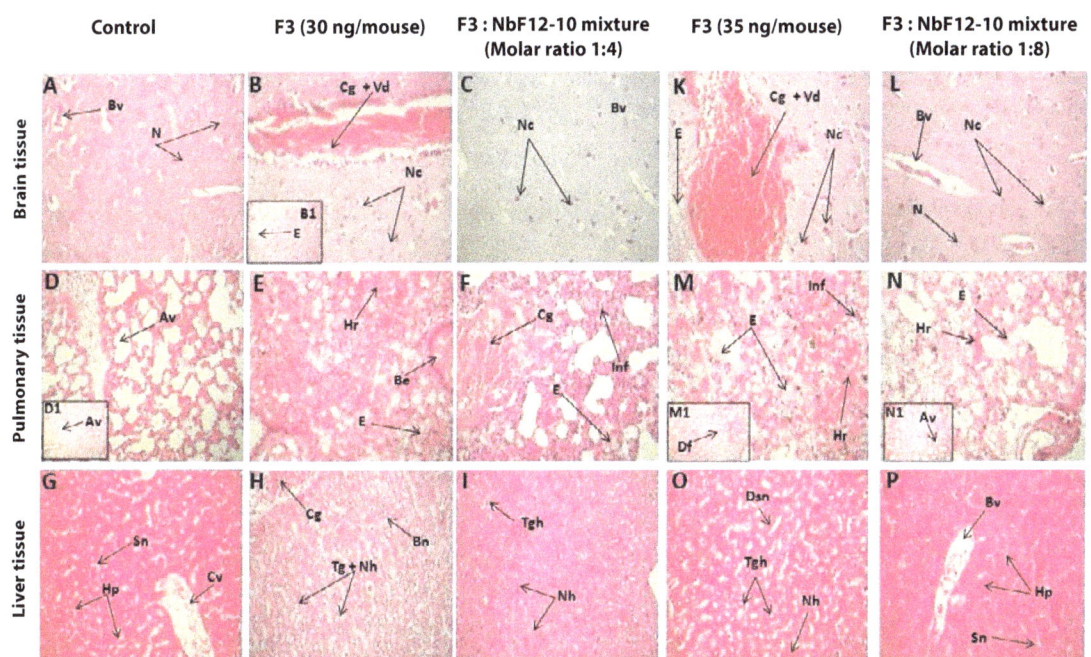

Figure 6: Histology of brain, pulmonary and liver tissues from mice envenomed with F3 fraction at 35 ng / mouse (Panels K, M-M1 and O) or receiving F3 mixed with 8 molar excess of NbF12-10 (Panels L, N-N1 and P). Histology of brain, pulmonary and liver tissues from mice envenomed with injection of F3 fraction at 30 ng / mouse (Panels B-B1, E and H) or receiving F3 mixed with 4 molar excess of NbF12-10 (Panels C, F and I) in comparison to tissues from control mice (Panels A, D-D1 and G).N: Neurons, Bv: Blood vessel, Cg + vd: congestion and vasodilatation, Nc: Neuronal constriction, Av: Alveole, Hr: hemorrhage, Be: Bronchial edema, E: Edema, Inf: Infiltration of inflammatory cells, Cg: Congestion, Hp: Hepatocyte; Sn: Sinusoids, Cv: Centrolobular vein, Tg + Nh: Turgescence + nuclear hypertrophy, Bn: Bi-nucleating, Fd: Fibrin deposit (X 40 magnifications). All injections were made via i.c.v injections.

15 ng/mouse, approximately. However, previous experiments were conducted using intra-peritoneal injection of the toxins or venoms. Here, we investigated for the first time the envenoming effect after injection of an Am toxic fraction (F3) via an i.c.v. route with 30 and 35 ng (equivalent to 2 LD_{50} and 2.3 LD_{50}). Histological examination showed that both doses provoked considerable tissue damage leading to significant structural changes in brain, lung and liver parenchyma.

It has been demonstrated that toxins from scorpion venom target to their specific receptors in sodium, potassium channels of nerve and muscle cells which disrupt the propagation of nerve impulses (activation or inactivation of channels) and cause the release of neurotransmitters and cellular mediators. Such changes is causing disturbance of metabolic parameters (glycemia, urea, creatinine, ...) and structural disorganization leading to dysfunction of vital organs have been described (i.e. brain, lungs, heart, liver, kidneys) [15,16], [43,44].

Indeed, cerebral alterations were assumed to be the consequence of neurotransmitter releases [43-51]. More recently, similar structural damage in brain tissue (i.e., edema, hemorrhage, neuronal darkness) were evoked by a small scorpion toxin called Kaliotoxin isolated from Aah [52].

Many studies showed similar results in pulmonary tissues [14-16], [53,54]. It was highlighted that scorpion envenomation is followed by an imbalance of pro-and anti-inflammatory response [55] and scorpion venom is able to affect parameters for pulmonary mechanisms [56]. The fibrin deposit was associated with disruption of blood coagulation process generated after scorpion envenomation [57]. The genesis of pulmonary edema can be attributed to a cardiogenic dysfunction [58]. Moreover, it may be non-cardiogenic origin [17,59] and consequently, pulmonary edema is in that case multifactorial.

In liver tissue, similar observations (i.e., hepatocytes with cytoplasm distended to nuclear hypertrophy and large vacuoles) were noticed after envenomation by *Tityus* genus [14]. Otherwise, hepatocyte cells may exhibit Mallory bodies resulting from hepatic steatosis [60].

Hence, to remove the circulating scorpion venom toxins, immunotherapy is the specific treatment to be applied. Currently, F (ab')$_2$ based therapy is the only anti-venom therapy available into market for clinical envenoming treatment. This so-called fabotherapy is based on administration of scorpion anti-venom serum produced in pre-immunized horses. As polyclonal product, F (ab')$_2$-based antivenom has potency to prevent histopathological injuries in tissue and to return into normal, metabolic parameters and electrocardiogram changes caused in patients after scorpion envenoming [61,62]. However, the efficiency of intra-muscular route for antivenom treatment of envenomed patients was not reported systematically in all cases [63]. Hence, avian anti-*Tityus cariptensis* (Tc) venom antibodies (isolated from chicken egg yolks) was recently applied as anti-venom alternative and was effective in neutralizing only 2 LD_{50} doses of Tc venom [64]. A mixture of antibody fragments F (ab')2/Fab is able to significantly reduce local leukocytosis, hemorrhage and inflammatory edema induced Aah venom and its toxins [25].

In this study, we first studied the para-specificity between Aah and Am venoms using polyclonal (anti-AahI and anti-AahII) and monoclonal (NbF12-10, NbAahI'F12 and NbAahII10) antivenom against Am venom and its fractions F2 and F3. Thereby, the immunological screening using polyclonal antibodies and Nbs favors the presence of several AahI, AahI' and AahII related or cross-reacting toxins within Am venom and F3 fraction. Indeed, Am venom

molecules (F3 fraction) could be detected easily by both, monospecific NbAahI'F12 and the bispecific NbF12-10 construct, which is suggestive for the presence of AahI related toxins or epitopes within the F3 fraction of Am venom. Similar results reported that human single chain fragment (scFv) recognized toxins of *Centruroides noxius Hoffmann* and *Centruroides suffuses* scorpion venom and rescue mice from severe envenomation by whole venom of *Centruroides suffuses* and *Centruroides noxius* [65]. Also, polyclonal anti-venom against *Hadruroides lunatus* displayed cross reactivity with venom from *Tityus serrulatus*, *Centruroides sculpturatus* and *Androctonus australis hector* scorpions [66]. Other study has explained that anti-AmmVIII (Anatoxin from Am venom) antibodies were also found to cross-react towards several of the peptides designed from the AahII structure [67]. Devaux et al. (2001) [68] reported that 9C2 (scFv), a murine monoclonal IgG, was able to neutralize AahI toxin from Aah scorpion venom.

Herein we demonstrated in the first time, the effectiveness of Aah-specific NbF12-10 nanotherapeutic to bind and neutralize Am venom related toxins and to prevent severe structural abnormalities at cerebral, pulmonary and hepatic parenchyma, provoked by i.c.v injection of Am venom F3 fraction. More interestingly, pre-incubation with NbF12-10 leads to less toxic mixture and therefore envenomed mice rescued from death. Similarly, F7Nb nanobody raised against Heminecrolysin (major known hemolytic and dermonecrotic fraction of *Hemiscorpus lepturus* scorpion) venom showed in vitro and *in vivo* neutralization of heminocrolysin activity [69]. Clearly, our data revealed that i.c.v route is very sensitive and associated with distant and significant structural lesions and confirms the importance of metabolic releases in severe and dramatic symptoms [70,71]. Further investigations are in progress to test additional nanobody candidates with sub-nanomolar affinity for the AahI' and AahII toxins, separately or in combination and to study the effect of NbF12-10 against whole Am venom. Indeed, study on large cohorts of animals and using classical pharmacokinetics/pharmacodynamics experiments is in progress.

Conclusion

In this study, we demonstrated a significant antigenic cross-reactivity ($p < 0.05$) of polyclonal antibodies and Nbs between the Tunisia Aah and Morocco Am scorpion venom components. Especially, the result with NbF12-10 is important, as this is our lead product (produced against the major toxins from Aah scorpion venom of Tunisia) with which we provided recently the proof-of-concept to neutralize the Aah envenoming. These promising data prompted us to further study it's *in vivo* neutralizing capacity against experimental Am envenoming. Our results with this bispecific Nb on the Am venom highlights its effectiveness to reduce pathophysiological effects of toxicity caused by the major toxic fraction of this Moroccan Am scorpion. Evidence is provided that this Nb construct might be seriously considered as promising anti-venom therapeutic to treat severe scorpion envenoming cases in the large Maghreb area. Further preclinical studies to include larger cohorts of mice and other experimental animals should be considered in the future.

Acknowledgments

This work was partially supported by International Pasteur Institute Network (RIIP), Islamic Bank for Development (BID), Pasteur Institute of Morocco (IPM) and Pasteur Institute of Tunis (IPT) grants. We would like to thank Prof. Serge Muyldermans for support in identifying Nanobodies. Our gratitude's are addressed to Professors Naima ELMdaghri Director of Pasteur Institute of Morocco, Hechmi Louzir General Director of Pasteur Institute of Tunis for encouraging this research project. Our thanks are extended to Dr. Zakaria Benlasfar (IPT) and Lotfi Boussada (IPM) for animal facilities; we also thanked Dr. Abderrahmane Belhouari, Faculty of Sciences, Ben M'sik, Casablanca, Morocco for assistance in statistical data analysis.

Author Contributions

Fatima Chgoury conducted biochemical and experimental studies. Rahma Ben Abderrazek and Naoual Oukkache contributed to technical and experimental work. Issam Hmila contributed in part to Nanobody production and purification; Haifa Tounsi and Samir Boubaker for design and analysis of histological sections; Rachid Saïle, Noreddine Ghalim and Mohamed El Ayeb for analysis and discussing results. Fatima Chgoury and Balkiss Bouhaouala-Zahar are responsible for writing this manuscript. Balkiss Bouhaouala-Zahar was responsible for designing experiments, result interpreting and the editorial corrections.

References

1. Goyffon M, Vachon M, Broglio N (1982) Epidemiological and clinical characteristics of the scorpion envenomation in Tunisia. Toxicon 20: 337-344.

2. Dehesa Dávila M, Possani LD (1994) Scorpionism and serotherapy in Mexico, Toxicon 32: 1015-1018.

3. Ismail M (1994) The treatment of the scorpion envenoming syndrome: the Saudi experience with serotherapy. Toxicon 32: 1019-1026.

4. Ghalim N, El-Hafny B, Sebti F, Heikel J, Lazar N, et al. (2000) Scorpion envenomation and serotherapy in Morocco. Am J Trop Med Hyg 62: 277-283.

5. Lira-da-Silva RM, Amorim AM, Brazil TK (2000) [Poisonous sting by Tityus stigmurus (Scorpiones; Buthidae) in the state of Bahia, Brazil]. Rev Soc Bras Med Trop 33: 239-245.

6. Touloun O, Slimani T, Boumezzough A (2001) Epidemiological survey of scorpion envenomation in Southwestern Morocco. J Venom Anim Toxins 7: 199-218.

7. Otero R, Navío E, Céspedes FA, Núñez MJ, Lozano L (2004) Scorpion envenoming in two regions of Colombia: clinical, epidemiological and therapeutic aspects. Trans R Soc Trop Med Hyg 98: 742-750.

8. Bouaziz M, Bahloul M, Kallel H, Samet M, Ksibi H, et al. (2008) Epidemiological, clinical characteristics and outcome of severe scorpion envenomation in South Tunisia: multivariate analysis of 951 cases. Toxicon 52: 918-926.

9. Soulaymani Bencheikh R, Faraj Z, Semlali I, Ouammi L, Badri M (2003) National strategy in the battle against scorpion stings and envenomations. Application and evaluation. Bull Soc Pathol Exot 96: 317-319.

10. Krifi MN, Miled K, Abderrazek M, El Ayeb M (2001) Effects of antivenom on Buthus occitanus tunetanus (Bot) scorpion venom pharmacokinetics: towards an optimization of antivenom immunotherapy in a rabbit model. Toxicon 39: 1317-1326.

11. El Hafny B, Chgoury F, Adil N, Cohen N, Hassar M, et al. (2002) Intraspecific variability and pharmacokinetic characteristics of Androctonus mauretanicus mauretanicus scorpion venom. Toxicon 40: 1609-1616.

12. Hammoudi-Triki D, Lefort J, Rougeot C, Robbe-Vincent A, Bon C, et al. (2007) Toxicokinetic and toxicodynamic analyses of Androctonus australis hector venom in rats: optimization of antivenom therapy. Toxicol Appl Pharmacol 218: 205-214.

13. Sofer S, Gueron M, White RM, Lifshitz M, Apte RN (1996) Interleukin-6 release following scorpion sting in children. Toxicon 34: 389-392.

14. Corrêa MM, Sampaio SV, Lopes RA, Mancuso LC, Cunha OAB, et al. (1997) Biochemical and histopathological alterations induced in rats by Tityus serrulatus scorpion venom and its major neurotoxin tityustoxin-I. Toxicon 35: 1053-1067.

15. Bessalem S, Hammoudi-Triki D, Laraba-Djebari F (2003) Effect of immunotherapy on metabolic and histopathological modifications after experimental scorpion envenomation. Bull. Société. Pathol. Exot 96: 110-114.

16. Adi-Bessalem S, Hammoudi-Triki D, Laraba-Djebari F (2008) Pathophysiological effects of Androctonus australis hector scorpion venom: tissue damages and inflammatory response. Exp. Toxicol. Pathol 60: 373-380.

17. Cavari Y, Lazar I, Shelef I, Sofer S (2013) Lethal brain edema, shock, and coagulopathy after scorpion envenomation. Wilderness Environ Med 24: 23-27.

18. Rosso JP, Rochat H (1985) Characterization of ten proteins from the venom of the Moroccan scorpion Androctonus mauretanicus mauretanicus, six of which are toxic to the mouse. Toxicon 23: 113-125.

19. Zerrouk H, Bougis PE, Céard B, Benslimane A, Martin-Eauclaire MF (1991) Analysis by high-performance liquid chromatography of Androctonus mauretanicus mauretanicus (black scorpion) venom. Toxicon 29: 951-960.

20. Oukkache N, Rosso JP, Alami M, Ghalim N, Saïle R, et al. (2008) New analysis of the toxic compounds from the Androctonus mauretanicus mauretanicus scorpion venom. Toxicon 51: 835-852.

21. Martin-Eauclaire MF, Alami M, Giamarchi A, Missimilli V, Rosso JP, et al. (2006) A natural anatoxin, Amm VIII, induces neutralizing antibodies against the potent scorpion alpha-toxins. Vaccine 24: 1990-1996.

22. Karlson-Stiber C, Persson H, Heath A, Smith D, al-Abdulla IH, et al. (1997) First clinical experiences with specific sheep Fab fragments in snake bite. Report of a multicentre study of Vipera berus envenoming. J Intern Med 241: 53-58.

23. Ismail M, Abd-Elsalam MA (1998) Pharmacokinetics of 125I-labelled IgG, F(ab')2 and Fab fractions of scorpion and snake antivenins: merits and potential for therapeutic use. Toxicon 36: 1523-1528.

24. Abroug F, ElAtrous S, Nouira S, Haguiga H, Touzi N, et al. (1999) Serotherapy in scorpion envenomation: a randomised controlled trial. Lancet 354: 906-909.

25. Sami-Merah S, Hammoudi-Triki D, Martin-Eauclaire MF, Laraba-Djebari F (2008) Combination of two antibody fragments F(ab')(2)/Fab: an alternative for scorpion envenoming treatment. Int Immunopharmacol 8: 1386-1394.

26. Sofer S, Gueron M (1988) Respiratory failure in children following envenomation by the scorpion Leiurus quinquestriatus: hemodynamic and neurological aspects. Toxicon 26: 931-939.

27. Cupo P, Hering SE (2002) Cardiac troponin I release after severe scorpion envenoming by Tityus serrulatus. Toxicon 40: 823-830.

28. Meki AR, Mohamed ZM, Mohey El-deen HM (2003) Significance of assessment of serum cardiac troponin I and interleukin-8 in scorpion envenomed children. Toxicon 41: 129-137.

29. Ismail M, Abd-Elsalam MA (1988) Are the toxicological effects of scorpion envenomation related to tissue venom concentration? Toxicon 26: 233-256.

30. Devaux C, Jouirou B, Naceur Krifi M, Clot-Faybesse O, El Ayeb M, et al. (2004) Quantitative variability in the biodistribution and in toxinokinetic studies of the three main alpha toxins from the Androctonus australis hector scorpion venom. Toxicon 43: 661-669.

31. Hamers-Casterman C, Atarhouch T, Muyldermans S, Robinson G, Hamers C, et al. (1993) Naturally occurring antibodies devoid of light chains. Nature 363: 446-448.

32. Muyldermans S, Atarhouch T, Saldanha J, Barbosa JA, Hamers R (1994) Sequence and structure of VH domain from naturally occurring camel heavy chain immunoglobulins lacking light chains. Protein Eng 7: 1129-1135.

33. Vu KB, Ghahroudi MA, Wyns L, Muyldermans S (1997) Comparison of llama VH sequences from conventional and heavy chain antibodies. Mol Immunol 34: 1121-1131.

34. Hmila I, Abdallah R BA, Saerens D, Benlasfar Z, Conrath K, et al. (2008) VHH, bivalent domains and chimeric Heavy chain-only antibodies with high neutralizing efficacy for scorpion toxin AahI'. Mol Immunol 45: 3847-3856.

35. Hmila I, Saerens D, Ben Abderrazek R, Vincke C, Abidi N, et al. (2010) A bispecific nanobody to provide full protection against lethal scorpion envenoming. FASEB J 24: 3479-3489.

36. Abderrazek RB, Hmila I, Vincke C, Benlasfar Z, Pellis M, et al. (2009) Identification of potent nanobodies to neutralize the most poisonous polypeptide from scorpion venom. Biochem J 424: 263-272.

37. Bradford MM (1976) A rapid and sensitive method for the quantitation of microgram quantities of protein utilizing the principle of protein-dye binding. Anal Biochem 72: 248-254.

38. El Ayeb M, Delori P, Rochat H (1983) Immunochemistry of scorpion alpha-toxins: antigenic homologies checked with radioimmunoassays (RIA). Toxicon 21: 709-716.

39. Bouhaouala-Zahar B, Ducancel F, Zenouaki I, Ben Khalifa R, Borchani L, et al. (1996) A recombinant insect-specific alpha-toxin of Buthus occitanus tunetanus scorpion confers protection against homologous mammal toxins. Eur. J. Biochem. FEBS 238: 653-660.

40. Miranda F, Kupeyan C, Rochat H, Rochat C, Lissitzky S, et al. (1970) Purification of animal neurotoxins. Isolation and characterization of eleven neurotoxins from the venoms of the scorpions *Androctonus australis hector*, *Buthus occitanus tunetanus* and *Leiurus quinquestriatus quinquestriatus*. Eur. J. Biochem. FEBS 16: 514-523.

41. Bouhaouala-Zahar B, Ben Abderrazek R, Hmila I, Abidi N, Muyldermans S, et al. (2011) Immunological aspects of scorpion toxins: current status and perspectives. Inflamm Allergy Drug Targets 10: 358-368.

42. Meddeb-Mouelhi F, Bouhaouala-Zahar B, Benlasfar Z, Hammadi M, Mejri T (2003) Immunized camel sera and derived immunoglobulin subclasses neutralizing *Androctonus australis hector* scorpion toxins. Toxicon 42: 785-791.

43. Oukkache N, Malih I, Chgoury F, El Gnaoui N, Saïle R, et al. (2009) Modifications histopathologiques après envenimation scorpionique expérimentale chez la souris. Medical Sciences Rev Médicopharmaceutique 53: 48-52.

44. Chgoury F, Oukkache N, El Gnaoui N, Benomar H, Saïle R, et al. (2011) Etude cinétique et biologique du venin de scorpion *Androctonus mauretanicus* chez le lapin. Toxins and ions transferts 19: 141-145.

45. Clot-Faybesse O, Guieu R, Rochat H, Devaux C (2000) Toxicity during early development of the mouse nervous system of a scorpion neurotoxin active on sodium channels. Life Sci 66: 185-192.

46. Nunan EA, Moraes MF, Cardoso VN, Moraes-Santos T (2003) Effect of age on body distribution of Tityustoxin from *Tityus serrulatus* scorpion venom in rats. Life Sci 73: 319-325.

47. Sandoval MRL, Lebrun I (2003) TsTx toxin isolated from *Tityus serrulatus* scorpion venom induces spontaneous recurrent seizures and mossy fiber sprouting. Epilepsia 44: 904-911.

48. Sampaio SV, Coutinho-Netto J, Arantes EC, Marangoni S, Oliveira B, et al. (1996) Isolation of toxin TsTX-VI from *Tityus serrulatus* scorpion venom. Effects on the release of neurotransmitters from synaptosomes. Biochem Mol Biol Int 39: 729-740.

49. Lourenço GA, Lebrun I, Dorce VA (2002) Neurotoxic effects of fractions isolated from *Tityus bahiensis* scorpion venom (Perty, 1834). Toxicon 40: 149-157.

50. Nencioni AL, Lourenço GA, Lebrun I, Florio JC, Dorce VA (2009) Central effects of *Tityus serrulatus* and *Tityus bahiensis* scorpion venoms after intraperitoneal injection in rats. Neurosci Lett 463: 234-238.

51. Ossanai LT, Lourenço GA, Nencioni AL, Lebrun I, Yamanouye N, et al. (2012) Effects of a toxin isolated from *Tityus bahiensis* scorpion venom on the hippocampus of rats. Life Sci 91: 230-236.

52. Ladjel-Mendil AL, Martin-Eauclaire MF, Laraba-Djebari F (2013) Neuropathophysiological effect and immuno-inflammatory response induced by kaliotoxin of *Androctonus* scorpion venom. Neuroimmunomodulation 20: 99-106.

53. De Matos IM, Rocha OA, Leite R, Freire-Maia L (1997) Lung oedema induced by *Tityus serrulatus* scorpion venom in the rat. Comp Biochem Physiol C Pharmacol Toxicol Endocrinol 118: 143-148.

54. D'Suze G, Salazar V, Díaz P, Sevcik C, Azpurua H, et al. (2004) Histopathological changes and inflammatory response induced by *Tityus discrepans* scorpion venom in rams. Toxicon 44: 851-860.

55. Petricevich VL (2010) Scorpion venom and the inflammatory response. Mediators Inflamm 1-16.

56. Paneque Peres AC, Nonaka PN, de Carvalho Pde T, Toyama MH, Silva CA, et al. (2009) Effects of *Tityus serrulatus* scorpion venom on lung mechanics and inflammation in mice. Toxicon 53: 779-785.

57. Suze GD, Moncada S, González C, Sevcik C, Aguilar V, et al. (2003) Relationship between plasmatic levels of various cytokines, tumor necrosis factor, enzymes, glucose and venom concentration following *Tityus* scorpion sting. Toxicon 41: 367-375.

58. Bahloul M, Chaari A, Dammak H, Bouaziz M (2012) "Pulmonary edema induced by scorpion venom: evidence of cardiogenic nature". Int J Cardiol 158: 292-293.

59. Deshpande SB, Akella A (2012) Non-cardiogenic mechanisms for the pulmonary edema induced by scorpion venom. Int J Cardiol 157: 426-427.

60. Tilg H, Diehl AM (2000) Cytokines in alcoholic and nonalcoholic steatohepatitis. N Engl J Med 343: 1467-1476.

61. Natu VS, Murthy RK, Deodhar KP (2006) Efficacy of species specific anti-scorpion venom serum (AScVS) against severe, serious scorpion stings (Mesobuthus tamulus concanesis Pocock) an experience from rural hospital in western Maharashtra. J Assoc Physicians. India 54: 283-287.

62. Zayerzadeh E, Koohi MK, Mirakabadi AZ, Fardipoor A, Kassaian SE, et al. (2012) Amelioration of cardio-respiratory perturbations following Mesobuthus eupeus envenomation in anesthetized rabbits with commercial polyvalent F (ab')2 antivenom. Toxicon 59: 249-256.

63. Jalali A, Bavarsad-Omidian N, Babaei M, Najafzadeh H, Rezaei S, et al. (2012) The pharmacokinetics of *Hemiscorpius lepturus* scorpion venom and Razi antivenom following intramuscular administration in rat. J Venom Res 3: 1-6.

64. Alvarez A, Montero Y, Jimenez E, Zerpa N, Parrilla P, et al. (2013) IgY antibodies anti-*Tityus caripitensis* venom: purification and neutralization efficacy. Toxicon 74: 208-214.

65. Riaño-Umbarila L, Contreras-Ferrat G, Olamendi-Portugal T, Morelos-Juárez C, Corzo G, et al. (2011) Exploiting cross-reactivity to neutralize two different scorpion venoms with one single chain antibody fragment. J Biol Chem 286: 6143-6151.

66. Costal-Oliveira F, Duarte CG, Machado de Avila RA, Melo MM, Bordon KC, et al. (2012) General biochemical and immunological characteristics of the venom from Peruvian scorpion Hadruroides lunatus. Toxicon 60: 934-942.

67. Alvarenga L, Moreau V, Felicori L, Nguyen C, Duarte C, et al. (2010) Design of antibody-reactive peptides from discontinuous parts of scorpion toxins. Vaccine 28: 970-980.

68. Devaux C, Moreau E, Goyffon M, Rochat H, Billiald P, et al. (2001) Construction and functional evaluation of a single-chain antibody fragment that neutralizes toxin AahI from the venom of the scorpion *Androctonus australis hector*. Eur J Biochem 268: 694-702.

69. Yardehnavi N, Behdani M, Pooshang Bagheri K, Mahmoodzadeh A, Khanahmad H, et al. (2014) A camelid antibody candidate for development of a therapeutic agent against *Hemiscorpius lepturus* envenomation. FASEB J Off Publ Fed Am Soc Exp Biol 28: 247-478.

70. Hmila I, Cosyns B, Tounsi H, Roosens B, Caveliers V, et al. (2012) Pre-clinical studies of toxin-specific nanobodies: evidence of *in vivo* efficacy to prevent fatal disturbances provoked by scorpion envenoming. Toxicol Appl Pharmacol 264: 222-231.

71. Mesquita MB, Moraes-Santos T, Moraes MF (2003) Centrally injected tityustoxin produces the systemic manifestations observed in severe scorpion poisoning. Toxicol Appl Pharmacol 187: 58-66.

9

Experimental IR and Raman Spectroscopy and DFT Methods based Material Characterization and Data Analysis of 2- Nitrophenol

Dixit V* and Yadav RA

Laser and Spectroscopy Laboratory, Department of Physics, Banaras Hindu University, Varanasi -221005, India

Abstract

Vibrational characteristics of 2- nitrophenol have been investigated using experimental IR and Raman data and computational data using DFT method employing the 6-311++G** basis set available on Gaussian-09 software for the most stableconformer C-1. Complete vibrational assignments of the experimental IR and Raman bands have been proposed in light of the results obtained from the DFT computations and the PEDs computed using GAR2PED software. The optimized geometrical parameters suggest that the overall symmetry of the most stablemolecule is Cs. The molecule is expected to have three conformers. In the present article all the characterizations and the analyses of the lowest energy conformer of 2-NP have been studied. The charge transfer occurring in the molecule has been shown by HOMO–LUMO energy orbitals the energy gap of HOMO LUMO orbitals have been found 4.03eV. The mappings of electron density iso-surface with the electrostatic potential (ESP), has been carried out to get the information about the size, shape, charge density distribution and site of chemical reactivity of 2-NP. Current density and magnetic shielding of C-1 have been investigated. Some essential thermo molecular characteristics, namely, enthalpy, Gibb's free energy, thermal energy, entropy, heat capacity, internal energy and the partition functions of the molecule have also been analyzed.

Keywords: Optimized structure; Conformers; Entropy; MESP; Magnetic shielding; 2-nitro-phenol

Introduction

Nitro phenols constitute a class of volatile organic compounds that is increasingly presented in urban as well as in natural environments [1-3]. These are important and versatile compounds in the industrial, agricultural and defence applications [4] and are frequently used as intermediates in the manufacture of explosives, pharmaceuticals, pesticides, pigments, dyes, rubber chemicals, lumber preservatives, photographic chemicals, etc. [5-8]. 2- Nitro-phenols (2-NP), in particular, poses significant health risks since it is a toxic to mammals, microorganisms and anaerobic bacteria. Its toxicity is thought to be due to the nitro group being easily reduced by the enzymes into nitro anion radical, nitroso and hydroxylamine derivatives [4]. Although extensive experimental and theoretical studies are reported on the structural and vibrational studies of mono-substituted phenols [9,10] dealing with their structural features, intra-molecular H-bonding parameters and the vibrational spectra [11-14], only few works of this kind exist on phenols [15-18]. In the present study we report the results of our probing into the application of the DFT based SQM method [19] to the vibrational analysis of hydrogen bonded systems. The main difficulty in such investigations is that the vibrational spectra of these compounds have not been completely analyzed even now and generally only rough assignments are available. Therefore, an investigation of the performance of the DFT-based SQM method has to be carried out simultaneously with a complete vibrational analysis of the molecule. This process was done successfully in the case of 2 6-difluorophenol earlier [20].

The 2-NP molecule, contains a strong intra-molecular (O) H......O(N) hydrogen bonding interaction which has been analyzed by various experimental and theoretical studies [21-31]. The extensive investigations corresponding to the vibrational description of **2**-NP is not complete. Most of the numerous spectroscopic studies [24,31-33] focused on the vibrations from which the information can be carried out about the hydrogen bonding interaction, first of all on the OH stretching and OH torsion.

In the present work calculations have been made for the optimized molecular geometries, APT and Mulliken atomic charges and the fundamental vibrational wave numbers along with their intensities in the IR spectrum, Raman activities and the depolarization ratios of the Raman lines using the DFT (B3LYP) method employing the 6-311++G** basis set [34-38] available with Gaussian-09 software [39] for the lowest energy conformer C-1 of 2- NP. The experimental IR and Raman spectral data have been analyzed in the light of the computed fundamentals and the corresponding PEDs calculated, using the GAR2PED software [40]. For the calculation of the PEDs the vibrational problem was set up in terms of the internal coordinates for the GAR2PED software. HOMO-LUMO, total density plots, electrostatic potential (ESP) surface and their arrays have been investigated. The essential NLO as well as thermo molecular parameters have been investigated and using NMR analysis employing Continuous Set of Gauge Transformation (CSGT) method electro-magnetic characteristics of 2-NP have been investigated.

Experimental Detail

One to two milligrams of the pure (98%), a yellow crystalline solid in powdered form, 2-nitro phenol, purchased from Sigma Aldrich Chemical Co. (USA), was used to record the Raman spectra using a home assembled micro-Raman spectrometer: Horiba Jobin-Yuon Spectrometer (iHR-320) system with an inverted microscope (Nikon Eclipse Ti-U, Japan). A Diode laser (Star bright Diode Laser, Torsana Laser Tech, Denmark) of λ=785 nm used as source to illuminate the

*Corresponding author: V. Dixit, Laser and Spectroscopy Laboratory, Department of Physics, Banaras Hindu University, Varanasi-221005, India, E-mail: vikazlmp@rediffmail.com, drvikasbhu@gmail.com

sample sandwiched between quartz cover slip and borosilicate glass slide. The sample was mounted on the microscope stage and a 60X microscope objective have been used to focus the laser beam and to record the Raman signals. A liquid Nitrogen cooled Symphony CCD detector have been utilized to collect the Raman scattered radiation. The spectral range of the micro-Raman have been kept 200-3100 cm^{-1} with resolution 5 cm^{-1}, accuracy 2 cm^{-1} at spectrometer slit width 100 μm. In order to record a better Raman spectrum, data were obtained using a laser power of 47mW with the acquisition times of 5 min.

FTIR spectrum of 2-NP sample was recorded using KBr pellet. The 10 mg of the 2-NP sample was weighed and properly mixed with 990 mg KBr. This mixture was then pelleted using KBr pellet maker by applying pressure using 8 tons weight for half an hour. FTIR spectrum was recorded using the above mentioned pellet at room temperature, using an FTIR spectrometer (Jasco 6300) with a standard source. The spectra have been recorded in the range of 400- 4000 cm^{-1}. The 200 scans have been taken with 2 cm^{-1} spectral resolution for all the three samples.

Computational Details

To optimize the structure of 2- NP the following procedure was adopted. Initially the benzene ring (including H atoms only) was optimized. After this an OH group was added to a carbon atom of benzene ring and the structure was optimized. With this structure a nitro group was added to the ortho position of phenolic group (Figure 1).

This structure was further optimized. In the optimized structure if hydrogen atom of the OH group faces the NO$_2$ group the structure remains planar. However, if the hydrogen atom of the OH group is kept away from the NO$_2$ group there are two possible conformers of 2-NP, in one conformer the plane of NO2 makes the angle -33.70 while in the other it makes an angle of 33.70 with the plane of phenyl ring (Figure 2).

Therefore total 3 possible conformers have been found to exist of the 2-NP molecule. The energies of all the three optimized conformers are -512.12911314 (C-1), -512.11232617 (C-2) and -512.10755721(C-3) a.u. (Table 1). In the present paper we have considered the vibrational characteristics of the most stableconformer C-1 only.

The optimized molecular geometries, APT charges and the fundamental vibrational wave numbers along with their corresponding intensities in IR spectrum, Raman activities and the depolarization ratios of the Raman bands for the present molecule were computed at the B3LYP/6-311++G** level using the Gaussian 09 program package. The unscaled B3LYP/6-311++G** vibrational frequencies are generally slightly larger than the experimental values. In order to achieve the reasonable frequency matching, the scale factors proposed by Rauhut and Pulay [42] were employed. The assignments of all the normal modes of vibration have been made on the basis of the computed PEDs. The experimental IR and Raman frequencies corresponding to the fundamental modes have been compared with the calculated fundamental frequencies in light of the PEDs. The molecular electrostatic potential (ESP) surface, used for the predicting sites and relative reactivity towards the electrophilic attack and in the studies of biological recognition and hydrogen bonding interactions, has been plotted and the complete thermo-molecular data analysis, complete

description of global reactivity parameters and essential features of electro-magnetism of 2-NP have been investigated.

Results and Discussions

Molecular geometries

The geometrical parameters of 2-NP computed at the B3LYP/6-311G** level of theory are compared with the experimental and MP2/6-31G* data in Table 2. The optimized geometrical structure of 2-NP has overall Cs symmetry for the lowest energy conformer. The computed O–H and N–O bond lengths are larger compared with the experimental values. At the same time, the C–O and C–N bond lengths seem to be somewhat shorter. These geometrical parameters are sensitive to hydrogen bonding [15]. Taking into account the above considerations, the data (Table 2) show good agreement between the experimental and theoretical geometries with some minor discrepancies. The computed O–H and N–O bond lengths are larger compared to the experimental values. The computed bond angles are consistent at both levels (Electron Diffraction and MP2/6-31G') of theory; the deviations from the experimental values are within or close to experimental error.

The bond lengths of C$_1$-C$_2$, C$_3$-O$_{11}$, C$_4$-N$_{13}$ and C$_5$-C$_6$ respectively are shorter while those lengths of C1-C$_6$, C$_2$-C$_3$, C$_3$-C$_4$, C$_4$-C$_5$ and O$_{11}$-H$_{12}$ respectively are found to be larger in the most stableconformer than both the C-1 and C-2 conformers. Also, angle α (C$_4$-C$_3$-O$_{11}$) is found to be larger while angle α (O$_{14}$-N$_{13}$-O$_{15}$) is found to be shorter in the most stableconformer than the other two (Table 2). These conformational discrepancies may be due to intra-molecular hydrogen bonding in the most stableconformer and also due to instability of conformers C-2 and C-3 respectively.

APT charges

Atomic polarizability tensor (APT) charge is interpreted as the sum of charge tensor and charge flux tensor, leading to a charge-charge flux model [43,44]. The APT atomic charges (in unit of e) at various atomic sites of 2-NP are collected in Table 3. The carbon atoms belonging to the ring have alternately positive and negative APT charges with different magnitudes. All the H and N atoms have positive APT charges with different magnitudes, while the O atoms possess negative and different magnitudes of APT charges. The N atom possesses the highest magnitude which is connected directly to the ring and the two O atoms. It is also noticeable that the magnitude of the APT charge on

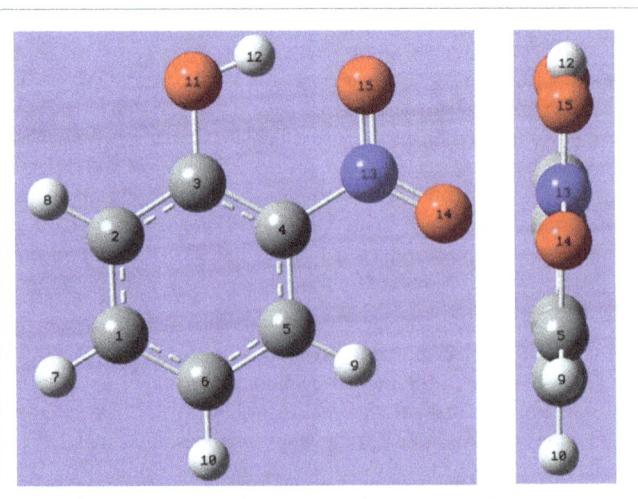

Figure 1: Optimized structure of 2-Nitro phenol (C-I).

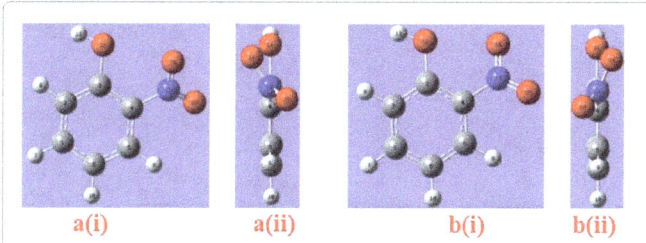

Figure 2: Front and side views of conformer C-2 {a(i) & a(ii)} and conformer C-3 {b(i) & b(ii)}of 2-NP.

C₃ attached to the OH group is the largest of all the C atoms. Also, it is interesting to note that the N atom possesses positive APT charge. The magnitude of the APT charge on H₁₂ is the largest of all the H atoms. The O atoms possess almost equal APT charges.

Mulliken atomic charges

Mulliken atomic charge calculation plays an important role in the application of quantum chemical calculation to molecular systems, because the atomic charges affect the dipole moment, polarizability, electronic structure, and much more properties of the molecular systems. Mulliken atomic charges (in unit of e) at various atomic sites of 2-NP are collected in Table 3 from which it can be noticed that all the carbon atoms except C₄ and C₅, have negative Mulliken atomic charges. One of the O atoms attached to the N atom with a single bond possesses positive Mulliken atomic charge. However, it is an electronegative atom like N and O atoms. The H atoms possess positive Mulliken atomic charge. The Mulliken atomic charge at the C atom attached to the OH group is the largest of all the C atoms and the H atom of the OH group possesses the largest Mulliken atomic charge of all the H atoms in the C-1 conformer.

ESP charges

The studies of effective atomic charges play a crucial role in the application of quantum mechanical computations to the molecular systems. Despite the conceptual problems associated with the dividing up overall molecular charge density in atomic contributions, and all the conventional problems related to the finding of convenient and robust algorithm applicable to a wide range of the systems [45]. The beauty of effective atomic charges as the parameters for the calculation of electrostatic interactions in a various molecular mechanics simulation packages is certainly one essential area of application. Partial atomic charges play a different, but even more important, role in the qualitative rationalization of organic and inorganic reactivity [46]. The molecular electrostatic potential (ESP) derived charges are those are reproduced by fitting the partial atomic charges to reproduce the molecular electrostatic potential (MEP) at a number of points around the molecule at a (large) number of grid points using Merge-Singh-Kollman (MK) scheme [47].

The molecular ESP derived charges at various atomic sites of 2-NP have been contained in the Table 3. Clearly, the ESP charges at all the

C atoms except C₃, have negative and small but different value while C₃ atom, attached to OH group of 2-NP, have positive and largest value amongst all the C atoms of 2-NP. All the H atoms on the ring possess smaller but positive ESP charges while H atom of OH group attains positive and largest value of all the H atoms in the molecule. The O atoms possess negative ESP charges. The O atom of OH group attains largest negative value (-0.590398 e) while N atom of NO₂ group attains largest positive value (0.681548 e) of ESP charges in 2-NP.

Vibrational assignments

The 2-NP molecule is a 15 atomic molecule with 39 normal modes of vibration in which 30 modes are associated with the benzene ring which are : 12 stretching modes -ν, 3 planar ring deformation -α(R), 3 non planar ring deformation -Φ(R), 6 planar deformation modes -β(C-H) and 6 non-planar deformation modes -γ(C-H),out of which 2 of each i.e. β(C-H) and γ(C-H) become β(C-N), β(C-O) and γ(C-N), γ(C-O) respectively. The three normal modes of OH-group are: OH stretching -ν(OH), OH torsion -τ(OH) and C-O-H angle bending. The six normal modes of the nitro group are: anti-symmetric NO₂ stretching -ν$_{as}$(NO2), symmetric NO₂ stretching -ν$_s$(NO₂), NO₂ rocking -ρ(NO₂), NO₂ wagging -ω(NO₂), NO₂ scissoring -δ(NO₂) and NO₂ torsion -τ(NO₂).

The calculated and observed vibrational frequencies along with the corresponding PEDs and vibrational assignments are collected in Table 4. The experimental and calculated IR and Raman spectra are reproduced in Figure 3-6. The normal mode assignments have been discussed under the following sections: (i) The phenyl ring modes (30), (ii) The OH group modes (3) and (iii) The NO₂ group modes (6).

Phenyl ring modes (30): The four C-H stretching modes ν (C-H) are assigned to the frequencies 3034 (ν₅), 3181(ν₄), 3186(ν₃) and 3205(ν₂) cm⁻¹ which correspond dominantly to the modes ν(C₁-H₇), ν(C₆-H₁₀), ν(C₂-H₈) and ν(C₅-H₉) respectively. The C-H stretching modes ν (C-H) were assigned to the frequencies 3070, 3088, 3096 and 3117 cm⁻¹ [41] and also to the frequencies 3208, 3229 and 3245 cm⁻¹ [48]. The C-H stretching vibrations are pure and highly localized modes. There are 6 C-C stretching modes ν(R) due to the phenyl ring which are identified as the computed frequencies 1002 (ν₁₉), 1051 (ν₁₈), 1306 (ν₁₂), 1420 (ν₁₀), 1547 (ν₇), 1586 (ν₆) cm⁻¹. These modes are strongly coupled with many other modes. These modes were assigned to the frequencies 1020, 1581 and 1620 cm⁻¹ [41] and also to the frequencies 1369, 1551, 1584 and 1612 cm⁻¹ [48]. The C-N and C-O stretching modes occur at frequencies 667 (ν₂₈), 1442 (ν₉) cm⁻¹ corresponding to the modes ν(C₄-N₁₃) and ν(C₃-O₁₁) respectively. These modes are also coupled with many other modes. The C-O stretching mode in the literature was found to be corresponding to the frequency 1269 [41] and 1464 cm⁻¹ [48].

There are three ring planar deformation modes which we assign as the frequencies 865(ν₂₂), 559(ν₃₀) and 373(ν₃₅) cm⁻¹. These modes are coupled with other modes as shown in the Table-4.The three ring non-planar deformation modes are correlated to the frequencies 657(ν₂₉), 413(ν₃₄) and 141(ν₃₈) cm⁻¹ corresponding to modes 4 and 16(a,b) of the

Conformers	Point group	Total energy (Hartree)	Relative energy		
			Hartree	Temp. (K)	kcal/mol
C-1	C$_s$	-512.12911314	0	0	0
C-2	C₁	-512.11232617	0.01678697	5300.9405365	10.533984965
C-3	C₁	-512.10755721	0.02155593	6806.868848	13.52655319

Table 1: Total and relative energies of all the possible conformers of 2- NP.

S.No.	Parameters	B3-LYP/6-311++G**			ED@	MP2(FC) / 6-31G*@
		C-1[s,#]	C-2[#]	C-3[#]		
1	r(C$_1$-C$_2$)	1.382	1.389	1.389	1.388	1.387
2	r(C$_1$-C$_6$)	1.404	1.396	1.396	1.399	1.402
3	r(C$_1$-H$_7$)	1.084	1.084	1.084	1.089	1.086
4	r(C$_2$-C$_3$)	1.404	1.400	1.400	1.406	1.405
5	r(C$_2$-H$_8$)	1.083	1.086	1.086	1.089	1.086
6	r(C$_3$-C$_4$)	1.415	1.405	1.405	1.411	1.410
7	r(C$_3$-O$_{11}$)	1.336	1.352	1.352	1.359	1.351
8	r(C$_4$-C$_5$)	1.402	1.393	1.393	1.402	1.401
9	r(C$_4$-N$_{13}$)	1.453	1.473	1.473	1.464	1.456
10	r(C$_5$-C$_6$)	1.380	1.387	1.387	1.387	1.386
11	r(C$_5$-H$_9$)	1.081	1.082	1.082	1.089	1.086
12	r(C$_6$-H$_{10}$)	1.082	1.082	1.082	1.089	1.086
13	r(O$_{11}$-H$_{12}$)	0.982	0.964	0.964	0.969	0.986
14	r(N$_{13}$-O$_{14}$)	1.219	1.221	1.221	1.225	1.239
15	r(N$_{13}$-O$_{15}$)	1.248	1.228	1.228	1.241	1.255
16	α(C$_2$-C$_1$-C$_6$)	121.031	120.5	120.5	122.9	120.5
17	α (C$_2$-C$_1$-H$_7$)	119.217	119.3	119.3	--	--
18	α (C$_6$-C$_1$-H$_7$)	119.752	120.2	120.2	--	--
19	α (C$_1$-C$_2$-C$_3$)	120.786	121.0	121.0	118.1	121.1
20	α (C$_1$-C$_2$-H$_8$)	121.644	120.2	120.2	--	--
21	α (C$_3$-C$_2$-H$_8$)	117.570	118.8	118.8	--	--
22	α (C$_2$-C$_3$-C$_4$)	117.659	117.8	117.8	119.4	117.4
23	α (C$_2$-C$_3$-O$_{11}$)	117.741	122.0	122.0	--	--
24	α (C$_4$-C$_3$-O$_{11}$)	124.600	120.2	120.2	123.9	125.6
25	α (C$_3$-C$_4$-C$_5$)	121.165	121.1	121.1	121.4	121.7
26	α (C$_3$-C$_4$-N$_{13}$)	120.816	121.5	121.5	120.8	121.0
27	α (C$_5$-C$_4$-N$_{13}$)	118.019	117.4	117.4	--	--
28	α (C$_4$-C$_5$-C$_6$)	119.999	120.3	120.3	119.0	119.6
29	α (C$_4$-C$_5$-H$_9$)	118.254	118.2	118.2	--	--
30	α (C$_6$-C$_5$-H$_9$)	121.747	121.5	121.5	--	--
31	α (C$_1$-C$_6$-C$_5$)	119.360	119.2	119.2	119.3	119.7
32	α (C$_1$-C$_6$-H$_{10}$)	120.505	120.7	120.7	--	--
33	α (C$_5$-C$_6$-H$_{10}$)	120.135	120.1	120.1	--	--
34	α (C$_3$-O$_{11}$-H$_{12}$)	107.393	109.5	109.5	104.4	106.8
35	α (C$_4$-N$_{13}$-O$_{14}$)	119.320	118.1	118.1	118.2	118.4
36	α (C$_4$-N$_{13}$-O$_{15}$)	117.914	116.9	116.9	118.6	118.8
37	α (O$_{14}$-N$_{13}$-O$_{15}$)	122.766	124.9	124.9	123.3	122.8
38	δ(C$_6$-C$_1$-C$_2$-C$_3$)	0.004	0.8	-0.8	--	--
39	δ(C$_6$-C$_1$-C$_2$-H$_8$)	179.999	-179.0	179.0	--	--
40	δ(H$_7$-C$_1$-C$_2$-C$_3$)	179.997	-179.6	179.6	--	--
41	δ(H$_7$-C$_1$-C$_2$-H$_8$)	-0.008	0.6	-0.6	--	--
42	δ(C$_2$-C$_1$-C$_6$-C$_5$)	-0.011	0.0	-0.0	--	--
43	δ(C$_2$-C$_1$-C$_6$-H$_{10}$)	180.001	179.9	-179.9	--	--
44	δ(H$_7$-C$_1$-C$_6$-C$_5$)	-180.004	-179.7	179.8	--	--
45	δ(H$_7$-C$_1$-C$_6$-H$_{10}$)	0.008	0.2	-0.2	--	--
46	δ(C$_1$-C$_2$-C$_3$-C$_4$)	-0.004	-0.4	0.4	--	--
47	δ(C$_1$-C$_2$-C$_3$-O$_{11}$)	-180.000	-178.4	178.4	--	--
48	δ (H$_8$-C$_2$-C$_3$-C$_4$)	-179.999	179.4	-179.4	--	--
49	δ (H$_8$-C$_2$-C$_3$-O$_{11}$)	0.004	1.4	-1.4	--	--
50	δ (C$_2$-C$_3$-C$_4$-C$_5$)	0.011	-0.8	0.8	--	--
51	δ (C$_2$-C$_3$-C$_4$-N$_{13}$)	-180.029	179.3	-179.3	--	--
52	δ (O$_{11}$-C$_3$-C$_4$-C$_5$)	180.007	177.3	-177.3	--	--
53	δ (O$_{11}$-C$_3$-C$_4$-N$_{13}$)	-0.033	-2.7	2.7	--	--
54	δ (C$_2$-C$_3$-O$_{11}$-H$_{12}$)	180.028	2.2	-2.1	--	--
55	δ (C$_4$-C$_3$-O$_{11}$-H$_{12}$)	0.032	-175.8	175.9	--	--
56	δ (C$_3$-C$_4$-C$_5$-C$_6$)	-0.018	1.5	-1.5	--	--
57	δ (C$_3$-C$_4$-C$_5$-C$_9$)	-180.007	-178.6	178.6	--	--
58	δ (N$_{13}$-C$_4$-C$_5$-C$_6$)	180.020	178.5	178.5	--	--
59	δ (N$_{13}$-C$_4$-C$_5$-H$_9$)	0.031	1.4	-1.4	--	--

60	δ (C$_3$-C$_4$-N$_{13}$-O$_{14}$)	180.052	-33.7	33.7	--	--
61	δ (C$_3$-C$_4$-N$_{13}$-O$_{15}$)	0.050	147.8	-147.8	--	--
62	δ (C$_5$-C$_4$-N$_{13}$-O$_{14}$)	0.013	146.3	-146.3	--	--
63	δ (C$_5$-C$_4$-N$_{13}$-O$_{15}$)	180.011	-32.1	32.1	--	--
64	δ (C$_4$-C$_5$-C$_6$-C$_1$)	0.017	-1.1	1.1	--	--
65	δ (C$_4$-C$_5$-C$_6$-H$_{10}$)	-179.994	179.0	-179.0	--	--
66	δ (H$_9$-C$_5$-C$_6$-C$_1$)	180.006	179.0	-179.0	--	--
67	δ (H$_9$-C$_5$-C$_6$-H$_{10}$)	-0.006	-0.9	0.9	--	--

$^\$$ Conformer C-1 is the lowest energy conformer of 2-NP; # Our Work; @ Ref. 1

Table 2: Computed and observed geometrical parameters of 2- NP.

Atoms	APT charges		Mulliken atomic charges		ESP charges		ESP Potentials	
	(C-1)	(C-2/C-3)	(C-1)	C-2/C-3	(C-1)	C-2/C-3	C-1	C-2/C-3
C$_1$	0.168082	0.109390	-0.251868	-0.187756	-0.087841	-0.070392	-14.73524	-14.73734
C$_2$	-0.168431	-0.166562	-0.165953	0.112368	-0.242264	-0.276459	-14.74573	-14.73986
C$_3$	0.617390	0.569682	-0.630033	-0.280495	0.387901	0.311740	-14.66298	-14.66522
C$_4$	-0.369569	-0.186726	0.559561	-0.248181	-0.069178	0.011254	-14.69304	-14.70101
C$_5$	0.098974	0.070105	0.139598	0.278052	-0.166961	-0.210985	-14.73417	-14.73785
C$_6$	-0.238821	-0.186101	-0.249269	-0.259811	-0.137599	-0.132966	-14.74581	-14.74815
H$_7$	0.051609	0.049260	0.175404	0.172879	0.138456	0.134908	-1.07628	-1.07627
H$_8$	0.067916	0.037818	0.205976	0.138330	0.181123	0.149018	-1.07645	-1.06388
H$_9$	0.102578	0.094642	0.239102	0.231315	0.166468	0.186660	-1.07216	-1.07586
H$_{10}$	0.049672	0.048614	0.185472	0.174564	0.136537	0.133989	-1.08086	-1.08272
O$_{11}$	-0.726207	-0.645764	-0.185498	-0.177027	-0.590398	-0.522159	-22.31645	-22.30600
H$_{12}$	0.390488	0.297918	0.290132	0.270747	0.471626	0.417133	-0.95701	-0.94374
N$_{13}$	1.350233	1.219919	-0.296760	-0.207132	0.681548	0.736291	-18.13866	-18.15683
O$_{14}$	-0.688853	-0.677157	0.004956	-0.034067	-0.388638	-0.452560	-22.32424	-22.34426
O$_{15}$	-0.705060	-0.635038	-0.020819	0.016214	-0.480781	-0.415470	-22.32304	-22.34320

*Charges are in the unit of e

Table 3: APT, Mulliken and ESP fitted (MK scheme) atomic charges and molecular electrostatic potentials at different atomic sites of 2-NP (C-I).

t	Calculated Frequencies (cm^{-1})		Observed Freq@. (cm^{-1})				PEDs	Mode Assigned
			Ref-[41]		Our work			
	Sc.	Unsc.	Raman	IR	Raman	IR		
ν_1	3453	3471(241,108)0.14	--	3253	--	3358	ν(O$_{11}$-H$_{12}$) (100)	ν(O-H)
ν_2	3205	3222(4,94)0.16	--	3115*	--	--	ν(C$_5$-H$_9$) (91) + ν(C$_6$-H$_{10}$) (8)	ν(C-H)
ν_3	3186	3203(2,170)0.12	--	3099	--	--	ν(C$_2$-H$_8$) (67) + (C$_1$-H$_7$) (17) + ν(C$_6$-H$_{10}$) (12)	ν(C-H)
ν_4	3181	3197(5,88)0.62	--	3091	--	3136	ν(C$_6$-H$_{10}$) (67) + (C$_2$-H$_8$) (23)	ν(C-H)
ν_5	3034	3178(4,73)0.65	3100	3060	--	3065	ν(C$_1$-H$_7$) (78)+ν(C$_6$-H$_{10}$) (13)+ ν(C$_2$-H$_8$) (9)	ν(C-H)
ν_6	1586	1661(133,9)0.75	1615	1625	--	1600	ν(C$_3$-C$_4$)(15) + (C$_1$-C$_6$)(13) + ν(C$_4$-C$_5$)(13) + ν(C$_1$-C$_2$)(13) +ν(N$_{13}$-O$_{14}$) (6)+ α_3(R)(9)	ν(R)
ν_7	1547	1620(81,31)0.56	1600	1603	1582	1559	ν(C$_5$-C$_6$)(21) + ν(C$_2$-C$_3$)(18) + ν(C$_1$-C$_2$)(7) + ν(C$_4$-C$_5$)(6) + ν(C$_3$-C$_4$)(6) + α(C$_3$-O$_{11}$-H$_{12}$)(10) + α_2(R)(9)	ν(R)
ν_8	1511	1582(163,37)0.60	1540	1550	1525	1501	ν_{as}(NO$_2$) (52) +(C$_1$-C$_2$)(8) + ν(C$_3$-C$_4$)(7) + β(C$_4$-N$_{13}$) (8) + ρ(NO$_2$) (8)	ν_{as}(NO$_2$)
ν_9	1442	1510(119,2)0.30	1465	1476	--	1462	ν(C$_3$-O$_{11}$) (13) + (C$_1$-C$_6$) (11) +ν(C$_2$-C$_3$)(9) + ν(C$_4$-C$_5$)(7) + β(C$_1$-H$_7$) (11) + β(C$_5$-H$_9$) (13) + β(C$_2$-H$_8$) (17)	ν(C-O)
ν_{10}	1420	1487(107,8)0.44	--	1460*	1453	1423	ν(C$_1$-C$_6$)(12) + ν(C$_4$-C$_5$)(4) + ν(C$_3$-C$_4$)(3) + ν_{as}(NO$_2$) (26) + β(C$_6$-H$_{10}$) (20)+ α(C$_3$-O$_{11}$-H$_{12}$) (6)	ν(R)
ν_{11}	1349	1413(68,40)0.16	1398	1380	1366	1404	α(C$_3$-O$_{11}$-H$_{12}$) (28)+ ν(C$_3$-C$_4$)(10) + ν(C$_1$-C$_2$)(9) + ν(C$_1$-C$_6$) (8) + ν(C$_2$-C$_3$)(6)+ ν_s(NO$_2$) (9) + β(C$_1$-H$_7$) (9) + β(C$_5$-H$_9$) (7)	α(C-O-H)
ν_{12}	1306	1368(86,3)0.53	1319	1333*		1348	ν(C$_3$-C$_4$)(15)+ν(C$_5$-C$_6$)(11)+ν(C$_1$-C$_2$) (10)+ν(C$_4$-C$_5$) (5)+ν(C$_2$-C$_3$)(4)+ν(C$_3$-O$_{11}$)(13)+ β(C$_2$-H$_8$) (13) + β(C$_6$-H$_{10}$) (8)	ν(R)
ν_{13}	1260	1319(218,77)0.30	1252	1325*	1234	--	β(C$_5$-H$_9$) (13) + ν(N$_{13}$-O$_{15}$) (22) +ν(C$_1$-C$_6$)(9) + ν(C$_5$-C$_6$) (9) + α(C$_3$-O$_{11}$-H$_{12}$) (12) + ν(C$_4$-N$_{13}$) (8) + δ(NO$_2$) (6) + ν(C$_3$-O$_{11}$) (6)	β(C-H)
ν_{14}	1226	1284(175,98)0.23	1198	1256*	1181	1284	ν_s(NO$_2$) (24) + ν(C$_3$-O$_{11}$) (22) +ν(C$_4$-C$_5$)(9) + ν(C$_1$-C$_6$)(7) + β(C$_1$-H$_7$) (7) + δ(NO$_2$) (7)	ν_s(NO$_2$)

ν_{15}	1177	1232(107,42)0.22	1160	1201	1158	1209	$\beta(C_2-H_8)$ (19) $+\nu(C_4-C_5)$(10) + $\nu(C_5-C_6)$(8) + $\nu(C_1-C_6)$(5) + $\alpha(C_{3-O_{11}}-H_{12})$ (17) + $\beta(C_5-H_9)$ (10) + $\nu(C_4-N_{13})$ (7)	β(C-H)
ν_{16}	1131	1185(10,3)0.61	1145	1165	1136	--	$\beta(C_6-H_{10})$ (43) + $\beta(C_5-H_9)$ (18) $+\nu(C_1-C_2)$(11) + $\nu(C_2-C_3)$(5) + $\beta(C_1-H_7)$ (12)	β(C-H)
ν_{17}	1106	1158(41,32)0.33	1113	1140	1117	1146	$\nu(C_3-C_4)$(9) + (C_1-C_6)(8) + $\nu(C_1-C_2)$(8)+$\beta(C_5-H_9)$ (25) + $\beta(C_2-H_8)$ (19) + $\nu(C_4-N_{13})$ (11)	ν(R)
ν_{18}	1051	1101(28,4)0.14	1094	1080	--	1092	$\nu(C_4-C_5)$(13) + (C_4-N_{13}) (22) + $\alpha_1(R)$(32) + $\beta(C_5-H_9)$ (9)	ν(R)
ν_{19}	1002	1049(14,26)0.04	1055	1030	1026	1040	$\nu(C_2-C_3)$(47) + (C_3-C_4)(13) + $\nu(C_1-C_2)$(7) + $\beta(C_2-H_8)$ (10) + $\beta(C_5-H_9)$ (8)	ν(R)
ν_{20}	978	1000(0,0)0.75	1022	981*	--	1002	$\gamma(C_1-H_7)$(51) + $\gamma(C_6-H_{10})$(18) + $\gamma(C_2-H_8)$ (14) + $\Phi_1(R)$ (11)	γ(C-H)
ν_{21}	956	977(2,0)0.75	998	954	--	973	$\gamma(C_5-H_9)$(53) + $\gamma(C_6-H_{10})$(21) + $\gamma(C_2-H_8)$(11) + $\Phi_2(R)$ (7) + $\gamma(C_1-H_7)$(6)	γ(C-H)
ν_{22}	865	884(17,4)0.18	883	871	867	882	$\alpha_1(R)$(37) + $\alpha_3(R)$(8) + $\delta(NO_2)$ (29) + $\nu(C_4-N_{13})$ (7) + $\nu(C_3-O_{11})$ (6)	α(R)
ν_{23}	849	868(0,0)0.75	--	860*	--	--	$\gamma(C_2-H_8)$(49)+$\gamma(C_5-H_9)$(17)+$\gamma(C_6-H_{10})$(9) + $\gamma(C_3-O_{11})$(7) + $\Phi_1(R)$ (6) + $\gamma(C_1-H_7)$(6)	γ(C-H)
ν_{24}	819	837(9,35)0.07	817	820	818	832	$\delta(NO_2)$ (32) $+\nu(C_5-C_6)$(12) + $\nu(C_4-C_5)$(10) + $\nu(C_1-C_6)$(5) + $\nu(C_3-O_{11})$ (11) + $\alpha_1(R)$(8) + $\alpha_3(R)$(6)	$\delta(NO_2)$
ν_{25}	760	777(48,0)0.75	--	780	--	773	$\gamma(C_6-H_{10})$(39) + $\gamma(C_5-H_9)$(20) + $\gamma(C_1-H_7)$(17) + $\gamma(C_2-H_8)$(10)	γ(C-H)
ν_{26}	720	736(43,1)0.75	--	690	--	712	$\tau(C_3-O_{11})$ (64) + $\omega(NO_2)$(24) + $\gamma(C_4-N_{13})$(7)	τ(C-O)
ν_{27}	683	698(83,0)0.75	--	697**	--	--	$\omega(NO_2)$(47) + $\tau(C_3-O_{11})$ (20) + $\Phi_1(R)$ (17) + $\gamma(C_1-H_7)$(7)	$\omega(NO_2)$
ν_{28}	667	682(9,4)0.20	667	669**	666	--	$\nu(C_4-N_{13})$ (9) $+\alpha_2(R)$(39) + $\alpha_3(R)$(16) $+\nu(C_5-C_6)$ (8)+$\nu(C_1-C_2)$(5) + $\delta(NO_2)$ (12)	ν(C-N)
ν_{29}	657	671(16,0)0.75	--	--	--	--	$\Phi_1(R)$ (53)+$\gamma(C_3-O_{11})$(23)+$\gamma(C_4-N_{13})$(11)	Φ(R)
ν_{30}	559	571(1,12)0.74	581	563*	561	--	$\alpha_2(R)$(25)+$\alpha_3(R)$(10)+$\beta(C_4-N_{13})$(22)+ $\rho(NO_2)$(16)+$\nu(C_4-C_5)$ (9) + $\beta(C_3-O_{11})$ (8)	α(R)
ν_{31}	542	554(8,3)0.14	549	546*	--	554	$\rho(NO_2)$ (24) + $\beta(C_3-O_{11})$ (20) + $\alpha_2(R)$(12) + $\alpha_3(R)$(11) + $\nu(C_4-N_{13})$ (6)	$\rho(NO_2)$
ν_{32}	522	533(8,0)0.75	--	531	--	536	$\gamma(C_3-O_{11})$(29) + $\Phi_3(R)$ (32) + $\Phi_1(R)$ (16) + $\gamma(C_6-H_{10})$(9) + $\Phi_2(R)$ (6)	γ(C-O)
ν_{33}	427	436(2,4)0.56	427	426*	424	437	$\beta(C_3-O_{11})$ (34)+$\rho(NO_2)$(33)+$\alpha_3(R)$(11) $+\nu(C_4-N_{13})$ (9)	β(C-O)
ν_{34}	413	422(1,0)0.75	--	--	--	401	$\Phi_2(R)$ (45)+ $\Phi_3(R)$ (15) + $\gamma(C_4-N_{13})$(28)	Φ(R)
ν_{35}	373	381(6,1)0.20	--	372*	--	--	$\alpha_3(R)$(24) + $\alpha_2(R)$(6)+$\beta(C_3-O_{11})$ (32) + $\nu(C_4-N_{13})$ (19) + $\rho(NO_2)$ (7)	α(R)
ν_{36}	285	291(5,3)0.44	297	285*	284	--	$\beta(C_4-N_{13})$ (73) + $\rho(NO_2)$ (9)	β(C-N)
ν_{37}	240	245(0,1)0.75	--	251*	--	--	$\gamma(C_4-N_{13})$(36) + $\Phi_3(R)$ (20) + $\Phi_2(R)$ (16) + $\Phi_1(R)$ (12) + $\gamma(C_2-H_8)$(9)	γ(C-N)
ν_{38}	141	144(0,1)0.75	159*		--	--	$\Phi_3(R)$ (44) + $\Phi_1(R)$ (4) + $\tau(C_3-O_{11})$ (24) + $\gamma(C_4-N_{13})$(20)	Φ(R)
ν_{39}	74	76(1,0)0.75	67	85	--	--	$\tau(C_4-N_{13})$ (74) + $\tau(C_3-O_{11})$ (17)	τ(C-N)

* Calculated wave numbers below 1000 cm-1 were scaled by the scale factor 0.9786 and those above 1000 cm-1 by the scale factor 0.9550.

* Number outside bracket is frequency in cm-1 unit, numbers within the bracket are IR intensity and Raman activity and number outside bracket is depolarization ratio.

* Gas-phase except where noted [41]. * in CCl4 solution [41]. **recorded in Ar-Matrix [41].

* The nos. after the modes are the % PED calculated using GAR2PED. The modes with contribution less than 5% are omitted, except ν(R), Φ(R) and α(R). ν = stretching, γ = out-of-plane deformation, β = in-plane deformation, α = planar ring deformation, Φ = non-planar ring deformation, $\rho(NO_2)$ = rocking of NO_2 group, δ (NO_2) = scissoring of NO_2 group , $\omega(NO_2)$ = wagging of NO_2 group, $\tau(NO_2)$ = torsion of NO_2 group

Table 4: Computed and observed vibrational fundamentals, PEDs and vibrational modes assignments for lowest energy conformer C-1 of 2-NP

benzene molecule. These modes were found to occur at frequencies 152, 297 and 565 cm-1 [48].

The four C-H planar deformations β(C-H) and four C-H non-planar deformations γ(C-H) are assigned at the frequencies 1106(ν_{17}), 1177(ν_{15}), 1260(ν_{13}), 1131(ν_{16}), 978(ν_{20}), 849(ν_{23}), 956(ν_{21}) and 760(ν_{25}) cm-1 corresponding to the modes $\beta(C_1-H_7)$, $\beta(C_2-H_8)$, $\beta(C_5-H_9)$, $\beta(C_6-H_{10})$, $\gamma(C_1-H_7)$, $\gamma(C_2-H_8)$, $\gamma(C_5-H_9)$ and $\gamma(C_6-H_{10})$ respectively. These modes are coupled with many other modes. The modes β(C-N), γ(C-N), β(C-O) and γ(C-O) correspond to the frequencies 285(ν_{36}), 240(ν_{37}), 427 (ν_{33}) and 522(ν_{32}) cm-1 respectively. These modes are strongly coupled modes. The modes β(C-N) and β(C-O) were assigned to the frequencies 298 and 432 cm-1 [41].

O-H group modes (3 modes): The OH stretching $\nu(O_{11}-H_{12})$ mode corresponds to the frequency 3453(ν_1) cm-1. The O-H stretching vibration is pure and highly localized mode. The O-H stretching

mode was found to correspond to the frequency 3255 [41] and to the frequency 3308 cm-1 [48]. The torsion of the OH group - $\tau(C_3-O_{11})$ occurs at frequency 720(ν_{26}) cm-1 in our work and at the frequency 711 cm-1 [41] and is strongly coupled with other modes of vibrations. The C-O-H angle bending- $\alpha(C_3-O_{11}-H_{12})$ mode is found to correspond to the frequency 1349(ν_{11}) cm-1 and also to the frequencies 1377 cm-1 [41] and 1266/1426 cm-1 [48], which is also strongly coupled with many modes.

NO_2 group modes (6 modes): There are six modes of vibrations due to the NO_2 group , namely, asymmetric NO_2 stretching -$\nu_{as}(NO_2)$, symmetric NO_2 stretching-$\nu_s(NO_2)$, NO_2 rocking-$\rho(NO_2)$, NO_2 wagging-$\omega(NO_2)$, NO_2 scissoring -$\delta(NO_2)$ and NO_2 torsion-$\tau(NO_2)$ which correspond to the frequencies 1511(ν_8), 1226(ν_{14}), 542(ν_{31}), 683(ν_{27}), 819(ν_{24}) and 74(ν_{39}) respectively. The NO_2 torsion-$\tau(NO_2)$ is slightly coupled with $\tau(C_3-O_{11})$ and the other five modes strongly coupled with various vibrational modes. The modes $\nu_{as}(NO_2)$,

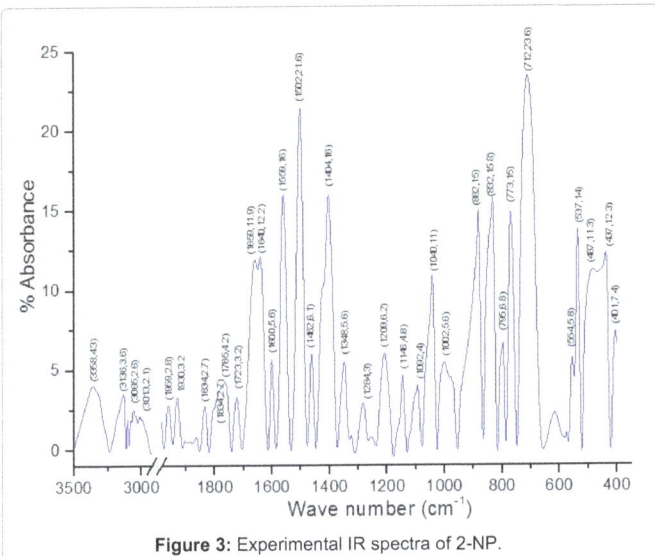

Figure 3: Experimental IR spectra of 2-NP.

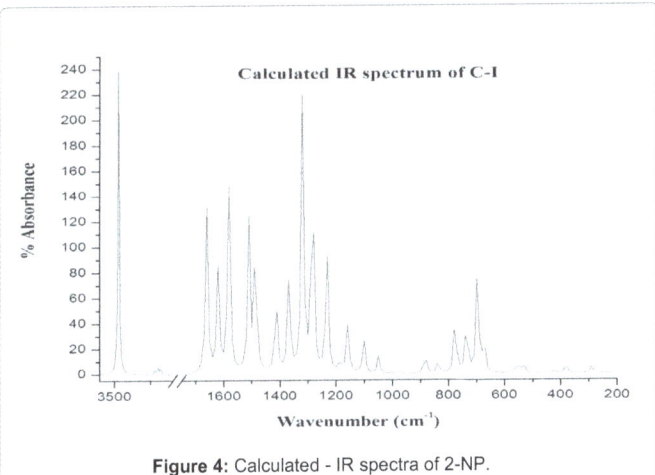

Figure 4: Calculated - IR spectra of 2-NP.

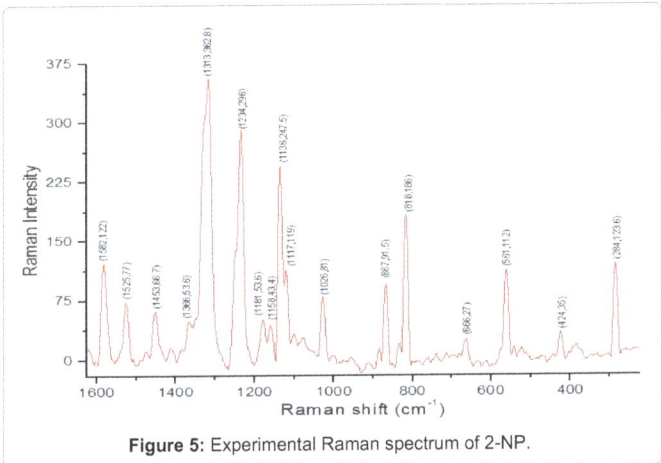

Figure 5: Experimental Raman spectrum of 2-NP.

$\nu_s(NO_2)$, $\omega(NO_2)$, $\delta(NO_2)$ and $\tau(NO_2)$ were found to correspond to the frequencies 1560, 1294, 741, 818 and 75 cm^{-1} [41] and also 1531, 1258, 702, 825 and 165 and also $\rho(NO_2)$ corresponds to the frequency 505 cm^{-1} [48].

Comparative study of vibrational modes for the three

conformers: The computed vibrational fundamentals of the three conformers of 2-NP together with their respective differences have been collected in Supplementary material (Table-S1). It could be seen that the modes $\tau(C\text{-OH})$ and $\nu(O\text{-H})$ of the OH group show very large frequency differences (in the range 350-400 cm^{-1}). Also, the modes $\tau(C_4\text{-}N_{13})$, $\beta(C_3\text{-}O_{11})$, $\omega(NO_2)$ $\alpha(C_3\text{-}O_{11}\text{-}H_{12})$ and $\nu_{as}(NO_2)$ show frequency differences of the order of a few tens of a wave number. Clearly, major contribution for this frequency difference is expected to come from H bonding between H_{12} and O_{15} atoms in the conformer C-1 which is absent in the conformers C-2 /C-3. The phenyl ring modes $\Phi_3(R),\alpha_3(R)$, $\Phi_2(R)$, $\gamma(C\text{-H})$ and $\nu(C\text{-H})$ in the C-1 conformer have higher magnitudes than the corresponding modes in the conformers C-2 / C-3. However, the modes $\omega(NO_2)$, $\beta(C_3\text{-}O_{11})$, $\nu(O_{11}\text{-}H_{12})$, $\Phi_1(R)$, $\nu(C_3\text{-}O_{11})$, $\nu(R)$ and $\beta(C_2\text{-}H_8)$ have higher frequencies in the conformers C-2 /C-3 than their corresponding modes in the most stable one.

The IR intensities and Raman activities for each of the three conformers are collected in Supplementary material (Table-S2). It is noticeable that the IR intensities for the C-1 conformer are much higher than those of the C-2/C-3 conformers for the modes $\nu(O_{11}\text{-}H_{12})$, $\nu(C_3\text{-}O_{11})$, $\nu s(NO_2)$, $\beta(C_2\text{-}H_8)$, $\beta(C_1\text{-}H_7)$, $\nu(R)$ $\omega(NO_2)$, $\rho(NO_2)$ and $\beta(C_4\text{-}N_{13})$ (S_2).

The IR intensities for the modes $\alpha(C3\text{-}O11\text{-}H12)$, $\nu as(N13\text{-}O14)$, $\tau(C3\text{-}O11)$, $\alpha1(R)$, $\nu(C_2\text{-}H_8)$, $\nu(C_5\text{-}H_9)$, $\nu(O_{11}\text{-}H_{12})$, $\nu s(NO_2)$, $\alpha_2(R)$, $\gamma(C_6\text{-}H_{10})$, $\beta(C_2\text{-}H_8)$, $\beta(C_5\text{-}H_9)$, $\delta(NO_2)$ $\beta(C_3\text{-}O_{11})$, $\nu(C_1\text{-}H_7)$ and $\gamma(C_4\text{-}N_{13})$ for the conformers C-2/C-3 are much higher than the conformer C-1. One could see the major differences in the Raman activities for the modes $\nu s(NO_2)$, $\nu(C_3\text{-}O_{11})$, $\alpha(C_3\text{-}O_{11}\text{-}H_{12})$, $\nu(C_2\text{-}H_8)$, $\nu(R)$ $\nu(C_5\text{-}H_9)$, $\nu as(NO_2)$, $\nu(O_{11}\text{-}H_{12})$, $\nu(C_1\text{-}H_7)$, $\delta(NO_2)$, $\beta(C_1\text{-}H_7)$, $\beta(C_6\text{-}H_{10})$ $\nu(C_6\text{-}H_{10})$, and $\beta(C_4\text{-}N_{13})$. Such discrepancies could be due to the hydrogen bonding in the conformer C-1and the non-planar geometry of the C-2/C-3 conformers of 2-NP. The highest IR intensity and Raman activity for C-1 occur for the modes $\nu(O_{11}\text{-}H_{12})$ and $\nu(C_2\text{-}H_8)$ respectively and those for C-2/C-3 for $\nu as(NO_2)$ and $\nu(C_2\text{-}H_8)$ respectively. From the above discussion it is clear that the intra-molecular H-bonding plays a crucial role in the molecular conformation.

HOMO–LUMO energy gap

The HOMO and LUMO studies are very important for quantum chemistry. These orbitals are also known by the name frontier orbitals, because they lie at the outermost boundaries of the electrons of the molecules. Both the HOMO and the LUMO are the main orbitals that take part in the chemical stability [49]. The kinetic stability of the molecule is measured in terms of energy gap DE [32,50] and the difference of the energies of the HOMO and LUMO is a measure of the excitability of the molecule, the smaller the energy, more easily it can be excited and vice versa. The lower HOMO and LUMO energy gap explains the eventual CT interaction taking place within the molecule, which is responsible for the bioactivity of the molecule. The larger the value of the energy gap the higher the kinetic stability and lower the chemical reactivity because it is energetically unfavorable to add electrons to a high lying LUMO, to remove electrons from a low lying HOMO and so to form the activated complex of any potential reaction [33]. The sketch of the atomic orbital compositions of the frontier MOs are shown in Figure 7. The green and red solid regions in Figure 7 represent the MOs with completely opposite phases. The present calculations predict that the energy gap (DE) of the 2-NP, i.e. the transition energy from HOMO to LUMO of the 2-NP is 0.148189 a.u. This electronic transition corresponds to the transition from the ground to the first excited state and is mainly described by an electron excitation from HOMO to LUMO.

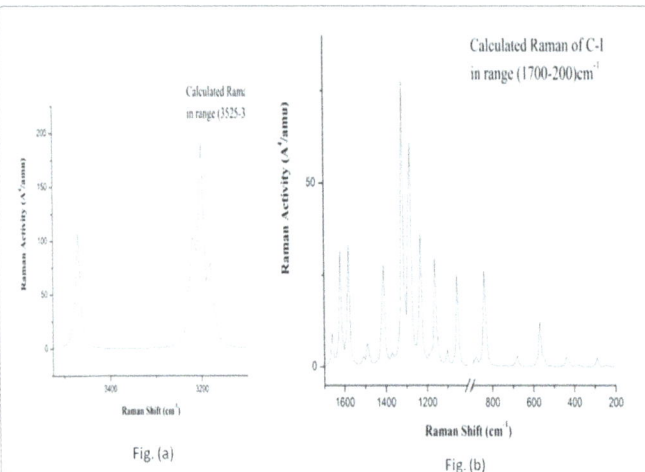

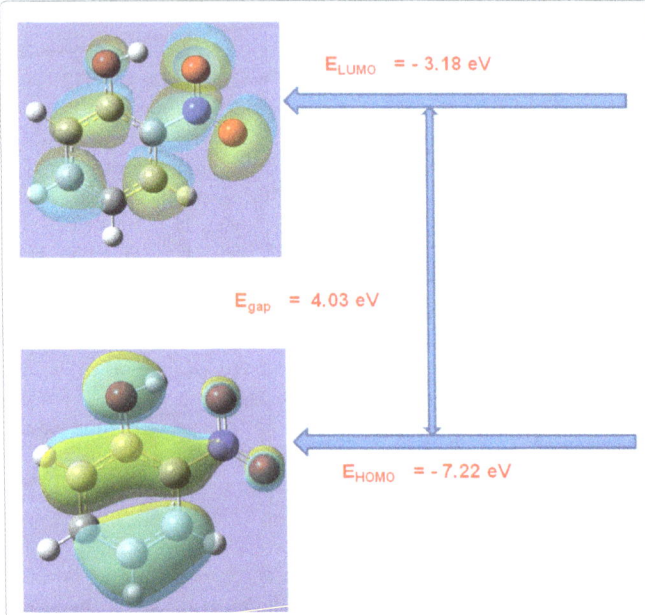

Figure 6: Calculated - Raman spectra of 2-nitrophenol in two parts of Raman shifts.

Figure 7: The atomic orbital compositions of the frontier MO of 2-NP (C-I).

Global reactivity descriptors

A molecule having high ionization potential (V_p) or electron affinity (V_A) loses or admits electron hardly [51,52]. By Koopmans' approximation [53,54], the ionization potential and electron affinity of any molecule can be calculated using the relations,

$$V_p = {}^- E_{HOMO}$$

$$V_A = {}^- E_{LUMO}$$

Koopmans` theorem for closed-shell molecules [54] results in the hardness of the molecule;

$$\eta = (V_p - V_A)/2$$

The chemical potential of the molecule;

$$\mu = -(V_p + V_A)/2$$

The softness of the molecule;

$$S = 1/2\eta$$

The electro negativity of the molecule;

$$\chi = (V_p + V_A)/2$$

The electro-philicity index of the molecule;

$$\omega = \mu^2 S$$

Using the above relations we find the electro molecular characteristics for 2-NP has been presented in Table-5.

NLO characteristics: Static polarizability and first order hyperpolarizability

Quantum chemical computational theory has been shown to be essential in the description of the relationship between the electronic structure of the systems and its NLO response [55]. The NLO activities provide the key functions for frequency shifting, optical switching, optical modulation and optical logic to develop the technologies for the communication, signal processing and optical interconnections [56]. The electric dipole moment (μ), the polarizability (α) and the hyper polarizability (β) of the 2-NP molecule have been calculated by finite field method using DFT-B3LYP method employing 6-311++G(d,p) basis set for the isolated molecule, the origin of the Cartesian coordinate system (x, y, z) = (0, 0, 0) was chosen at own centre of mass of 2-NP. In the presence of an external electric field, the energy of a system is a function of the field and the first hyperpolarizability is a third rank tensor that can be described by a 3x3x3 matrix. The 27 components of the 3D matrix can be reduced to 10 components using the Klein man symmetry [57]. The matrix can be given in the lower tetrahedral format. Clearly, the lower part of the 3x3x3 matrices is a tetrahedral. The components of β are defined as the coefficients in the Taylor series expansion of the energy in the external electric field. If the external field is weak and homogeneous, this expansion is as given below,

$$E = E^o - \mu_i F_i - 1/2(\alpha_{ij}F_iF_j - 1/6(\beta_{ijk}F_iF_jF_k) + - - - -$$

Here, E^o is the energy of the unperturbed molecules, F_i is the field at the origin, μ_i, α_{ij} and β_{ijk} are the components of dipole moment, polarizability and first hyperpolarizability, respectively.

The total static dipole moment μ, the mean polarizability α_0, the anisotropy of the polarizability $\Delta\alpha$ and the mean first hyperpolarizability β_0, using the x, y and z components are defined as;

Dipole moment;

$$\mu = \left(\mu_x^2 + \mu_y^2 + \mu_z^2\right)^{1/2}$$

Static polarizability;

$$\alpha_0\alpha_0 = \left(\alpha_{xx} + \alpha_{yy} + \alpha_{zz}\right)/3$$

The total polarizability;

$$\Delta\alpha = \left(1/\sqrt{2}\right)\sqrt{[(\alpha_{xx} - \alpha_{yy})2 + (\alpha_{yy} - \alpha_{zz})2 + (\alpha_{zz} - \alpha_{xx})2 + 6\{\alpha_{xy}^2 + \alpha_{yz}^2\alpha_{zx}^2\}]}$$

First order hyperpolarizability;

$$\beta = \sqrt{\left[\Sigma\beta_x^2\right]} ,$$

Where

$$\beta_x = (\beta_{xxx} + \beta_{xyy} + \beta_{xzz})$$

$$\beta_y = (\beta_{yxx} + \beta_{yyy} + \beta_{yzz})$$

$$\beta_z = (\beta_{zxx} + \beta_{zyy} + \beta_{zzz})$$

The static polarizability α_0 (91.966 au) and total polarizability $\Delta\alpha$ (9483.787 au) of the 2-NP together with all its components and perturbation to all its components, first order hyperpolarizability (β = 426.118 au) and its components and the total as well as components of the dipole moment have been tabulated in the Table-5.

Electrostatic potential

The electrostatic potential (ESP) is the tool which is used to study the intermolecular association and molecular properties of small molecules, actions of drug molecules and their analogues, the biological function of haemoglobin and enzyme catalysis [33,58-61]. ESP is widely used as the reactivity map displaying most probable regions for the electrophilic attack of charged point-like reagents on organic molecules [62]. The values and spatial distribution of ESP are in fact responsible for the chemical behaviour of an agent in a chemical reaction. They strongly influence the binding of a substrate to its active site. ESP is typically visualized through mapping its values onto the molecular ED. The different values of the electrostatic potential at the surface are represented by different colors; the red represents regions of the most negative electrostatic potential, the blue represents regions of the most positive electrostatic potential and the green represents regions of zero potential. Potential increases in the order red, orange, yellow, green and blue. While the negative electrostatic potential corresponds to an attraction of the proton by the concentrated ED in the molecule (and is colored in shades of red), the positive electrostatic potential corresponds to the repulsion of the proton by atomic nuclei in regions where a low ED exists and the nuclear charge is incompletely shielded (and is colored in shades of blue). The total density plot and its array of the 2-NP are shown in the Figure 8. The molecular ESP values, corresponding to Merge-Singh-Koll man scheme [47], of the 2-NP molecule have been arranged in the Table 3. Also, the diagrammatic demonstration of the MESP via map and its contour has been shown in Figure 9. These Figs provide a visual representation of the chemically active sites and comparative reactivity of atoms. The ESP plots and the value arranged in the Table 3 predict that there are no regions of positive and zero potential present in the molecule. Also, the Figure 9 and the data in the Table 3 predict that the sites associated with the functional groups, namely, OH and NO_2 groups are most reactive sites for the neucleophilic reactions.

Thermo molecular characteristics

The studies of some thermo molecular characteristics, namely, zero point vibrational energy, enthalpy, Gibb's free energy, internal energy, entropy, heat capacity, thermal energy and the partition functions etc. have been found to play crucial role in the material characterization. We have presented some thermal parameters in Table 6. It can be noticed that all of the analysed thermodynamic parameters are increasing with the temperature but G is found to decrease with T [Figure 10(a)-10(h)] while the zero point vibrational energy remains constant (67.226 Kcal/mol) at all the temperature because it is a characteristic property of the molecule. All the fitting parameters and other essential statistical data have been demonstrated together with the fitted graphs of these parameters. All of the characteristic thermal properties of crystalline 2- NP solid have been found to be in agreement with the explanation of Dulong-Pettit law as well as of Einstein's thermo dynamical theory of crystalline solids. The fitting equations of the thermal parameters of 2-NP are as given below;

$$\left[Log_e q(t,e,r,v)\right]_{Ref.-Bottom\ of\ Well} = 51.2676 - 837.243exp\left(-\frac{T}{43.5306}\right) - 311.0166exp\left(-\frac{T}{124.5469}\right) - 162.7858exp\left(-\frac{T}{622.2405}\right)$$

$$\left(R^2 = 1,\ \chi^2 = 1.7599\ x\ 10^{-5}\right)$$

$$\left[Log_e q(t,e,r,v)\right]_{Ref.-1st\ Vib\ state} = 23.9202 + (0.0388)\ T - (11.04)\ T^2 \quad \left(R^2 = 0.999\right)$$

$$S_{m^0} = 52.5299 + (0.1240)\ T - \left(2.8791\ x\ 10^{-5}\right)\ T^2 \quad \left(R^2 = 0.99999\right)$$

$$c_{p,m^0} = -0.9985 + (0.1195)T - (5.4209)T^2 \quad \left(R^2 = 0.999\right)$$

$$H_{m^0} = 66.321 + (0.0120)\ T + (3.3350)\ T^2 \quad \left(R^2 = 0.9993\right)$$

$$U_{m^0} = 65.7785 + (0.0120)\ T + (3.3350)\ T^2 \quad \left(R^2 = 0.9993\right)$$

$$Q_{m^0} = 66.3222 + (0.0100)\ T + (0.3335)\ T^2 \quad \left(R^2 = 0.9993\right)$$

$$G_{m^0} = 68.2813 - (0.0586)\ T - (4.7655)\ T^2 \quad \left(R^2 = 0.9999\right)$$

All the thermo molecular data provide the crucial and helpful information for the further study on the 2-NP. They can be applied to compute the other thermodynamic characteristics according to relationships of thermo dynamical parameters and estimate directions of chemical reactions according to the second law of thermodynamics in thermo chemical fields. It should be noticeable that all calculations of thermo dynamical parameters have been done in gas phase and they could not be used in solution phase.

NMR characterization: Magnetic susceptibility, shielding and current density tensors

The NMR analysis plays an essential part in material characterization in presence of magnetic fields. This type investigation provides chemical shifts and magnetic shielding tensors to each atomic site of the molecule as well as magnetic susceptibility and the current density tensor for the material being investigated. We have applied Continuous Set Gauge of Transformation (CSGT) method for NMR investigation of the 2-NP molecule. The magnetic susceptibility tensor of 2-NP has been computed as

$$X_{ij} = \begin{bmatrix} -41.82 & -3.21 & -0.01 \\ -3.06 & -40.23 & 0.01 \\ -0.01 & 0.01 & -111.72 \end{bmatrix}$$

Having the Eigen values λ_1 = -111.7209, λ_2 = -44.2576 and λ_3 = -37.7896 and the value of magnetic susceptibility χ is found to be -64.5893 cgs-ppm, the negative sign of χ shows the diamagnetic nature of the 2-NP molecule.

Also, the magnetic shielding tensors together with their corresponding Eigen values at different atomic sites computed are depicted as below;

$$C_1: \sigma_{ij}^{C_1} = \begin{bmatrix} -71.44 & 8.10 & 0.11 \\ 9.44 & 23.35 & -0.04 \\ 0.09 & -0.04 & 169.96 \end{bmatrix} \quad C_2: \sigma_{ij}^{C_2} = \begin{bmatrix} 29.73 & 29.20 & 0.06 \\ 33.52 & -9.23 & -0.06 \\ 0.08 & -0.03 & 158.67 \end{bmatrix}$$

$$\lambda_1 = -72.25, \lambda_2 = 24.16\ and\ \lambda_3 = 169.9 \quad \lambda_1 = -26.67, \lambda_2 = 47.17\ and\ \lambda_3 = 158.67$$

$$C_3: \sigma_{ij}^{C_3} = \begin{bmatrix} -21.45 & -23.40 & 0.04 \\ 3.26 & -37.00 & 0.01 \\ -0.02 & 0.04 & 119.98 \end{bmatrix} \quad C_4: \sigma_{ij}^{C_4} = \begin{bmatrix} 3.97 & 14.74 & -0.02 \\ -7.92 & 16.60 & -0.02 \\ 0.09 & 0.01 & 117.78 \end{bmatrix}$$

$$\lambda_1 = -41.94, \lambda_2 = -16.50\ and\ \lambda_3 = 119.98 \quad \lambda_1 = 3.11, \lambda_2 = 17.46\ and\ \lambda_3 = 117.78$$

$$C_5: \sigma_{ij}^{C_5} = \begin{bmatrix} 21.47 & 31.27 & 0.03 \\ 12.38 & -31.99 & -0.02 \\ 0.05 & 0.00 & 172.29 \end{bmatrix} \quad C_6: \sigma_{ij}^{C_6} = \begin{bmatrix} 26.49 & -35.07 & 0.02 \\ -39.51 & -16.53 & -0.04 \\ 0.04 & -0.01 & 172.56 \end{bmatrix}$$

$$\lambda_1 = -39.76, \lambda_2 = 29.24\ and\ \lambda_3 = 172.29 \quad \lambda_1 = -38.07, \lambda_2 = 48.03\ and\ \lambda_3 = 172.56$$

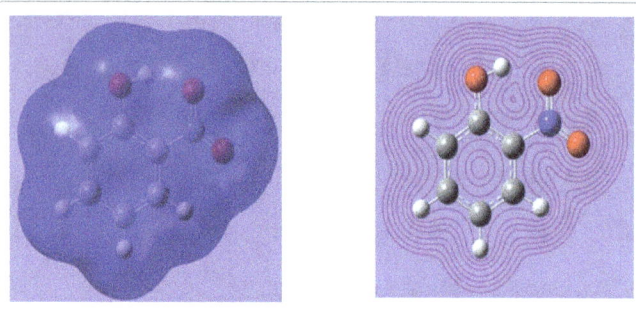

Figure 8: (a) Total density (b) total density array of 2-NP (C-I).

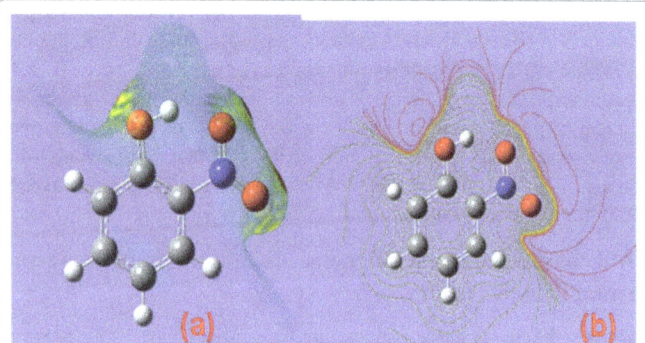

Figure 9: (a) Electrostatic potential (ESP) of 2-NP (C-I). (b) Electrostatic potential array of 2-NP.

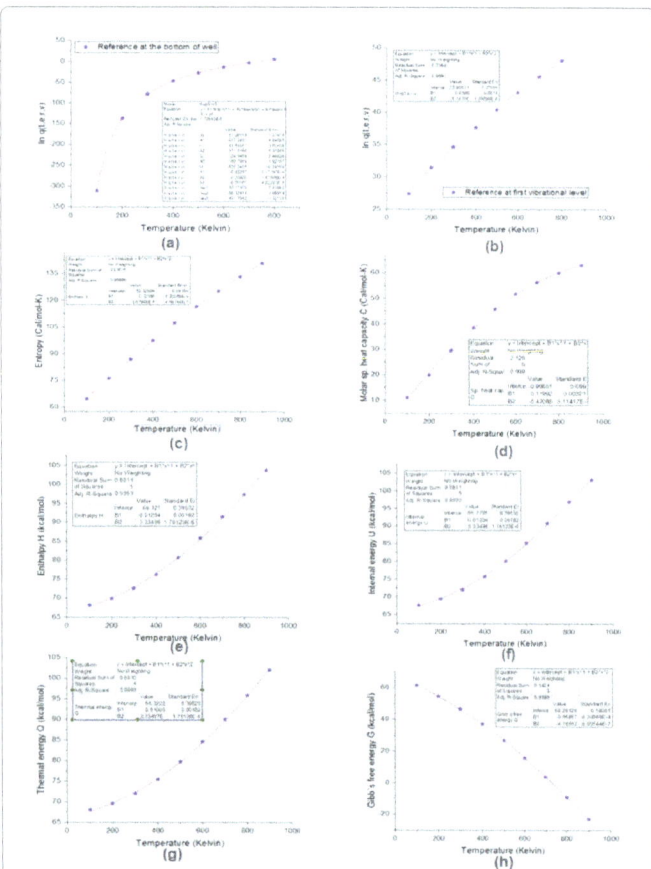

Figure 10: Graphical demonstration of essential thermodynamic parameters of 2-NP.

$$H_7 : \sigma_{ij}^{C_7} = \begin{bmatrix} 22.75 & 0.52 & 0 \\ 0.74 & 24.26 & 0 \\ -0.002 & 0 & 21.83 \end{bmatrix} \quad H_8 : \sigma_{ij}^{H_8} = \begin{bmatrix} 27.52 & 1.41 & -0.001 \\ 2.28 & 24.35 & -0.002 \\ -0.004 & 0.002 & 21.37 \end{bmatrix}$$

$$\lambda_1 = 21.83, \lambda_2 = 22.70 \text{ and} \lambda_3 = 27.88 \quad \lambda_1 = 21.37, \lambda_2 = 23.50 \text{ and} \lambda_3 = 28.37$$

$$H_9 : \sigma_{ij}^{H_9} = \begin{bmatrix} 26.74 & 1.36 & 0 \\ 0.74 & 24.26 & 0 \\ -0.001 & -0.003 & 20.34 \end{bmatrix} \quad H_{10} : \sigma_{ij}^{H_{10}} = \begin{bmatrix} 27.07 & -1.38 & -0.002 \\ -1.59 & 25.46 & 0 \\ -0.0004 & 0.003 & 22.21 \end{bmatrix}$$

$$\lambda_1 = 20.34, \lambda_2 = 23.87 \text{ and} \lambda_3 = 27.12 \quad \lambda_1 = 22.21, \lambda_2 = 24.58 \text{ and} \lambda_3 = 27.96$$

$$O_{11} : \sigma_{ij}^{O_{11}} = \begin{bmatrix} 98.07 & -1.38 & -0.002 \\ 9.71 & 161.51 & -0.002 \\ 0.16 & 0.12 & 286.79 \end{bmatrix} \quad H_{12} : \sigma_{ij}^{H_{12}} = \begin{bmatrix} 33.34 & -1.38 & -0.002 \\ -1.08 & 20.94 & -0.001 \\ 0.02 & -0.06 & 10.39 \end{bmatrix}$$

$$\lambda_1 = 85.06, \lambda_2 = 174.53 \text{ and} \lambda_3 = 286.79 \quad \lambda_1 = 10.39, \lambda_2 = 20.50 \text{ and} \lambda_3 = 33.78$$

$$N_{13} : \sigma_{ij}^{N_{13}} = \begin{bmatrix} -274.04 & -14.18 & -0.16 \\ -7.61 & -209.55 & -0.04 \\ -0.13 & -0.04 & 41.91 \end{bmatrix} \quad O_{14} : \sigma_{ij}^{O_{14}} = \begin{bmatrix} -450.67 & 153.53 & -0.28 \\ -0.51 & -682.72 & -0.09 \\ -0.31 & 0.08 & 154.15 \end{bmatrix}$$

$$\lambda_1 = -275.83, \lambda_2 = -207.76 \text{ and} \lambda_3 = 41.91 \quad \lambda_1 = -705.68, \lambda_2 = -427.72 \text{ and} \lambda_3 = 154.15$$

$$O_{15} : \sigma_{ij}^{O_{15}} = \begin{bmatrix} -398.51 & -79.71 & -0.27 \\ 128.83 & -506.31 & 0.01 \\ -0.17 & -0.04 & 113.76 \end{bmatrix}$$

$$\lambda_1 = -511.64, \lambda_2 = -393.18 \text{ and} \lambda_3 = 113.76$$

The magnetic shielding at the atomic sites, namely, C_1, C_2, C_3, C_4, C_5, C_6, H_7, H_8, H_9, H_{10}, O_{11}, H_{12}, N_{13}, O_{14} and O_{15} have been computed 40.625, 59.723, 20.510, 46.115, 53.924, 60.840, 24.138, 24.414, 23.778, 20.340, 182.124, 21.558, -147.229, -326.418 and -263.685 ppm. respectively. It is noticeable that the shielding at every sites associated to NO_2 group is negative and attaining higher values [Figure 11(a, b)]. From the Figure 11 it is obvious that the effect of the magnetic field is least nearby the NO_2 group of 2-NP molecule.

The current density tensor (J) for the 2-NP have been computed and depicted in matrix form as;

$$J_{ij} = \begin{bmatrix} 0.0002 & 0.0001 & 0.0139 \\ 0.0004 & 0 & 0.3173 \\ 0.0084 & -0.2080 & 0.0001 \end{bmatrix}$$

The two Eigen values of the current density tensor have been found imaginary while one Eigen value of J is λ=0.0002 for 2-NP molecule. The value of the J (~ 1.231x10⁻⁵ a.u.) has been found to be negligibly small, which reveals that the electrical conductivity of 2-NP molecule is negligibly small. The mapping and corresponding contour of J for the title molecule have been demonstrated diagrammatically (Figure 12). Figure 12 also represents that the current density is extremely weak for the 2-NP molecule.

Conclusions

For the first time; complete material characterization, complete vibrational mode assignment, conformational analysis, HOMO – LUMO analysis, complete data analysis on thermo-dynamical parameters, data analysis on reactivity parameters and on NMR parameters, potential energy distribution and investigations of APT, Mulliken atomic charges and ESP derived charge of 2-NP has been carried out. The 2-NP molecule has been expected to possess three conformations out of which lowest energy conformer is planar possessing C_s symmetry while other two are non-planar possessing

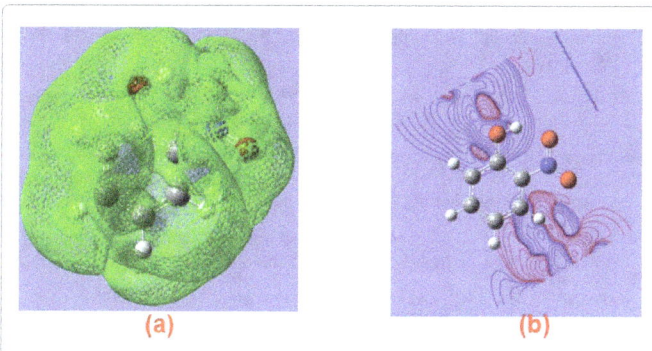

Figure 11: Map (left) and contour (right) of magnetic shielding on 2-NP.

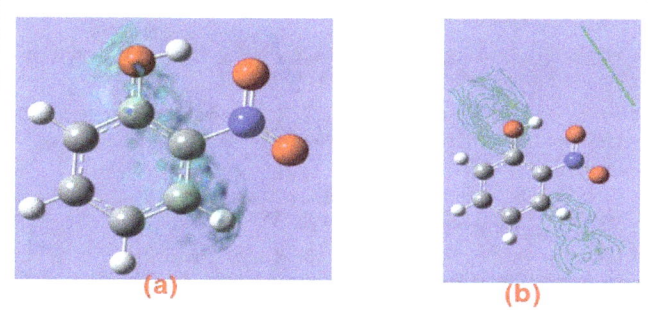

Figure 12: Current density demonstration through map (left) and contour (right) for 2-NP.

C_1 symmetry. Conformer C-1 is planar, in which NO_2 group is in the plane of phenyl ring while in conformers C-2 and C-3 the plane of NO_2 group makes the angle -33.7^0 and 33.7^0 respectively. The Nitrogen atom of NO_2 group attains highest APT charge while carbon atom directly attached to OH group bears highest Mulliken charge. For lowest energy conformer α (C_4-C_3-O_{11}) is largest (124.6^0) and $\alpha(C_3$-O_{11}-$H_{12})$ is smallest (107.3^0) respectively. For the modes $\tau(C_3$-$O_{11})$ and $\nu(O_{11}$-$H_{12})$ are found to have very large frequency differences 394 and -352 cm^{-1} respectively among the conformers C-1 and C-2/C-2. $\nu(O_{11}$-$H_{12})$ is of largest IR intensity and $\nu(C_2$-$H_8)$ is found to be largest Raman activity mode. All the modes of vibrations are precisely assigned to the corresponding appropriate frequencies and also the experimental work has been compared with the computational work as well as the work already been carried out, which found to be in agreement with our work. The HOMO–LUMO transition clearly explicates CT interaction involving donor and acceptor groups. The ESP plots and corresponding values show that there are neucleophilic most reactive regions are found nearby OH and NO_2 groups while no regions of positive and zero potential present in the molecule. The HOMO – LUMO energy gap is found to be $\Delta E = 0.148189$ a.u. In conformer C-1 intramolecular hydrogen bonding O_{15}......H_{12} is expected in 2-NP molecule. NMR investigations as well as HOMO- LUMO theory reveal that the conductivity of the title molecule is extremely low and the molecule is diamagnetic in nature.

Reactivity Descriptor		Dipole Moment(μ)		Polarizability (α)						1st order Hyperpolarizability(β)		
					Exact		Perturbation to α					
Para.	Value	Para.	Debye	Para.	(a.u.)	esu *10^{-24}	(a.u.)	esu *10^{-24}		Para.	a.u.	esu *10^{-32}
V_p	6.635	$(\mu_x)_{Fl}$	-3.951	α_{xx}	123.434	18.268	74.308	10.998		β_{xxx}	524.773	4534.563
V_A	0.881	$(\mu_y)_{Fl}$	-0.611	α_{xy}	-0.198	-0.029	-1.208	-0.179		β_{xxy}	-125.223	-581.160
η	2.877	$(\mu_z)_{Fl}$	-0.001	α_{yy}	105.178	15.566	95.758	14.172		β_{xyy}	-102.311	-884.069
μ	- 3.758	$(\mu)_{Fl}$	3.998	α_{xz}	-0.005	-0.001	-0.002	-0.0003		β_{yyy}	-95.389	-824.256
S	0.174	$(\mu_x)_{esp}$	-3.964	α_{yz}	0.012	0.002	0.023	0.003		β_{xxz}	-0.080	-0.691
χ	3.758	$(\mu_y)_{esp}$	-0.603	α_{zz}	47.285	6.998	23.282	3.446		β_{xyz}	-0.023	-0.199
ω	2.457	$(\mu_z)_{esp}$	-0.003	α_0	91.966	13.612	64.449	9.538		β_{yyz}	-0.014	-0.121
E_g	4.03	$(\mu)_{esp}$	4.010	$\Delta\alpha$	9483.787	1403.600	8325.284	1232.142		β_{xzz}	-75.942	-656.215
										β_{yzz}	-27.380	-236.590
										β_{zzz}	-0.013	-0.112
										β_{total}	426.118	3681.229

* V_p= Ionization potential, V_A= Electron affinity, η = Hardness, μ= Chemical potential, S= Softness, χ= Electro-negativity, ω= electro-philicity of the molecules.

Table 5: Molecular reactivity and NLO parameters of C-1 conformer of 2-NP.

T (K)	G Kcal/mol	H Kcal/mol	Q Kcal/mol	C cal/mol-K	S cal/mol-K	U Kcal/mol	ZPE Kcal/mol	LnQ$_{V=0}$	LnQ$_{Bot}$
100	61.7744	68.2344	68.037	11.236	64.604	67.6919	67.226	27.427241	-310.866945
200	54.7113	69.9739	69.578	19.973	76.312	69.4314	67.226	31.484367	-137.662726
298.15	46.7007	72.6006	72.010	29.552	86.870	72.0581	67.226	34.641248	-78.823178
300	46.5394	72.6589	72.064	29.728	87.066	72.1164	67.226	34.697505	-78.067224
400	37.3109	76.2864	75.493	38.613	97.440	75.7439	67.226	37.633424	-46.940123
500	27.0689	80.7254	79.734	45.928	107.316	80.1829	67.226	40.415236	-27.243602
600	15.8687	85.8181	84.628	51.726	116.585	85.2756	67.226	43.073074	-13.309290
700	3.7721	91.4280	90.039	56.315	125.223	90.8855	67.226	45.615146	-2.712595
800	-9.1554	97.4488	95.861	60.001	133.258	96.9063	67.226	48.045839	5.759065
900	-22.8595	103.8028	102.017	63.013	140.739	103.2603	67.226		

* T= Temperature, G = Gibb's free energy, H = Enthalpy, Q = Thermal energy, C= Molar heat capacity, S = Entropy, U= Internal energy, ZPE = Zero point vibrational energy, Q$_{V=0}$ = Total partition function taking reference 1st vibrational level, Q$_{Bot}$ = Total partition function taking reference at bottom of the well.

Table 6: Some crucial molecular thermodynamic parameters of C-1 conformer of 2-NP.

Reference

1. Leuenberger C, Ligocki MP, Pankow JF (1985) Trace organic compounds in rain. 4. Identities, concentrations, and scavenging mechanisms for phenols in urban air and rain. Environ Sci Technol 19: 1053-1058.

2. Tremp J, Mattrel P, Fingler S, Giger W (1993) Phenols and Nitrophenols as tropospheric pollutants: emissions from automobile exhausts and phase transfer in the atmosphere. Water Air Soil Pollut. 68: 113-123.

3. Luttke J, Levsen K (1997) Phase Partitioning of Phenol and Nitrophenols in clouds. Atmos. Environ. 31: 2649-2655.

4. Zhang DP, Wu WL, Long HY, Liu YC, Yang ZS (2008) Voltammetric Behavior of o-Nitrophenol and Damage to DNA. Int J Mol Sci 9: 316-326.

5. Pedrosa VA, Codognoto L, Avaca LA (2003) Electroanalytical Determination of 4-Nitrophenol by Square Wave Voltammetry on Diamond Electrodes. J. Braz. Chem. Soc. 14: 530-536.

6. Uberoi V, Bhattacharya SK (1997) Toxicity and degradability of nitrophenols in anaerobic systems. Water. Environ. Res. 69: 146-156.

7. Zaggout FR, Abu Ghalwa N (2008) Removal of o-nitrophenol from water by electrochemical degradation using a lead oxide/titanium modified electrode. J Environ Manage 86: 291-296.

8. Canizares P, Lobato J, Paz R, Rodrigo MA, Sáez C (2005) Electrochemical oxidation of phenolic wastes with boron-doped diamond anodes. Water Res 39: 2687-2703.

9. Qin Y, Wheeler RA (1996) Density-Functional-Derived Structures, Spin Properties, and Vibrations for Phenol Radical Cation. J. Phys. Chem. 100: 10554-10563.

10. Lampert H, Mikenda W, Karpfen A (1996) Intramolecular Hydrogen Bonding in 2-Hydroxybenzoyl Compounds: Infrared Spectra and Quantum Chemical Calculations. J. Phys. Chem. 100: 7418-7425.

11. De Heer MI, Korth HG, Mulder P (1999) Poly Methoxy Phenols in Solution: OH Bond Dissociation Enthalpies, Structures, and Hydrogen Bonding. J. Org. Chem. 64: 6969-6975.

12. De Heer MI, Mulder P, Korth HG, Ingold K, Lusztyk J (2000) Hydrogen Atom Abstraction Kinetics from Intramolecularly Hydrogen Bonded Ubiquinol-0 and Other (Poly) methoxy Phenols. J. Am. Chem. Soc. 122: 2355-2360.

13. Bene JED, Person WB, Szczepaniak K (1995) Properties of Hydrogen-Bonded Complexes Obtained from the B3LYP Functional with 6-31G (d,p) and 6-31+G (d,p) Basis Sets: Comparison with MP2/6-31+G(d,p) Results and Experimental Data. J. Phys. Chem. 99: 10705-10707.

14. Zierkiewicz W, Michalska D, Matusewicz BC, Raspenk M (2003) Molecular Structure and Infrared Spectra of 4-Fluorophenol: A Combined Theoretical and Spectroscopic Study. J Phys Chem. A 107: 4547-4554.

15. Borisenko KB, Bock CW, Hargittai I (1994) Intramolecular Hydrogen Bonding and Molecular Geometry of 2-Nitrophenol from a Joint Gas-Phase Electron Diffraction and ab Initio Molecular Orbital Investigation. J. Phys. Chem. 98: 1442-1448.

16. Kovacs A, Izvekov V, Keresztury G, Pongor G (1998) Vibrational analysis of 2-nitrophenol: A joint FT-IR, FT-Raman and scaled quantum mechanical study. Chem. Phys. 238: 231-243.

17. Abkowicz-Bienko AJ, Latajka Z, Bienko D, Michalska D (1999) Theoretical infrared spectrum and revised assignment for para-nitrophenol. Density functional theory studies. Chem. Phys. 250: 123-129.

18. Korth HG, de Heer MI, Mulder P (2002) A DFT Study on Intramolecular Hydrogen Bonding in 2-Substituted Phenols: Conformations, Enthalpies, and Correlation with Solute Parameters. J. Phys. Chem. 106: 8779-8789.

19. Rauhut G, Pulay P (1995) Transferable Scaling Factors for Density Functional Derived Vibrational Force Fields. J. Phys. Chem. 99: 3093-3100.

20. Macsari I, Izvekov V, Kovacs A (1997) Scaled quantum mechanical study of 2,6-difluorophenol: a fluorine-containing weak hydrogen-bonded system. Chem. Phys. Lett. 269: 393-400.

21. Behringer J (1958) The connection of Raman dispersion, adsorption and fluorescence (resonance Raman effect). Z. Elektrochem. 62: 544-567.

22. Green JHS, Kynaston W, Lindsey AS (1961) The vibrational spectra of benzene derivatives-I Nitrobenzene, the benzoate ion, alkali metal benzoates and salicylates. Spectrochim. Acta 17: 486-502.

23. Horak M, Smolikova J, Pitha J (1961) Spectroscopic study of the hydrogen bond in substituted 2-nitrophenols. Coll. Czech. Chem. Commun. 26: 2891-2896.

24. Robinson EA, Schreiber HD, Spencer JN (1971) Solvent and temperature effects on the hydrogen bond. J. Phys. Chem. 75: 2219-2222.

25. Bedarek V, Janu I, Jirkovszky J, Socha J, Klicnar J (1972) Influence of substitution of aromatic nucleus on frequency of valence vibrations of groups bonded by hydrogen bond. Coll. Czech. Chem. Commun. 37: 3447-3450.

26. Leavell S, Curl Jr. R (1973) Microwave spectrum of 2-nitrophenol: Structure of the hydrogen bond. J. Mol. Spectrosc. 45: 428-442.

27. Kishore Y, Sharma NS, Dwiredi CPD (1974) Indian J. Phys. 48 412.

28. Dietrich SW, Jorgensen EC, Kollman PA, Rothenberg S (1976) A theoretical study of intramolecular hydrogen bonding in ortho-substituted phenols and thiophenols. J. Am. Chem. Soc. 98: 8310-8324.

29. Canadell E, Catalan J, Fernandez-Alonso JI (1978) Adv. Mol. Relaxation Interact. Process. 12 265.

30. Iwasaki F, Kawano Y (1978) The crystal and molecular structure of o-nitrophenol. Acta Crystallogr. B34: 1286-1290.

31. Schreiber V, Koll A, Kulbida A, Majerz I (1995) IR matrix isolation and MNDO/PM3 studies of ortho-substituted phenols with intramolecular H-bonds. J. Mol. Struct. 348: 365-368.

32. Foresman JB, Frisch AE (1996) Exploring Chemistry with Electronic Structure Methods, (2nd ed), Gaussian, Pittsburgh, PA.

33. Manolopoulos DF, May JC, Down SE (1991) Theoretical studies of the fullerenes: C34 to C70 Chem. Phys. Lett. 181: 105-111.

34. Seminario JM, Politzer P (1995) Modern Density Functional Theory: A Tool for Chemistry, Elsevier, Amsterdam.

35. Becke AD (1993) Density-functional thermochemistry. III. The role of exact exchange. J. Chem. Phys. 98: 5648-5652.

36. Becke AD (1988) Density-functional exchange-energy approximation with correct asymptotic behavior. Phys Rev A 38: 3098-3100.

37. Lee C, Yang W, Parr RG (1988) Development of the Colle-Salvetti correlation-energy formula into a functional of the electron density. Phys Rev B Condens Matter 37: 785-789.

38. Vosko SH, Wilk L, Nusair M (1980) Accurate spin-dependent electron liquid correlation energies for local spin density calculations: a critical analysis. Can. J. Phys. 58: 1200-1211.

39. Frisch MJ, Trucks GW, Schlegel HB, Scuseria GE (2010) Gaussian 09, Revision C.01, Gaussian, Inc., allingford, CT.

40. Martin JML, Van Alsenoy C (1995) GAR2PED, A Program to Obtain a Potential Energy Distribution from a Gaussian Archive Record, University of Antwerp, Belgium.

41. Ferreira MMC, Suto E (1992) Atomic Polar Tensor Transferability and Atomic Charges kr the Fluoro-methane Series CHxF4-x. J. Phys. Chem. 96: 8844-8849.

42. Dixit V, Yadav RA (2015) Asian J Phys, 24, in press.

43. Martin F, Zipse H (2005) Charge distribution in the water molecule--a comparison of methods. J Comput Chem 26: 97-105.

44. Besler BH, Merz KM, Kollman PA (1990) Atomic charges derived from semi-empirical methods. J Comput Chem, 11: 431-439.

45. Sing UC, Kollman PA (1984) An approach to computing electrostatic charges for molecules. J Comput Chem, 5: 129-145.

46. Chis V (2004) Molecular and vibrational structure of 2,4-dinitrophenol: FT-IR, FT-Raman and quantum chemical calculations. Chemical Physics 300: 1-11.

47. Dixit V, Yadav RA (2015) DFT-B3LYP computations of electro and thermo molecular characteristics and mode of action of fungicides (chlorophenols). Int J Pharm 491: 277-284.

48. Lewars E (2003) Computational Chemistry Introduction to the Theory and Applications of Molecular and Quantum Mechanics, Kluwer Academic Publishers, Norwell, MA.

49. Chang R (2001) Chemistry, (7th ed) McGraw-Hill, New York.

50. Koopmans TA (1934) Uber die zuordnung von wellenfunk- tionen und eigenwerten zu den, einzelnen elektronen eines atoms. Physica 1: 104-113.

51. Govindarasu K, Kavitha E (2014) Molecular structure, vibrational spectra, NBO, UV and first order hyperpolarizability, analysis of 4-Chloro-DL-phenylalanine by density functional theory. Spectrochimica Acta Part A 133: 799-810.

52. Burland DM, Miller RD, Walsh CA (1994) Second-order nonlinearity in poled-polymer systems. Chem. Rev. 94: 31-75.

53. Geskin VM, Lambert C, Brédas JL (2003) Origin of high second- and third-order nonlinear optical response in ammonio/borato diphenylpolyene zwitterions: the remarkable role of polarized aromatic groups. J Am Chem Soc 125: 15651-15658.

54. Kleinman DA (1977) Nonlinear Dielectric Polarization in Optical Media. Phys. Rev. 126: 1962-1979.

55. Tomasi J, Politzer P, Truhlar D (Eds.) (1981) Chemical Application of Atomic and Molecular Electrostatic Potentials, Plenum, New York 257-294.

56. Moro S, Bacilieri M, Ferrari C, Spalluto G (2005) Autocorrelation of molecular electrostatic potential surface properties combined with partial least squares analysis as alternative attractive tool to generate ligand-based 3D-QSARs. Curr Drug Discov Technol 2: 13-21.

57. Murray JS, Sen K (1996) Molecular Electrostatic Potentials, Concepts and Applications, Elsevier, Amsterdam.

58. Weiner PK, Langridge R, Blaney JM, Schaefer R, Kollman PA (1982) Electrostatic potential molecular surfaces. Proc Natl Acad Sci U S A 79: 3754-3758.

59. Politzer P, Truhlar DG (1981) Chemical Application of Atomic and Molecular Electrostatic Potentials, Plenum, New York.

60. JS Murray, K Sen (1996) Molecular Electrostatic Potentials, Concepts and Applications, Elsevier, 558 Amsterdam.

61. Weiner PK, Langridge R, Blaney JM, Schaefer R, Kollman PA (1982) Electrostatic potential molecular surfaces. Proc Natl Acad Sci U S A 79: 3754-3758.

62. P Politzer, DG Truhlar (1981) Chemical Application of Atomic and Molecular Electrostatic Potentials, Plenum, New York.

10

Full Scale Evaluation of Phytoattenuation

Yeh TY *, Peng YP and Chen KF

Department of Civil and Environmental Engineering, National University of Kaohsiung, Taiwan

Abstract

The biosorption mechanism of metal removal (copper, Cu and zinc, Zn) by four phytoremediation macrophytes biomasses including sunflower (*Helianthus annuus*), Chinese cabbage (*Brassica campestris*), cattail (*Typha latifolia*), and reed (*Phragmites communis*) was investigated in this study. The primary objectives were exploring the potential of reusing these bio-wastes after harvesting from phytoremediation operations. Based on the surface area, zeta potential, scanning electron microscopy (SEM), and energy dispersive X-ray (EDX) investigations, Chinese cabbage biomass presented the highest metal adsorption property while both cattail and reed revealed a lower adsorption capability for both metals tested. The equilibrium adsorption rate between biomass and metal occurred very fast during the first 10min. The metal adsorption data were fitted with the Langmuir and Freundlich isotherms and presented that the Langmuir isotherm was the best fitted model for all biomass tested. All tested biomasses are fast growing plants with fairly high biomass production that are able to accumulate metals. The Langmuir model was used to calculate maximum adsorption capacity and related adsorption parameters in this study. The results revealed that the maximum metal adsorption capacity Qmax was in the order of Chinese cabbage (Cu: 2000; Zn: 1111 mg/kg) > sunflower (Cu: 1482; Zn: 769 mg/kg) > reed (Cu: 238; Zn: 161 mg/kg) > cattail (Cu: 200; Zn: 133mg/kg). The harvested sunflower, Chinese cabbage, cattail, and reed biomass possess the potential to be employed as biosorbents to remove Cu and Zn from aqueous solutions. Adsorption isotherms derived in this study might be crucial information for practical design and operation of adsorption engineering processes and prediction of relation between reused macrophyte biosorbents and heavy metal adsorbates.

Keywords: Heavy metals; Biosorbent; Macrophyte; Adsorption; Phytoremediation

Introduction

The wastewater generated from confined swine operations is one of the primary pollution sources in Taiwan [1,2]. The effluent is discharged in the surrounding waterways containing significant amounts of heavy metals such as copper (Cu) and zinc (Zn). These metals are intentionally added in fodder to prevent diarrhea and to enhance immune systems of swine. Conventional physical-chemical technologies employed for heavy metals removal for contaminated water include chemical precipitation, ion-exchange, however, they are usually quite costly and energy consumed. Phytoremediation using green plants in constructed wetlands and soil decontamination recently has drawn great attention in Taiwan and worldwide [3-5].

The biomass can be harvested and used for various purposes such as biosorbents for metal removal in water treatment [6,7]. The use and evaluation of recycled biosorbents is very important to compare and analyze the adsorption mechanism and optimize the purification techniques that are based on biosorption. Several studies were published recently using recycled bio-wastes to remove pollutants [8-10]. The use of recycled and dried plants for metal removal as a simple biosorbent material has advantages in its efficiency in detoxifying dilute effluents and has been viewed as a cost-effective and energy-efficient wastewater treatment approach. The reuse of harvested macrophytes in wastewater engineering can also benefit waste disposal management and save waste treatment costs. The adsorption properties of phytoremediation macrophytes have been investigated for the removal of metals in polluted effluent. The results revealed that the extent of metal adsorption onto biomass seems to have important consequences in the capacity of metal removal [11]. Therefore, it is important to investigate the biosorption mechanism and related sorption parameters of harvested macrophytes to facilitate future biosorbent water purification operation. Metal cations in polluted effluent can be adsorbed by the negative charge of the macrophyte biomass surface. The process of metal removal by plants involves a combination of rapid sorption on the cell wall surface and slow accumulation and possibly translocation into the biomass [12]. The rapid sorption may include chelation and ion exchange. Carboxylic group, one of the functional groups on the plant biomass surface, provides binding sites with metals [13].

Research results indicated that all plant parts might accumulate heavy metals, and the ability to concentrate metals from the external solution varied between both plant parts and metals. Between 24% and 59% of the metal content was adsorbed onto the cell walls of the plants [14]. The biomasses of plants, both living and dead, were heavy metal accumulators. The mechanisms of metal biosorption included extracellular accumulation, cell surface sorption, and intracellular accumulation. These mechanisms resulted from complexation, ion exchange, precipitation, and adsorption [15]. The main mechanism involved in biosorption was reported as ion exchange between metal cations and counterions presented in the macrophytes biomass. The investigation revealed that no significant difference was observed in the exchange amounts while using muti-metal or individual metal solutions [16]. Sunflower (*Helianthus annuus*) and Chinese cabbage (*Brassica campestris*) are fast-growing crops that have been commonly used for phytoextraction of metal contaminated soils, while reed (*Phragmites communis*) and cattail (*Typha latifolia*) are predominant

*****Corresponding author:** Yeh TY, Department of Civil and Environmental Engineering, National University of Kaohsiung, Kaohsiung 811, Taiwan, E-mail: tyyeh@nuk.edu.tw

macrophytes that have been employed for water purification within constructed wetlands. These plants contain high amount of lignin and cellulose which may adsorb heavy metal cations from aqueous solution. After harvesting, these plant biomasses could be used as biosorbents for metal adsorption. *Brassica* family has been reported for its prominent ability to remove heavy metals from contaminated soils [17]. B. *campestris* and H. *annuus* have the potential as biofuel to become the substitute of fossil fuels, especially the increasing oil prize in recent years. The higher biomass production of these economic crops, namely sunflower and Chinese cabbage, contribute them being the candidates of phytoextration contaminant and then harvested as potential biosorbents. Reed and cattail, commonly used macrophytes in constructed wetlands for water pollution mitigation, have been reported as a very high adsorption affinity value, which assist to predict its high ability to adsorb heavy metals in aqueous solutions [18]. This study focused on the biosorption characteristics of the harvested biomass of plants may provide information for enhancing phytoremediation processes to remove metals both in soil and water. The aim of this study was to investigate the biosorption performance and mechanisms of four macrophyte biomasses.

The benefits from this study were two folds: to highlight the metal adsorption capability of plant biomass for environmental decontamination, and to test the possibility to recycle the harvested biomass for biosorbents.

Materials and Methods

The preparation of harvested macrophytes for metal adsorption experiments

The plant biomasses collected from local soil contaminated sites and constructed wetlands were rinsed with deionized water. Fresh biomass was dried in an oven at 104°C for 24 h and grinded. The grinded biomass was passed through 200 and 250 mesh (74 - 62 μm) of filters for the surface area determination, zeta potential measurement, and sorption experiments. Analytical grade chemicals were used to prepare metal stock solutions. The natural pH of the synthetic solutions was measured to be 5.3. This pH was maintained throughout for all the experiments except for zeta potential measurement. The zeta potential were conducted at pH 2 to 10 varied with NaOH and HCl. Triplicates of 0.2 g grinded biomass and 25 mL

metal solution of intended concentration were performed in 50 mL flask. Adsorption tests were conducted at room temperature (24±2ºC). Flasks were shaken on a rotary shaker under various contact time (e.g. 10, 30, 60, 120, 180, and 360 min) to evaluate the metal adsorption capacity. The solution was separated by centrifugation with 4000 rpm for 20 min. The supernates were then collected and analyzed for metal contents by an atomic adsorption spectrophotometer.

The feasible adsorption isotherms fitting

Adsorption experiments were conducted to determine the adsorption of Cu and Zn by the studied plants. The adsorption capacity Q, the amounts of total metals adsorbed per biomass unit was evaluated using the following formula:

$$Q = \left(C_o - C_e\right)V / M$$

Where C_0 is the initial metal concentration (mg/L), C_e is the equilibrium concentration (mg/L), V is the volume (L) of metal solution, and M is the biomass (g) of the plant tested. The adsorption of metals by biosorbents was further evaluated using the Freundlich

and Langmuir adsorption isotherms. The Freundlich equation can be written as

$$Q_e = K_f \times C_e^{1/n}$$

In the aforementioned equation, Q_e is the metal content onto the adsorbent material, mg/kg; K_f is an empirical constant related to the adsorption capacity; C_e is the equilibrium metal concentration in solution; and n is a constant related to the intensity of adsorption. The Langmuir equation can be written as

$$Q_e = \frac{Q_{max} \times b \times C_e}{1 + b \times C_e}$$

In the equation, Q_{max} is the maximum metal capacity, mg/kg; and b is a parameter related to the binding strength of metals.

Scanning electron microscopy (SEM)-energy dispersive X-ray (EDX) spectroscopy

Pretreated macrophyte samples were gold-coated for SEM observation with qualitative EDX analysis. Specifically, grinded and dried samples were mounted on carbon tape and sputter coated in gold. A Hitachi S-4300 SEM (Tokyo, Japan) was used to capture micrographs. The elements C, O, Cu, and Zn were detected using a SEM coupled with an EDX spectroscopy at an acceleration voltage of 15 kV.

Results and Discussion

The properties of tested macrophytes

The surface areas of four studied biomasses were 2.75 ± 0.48, 3.71 ± 0.13, 2.30 ± 0.03, and 2.43 ± 0.17 m²/g, for sunflower, Chinese cabbage, cattail, and reed, respectively, analyzed by the BET method with liquid N_2. Chinese cabbage, the *Brassica* family, has the largest surface area in this study rendering for better metal adsorption. The adsorption capacity can be further illustrated via comparing the electrokinetic potential (zeta potential) as shown in Figure 1. The effect of pH on the zeta potential of all tested macrophytes was examined. The zeta potential had negative charge for all studied macrophytes rendering for the potential of metal adsorption. The increase in negative charge of the zeta potential was observed while the pH increased. This result indicated that the degree of metal biosorption may increase as the pH increased. The biomass Chinese cabbage was recorded as the negative zeta potential around neutral pH while the lowest recorded was at pH 10. This result revealed that Chinese cabbage had better metal adsorption capability compared to other macrophytes tested. The rest of tested plants also presented negative charge of zeta potential following the order sunflower < reed < cattail. The lower negative zeta potential also indicated better metal cations adsorption.

The metal adsorption rate and isotherms

The adsorption rate of Cu and Zn by four studied biomasses is depicted in Figure 2. Most of metal biosorption occurred during first 10 min. This adsorption result revealed that a contact time of 120 min for both Cu and Zn was sufficient to achieve equilibrium for four tested macrophytes. Similar rapid metal biosorption has been reported by other researcher [19]. Several factors including the structure of biosorbent and existence of metal species have also been presented to influence adsorption rates. In order to obtain basic information of tested macrophytes as biosorbents, the equilibrium metal concentration (C_e) and the concentration adsorbed onto the surface of the biomass (Q) were linearized and fitted to the Langmuir and Freundlich equations. The Langmuir and Freundlich isotherm models were calculated to

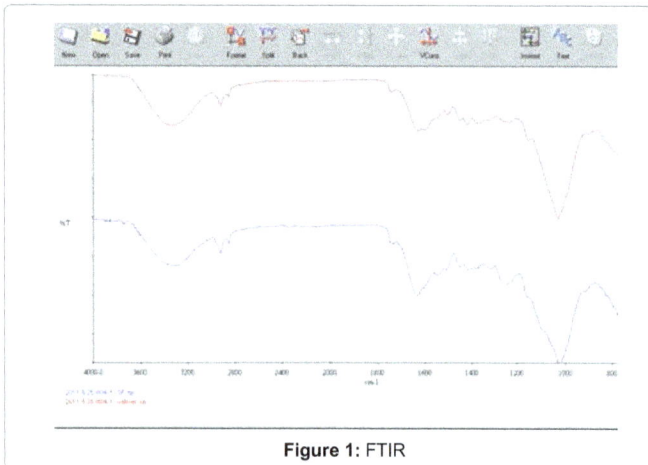

Figure 1: FTIR

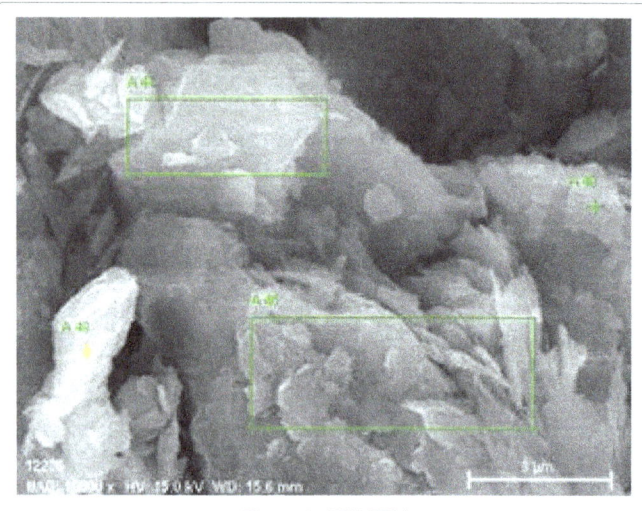

Figure 2: SEM/EDX

(a)	Langmuir			Freundlich		
Copper	Q_{max}	b	R^2	K_r	N	R^2
Sunflower	1482.57	3.00	0.99	297.85	1.33	0.95
Chinese cabbage	2000.00	3.80	0.99	350.91	1.29	0.96
Cattail	200.00	0.42	0.92	92.96	4.29	0.72
Reed	238.10	0.46	0.90	103.23	4.20	0.70
(b) Zinc						
Sunflower	769.23	2.92	0.99	145.21	1.58	0.96
Chinese cabbage	1111.11	5.11	0.99	143.91	1.38	0.97
Cattail	133.33	0.51	0.98	66.65	4.18	0.80
Reed	161.29	0.54	0.94	82.57	4.41	0.67

Table 1: The adsorption parameters of linearized Langmuir and Freundlich isotherms for four macrophyte biomasses.

that the Langmuir isotherm was best fit model and the maximum adsorption capacity was 13.98 mg/g for Zn and 6.17 free floating macrophyte *Lemna minor* biomass regarding its adsorption of metals from aqueous solutions. The equilibrium adsorption was reached within 40-60 min. The maximum adsorption capacities of biomass was determined as 83 mg/g for Cu based on the best fitted Langmuir equation [21]. The maximum adsorption capacity might vary with the biomass investigated and adsorption experimental conditions. The equilibrium metal concentration (C_e) after a contact time of 5 h was lower than the initial concentration (C_i). Five hours was assumed to be adequate for the adsorption system to achieve equilibrium which was longer than the time (60 min) to reach equilibrated condition in the aforementioned adsorption rate experiment. The removal efficiency of metals from solutions can be expressed as the fraction of metals adsorbed by studied biomasses which was related to the reciprocal value of the ratio of the metal concentration in the solution at equilibrium to that in the initial solution. In general, the fraction of metals adsorbed onto biomass decreased as the initial concentration C_i increased. At high initial Cu concentration (10 mg/L), the percentage of Cu that was adsorbed by the biomass decreased to around 20% then gradually leveled off for both cattail and reed while sunflower and Chinese cabbage continued to drop. At high initial Zn concentration (5 mg/L), the percentage of Zn that was adsorbed by the biomass decreased to around 18% then gradually leveled off for both cattail and reed while sunflower and Chinese cabbage gradually decrease. At low initial Cu concentration (1 mg/L), the metals adsorbed by the biomass ranged 72% for sunflower, 73% for Chinese cabbage, 61% for cattail, and 67% for reed, respectively, while at low initial Zn concentration (1 mg/L), the metals adsorbed by the biomass ranged 50% for sunflower, 54% for Chinese cabbage, 35% for cattail, and 40% for reed, respectively. The biosorption efficiency was high at a low metal concentration, especially for Chinese cabbage and sunflower. At a low metal concentration, the ratio of available adsorbent surface area to the metal in solution was high indicating a great metal removal. As metal initial concentration increased, the efficiency was gradually decreased. This result might be attributed to the saturation of the adsorption sites on the biomass.

The microstructure investigation

The microstructures of the tested biosorbents and adsorbed metal determinations onto biomass surface were performed by the scanning electron microscopy (SEM) and energy dispersive X-ray (EDX). The biomass treated with metals revealed several small bulges that were not observed before the metal sorption experiment. Further EDX observations indicated that small bulges are higher in Cu and Zn. There were more bulges on the surface of Chinese cabbage compared to other

determine the adsorption capacities and related parameters. The calculation results and related Langmuir and Freundlich sorption parameters are listed in Table 1. The sorption process for Cu and Zn by four tested biomasses was better described by the Langmuir equation ($R^2 = 0.90$-0.99) compared to the Freundlich model ($R^2 = 0.67$-0.97). The linear regression was calculated to demonstrate that the Langmuir equation was best fitted, therefore, the sorption as a monolayer can be assumed. The maximum sorption capacity Q_{max} of Cu was 1482, 2000, 200, and 238 mg/kg while the Q_{max} of Zn was 769, 1111, 133, and 161 mg/kg for biomass sunflower, Chinese cabbage, cattail, and reed, respectively, predicted by the Langmuir model. The aforementioned maximum sorption capacity was comparable with that of the activated carbon and less than that of the tested biosorbent peanut hulls [20]. The related adsorption parameters were also calculated through the Langmuir equation. For Cu, the binding constant b was 3.00, 3.80, 0.42, and 0.46 for biomass sunflower, Chinese cabbage, cattail, and reed, respectively. For Zn, the binding parameter b was 2.92, 5.11, 0.51, and 0.54 for biomass sunflower, Chinese cabbage, cattail, and reed, respectively. The high b value of Chinese cabbage biomass is reflected by the steep initial slope of the adsorption isotherm which indicated a high affinity for the adsorbate in dilute metal solutions. Research has presented that wetland macrophyte, *Ceratophyllum demersum*, was an effective biosorbent for Zn and Cu removal under dilute metal conditions. Batch adsorption experiments showed

three studied macrophytes. The results also suggested that Chinese cabbage might have better metal sorption capacity.

Conclusion

The harvested biomass of sunflower, Chinese cabbage, cattail, and reed possesses the potential to be used as biosorbents to remove metals from aqueous solutions. Adsorption experiment results showed that Cu and Zn adsorptions were fairly rapid occurring within first 10min. The adsorption capability of four tested biomasses can be well predicted by the Langmuir adsorption model. The surface area, zeta potential, SEM, and EDX results revealed that Chinese cabbage biomass presented the highest metal adsorption property while both cattail and reed presented lower adsorption capability for both metals tested. Further study (e.g. FT-IR) might be required to scrutinize the chemical functionalities responsible for the adsorption of the heavy metals. These studied plant biomasses are natural abundant and can be recycled from environmental decontamination operations, namely phytoremediation of metal polluted soil and water purification within constructed wetlands. This research results can benefit adsorption process engineering for mitigation of polluted metal water by reusing harvested macrophytes.

References

1. Lee CY, Lee CC, Lee FY, Tseng SK, Liao CJ (2004) Performance of subsurface flow constructed wetland taking pretreated swine effluent under heavy loads. Bioresour Technol 92: 173-179.

2. Yeh TY, Chou CC, Pan CT (2009) Heavy metal removal within pilot-scale constructed wetlands receiving river water contaminated by confined swine operations. Desalination 249: 368-373.

3. Dhote S, Dixit S (2009) Water quality improvement through macrophytes--a review. Environ Monit Assess 152: 149-153.

4. Yeh TY, Wu CH (2009) Pollutant removal within hybrid constructed wetland systems in tropical regions. Water Sci Technol 59: 233-240.

5. Yeh TY, Pan CT, Ke TY, Kuo TW (2010) Organic matter and nitrogen removal within field-scale constructed wetlands: Reduction performance and microbial identification studies. Water Environ Res 82: 27-33.

6. Jang A, Seo Y, Bishop PL (2005) The removal of heavy metals in urban runoff by sorption on mulch. Environ Pollut 133: 117-127.

7. Tsui M, Cheung KC, Tam NF, Wong MH (2006) A comparative study on metal sorption by brown seaweed. Chemosphere 65: 51-57.

8. Bansal M, Singh D, Garg VK (2009) Chromium (VI) uptake from aqueous solution by adsorption onto timber industry waste. Desalination and Water Treatment 12: 238-246.

9. Hannachi Y, Shapovalov NA, Hannachi A (2009) Adsorption of nickel from aqueous solution by the use of low-cost adsorbents. Desalination and Water Treatment 12: 276-283.

10. Okoronkwo AE, Aiyesanmi AF, Olasehinde EF (2009) Biosorption of nickel from aqueous solution by Tithonia diversifolia. Desalination and Water Treatment 12: 352-359.

11. Miretzky P, Saralegui A, Cirelli AF (2004) Aquatic macrophytes potential for the simultaneous removal of heavy metals (Buenos Aires, Argentina). Chemosphere 57: 997-1005.

12. Lesage E, Mundia C, Rousseau DPL, Van de Moortel AMK, Du Laing G, et al. (2007) Sorption of Co, Cu, Ni and Zn from industrial effluents by the submerged aquatic macrophyte Myriophyllum spicatum L. Ecological engineering 30: 320-325.

13. Sune N, Sánchez G, Caffaratti S, Maine MA (2007) Cadmium and chromium removal kinetics from solution by two aquatic macrophytes. Environ Pollut 145: 467-473.

14. Fritioff , Greger M (2006) Uptake and distribution of Zn, Cu, Cd, and Pb in an aquatic plant Potamogeton natans. Chemosphere 63: 220-227.

15. Keskinkan O, Goksu MZ, Basibuyuk M, Forster CF (2004) Heavy metal adsorption properties of a submerged aquatic plant (Ceratophyllum demersum). Bioresour Technol 92: 197-200.

16. Miretzky P, Saralegui A, Fernández Cirelli A (2006) Simultaneous heavy metal removal mechanism by dead macrophytes. Chemosphere 62: 247-254.

17. Grispen VM, Nelissen HJ, Verkleij JA (2006) Phytoextraction with Brassica napus L.: a tool for sustainable management of heavy metal contaminated soils. Environ Pollut 144: 77-83.

18. Southichak B, Nakano K, Nomura M, Chiba N, Nishimura O (2006) Phragmites australis: a novel biosorbent for the removal of heavy metals from aqueous solution. Water Res 40: 2295-2302.

19. Bunluesin S, Kruatrachue M, Pokethitiyook P, Upatham S, Lanza GR (2007) Batch and continuous packed column studies of cadmium biosorption by Hydrilla verticillata biomass. J Biosci Bioeng 103: 509-513.

20. Oliverira FD, Paula JH, Freitas OM, Figueiredo SA (2009) Copper and lead removal by peanut hulls: Equilibrium and kinetic studies. Desalination 248: 931-940.

21. Saygideger S, Gulnaz O, Istifli ES, Yucel N (2005. Adsorption of Cd(II), Cu(II) and Ni(II) ions by Lemna minor L.: effect of physicochemical environment. J Hazard Mater 126: 96-104.

Identification and Qualitative Analysis of β-Sitosterol and Some Phytoestrogens in *In Vivo* and *In Vitro* Samples of *Lepidium sativum:* A Semi-Arid Bone Healing Plant

Raghunandan S Nathawat, Preeti Mishra* and Vidya Patni

Plant Pathology, Tissue Culture and Biotechnology Laboratory, Department of Botany, University of Rajasthan, Jaipur, India

Abstract

Dry powder of different plant parts of *Lepidium sativum* (Garden Cress) are known to be used for treatment of fracture (bone healing) from ancient times. Seeds as *in vivo* plant part and callus as *in vitro* plant parts were chromatographically tested to identify and estimate β-sitosterol and various phytoestrogens. Plant-derived sterols and estrogens in tissues and oilseeds of *Lepidium sativum* were isolated by solvent extraction method. β-sitosterol, diadzein and formononetin were estimated qualitatively and quantitatively through TLC and HPTLC techniques. *In vitro* grown callus was compared biochemically with *in vivo* plant parts. CAMAG HPTLC was used and the developed plates were photo-documented using UV and white light. The amount of β-sitosterol was estimated to be about 0.20% w/w for seed powder and 0.024% w/w for callus powder. Daidzein and formononetin isolated from the samples of *Lepidium sativum* showed Rf values 0.73 and 0.67 and peak areas were 546.8 and 1033.5, respectively. Chloroform: methanol (8:2) gave excellent results in the present investigation for all samples. Results indicated that applied assay is accurate and reliable for the determination of phytoestrogens in the plant.

Keywords: *Lepidium sativum*; HPTLC; Diadzein; Formononetin

Abbreviations

β: Betasitosterol; Stg: Stigmasterol; Ln: Lanosterol; D: Daidzein; G: Genistein; Fr: Formononetin; Sp: Sprout; C: Callus; S: Seed

Introduction

The plant species *Lepidium sativum* L. belongs to family Brassicaceae (Synonym: *Nasturtium sativum* Medik) is also known as Garden Cress, Pepper Cress in English, Chandrasoora (/ˈtʃɑː.də-səˈrɑ, -ˈrɔ/), Chandrika (/ˈtʃɑː.də rɪk.ə/) in Sanskrit, and vernacularly as Haim (/hæɪm/), Hin-Chansur (/hɪn ˈtʃɑːn.sɝ r/) etc. It is cultivated throughout India and Tibet as a culinary vegetable and grows as a wild plant. It is also found distributed in North Africa, Palestine, Syria, Mesopotamia, Iran, ex-USSR, Southern and middle European Part, New Caledonia and in Australia and Indonesia. In Rajasthan (Mewar region, India), this plant has been studied under exploited fodder species [1]. The plant demonstrates weedy habit, grows on waste land and cultivated places. It is an erect, annual herb, up to 50 cm height. The plant extract is bitter, used as tonic, galactogogue, and aphrodisiac, in the treatment of dysentery, pain in abdomen, blood and skin disorders, injuries, tumors, eye diseases, asthma, cough, and bleeding piles. Seeds of *L. sativum* are useful in the treatment of fracture [2] and induce production of breast milk. Garden cress seed oil is rich in omega-3 fatty acid [3]. Seed powder has been proved useful in the treatment of fracture healing [4]. *Lepidium sativum* is one of the herbs mentioned in ancient scriptures of Ayurveda. Anti-osteoporotic effect of the plant has been discussed by many authors [5]. **Sudard** is an herbal formulation containing extracts of 11 medicinal plants including *Lepidium sativum* seeds. **Bio-Trib** is a synergic preparation including *L. sativum* roots-effective, safe and useful for successful treatment of a wide range of male sexual health disorders. **Delentigo** (made up of *Lepidium sativum* sprout extract) is an efficient and targeted solution for reducing age spots. **Flex, Laksha gogglu, painmukti** etc. are other formulations of Lepidium. Phytosterols and phytoestrogens are some important compounds present in higher quantities in this medicinal plant. Phytoestrogens have been suggested as cancer preventatives and as treatments for menopausal symptoms and osteoporosis. Phytoestrogens like Diadzein, formononetin containing diet can be useful for the prevention and treatment of many diseases including osteoporosis [6]. The widely distributed C-29 sterols are formed from acetate via melvaonic acid pathway by higher plants. Phytosterols have been reported in many plants by several workers [4,7-9].

Separation of phytoestrogens by chromatography is particularly very useful, since it permits their identification, confirmation and/or quantification. The focus of this study was to simplify the extraction procedure and to qualitatively analyze various *in vivo* and *in vitro* parts of *Lepidium sativum* for relative determination of phytoestrogens.

Materials and Method

Seeds of mature plant of *Lepidium sativum* were collected locally from different regions of Rajasthan (India). *In vitro* grown hypocotyls of *Lepidium sativum* were inoculated after several rinses with sterile distilled water on MS medium supplemented with various combinations of growth regulators. Ideal medium for callus establishment through nodal stem segment explant was MS-medium supplemented with NAA (1.0 mg/l) in combination with BAP (5.0 mg/l). Callus tissues thus grown were harvested periodically (2, 4, 6 and 8 weeks), dried and calculated for growth indices separately. Five such replicates of seeds and callus were examined and the mean values were recorded.

Extraction procedure

Plant derived sterols in tissues and oilseeds of *Lepidium sativum* can be isolated by solvent extraction with diethyl ether followed by saponification and chromatographic purification to obtain total sterols.

*Corresponding author: Preeti Mishra, Plant Pathology, Tissue Culture and Biotechnology Laboratory, Department of Botany, University of Rajasthan, Jaipur, India, E-mail: drpreetipathak@gmail.com

In vitro grown callus tissue and selected plant seeds were striped and milled before they were extracted by diethyl ether in a soxhlet extractor. After removal of solvent using evaporator, 30 ml of extracts were saponified with 9% alcoholic potassium hydroxide for 5 hrs. The resulting solution was then diluted two times by distilled water and extraction procedure followed five times with diethyle ether. The ether solution was dried to obtain unsaponifiable matters of plant seed oils and dried *in vitro* cultured callus. Five replicates were analyzed in each case. Identification of sterols was carried out by TLC, IR spectra, and HPTLC studies. Methanolic extracts of seed powder and callus were used in case of phytoestrogen studies.

Thin layer chromatography

The crude extracts were applied separately on silica gel 'G' coated and activated thin glass plates along with standard reference sample of sterols (β-sitosterol, stigmasterol, lanosterol, cholesterol). The plates were developed in different organic solvent mixturers of Benzene: Ethyl acetate (3:1) and Hexane: Acetone (8:2) [10]. The developed plates were air dried, sprayed with 50 % sulphuric acid or Anisaldehyde reagent and subsequently heated at 100°C for 10 minutes. To quantify phytoestrogens-diadzein, genistein and formononetin, different organic solvents like chloroform: methanol (8:2); chloroform: acetone: formic acid (75:16.5:8.5) were tested. Five to ten replicates were run and average Rf values were calculated for the standard and plant parts' extracts (*in vivo* and *in vitro*).

Preparative thin layer chromatography (PTLC)

The extracts along with standard reference β-sitosterol, stigmasterol, lanosterol, cholesterol were applied separately on thick (0.3 mm to 0.4 mm) silica gel 'G' coated and activated glass plates. The plates were developed in an organic solvent mixture of Hexane: Acetone (8:2). The developed plates were air dried and visualized by spraying 50% sulphuric acid and anisaldehyde reagent to mark the steroidal bands. Each of the mixture was eluted with chloroform, elutes were dried in vacuo, crystallized separately with acetone and methanol. The purified material was subjected for IR spectrum and HPTLC analysis.

HPTLC studies

The TLC spots corresponding to sterols were eluted by methanol (1/1 v/v). The separation was made on HPTLC system equipped with a sample applicator device CAMAG lino mate 5, CAMAG twin through chamber, CAMAG TLC scanner and integration software (Win CATS), stationary phase for the sample was pre washed HPTLC silica gel plates 60 F254, mobile phase for the samples was Hexane: Diethyl Ether (6.5:3.5). The developed bands were analyzed on 520 nm (β-sitosterol) and on 380 nm (Diadzein and formononetin). Peaks of standard sterols were compared with the peaks of *in vitro* callus tissue and with the peaks of *in vivo* plant parts. The plates were photo-documented by using UV and white light.

Results

Qualitative analysis showed the presence of β-sitosterol in all *in vivo* (seeds) and *in vitro* (callus) samples of *Lepidium sativum*. The developed TLC plates showed coloured spots for isolated β-sitosterol of seeds (Rf- 0.62) and callus (Rf-0.63) samples which coincided with that of the reference β-sitosterols (Rf- 0.64, purple). The Rf value of standard β-sitosterol in HPTLC analysis was found to be 0.18 and peak area recorded was 3580.50. Callus and seed extracts of the plant showed Rf value 0.18 and 0.20 respectively; which coincided with standard Rf value and peak area was 176.10 and 1449.1 respectively. The amount of

β-sitosterol was estimated to be about 0.20 % w/w for seed powder and 0.024 % for callus powder (Figure 1A-1D). The 3D spectra of all tracks scanned at 520 nm are shown in (Figure 2).

Daidzein and formononetin isolated from the samples of *Lepidium sativum* showed Rf value 0.73 (for seeds) and 0.67 (for callus) and peak area was 546.8 and 1033.5 respectively (Figure 3A-3C) (Figure 4A-4D). Chloroform: methanol (8:2) gave excellent results in the present investigation for all samples. During HPTLC analysis the amount of daidzein was estimated to be about 18.81 % w/w in seed and minimum in callus (9.99 % w/w) by using the HPTLC values. The 3D spectra of all tracks scanned at 380 nm (Figure 5).

Discussion

β-sitosterols have antifungal, antibacterial and anti-inflammatory activity [11,12]. In the present investigation Chloroform: methanol (8:2) combination showed best results and exhibited coherence with the results of [13,14]. HPTLC technique with other biochemical assays supplemented evidence to confirm the presence of some bioactive compounds, which have provided the plants an important position in folkloric usage [15] In the present study, quantitative and qualitative biochemical methods can be employed as a stability indicator [16] that can be used for the routine quality control analysis and quantitative determination of β-sitosterol from *Lepidium sativum*. Results obtained by HPTLC for diazdzein and formononetin were coincided with the results of [17-19]. Although originally identified in cementum, PTPLa/ CAP is very effective at inducing bone repair and healing and therefore this novel molecule has a great potential to be used for mineralized tissue bioengineering and tissue regeneration studied by [20]. *Lepidium* sativum seeds have been used in traditional folk medicine to heal fractured bones especially in cases of glucocorticoilds induced osteoporosis [21,22]. Results thus obtained provided a chromatographic fingerprint of specific phytochemicals and are suitable for identify and purify raw materials from such medicinal plants.

Conclusion

These results indicate that, the assay is accurate and reliable for the determination of phytoestrogens in *Lepidium sativum*. This technique

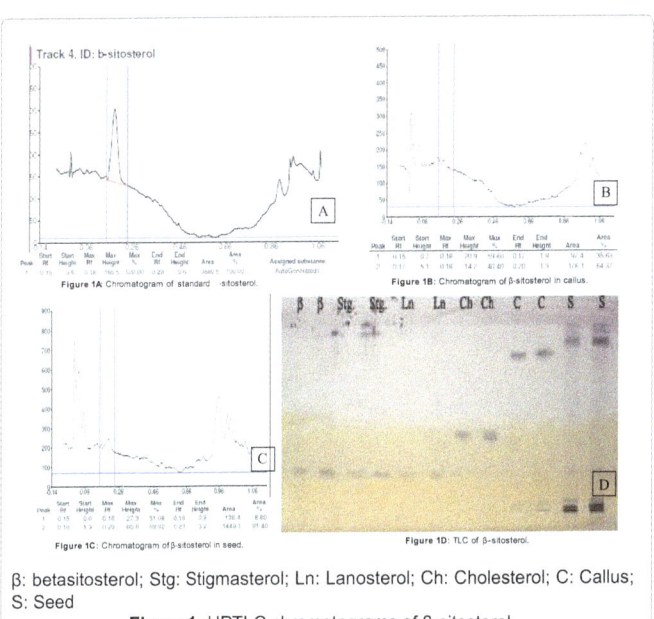

β: betasitosterol; Stg: Stigmasterol; Ln: Lanosterol; Ch: Cholesterol; C: Callus; S: Seed

Figure 1: HPTLC chromatograms of β-sitosterol.

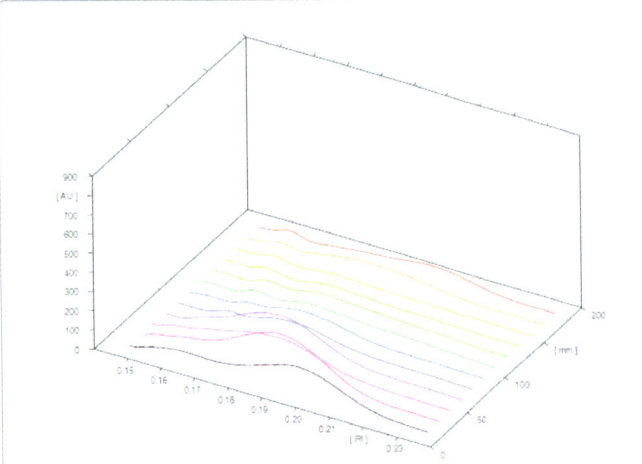

Figure 2: 3D spectra of all tracks of phytosterol (β-sitosterol) samples and standard at 520 nm.

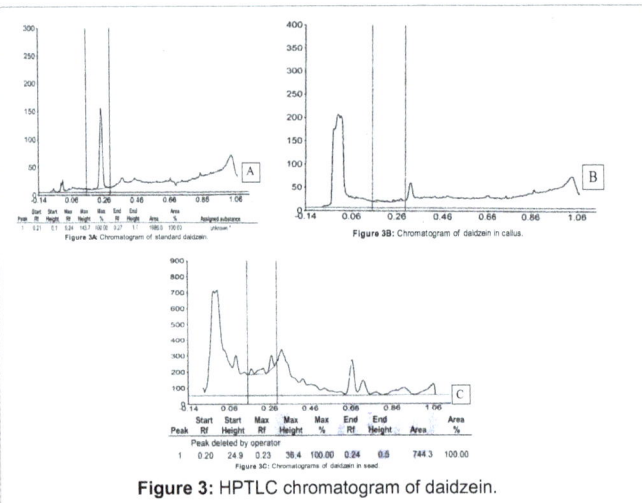

Figure 3: HPTLC chromatogram of daidzein.

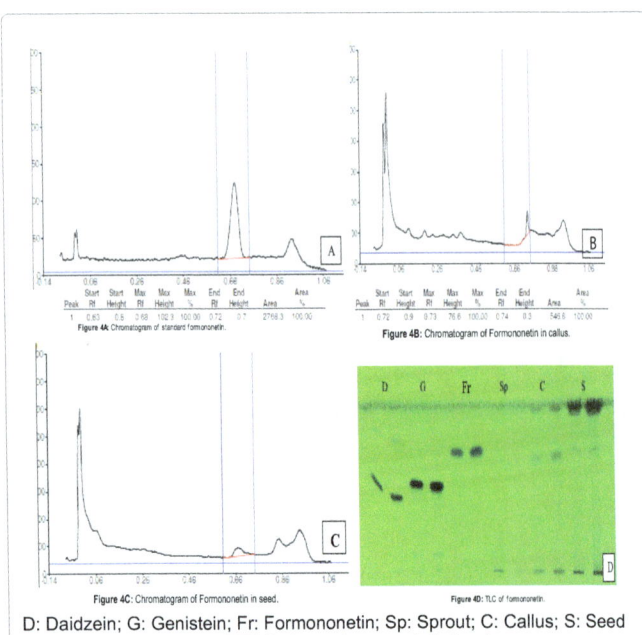

D: Daidzein; G: Genistein; Fr: Formononetin; Sp: Sprout; C: Callus; S: Seed
Figure 4: HPTLC chromatogram of phytoestrogen.

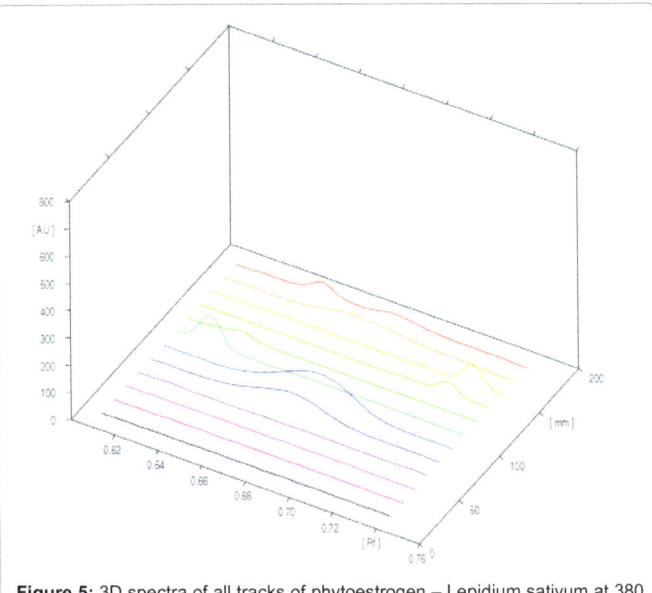

Figure 5: 3D spectra of all tracks of phytoestrogen – Lepidium sativum at 380 nm.

greatly simplifies the analysis of phytoestrogens. The HPTLC method provided a quick and easy approach for detection and quantitation of biomarker β-sitosterol in *Lepidium sativum*.

Aknowledgements

We are thankful to Rajasthan State Department of Science and Technology for the financial support to complete the research project, the part of which is presented here.

References

1. Gokavi SS, Malleshi NG, Guo M (2004) Chemical composition of garden cress (*Lepidium sativum*) seeds and its fractions and use of bran as a functional ingredient. Plant Foods Hum Nutr 59: 105-111.

2. Krishnaraju AV, Rao TVN, Dodda S, Vanisree M, Tsay HS, et al. (2005) Assessment of bioactivity of Indian medicinal plant using brin shrimp (*Artemia salina*) lethality assay. Int. J. Appl. Sci Eng 3: 125-134.

3. Umesha SS, Manohar RS, Indiramma AR, Naidu AK (2015) Enrichment of biscuits with microencapsulated omega-3 fatty acid (Alpha-linoleinic acid) rich Garden cress (*Lepidium sativum*) seed oil: Physical, sensory and storage quality characteristics of biscuits. LWT- Food Sci. Tech 62: 654-661.

4. MilovanoviÄ M, Banjac N, RadoviÄ BV (2009) Functional food: rare herbs, seeds and vegetable oils as sources of flavors and phytosterols. J Agri Sci 54: 80-93.

5. Juma Ab (2007) The effects of *Lepidium sativum* seeds on fracture-induced healing in rabbits. MedGenMed 9: 23.

6. Sirotkin AV, Harrath AH (2014) Phytoestrogens and their effects. Eur J Pharmacol 741: 230-236.

7. Shirwaikar A, Khan S, Kamariya YH, Patel BD, Gajera FP, et al. (2010) Medicinal plants for the management of post-menopausal osteoporosis: A review. The Open Bone J 2: 1-13.

8. Ye JC, Chang WC, Hsieh DJY, Hsiao MW (2010) Extraction and analysis of Î²-sitosterol in herbal medicines. J Med Plants Res 7: 522-527.

9. Shareef H, Rizwani GF, Haq MH, Ahmad S, Zahid H, et al. (2012) Tocopherol and phytosterol profile of *Sesbania grandiflora* (Linn.) seed oil. J Med Plants Res 6: 3478-3481.

10. Senthilmanickam J, Bhavani AL, Venkatramlingam K, Chandra G (2012) The role of 2, 4-D and NAA in callus induction of *Achyranthes aspera* and its secondary metabolite studies. Jamonline (J. Atoms Mol.) 2: 232-243.

11. Sathishkumar T, Baskar R, Rajeshkumar M (2012) In vitro antibacterial and antifungal activities of *Tabernaemontana heyneana* Wall. Leaves. J Appl. Pharm. Sci 2: 107-111.

12. Jasuja ND, Choudhary J, Sharama P, Sharma N, Joshi SC, et al. (2012) A review on bioactive compounds and medicinal uses of *Commiphora mukul*. J. Plant Sci 7: 113-137.

13. Liew R, Macleod KT, Collins P (2003) Novel stimulatory actions of the phytoestrogen genistein: Effects on the gain of cardiac excitation-contraction coupling. FASEB J 17: 1307-1309.

14. Ercetin TG, Toker M Kartal, Colgecen H, Toker MC (2012) *In vitro* isoflavonoid production and analysis in natural tetraploid *Trifolium pratense* (red clover) calluses. Rev Bras Farmacogn 22: 964-970.

15. Mariswamy Y, Gnaraj E, Antonisamy JM (2011) Chromatographic fingerprint analysis on flavonoids constituents of the medicinally important plant *Aerva lenata* L. by HPTLC technique. Asia-Pac. J. Trop. Biomed S8-S12.

16. Genetea G, Hymete A, Bekhi AAA (2012) Development and validation of HPTLC assay method for simultaneous quantification of hydrocortisone and clotrimazole in cream and applying for stability indicating test. J chil chem Soc 57: 1199-1203.

17. Fang C, Wan X, Jiang C, Cao H (2005) Comparison of HPTLC and HPLC for determination of isoflavonoids in several kudzu samples. J. Plant Chrmatogr 18: 73-77.

18. Shirke SS, Jadhav SR, Jagtap AG (2008) Methanolic extract of *Cuminum cyminum* inhibits ovariectomy-induced bone loss in rats. Exp Biol Med (Maywood) 233: 1403-1410.

19. Rakesh SU, Patil PR, Salunkhe VR, Dhabale PN, Burade KB (2009) HPTLC method for quantitative determination of quercetin in hydroalcoholic extract of dried flower of *Nymphaea stellata* willd. Inter J Chem Tech Res 1: 931-936.

20. Montoya G, Arenas J, Romo E, Zeichner-David M, Alvarez M, et al. (2014) Human recombinant cementum attachment protein (hrPTPLa/CAP) promotes hydroxyapatite crystal formation *in vitro* and bone healing *in vivo*. Bone 69: 154-64.

21. Elshal MF, Almalki AL, Hussein HK, Khan JA (2013) Synergistic antiosteoporotic effect of *Lepidium sativum* and alendronate in glucocorticoid-induced osteoporosis in Wistar rats. Afr J Tradit Complement Altern Med 10: 267-73.

22. Wu YB, Zheng CJ, Qin LP, Sun LN, Han T, et al. (2009) Antiosteoporotic activity of anthraquinones from *Morinda officinalis* on osteoblasts and osteoclasts. Molecules 14: 573-583.

12

In-Silico Structural and Functional Analysis of Hypothetical Proteins of *Leptospira Interrogans*

Anil P Bidkar[1]*, Krishan K Thakur[1], Nityanand B Bolshette[1], Jyotibon Dutta[1] and Ranadeep Gogoi[2]

[1]*Laboratory of Biotechnology, Department of Biotechnology, National Institute of Pharmaceutical Education and Research (NIPER), Guwahati Medical College, Guwahati-781032, Assam, India*

[2]*Department of Biotechnology & Bioengineering, Institute of Science and Technology, Guwahati University, Guwahati-781014, Assam, India*

Abstract

Though after a start of genome sequencing most of the protein sequences are deposited in databases, some proteins remain to be annotated and functionally characterized. Analyzing and annotating the function of Hypothetical proteins of Leptospira interrogans is very important which is a pathogenic spirochete causes various complications in human and animals. Randomly we have selected 12 sequences of hypothetical proteins and were analyzed through web tools as Pfam, CD Blast, Expasy's to determine physicochemical properties and protein family information based on conserved domains. Proteins from families AdoMetDC, LRR, and PilZ are most conserved in many microorganisms can be targeted to develop efficacious drug molecules. Ligand binding site and protein structure prediction was done by using Qsite finder and PS2 server which will help to develops therapeutic molecules in docking studies. Present study has shown intracellular interactions of proteins involved in drug resistance, transcription factors, and transport channels.

Keywords: Hypothetical protein; *Leptospira interrogans*; Bioinfor-matics tools; Functional analysis

Introduction

Genome sequencing projects and genetic engineering has revealed many aspects of complex cellular environment containing large number of proteins. Despite sequences of most of organisms are available and proteins coded are studied experimentally, there are some proteins whose functions are unknown, need to be characterised [1]. Such proteins are known as Hypothetical Proteins (HP) sequences [2] of which are known but there is no evidence of experimental study [3]. There is extensive need to study and classify these hypothetical proteins which can open new way to design drug molecules against infectious organisms. Functional annotation of HPs involved in infection, drug resistance, and essential biosynthetic pathways is important for development of the potent antibacterial against infectious agents. Improved understanding of these proteins may make them potential targets of antimicrobial drugs [4]. *Leptospira interrogans* is gram negative spirochete, having an internal flagella is pathogenic which causes Leptospirosis [5-7], other serovars (strains) are distinguished on the basis of cell surface antigens. These are infectious to animals, but through animal urine can be spread to human [8]. Leptospira enters in body via broken skin, mucosa and spreads in body, if immune system fails to stop the growth of bacteria it cause severe hepatic and renal dysfunctions [9,10]. This present study highlights the *in silico* studies to characterize HPs from *Leptospira interrogans*.

Methods

Sequence retrieval

KEGG (Kyoto Encyclopedia of Gene and Genomes) is a large collection of databases having entries of genes, proteins, pathways in metabolism and diseases, drug and ligands of organism [11]. We have selected the Sequences of 12 hypothetical proteins of *Leptospira interrogans* randomly from KEGG database (www.genome.jpg/kegg).Gene IDs for selected proteins are gi|24214908, gi|24215649, gi|24215664, gi|24215909, gi|24216444, gi|24217373, gi|24213620, gi|24214752, gi|24214753, gi|294827583, gi|294827687, gi|24213945.

Pfam

Pfam is curated Protein families database, it uses jackhmmer programme (HMMR3). To give profile HMM (Hiden Markov Model) with PSI-BLAST, which were searched against UniProt [12]. However, to include protein in a family its domain and sequence bit scores must be equal or above the Gathering Thresholds (GA). Pfam gives Pfam A families which are manually curated and Pfam B families generated automatically [13].

Batch CD search

Hypothetical Protein sequences were searched for conserved domains at batch CD search, which gives results by using MSA and 3D structures for homologous domains available on Pfam and SMART [12,14].

ExPASy-ProtParam tool

ProtParam tool (www.expasy.org/tools/protparam.html) was used to estimate physicochemical parameters of hypothetical proteins [15]. Query protein can be submitted in form of SWISS/TrEMBL ID or protein sequence. Server provides directly calculated values of pI/MW (Isoelectric point, Molecular Weight), Percentage of each amino acid, Extinction Coefficient (EC), Instability Index (II) [16], Aliphatic Index (AI) and GRAVY (Grand Average of Hydrophobicity).

---

*Corresponding author: Anil P Bidkar, Department of Biotechnology, National Institute of Pharmaceutical Education and Research (NIPER), Gauhati Medical College, Guwahati-781032, Assam, India, E-mail: anilbidkar1@gmail.com, nbolshette@gmail.com

SOSUI server

Amphiphilicity index and Hydropathy index of query protein sequences were calculated by SOSUI server which categorises protein into cytoplasmic or transmembrane nature [17].

Protein-Protein Interaction network

Protein in the cell environment interacts with other proteins, *in silico* these interactions were studied by STRING v9.1 (Search Tool for Retrieval of Interacting Genes). STRING is a large repository of protein-protein interactions involving functional interactions, stable complexes, and regulatory interactions among proteins [18,19]. Figure 1 Shows resulting protein-protein interaction network of selected hypothetical proteins, for better understanding interaction networks should be seen on server site.

Disulfide-Bonding in protein

Disulfide bonds among cysteine residues in protein plays an important role in folding it into functional and stable conformation. DISULFIND server utilizes SVM binary server to predict bonding state of cysteins, these cysteins are paired by Recursive Neural Network to show disulfide bridges [18]. Information about disulphide bonding helps in experimental structure determination and defining stability of the proteins.

Protein structure prediction

Protein structure prediction server (PS)^2 [20] requires query sequence in fasta format to generate 3D structure by comparative

modelling. Server utilizes consensus strategy to find template using PSI-BLAST and IMPALA. Query sequence and template aligned by T-coffee, PSI-BLAST, and IMPALA [17]. 3D structures are predicted from template using MODELLER and visualised by CHIME, Raster3D. Resulting 3D structural model of selected hypothetical proteins are shown in Figure 2.

Ligand binding site prediction

Q-site finder server was used for binding site prediction in selected proteins [21]. Server uses energy based methods to find clefts on protein surface for ligands [22]. These hot spots for ligand binding have predicted after ranking their physicochemical properties as hydrophobicity, desolvation, electrostatic & van der waal potentials.

Discussion

ProtParam tool computes different physicochemical parameters depending on the queries submitted to the databases. Isoelectric focusing separates proteins according to pI where pH gradients are developed [23]. Predicted pI via server may not be adequate because

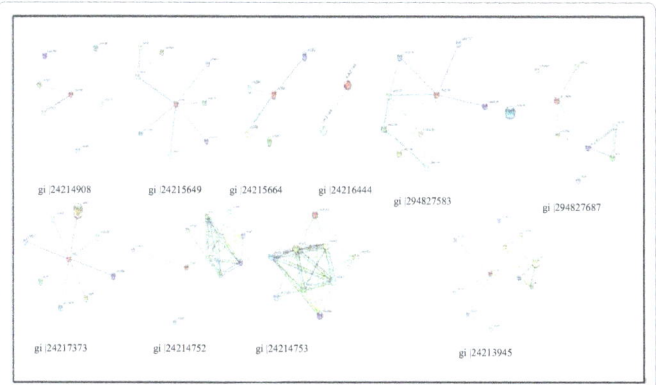

Figure 1: Showing Protein-protein Interaction of hypothetical proteins generated by STRING tool

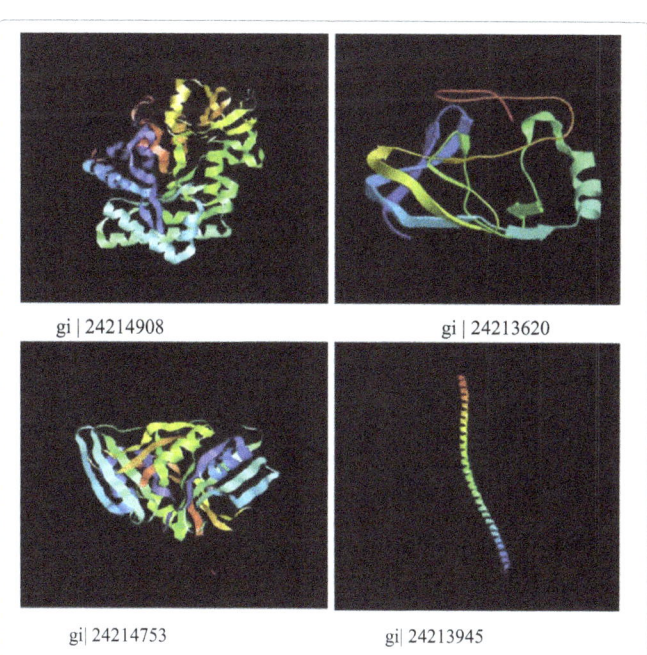

Figure 2: Predicted structures of hypothetical proteins of Leptospira interrogans by PS2 server

Sequence ID	No of AA	MW	pI	EC	II	AI	GRAVY
gi| 24214908	535	61891	8.27	100980	42.45	69.66	-0.761
gi| 24215649	445	50918	9.20	43445	39.23	79.26	-0.396
gi| 24215664	426	49102	8.7	13535	60.67	124.98	-0.460
gi| 24215909	251	26175.9	5.24	17795	28.55	65.58	-0.161
gi| 24216444	241	28062	8.74	11920	47.89	93.44	-0.297
gi| 24217373	288	32486.7	5.49	26275	36.72	83.30	-0.267
gi| 24213620	428	50351.8	5.13	31290	45.52	106.73	-0.065
gi| 24214752	399	46207.3	6.71	112550	34.23	121.93	0.631
gi| 24214753	182	20886.2	8.6	19285	37.95	95.33	-0.276
gi| 294827583	309	33712.5	8.68	11710	36.34	88.61	-0.358
gi| 294827687	199	22228.3	9.62	13075	33.11	116.03	0.323
gi| 24213945	212	23671.6	3.90	1490	51.06	90.71	-0.743

Table 1: Physicochemical properties of proteins using Protparam tool.

in case of high number of basic amino acids and lower buffer capacity. By using pH gradients and calculated pI, proteins can be separated experimentally. MW of proteins along with pI is used for the 2D gel electrophoresis. EC shows a light absorbed by a protein relative to their composition at a specific wavelength. EC given (Table 1) are calculated with reference to Tryptophan, Cysteine, Tyrosine [17]. Instability Index (II) refers to the stability of the protein in test tube [24]. Among studied proteins gi|24214908, gi|24215664, gi|24216444, gi|24213620, gi|24213945 were found to be unstable, and rest are stable (proteins with II above 40 are unstable). Aliphatic amino acid constitutes the aliphatic index (a relative volume of aliphatic side chains). Increased AI results into a hydrophobic interactions and thus gives thermostatic stability to protein, predicted AI and II shows inverse relation for stability except these two proteins gi|24215664 andgi|24215909. GRAVY [26] values are a ratio of all hydropathy values of amino acids

to the number of residues in sequence. Smaller the GRAVY [25] more hydrophilic is protein, gi|24214908 and gi|24213945 proteins found the most hydrophilic. In case of 3D structure hydrophilic domains tends to be on exterior surface, while hydrophobic domains avoids external environment and forms internal core of the protein. Search of family for hypothetical proteins based on conserved domains having consensus sequence in their structure is given in Table 2. Hypothetical protein gi|24214908 found to be a member of GH18_CFLE_spore_hydrolase, Cortical fragment Lytic Enzyme bearing a catalytic domain from glycosylhydrolase, an enzyme used in breaking spore peptidoglycans so as to activate it for germination when favourable conditions are available. Hypothetical protein gi|24215649 from PDZ_serine_ protease involved in protein reassembly and work as a heat shock protein. Protein gi|24215664 belongs to Leucine-Rich Repeats (LRR), ribonuclease inhibitor like family. LRR are motifs having role in protein interactions in complex networks (Table 3). S-adenosylmethionine decarboxylase (AdoMetDC) enzyme for biosynthesis of spermine and spermidine by decarboxylation of SAM belongs to Ado_Met_dc family (gi|24217373). Pilz domain in gi|24213620 is found in bacterial cellulose synthase and other proteins that forms biofilm around a bacterium and involve in effluxing drug [26]. Hypothetical protein gi|294827583 (FecR superfamily) is involved in Iron transport system in bacterial membranes, Fe^{3+} (insoluble) loaded on citrate carrier is sensed by FecR protein found in periplasmic space in bacterial membrane [27]. Protein sites are predicted as cytoplasmic, host associated, extracellular, cytoplasmic membrane proteins (Table 4). SOSOI server predictions (Table 5) shows that positively charged amino acids are more at the end of transmembrane region. Analysis by DISULFIND server (Table 6) shows the Cysteine residues involved in disulphide

Sequence ID	Family
gi|24214908	GH18_CFLE_spore_hydrolase,GH18_chitinase-like superfamily
gi|24215649	PDZ_serine_protease
gi|24215664	LRR_RI superfamily
gi|24216444	Macro superfamily
gi|24217373	AdoMet_dc superfamily, SET superfamily
gi|24213620	DUF1577 superfamily, PilZ superfamily
gi|24214752	DUF2157 superfamily
gi|24214753	GDYXXLXY superfamily
gi|294827583	FecR superfamily
gi|294827687	DUF2179 superfamily
gi|24213945	DUF904 superfamily

Table 2: Family distributions of HP's by Batch CD-BLAST analysis.

Protein	Site Volume (cubic A⁰)	Amino acid involved
gi|24214908	548	TYR 6, TRP 10, PHE 37, ALA 38, GLY 39,THR 48, GLY 76, GLY 77, TRP 78, LYS 79, PHE 80, ASP 117, GLN 119, TYR 120, THR 162, ALA 164, GLY 165, ILE 166, MET 189, TYR 191, ASP192, LEU 193.
gi|24213620	465	PRO 34, ALA 35, LYS 134, LYS 135, GLY 136, TRP 137, GLY 138, ASP 175, SER 176, ASN 177, TYR 178, ARG 206, PHE 207, LEU 208, ASN 209, HIS 210, SER 211.
gi|24214753	201	ARG 9, VAL 10, GLY 11, ARG 15, ASP 64, LYS 65, TYR 66, GLU 67, LEU 68, PRO 116, ASP 117, GLY 118, TYR 119.
gi|24213945	73	ASN 42, ASP 43, GLN 44, LYS 46, LEU 47, GLU 50

Table 3: Prediction of Amino acids involved in Ligand binding (Q-site finder).

Sequence ID	Protein Localization
gi|24214908	Unknown
gi|24215649	Extracellular
gi|24215664	Cytoplasmic
gi|24216444	Cytoplasmic
gi|24217373	Cytoplasmic
gi|24213620	Cytoplasmic Membrane
gi|24214752	Cytoplasmic
gi|24214753	Unknown
gi|294827583	Cytoplasmic Membrane
gi|294827687	Cytoplasmic
gi|24213945	Unknown

Table 4: Protein localisation by PSORTB.

Gene ID	N- Terminal	Trans membrane region	C-Terminal	Type	Length
gi|24215649	60	FYFFKIFVLVLCSLTISVPLKAE	82	PRIMARY	23
	130	AIVADQDFLLALLLPGEFPLFS	109	SECONDARY	22
gi|24215664	71	LMILLILICFSCKLQAQ	87	PRIMARY	17
gi|24214752	94	YYSFLILGVVIIGIGVLAIIAAN	116	PRIMARY	23
	121	DDLVKLGFSFIVLTFVAGLSFW	142	PRIMARY	22
	149	LFTVFIVLYSILILGMIGLISQV	171	PRIMARY	23
	188	LSCLFLITTDSKTFLHLWILGFQ	210	PRIMARY	23
	303	FSFPWVIMICRLLILTPIFYLLI	325	PRIMARY	23
gi|24214753	62	KLILPIALVFPILFFVSEIITLE	84	PRIMARY	23
gi|294827583	61	YLSIVILCTFAMLLLVC	77	PRIMARY	17
gi|294827687	73	VLLPCFIFLSRVTDVSIGTIRVI	95	PRIMARY	23
gi|294827687	103	GIAASLGFLEVLLWVVVITQVIK	125	PRIMARY	23
gi|294827687	138	GGFATGTFIGMILEEKLAIGFSL	160	SECONDARY	23

Table 5: SOSOI results for proteins.

Sequence ID	Bonded Cysteines
gi| 24215909	55-210, 192-217, 200-236
gi| 24214753	69-107, 87-118, 89-126

Table 6: Cysteine residues involved in disulphide bonding.

bonding of hypothetical proteins. Protein-protein interaction study has shown some hypothetical proteins are involved in essential cellular process such as transport across membrane, biosynthesis of molecules, translational regulation. Hypothetical protein gi\| 24214908 (Figure 1) interacts with SUA5 protein which is known as one of translational regulator from YrdC/SUA5 family. Search for gi\| 24215909 shown to be involved in chloride transport with chloride channel protein (EriC gene). Protein gi\| 24217373 found to be interacted with S-layer like protein (slpM) which forms layer around bacteria to attach other surfaces and protect it from environment. Additionally it involves in cell dividing processes and transport across membrane. Protein gi\| 294827687 had shown interaction with proteins for bleomycin resistance, chorismatesynthase (Trp biosynthesis) and Mammalian Cell Entry (MCE) like proteins. Figure 2 shows 3D structures of proteins gi\| 24214908, gi\| 24213620, gi\| 24214753, gi\|24213945 predicted from amino acid sequence on PS^2 server by using templates 1vf8A, 3bo5A, 1f9zA, and c2efsA respectively.

Conclusion

Development of potential bioinformatics tools and databases has opened new platform for in-silico study. Currently it is very needful to annotate and characterize hypothetical proteins in *Leptospira interrogans serovar*. These hypothetical proteins may have an imperative role in producing many virulence factors and cause serious infection or disease.We have analyzed 12 hypothetical proteins from KEGG database and categorized its physicochemical properties and recognized domains and families using various bioinformatics tools and databases. The structures were modeled and their ligand binding sites were identified.Physicochemical predictions made for hypothetical proteins, which can be used to find therapeutic agents against infections caused by *Leptospira interrogans*. Some of hypothetical proteins serves as channel proteins, ribosomal proteins or are involved in cell cycle process. Families which were identified for these hypothetical proteins are involved in normal cellular processes and the resistance against drugs. Ligand binding hotspots were found with Q-sitefinder which shown amino acids involved in interaction with ligands. It will help in study of molecular docking for development of potent and effective target against Leptospira infection.

Acknowledgement

This study was supported by NIPER Guwahati academic staff. We are very grateful for their excellent support in every manner.

References

1. Adinarayana KP, Sravani TS, Hareesh C (2011) A database of six eukaryotic hypothetical genes and proteins. Bioinformation 6: 128-130.

2. Shahbaaz M, Hassan MI, Ahmad F (2013) Functional annotation of conserved hypothetical proteins from Haemophilus influenzae Rd KW20. PLoS One 8: e84263.

3. Hsieh WJ, Pan MJ (2004) Identification Leptospira santarosai serovar shermani specific sequences by suppression subtractive hybridization. FEMS Microbiol Lett 235: 117-124.

4. Galperin MY, Koonin EV (1999) Searching for drug targets in microbial genomes. Curr Opin Biotechnol 10: 571-578.

5. Chou LF, Chen YT, Lu CW, Ko YC, Tang CY, et al. (2012) Sequence of Leptospira santarosai serovar Shermani genome and prediction of virulence-associated genes. Gene 511: 364-370.

6. Langston CE, Heuter KJ (2003) Leptospirosis. A re-emerging zoonotic disease. Vet Clin North Am Small Anim Pract 33: 791-807.

7. Tubiana S, Mikulski M, Becam J, Lacassin F, Lefèvre P, et al. (2013) Risk factors and predictors of severe leptospirosis in New Caledonia. PLoS Negl Trop Dis 7: e1991.

8. Kohn B, Steinicke K, Arndt G, Gruber AD, Guerra B, et al. (2010) Pulmonary abnormalities in dogs with leptospirosis. J Vet Intern Med 24: 1277-1282.

9. Picardeau M, Brenot A, Saint Girons I (2001) First evidence for gene replacement in Leptospira spp. Inactivation of L. biflexa flaB results in non-motile mutants deficient in endoflagella. Mol Microbiol 40: 189-199.

10. Ko AI, Goarant C, Picardeau M (2009) Leptospira: the dawn of the molecular genetics era for an emerging zoonotic pathogen. Nat Rev Microbiol 7: 736-747.

11. Kanehisa M, Goto S, Kawashima S, Okuno Y, Hattori M (2004) The KEGG resource for deciphering the genome. Nucleic Acids Res 32: D277-280.

12. Punta M, Coggill PC, Eberhardt RY, Mistry J, Tate J, et al. (2012) The Pfam protein families database. Nucleic Acids Res 40: D290-301.

13. http://pfam.sanger.ac.uk/search/

14. Letunic I, Doerks T, Bork P (2012) SMART 7: recent updates to the protein domain annotation resource. Nucleic Acids Res 40: D302-305.

15. Wilkins MR, Gasteiger E, Bairoch A, Sanchez JC, Williams KL, et al. (1999) Protein identification and analysis tools in the ExPASy server. Methods Mol Biol 112: 531-552.

16. Mohan R, Venugopal S (2012) Computational structural and functional analysis of hypothetical proteins of Staphylococcus aureus. Bioinformation 8: 722-728.

17. Mitaku S, Hirokawa T, Tsuji T (2002) Amphiphilicity index of polar amino acids as an aid in the characterization of amino acid preference at membrane-water interfaces. Bioinformatics 18: 608-616.

18. Lewis AC, Saeed R, Deane CM (2010) Predicting protein-protein interactions in the context of protein evolution. Mol Biosyst 6: 55-64.

19. Franceschini A, Szklarczyk D, Frankild S, Kuhn M, Simonovic M, et al. (2013) STRING v9.1: protein-protein interaction networks, with increased coverage and integration. Nucleic Acids Res 41: D808-815.

20. Chen CC, Hwang JK, Yang JM (2006) (PS)2: protein structure prediction server. Nucleic Acids Res 34: W152-157.

21. Laurie AT, Jackson RM (2005) Q-SiteFinder: an energy-based method for the prediction of protein-ligand binding sites. Bioinformatics 21: 1908-1916.

22. Burgoyne NJ, Jackson RM (2006) Predicting protein interaction sites: binding hot-spots in protein-protein and protein-ligand interfaces. Bioinformatics 22: 1335-1342.

23. Bjellqvist B, Hughes GJ, Pasquali C, Paquet N, Ravier F, et al. (1993) The focusing positions of polypeptides in immobilized pH gradients can be predicted from their amino acid sequences. Electrophoresis 14: 1023-1031.

24. Guruprasad K, Reddy BV, Pandit MW (1990) Correlation between stability of a protein and its dipeptide composition: a novel approach for predicting in vivo stability of a protein from its primary sequence. Protein Eng 4: 155-161.

25. Kyte J, Doolittle RF (1982) A simple method for displaying the hydropathic character of a protein. J Mol Biol 157: 105-132.

26. Amikam D, Galperin MY (2006) PilZ domain is part of the bacterial c-di-GMP binding protein. Bioinformatics 22: 3-6.

27. Van Hove B, Staudenmaier H, Braun V (1990) Novel two-component transmembrane transcription control: regulation of iron dicitrate transport in Escherichia coli K-12. J Bacteriol 172: 6749-6758.

13

Investigation of a Quality Check for Plasma Samples

Katsutoshi Shoda, Hirotaka Konishi*, Daisuke Ichikawa, Yuji Fujita, Hidekazu Hiramoto, Junichi Hamada, Tomohiro Arita, Toshiyuki Kosuga, Shuhei Komatsu, Atsushi Shiozaki, Kazuma Okamoto and Eigo Otsuji

Division of Digestive Surgery, Department of Surgery, Kyoto Prefectural University of Medicine, 465 Kajii-cho, Kamigyo-ku, Kyoto 6028566, Japan

Abstract

Background: MicroRNA (miRNA) molecules have been detected in many body fluids and used as biomarkers. However, blood cell-derived miRNA molecules due to hemolysis have been shown to affect the amounts of plasma miRNAs. It is important to check the quality of plasma samples for clinical applications. In the present study, an objective method for quality checking plasma samples was investigated using permitted color tone level and the absorbance at 414 nm.

Material and method: An ROC analysis of the macroscopic color tone and the absorbance in 1213 clinical samples was performed. The optimal cut-off absorbance value was validated using the amount of plasma miRNA.

Results: AUC for detecting hemolyzed samples was very high (0.986) at a cut-off absorbance value of 1.664. A sensitivity and specificity were 99% and 92%, respectively. For validation study, 3 candidate miRNAs were selected by a miRNA microarray between fresh and hemolyzed plasma samples; the amounts of miR-16 and miR-19b increased in hemolyzed samples, whereas that of miR-223 remained unchanged. The amounts of plasma miR-16 and miR-19b were significantly increased in 5 clinical samples with higher absorbance values (p=0.0001 and p=0.0003, respectively), while the amounts of these miRNAs were not increased in samples with lower absorbance values.

Conclusions: A simple method for quality checking plasma samples using color tone and absorbance is very useful and significant.

Keywords: Plasma sample; Quality check; Color tone; Absorbance, miRNA

Introduction

MicroRNAs (miRNAs) are small non-coding RNA molecules that play important roles in a variety of normal and disease-related biological processes by post-transcriptionally regulating the expression of target mRNAs [1,2]. They have been detected in many body fluids, because circulating or extracellular miRNAs that bind to protein complexes or are contained within membranous particles such as exosomes or micro-vesicles are protected from degradation by RNase [3-7]. Therefore, plasma miRNA molecules are stable and a potential source of novel biomarker for a number of diseases, including cancer [8,9].

However, the amount of plasma miRNA molecules is known to be markedly affected by sample collection or storage methods. For example, hemolysis, which is caused by negative pressure during sample extraction, results in reddish color tone and marked increase in the amounts of plasma miRNA, whereas the freeze-thaw process decreases the amounts. Thus, although circulating miRNAs are useful biomarkers for many diseases, objective quality checks on plasma samples should be performed carefully.

In the present study, a potential objective method for quality checking plasma samples was examined using the macroscopic color tone and absorbance. And the optimal absorbance cut-off values for a quality check of plasma samples were validated using the amounts of plasma miRNA molecules.

Materials and Methods

Clinical samples

A total of 1213 plasma samples were collected from patients who had been diagnosed with digestive cancer and underwent surgery between January 2012 and April 2015 at Kyoto Prefectural University of Medicine. Written informed consent was obtained from all patients.

Control samples were also collected from 10 adult healthy volunteers by standard cubital vein puncture.

Storage of plasma samples

Immediately after the collection of blood samples in sodium heparin tubes (BD Vacutainer, Franklin Lakes, NJ, USA), cell-free nucleic acids were isolated using a three-spin protocol (1500 rpm for 30 min, 3000 rpm for 5 min, and 4500 rpm for 5 min) in order to prevent contamination by cells or cellular nucleic acids. 120 μl of each plasma sample was added to the well of a 96-well plate and stored at -80°C until the absorbance was measured. The remainder of each plasma sample was stored at -80°C until further processing.

RNA extraction

Total RNA was extracted from 400 μl of plasma samples using a miRVana PARIS kit (Ambion, Austin, TX, USA) and eluted into 100 μl of pre-heated (95°C) elution solution according to the manufacturer's instructions. After plasma samples were thawed on ice and treated with Qiazol, synthetic *Caenorhabditis elegans* miRNA oligonucleotides, cel-miR-39 (a mixture of 25 fmol of each oligonucleotide in a total volume of 5 μl) were added to each plasma sample in order to normalize the efficacy of RNA extraction. RNA samples were stored at -80°C until further processing.

---

*Corresponding author: Hirotaka Konishi, Division of Digestive Surgery, Department of Surgery, Kyoto Prefectural University of Medicine, 465 Kajii-cho, Kamigyo-ku, Kyoto 6028566, Japan,
E-mail: h-koni7@koto.kpu-m.ac.jp

Study design

The study design is summarized in Figure 1. This study was divided into five steps: (1) Determination of the permitted color tone using intentionally hemolyzed plasma samples; i.e., to determine whether the samples were reddish or not, and (2) Examination of absorbance at 414 nm of the clinical plasma samples. (3) Decision of the optimal cut-off absorbance value for a quality check. (4) miRNA microarray analysis between fresh and intentionally hemolyzed plasma samples from a healthy volunteer, in order to select candidate miRNAs for validation. (5) Validation study of the optimal cut-off absorbance value in clinical plasma samples using the amounts of candidate miRNAs.

Measurement of absorbance in plasma samples

The absorbance values of plasma samples were measured using a fluorescent microplate reader with XFLUOR4 (TECAN, Mannedorf, Switzerland) at a wavelength of 414 nm (reference wavelength: 595 nm) according to the previous study [10].

MicroRNA microarray analysis

Plasma samples from healthy volunteers were analyzed by a microRNA microarray. The fresh sample and intentionally hemolyzed one due to negative pressure were examined [11-13]. Microarray analyses were performed using the 3D-Gene microRNA microarray platform (TORAY, Kamakura, Japan) [14,15], and RNA extraction was conducted according to the manufacturer's instructions. Only a very small amount of total RNA was present in the plasma samples; therefore 2 out of the 4 μl of total RNA extracted from 300 μl of plasma samples were used in microarray experiments. RNA was labeled with Hy5 and hybridized at 32°C for 16 h on the 3D-Gene chip. The 3D-Gene miRNA microarray contained more than 1000 miRNA molecules based on the Human miRNA Version 15 of MirBase (http://

microrna.sanger.ac.uk/). We analyzed microarray analysis data and selected three candidate miRNA molecules, the levels of which were significantly higher in hemolyzed samples than in fresh samples or similar between both samples.

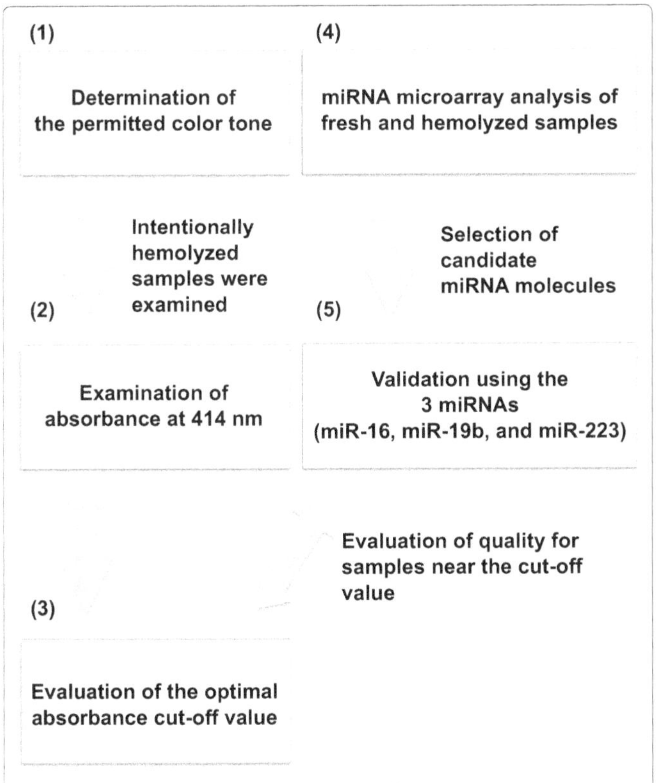

MicroRNA detection protocol

The amounts of target miRNA molecules in plasma were measured by RT-PCR. A reverse transcription reaction was carried out using the TaqMan MicroRNA Reverse Transcription Kit (Applied Biosystems, Foster City, CA, USA), and the amount of each miRNA molecule was quantified in duplicate by quantitative RT-PCR (qRT-PCR) with the human TaqMan MicroRNA Assay Kit (Applied Biosystems) in accordance with previously described protocols [16]. These assays were run on a Step One Plus PCR system v2.1 (Applied Biosystems). The primers for human miRNA (i.e., hsa-miR-16, hsa-miR-19b, and hsa-miR-223) and *C. elegans* miRNA (i.e., cel-miR 39) used in the TaqMan assays were obtained from Applied Biosystems. Changes in the plasma miRNA levels were calculated using the $2^{-\Delta\Delta Ct}$ method [17,18].

Statistical analysis

The paired *t*-test was used to compare the results obtained for fresh and hemolyzed plasma samples. *P*-values of <0.05 were considered significant. ROC curves and the AUC were used to assess the most appropriate absorbance cut-off value for detecting hemolyzed plasma samples, which was determined with the Youden index [19]. Spearman's correlation co-efficient was used to investigate the relationship between absorbance and miRNA levels.

Results

Examination of the permitted color tone and absorbance in control sample

The color series of intentionally hemolyzed plasma samples were shown in Figure 2a. The macroscopic color tone gradually became dense, and the permitted color tone as the not-hemolyzed plasma sample was determined. A borderline of absorbance value at 414 nm, whether the samples were hemolyzed or not, was between 1.363 and 1.761.

Evaluation of the most appropriate absorbance cut-off value for detecting damaged plasma sample

Absorbance value at 414 nm and macroscopic color tone were assessed in 1213 plasma samples. The mean and standard deviation of absorbance value were 1.086 and 0.662. A receiver operating characteristic (ROC) analysis of absorbance value and color tone of each sample revealed the optimal absorbance cut-off value for detecting damaged plasma sample. The area under the ROC curve (AUC) was very high (AUC=0.986) at an absorbance cut-off value of 1.664 (Figure 2b).

Results of the miRNA microarray analysis and validation study

Table 1 shows a list of miRNA molecules whose levels were higher in hemolyzed samples than in fresh samples, or similar in both samples. The miRNAs that were not detectable in fresh samples were not listed in Table 1. Three miRNA molecules, miR-16, miR-19b, and miR-223, were selected for the validation study of this quality checking method, because these miRNAs were present at high amounts in plasma and markedly different between hemolyzed and normal samples (Table 1, squarish marks).

(1)

Determination of the permitted color tone

(2)

Intentionally hemolyzed samples were examined

Examination of absorbance at 414 nm

(3)

Evaluation of the optimal absorbance cut-off value

(4)

miRNA microarray analysis of fresh and hemolyzed samples

Selection of candidate miRNA molecules

(5)

Validation using the 3 miRNAs (miR-16, miR-19b, and miR-223)

Evaluation of quality for samples near the cut-off value

Figure 1: Study design.

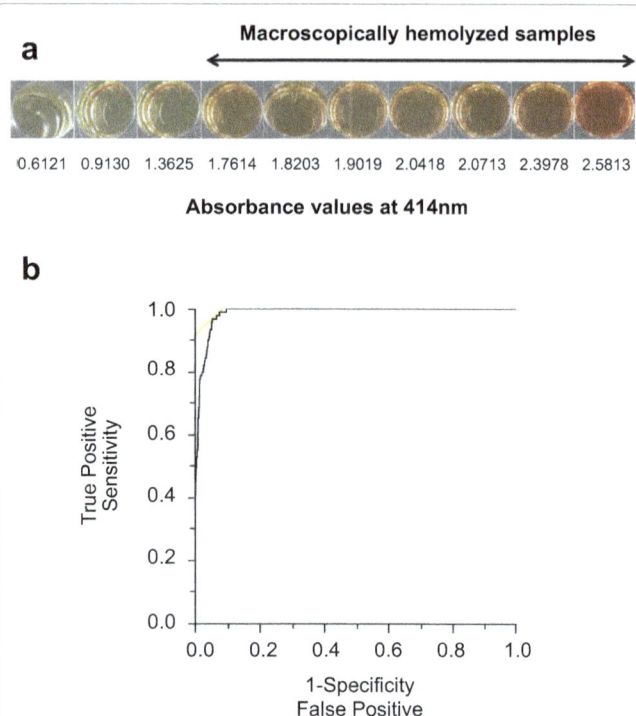

Figure 2: Evaluation of the most appropriate absorbance cut-off value for detecting damaged plasma sample. (a) Determination of the permitted color tone level using intentionally hemolyzed plasma samples. (b) Evaluation of the optimal plasma absorbance cut-off value in 1213 clinical plasma samples. Absorbance at 414 nm and the macroscopic color tone of the plasma samples were assessed. An analysis was performed based on these data, and the Youden index was used to determine the optimal absorbance cut-off value for detecting hemolyzed samples.

Increased				
Name	ID	Hemolyzed (A)	Fresh (B)	Ratio (A/B)
has-miR-4484	MIMAT0019018	4612.381617	231.3811	19.93413
has-miR-20b	MIMAT0001413	328.401954	17.35625	18.92125
has-miR-16	MIMAT0000069	2716.468946	144.752	18.76636
has-miR-15a	MIMAT0000068	373.143256	45.38332	8.222035
has-miR-19b	MIMAT0000074	767.425979	93.79371	8.182062
has-miR-20a	MIMAT0000075	371.74509	47.93124	7.7558
has-miR-4417	MIMAT0018929	1816.050244	236.477	7.679607
has-let-7b	MIMAT0000063	230.530356	30.09583	7.659877
has-miR-3135b	MIMAT0018985	129.862426	17.35625	7.482169
has-miR-26b	MIMAT0000083	71.139468	9.712508	7.324521
Not changed				
Name	ID	Hemolyzed (A)	Fresh (B)	Ratio (A/B)
has-miR-223	MIMAT0000280	451.440534	379.1602	1.190663
has-miR-4745-5p	MIMAT0019878	4397.064101	3693.998	1.190327
has-miR-4513	MIMAT0019050	163.418403	149.8479	1.090562
has-miR-3187-5p	MIMAT0019216	79.528462	81.05414	0.981177
has-miR-3925-5p	MIMAT0018200	82.324793	73.41039	1.121432
has-miR-4496	MIMAT0019031	59.954142	60.67082	0.988188
has-miR-3137	MIMAT0015005	55.759645	55.57498	1.003323
has-miR-4299	MIMAT0016851	52.963314	53.02707	0.998798
has-miR-513a-5p	MIMAT0002877	51.565148	47.93124	1.075815
has-miR-4514	MIMAT0019051	43.176154	40.28749	1.071701

Table 1: Results of the miRNA microarray analysis. MicroRNA molecules whose concentrations were increased or unchanged in hemolyzed plasma samples.

The amounts of miR-16 and miR-19b were significantly increased with approximately 100- and 60-times in hemolyzed plasma samples, respectively ($p<0.0001$ in both cases; paired t-test; Figures 3a and 3b), whereas that of miR-223 remained unchanged in fresh and hemolyzed samples ($p=0.169$, Figure 3c). The absorbance of these plasma samples at 414 nm was also examined, and it was found that the absorbance value correlated with the amounts of miR-16 or miR-19b ($p<0.001$; Spearman's correlation co-efficient; Figure 3d, data for only miR-16 was shown).

Absorbance values and miRNA amounts in clinical plasma samples

The absorbance values and amounts of plasma miR-16 and miR-19b were examined in 10 clinical plasma samples obtained from gastric or pancreatic cancer patients (Table 2). Tumor progression of these 10 randomly selected patients was various degree. The samples obtained from 5 patients were macroscopically reddish, and the others were not. The absorbance values at 414 nm of 5 reddish samples were more than 1.664, while those of the others were less than 1.664. The amounts of miR-16 and miR-19b were also increased in the samples with higher absorbance values regardless of their tumor progression ($p=0.0001$ and $p=0.0003$ for miR-16 and miR-19b, respectively; Figures 4a and 4b), however no significant difference was observed in the amounts of miR-223 between both groups ($p=0.241$, data was not shown).

Discussion

The quality of clinical sample is extremely important when researching new plasma biomarkers. Although many studies identified plasma miRNAs as disease biomarker and previous studies reported a relationship between hemolysis and the increase of plasma free nucleic acid [10], only a few studies have examined the effects of hemolysis and other damaging processes on clinical plasma researches. We also previously identified some plasma miRNA biomarkers, however only macroscopic color tone was mainly checked for the quality of clinical plasma samples. In the present study, we confirmed a more objective method for quality checking plasma samples based on their color tone and absorbance values.

During hemolysis, the cell membranes of red corpuscles are damaged physically, chemically, or biologically by various factors, and their protoplasm leaks into the bloodstream. Thus, when clinical blood samples are extracted, clinicians need to be aware that surplus negative pressure may cause hemolysis. Michaela et al. reported that plasma miRNA concentration was affected by hemolysis, and the degree of hemolysis in a particular plasma sample was able to be determined from its macroscopic color tone or absorbance at 414 nm [10]. Colin CP et al. also showed that blood cells were a major contributing factor to circulating miRNA levels and that blood cell count or hemolysis markedly altered plasma miRNA levels. Therefore, plasma miRNA-based data should be carefully interpreted, because the majority of the reported plasma miRNA biomarkers of cancer are strongly expressed in blood cells. The change of a particular miRNA biomarker may reflect the blood cell-based changes rather than cancer-specific ones [11,12]. Thus, clinical samples need to be handled very carefully when blood cell-derived miRNA molecules are examined as plasma biomarkers [13].

Some difficulties were associated with quality checking plasma samples. Chyle-containing samples were sometimes found, and the absorbance of these samples was slightly higher than that without hemolysis or chyle (data not shown). The chyle contained in plasma samples originates from various sources including chylomicrons, neutral fats, very low-density lipids, and intravenously administered fat tablets. Further studies are needed to confirm whether these samples are suitable for biomarker-based experiments. On the other hand, cancer and other diseases may affect the amounts of plasma miRNAs. If cancer-specific miRNAs are used to quality check of plasma samples, we may inappropriately exclude suitable samples and miss the cancer-specific changes. Therefore, the candidate miRNA molecules used for quality checking should be selected carefully, and some miRNAs should be examined repeatedly.

In the present study, the samples which showed higher absorbance more than the cut-off value contained significantly larger amounts of miR-16 and miR-19b than those showed lower absorbance value. These results may indicate that the amounts of these miRNAs are influenced

Cases	Age	Gender	Stage	Absorbance*	Macroscopic color
PK1	86	Female	Pancreas cancer, Stage III	0.998	Not reddish
PK2	72	Female	Pancreas cancer, Stage IA	1.112	Not reddish
MK1	72	Male	Gastric cancer, Stage III	1.227	Not reddish
MK2	70	Male	Gastric cancer, Stage IA	1.035	Not reddish
MK3	55	Male	Gastric cancer, Stage IA	1.297	Not reddish
PK3	39	Male	Pancreas cancer, Stage III	2.259	Reddish
PK4	80	Male	Pancreas cancer, Stage IA	1.916	Reddish
MK4	73	Male	Gastric cancer, Stage IB	1.67	Reddish
MK5	63	Male	Gastric cancer, Stage IA	1.861	Reddish
MK6	51	Male	Gastric cancer, Stage IB	1.9	Reddish

*414 nm absorbance

Table 2: Clinical features and absorbance values of clinical plasma samples. These ten random samples exhibited various degree of tumor progression. Five samples were macroscopically reddish, and the other five were not.

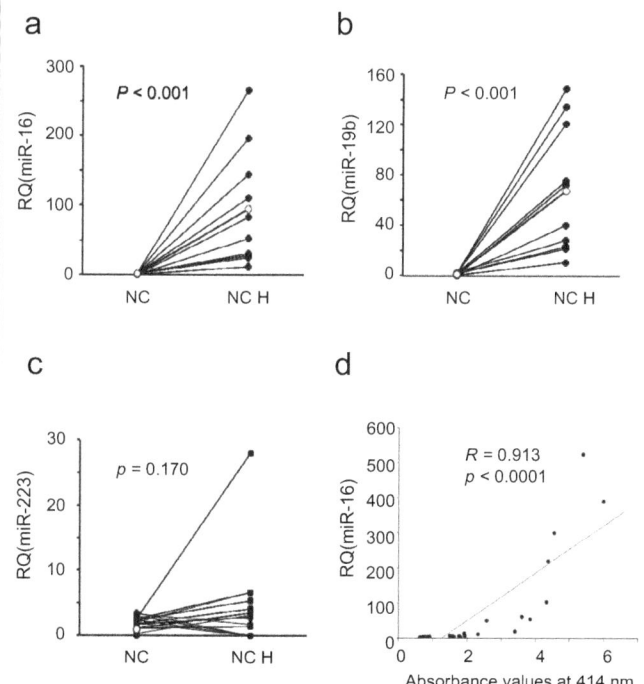

Figure 3: Validation study of paired fresh and hemolyzed plasma samples. The amounts of plasma miR-16, miR-19b, and miR-223 were examined by RT-PCR (a, b, and c). Differences between fresh and hemolyzed samples were analyzed using the paired *t*-test. NC: fresh samples, NC H: hemolyzed samples. (d) The relationship between 414 nm absorbance value and the amount of plasma miR-16 was analyzed in intentionally hemolyzed samples obtained from healthy volunteers.

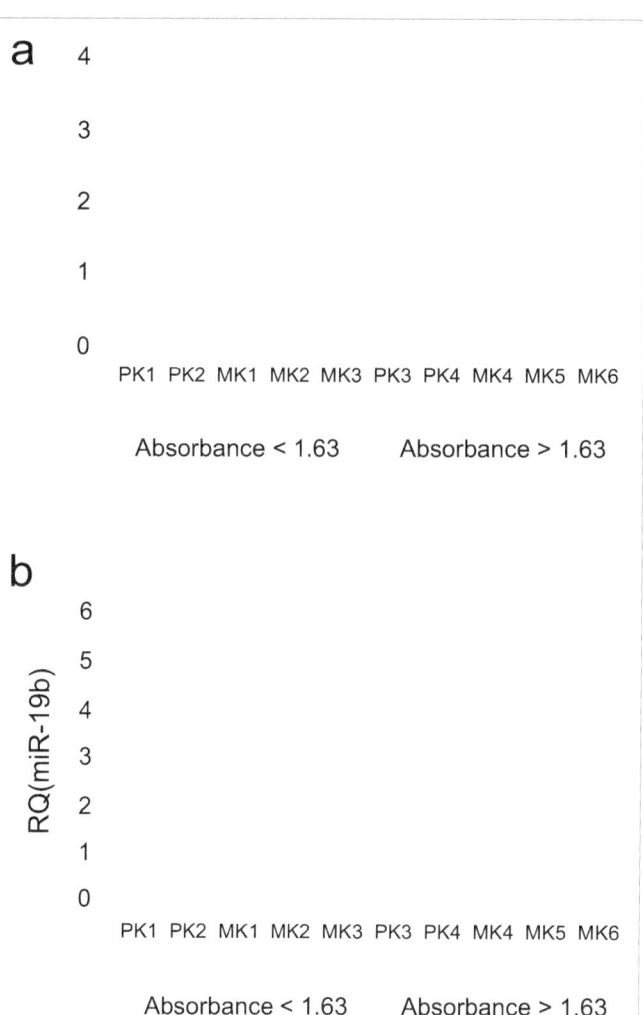

Figure 4: Comparison of plasma miRNA levels in cancer patients according to absorbance value. Plasma miR-16 (a) and miR-19b (b) levels of cancer patients are shown relative to the level of PK1. PK1, PK2, MK1, MK2, and MK3 exhibited absorbance values of less than 1.664 at 414 nm. PK3, PK4, MK4, MK5, and MK6 exhibited absorbance values of more than 1.664 at 414 nm.

by hemolysis rather than tumor progression, and support the accuracy and reproducibility of this cut-off absorbance value. The measurement of absorbance is an easy and objective method for quality checking plasma samples. Although plasma samples are very useful for a range of biomarker analyses, it may be better to discard samples with higher absorbance.

Conclusion

A simple method for quality checking plasma samples using color tone and absorbance is very useful and significant.

Competing Interests

None of the authors have any conflict of interest to disclose.

References

1. Umbach JL, Kramer MF, Jurak I, Karnowski HW, Coen DM, et al. (2008) MicroRNAs expressed by herpes simplex virus 1 during latent infection regulate viral mRNAs. Nature 454: 780-783.

2. Martinez NJ, Gregory RI (2013) Argonaute2 expression is post-transcriptionally coupled to microRNA abundance. RNA 19: 605-612.

3. Ichikawa D, Komatsu S, Konishi H, Otsuji E (2012) Circulating microRNA in digestive tract cancers. Gastroenterology 142: 1074-1078.

4. Weber JA, Baxter DH, Zhang S, Huang DY, Huang KH, et al. (2010) The microRNA spectrum in 12 body fluids. Clin Chem 56: 1733-1741.

5. Munch EM, Harris RA, Mohammad M, Benham AL, Pejerrey SM, et al. (2013) Transcriptome profiling of microRNA by Next-Gen deep sequencing reveals known and novel miRNA species in the lipid fraction of human breast milk. PLoS One 8: e50564.

6. Wang M, Zhao C, Shi H, Zhang B, Zhang L, et al. (2014) Deregulated microRNAs in gastric cancer tissue-derived mesenchymal stem cells: novel biomarkers and a mechanism for gastric cancer. Br J Cancer 110: 1199-1210.

7. Rani S, O'Brien K, Kelleher FC, Corcoran C, Germano S, et al. (2011) Isolation of exosomes for subsequent mRNA, MicroRNA, and protein profiling. Methods Mol Biol 784: 181-195.

8. Konishi H, Ichikawa D, Komatsu S, Shiozaki A, Tsujiura M, et al. (2012) Detection of gastric cancer-associated microRNAs on microRNA microarray comparing pre- and post-operative plasma. Br J Cancer 106: 740-747.

9. Cheng HH, Mitchell PS, Kroh EM, Dowell AE, Chéry L, et al. (2013) Circulating microRNA profiling identifies a subset of metastatic prostate cancer patients with evidence of cancer-associated hypoxia. PLoS One 8: e69239.

10. Kirschner MB, Kao SC, Edelman JJ, Armstrong NJ, Vallely MP, et al. (2011) Haemolysis during sample preparation alters microRNA content of plasma. PLoS One 6: e24145.

11. Pritchard CC, Kroh E, Wood B, Arroyo JD, Dougherty KJ, et al. (2012) Blood cell origin of circulating microRNAs: a cautionary note for cancer biomarker studies. Cancer Prev Res (Phila) 5: 492-497.

12. McDonald JS, Milosevic D, Reddi HV, Grebe SK, Algeciras-Schimnich A (2011) Analysis of circulating microRNA: preanalytical and analytical challenges. Clin Chem 57: 833-840.

13. Blondal T, Jensby Nielsen S, Baker A, Andreasen D, Mouritzen P, et al. (2013) Assessing sample and miRNA profile quality in serum and plasma or other biofluids. Methods 59: S1-S6.

14. Giovannetti E, van der Velde A, Funel N, Vasile E, Perrone V, et al. (2012) High-throughput microRNA (miRNAs) arrays unravel the prognostic role of MiR-211 in pancreatic cancer. PLoS One 7: e49145.

15. Hisaoka M, Matsuyama A, Nagao Y, Luan L, Kuroda T, et al. (2011) Identification of altered MicroRNA expression patterns in synovial sarcoma. Genes Chromosomes Cancer 50: 137-145.

16. Komatsu S, Ichikawa D, Takeshita H, Tsujiura M, Morimura R, et al. (2011) Circulating microRNAs in plasma of patients with oesophageal squamous cell carcinoma. Br J Cancer 105: 104-111.

17. Livak KJ, Schmittgen TD (2011) Analysis of relative gene expression data using real-time quantitative PCR and the 2(-Delta Delta C(T)) Method. Methods 25: 402-408.

18. Pfaffl MW (2011) A new mathematical model for relative quantification in real-time RT-PCR. Nucleic Acids Res 29: e45.

19. Akobeng AK (2007) Understanding diagnostic tests 3: Receiver operating characteristic curves. Acta Paediatr 96: 644-647.

14

Lithium Toxicity Effects on Oxidative Stress, Dyslipidemia and Apoptosis in the Aged Rats

Katiucha KHR Rocha[1], Rodrigo P Ureshino[1], Janaína Peixoto[1], Fernanda Mani[2] and Soraya S Smaili[1]*

[1]*Department of Pharmacology, Institute of Pharmacology, Federal University of São Paulo, São Paulo, Brazil*
[2]*Department of Chemistry and Biochemistry, Institute of Biological Sciences, São Paulo State University, Botucatu, São Paulo, Brazil*

Abstract

Aging is associated with metabolic changes and the development of diseases, due to the reduction of antioxidant defenses and alteration in apoptosis process. The lithium is used to treat bipolar disorder and neuroprotector; it also can be used as an antioxidant, but its function in aging has not been elucidated. The alterations in apoptosis could be associated with development oxidative stress in several tissues, although this information is unclear to aged rats. Disorders in apoptosis process and/or oxidative stress development impair the health of aged rats. The association between apoptosis with hepatic metabolism changes and oxidative stress disorder in aging is also unclear. Therefore, the objective of this work was to determine the effects of lithium on the lipid profile in serum and oxidative stress as well as apoptosis in the liver of aged rats. Twenty female Wistar rats were divided into 4 groups (n=5): the C group, with 3- month-old rats that received only water; the L group, with 3- month-old rats that received a lithium solution in drinking water; the S group, with 22- month-old rats that received water; and the SL group, with 22- month-old rats that received lithium in drinking water. The total experimental period was 30 days. All animals received standard diet *ad libitum*. The lithium dose took was according to neuroprotective dose and carefully monitored daily. The dyslipidemia studies were made through TC, HDL, LDL, VLDL, TG and glucose in serum. Oxidative stress analyses involved experiments with LH, TAS and ATP-SA. The apoptotic proteins analyses were made by western blot. Oxidative stress and apoptotic proteins were studied in the liver rats. The results showed that the lithium treatment reduced energy intake, aqueous solution intake and palatability in both, young and aged rats. This treatment increased TG and VLDL in the serum of animals in both groups. The treatment promoted hyperglycemia in young group, and in aged group, induced LDL enhanced as well as decreased HDL. Lithium induced enhanced Sirt 1 in livers of young and aged rats. TAS were higher in young group submitted lithium treatment. The livers of aged rats supplemented with lithium exhibited raised ATP- SA and Bax. In conclusion, the lithium induced dyslipidemia and hyperglycemia in the young, but this treatment also acted as a possible antioxidant agent, associated with Sirt 1 enhanced to protect this tissue of damages. In the aged rats, lithium promoted dyslipidemia and could induce cell death. Therefore, the supplementation could exert toxic effects in the livers of aged rats.

Keywords: Aging; Lithium; Mitochondria; Apoptosis; Liver; Dyslipidemia; Hyperglycemia

Abbreviations: C: Control Group; L: Young Group Treated With Lithium; SC: Senescent Group; SL: Senescent Group Treated With Lithium; ATP (SA): Atp Synthetase Activity; GSK-3: Glycogen Synthase Kinase 3; TC: Total Cholesterol; HDL: High Density Lipoprotein Cholesterol; VLDL: Very Low Density Lipoprotein Cholesterol; LDL: Low Density Lipoprotein Cholesterol; TG: Triacylglycerol; LH: Lipid Hydroperoxide; PDH: Pyruvate Dehydrogenase; TAS: Total Antioxidant Substances; ROS: Reactive Oxygen Species

Introduction

The aging process promotes decline in cellular function and the accumulation of damages to macromolecules and organelles [1]. The liver diseases incidence increases during aging, while decreased the ability to resist injuries changes [2]. This fact is associated with a reduction in organs functions [3] due mainly oxidative damage and oxidative stress development [4]. Oxidative stress had been associated with damages, such as cells degeneration, membrane lipid peroxidation or LH higher, cell death by apoptosis pathway p53, Bax, Bcl2 concentration changes. Sirt 1 (nicotinamide adenine dinucleotide (NAD⁺)-dependent class III histone deacetylases) affected oxidative stress in aged animals. Aged animals showed less active of these molecules in the liver, heart and lung [5].

The mitochondria have been involved in the production of ROS and development of oxidative stress. These organelles represents the main producer of ROS and presented the higher impaired by ROS during aging [6]. Dysfunction of the mitochondria affects the liver and central nervous system striatum functions [7], reduced ATP production and inducing apoptosis or cell death [8]. The liver function changes could be responsible for the metabolic alterations in this tissue, which probably modify the lipid profile (represented by TG and lipoproteins concentrations presents in blood), being associated with triggering diseases during aging. The lipid profile alteration could induce dyslipidemia condition; this fact is associated with development cardiovascular diseases [9].

Studies about substances with antioxidant capacity are important to prevent damages in the aged organisms and regulate the apoptotic process. Lithium has been described by acts as a neuroprotective agent due its capacity to modulate inflammation, mitochondrial function, and oxidative stress, thus preventing neurodegenerative diseases [10]. However, the neuroprotective role of lithium [11] was not associated

***Corresponding author:** Katiucha Rocha, Department of Pharmacology, Institute of Pharmacology, Federal University of São Paulo, São Paulo, Brazil, E-mail: katikaroll@yahoo.com.br; soraya.smaili23@gmail.com

with studies involving cell death, hepatic and serum metabolism in aging rats. The lithium is a monovalent cation that has been used for more than 60 years to treat bipolar disorder and depressive disorders [12]. This drug was reported to protect against Alzheimer's disease development after chronic treatment [13].

Lithium treatment either has beneficial or can have harmful effects, depending on the dose used, duration of treatment and age of the patient [14]. Chronic treatment with lithium carbonate and aged animals were used in this work. Lithium treatment in aged rat's livers could be prevented metabolic changes and oxidative stress as well as improving ATP production. The improvement of metabolic changes possibly may prevent the apoptosis process, avoiding diseases development in this organ. This work attempts to answer the following questions about alterations in lipid profile, oxidative stress and ATP production, associated with apoptosis process after lithium treatment in the liver, during the aging.

Methods

Animals

This work used 20 female Wistar 2BAW rats from the Federal University of Sao Paulo. This work was subjected to approval by the Ethical Committee for the Conduct of Animal Studies for this University (protocol 0311/12), and all the experiments and procedures were performed in accordance with the Guide for the Care and Use of Laboratory Animals published by the U.S. National Institutes of Health. Male Wistar rats show oxidative damage to mitochondrial DNA being 4-fold superior than in female. Therefore female rats have higher protection against oxidative damage, and consequently live longer than male rats [15]. The animals were divided into two large groups (n=10) of young and aged rats, and then subdivided into four groups (n=5). The initial body weight of the rats was 206 ± 10.49 g in the young group, and 218.46 ± 28.72 g in the aging group. The young groups aged 3 months were subdivided into the C groups that received drinking water, and the L groups that received lithium (1.05 g/L) solution in drinking water *ad libitum*. Animals aged 22 months were also subdivided into two groups: the SC received the same solution as the C group, and the SL group received lithium as well as the L group. All animals were fed standard chow diet, and it was kept individually housed in polypropylene cages. The animals were maintained in controlled clean-air rooms, with a temperature of 22 ± 3°C a 12- h light/dark cycle, and a relative humidity of 60 ± 5%. The total experiment period was 30 days.

The daily lithium intake was 0.068 ± 0.007 and 0.057± 0.09 g/kg/day in young and aging rats, respectively (L and SL). The lithium dose was determinate according to the neuroprotective dose described by Valdés and coworkers [16], and the dilution was made in water. The administrated lithium dose (g/Kg/day) was carefully evaluated, and calculated from amount of aqueous solution ingestion [17, 18]. The drinking solutions and food intake were determinate as the difference between what was given and the leftover. The food consumption and drinking solutions were measured daily at the same time (9:00-11:00 h), and the body weight was determined once a week (9:00-11:00 h) [19]. The nutrition parameters, such as energy intake and palatability, were analyzed in this work [17-19].

Experimental procedures

All animals were sacrificed by decapitation; the blood was collected into a centrifuge tube; it was centrifuged at 1400 g for 10 minutes to acquire the serum. The serum was use to the lipid profile

analysis through assays included glucose, TC, TG, LDL, VLDL, HDL concentrations. After finished the blood collected, samples (100 mg each) of livers from the rats were separated, placed in liquid nitrogen and stored in a -80°C freezer until Western blot analysis. Also were collected samples (200 mg each) that were used in the biochemical analysis of oxidative stress through LH, TAS and ATP-SA methods.

The samples of liver were homogenized in 5 mL of cold 0.1 M phosphate sodium buffer (pH 7.4). The homogenate was acquired through a motor driven Tefflon glass Potter and centrifuged at 10.000g for 15 minutes. After centrifugation, the supernatant was used to analyze lipid hydroperoxide (LH) and TAS. The resulting-pellets were suspended and used in the ATP-SA method.

Biochemical analysis in the serum

The following substances present in the serum as glucose, TG, TC, LDL and HDL concentration were analyzed with enzymatic methods (test kit Labtest Diagnostics Incorporated, Minas Gerais, Brazil). The VLDL concentration was analyzed in serum by Friedwald [20] method. The analyses were performed in the Pharmacia Biotech spectrophotometer at a controlled temperature within the cuvette chamber (UV/ Visible Ultropec 5000 with Swift II applications software to computer system control, 974212, Cambrigde, England, UK).

Hepatic oxidative stress analysis

LH was measured in the liver through the hydroperoxide-mediated oxidation of Fe^{2+}, with 100 µL of sample and 900 µL of a reaction mixture containing 250, l M FeSO4, 2 5mM H2SO4, 100 µM xylenol orange and 4 mM BHT in 90% (v/v) methanol. This analyze involved the oxidation of Fe^{2+} by lipid hydroperoxides presents in the liver samples at low pH in the presence of the Fe^{3+}-complexing dye xylenol orange [o-cresolsulfonphthalein-3',3''-bis(methyliminodiacetic acid sodium salt)]. This method used the ferrous oxidation Fe^{3+}-complexing xylenol orange in a study of nanomolar lipid hydroperoxyde formation during transition metal-catalyzed glucose oxidation [21]. Antioxidant capacity of the liver, or total antioxidant substances (TAS), were analyzed through assay kit (test kit Randox Laboratories Ltd., Crumlin, Co., Antrim, UK).

The resulting-pellets homogenate resulted of liver samples were suspended at 1ml of 0.1 mol/l phosphate buffer, pH 7.4 containing 250 mmol/l mannitol, 70 mmol/l sucrose, and 1 mmol/l EDTA Adenosine triphosphate (ATP)-synthetase activity or ATP-SA (ATP-ase, E.C. 2.7.1.20.) [9]. ATP-SA assay is used to analyze mitochondrial dysfunction. Alteration in ATP-SA could harm ATP synthesis and induce ROS production [22]. The analyses were made-in the microplate reader (Dcom Micro-injection Automatic, Flex Station 3, Molecular Devices Microplate, California, USA) with the software SoftMax Pro (Molecular Devices, California, USA).

Western blot analyses

Western blot analyses were used to determined apoptotic proteins concentration in the livers. The tissue samples were lysed to release the proteins. Liver samples of 100 mg were homogenized in ultra Turrax equipment in the lysis buffer containing 50 mM Tris (pH7.5), 150 mM NaCl, 1 mM EDTA, 0.05% deoxicolate, 1% NP-40, 0.1% SDS (detergent sodium dodecyl sulfate). The total protein concentration was determined through Bradford method [23]. The next step involved the reduction and denaturation of livers samples, adding SDS and beta-mercaptoethanol, and submitted this samples to heat (95°C) for 5 minutes. After, the samples were applied to the gel of polyacrylamide

(8-15%) followed by SDS-PAGE protocol (sodium dodecyl sulfate-polyacrylamide). The electrophoreses was made with running buffer containing 100 mM Tris, 768 mM Glycine at 100 V with 60 mA for 2 h, and the proteins were separated according to size. The protein's transfer process to PVDF membranes (Millipore, Billerica, MA) was made in a transfer buffer containing 0.15 M Tris and 1.2 M Glycine; the electrophoresis in this case was made at 100V with 60 mA for 30 minutes. The membranes were blocked in 5% non-fat milk in TBS-T buffer (20 mM Tris, 500 mM NaCl and 0.2% Tween) for 1 h at 4°C to prevent non-specific background binding of primary and/or secondary antibodies in these membranes.

The membranes were incubated with primary antibodies to studies of proteins involving apoptosis. These antibodies were made with diluted 1:200 to p53 and Bax antibodies. The diluted antibody to anti-apoptotic protein Bcl2 was 1: 200 as well as anti-aging protein Sirt 1. All membranes were incubated with primary antibodies overnight at 4°C. These membranes were washed to 4 times in TBS-T by 5 minutes each, and incubated with HRP-linked anti rabbit IgG, diluted 1:10000 for 2 hrs at 4°C. The membranes were exposed to ECL-plus reagent chemiluminescence detection (GE Healthcare, Waukesha, WI) and placed into gel documentation equipment which included the analysis system by software Gel Capture, Gel Quant (DNR Bio- Imaging Systems Ltd, Jerusalem, Israel). The antibodies for Bcl2 and Sirt 1 were from Santa Cruz (Dallas, Texas, USA). The p53, Bax antibodies and secondary antibody were from Cell Signaling (Danvers, Massachusetts, USA).

Statistical analyses

The analyses were expressed as the average ± the standard deviation (SD) in the tables and figures. Statistical comparisons were carried out by two-way analysis of variance (ANOVA), and Turkey's post-roc test, with significant set as $p < 0.05$ (SigmaStat software for Windows, Jandel Corporation, San Rafael, CA, USA).

Results

Alteration in nutritional and biochemical parameters

Aged rats (SC group) presented a decreased energy intake and palatability, compared to the C group, and enhanced parameters in relation to the L group. Lithium supplementation in aged animals reduced food consumption and aqueous solution intake compared to the C group, in addition to showing reduced energy intake and palatability in comparison to animals without supplementation. Young animals treated with lithium showed a reduction in energy intake, aqueous solution intake and palatability in comparison with the control group, similar to the aged rats treated with this cation. There was not any significant change in the final body weight between the groups (Table 1). These results were important to determine comparisons between the young and aged rats. The nutritional parameters provide results to understanding the use of energy by animals and possible lipid profile or glucose disorders.

Senescent rats, the SC group, did not show alterations in TG and VLDL; but, did show reduced glucose, cholesterol and LDL, compared to the young group. The SL group presented normalization glucose, LDL and VLDL in comparison with the C group. Lithium supplementation in the aged group raised TG, VLDL and LDL, as well as reduced HDL compared to the senescent animals without treatment. The lithium enhanced glucose, TG and VDL, as well as reduced LDL and cholesterol without altering HDL in the serum of the young animals (Table 2). These results indicated that lithium induced hyperglycemia

in the young group and dyslipidemia in young and aged rats, which could be associated with oxidative stress parameters.

Aged rats treated with lithium presented higher LH liver levels and decreased TAS in relation to the L group. LH liver concentration was enhanced in the SL group compared to the L group; however, the L group showed raised TAS in the liver of young rats (Table 3). The increase of LH liver concentration could be associated with possible development of oxidative stress while TAS represents protection against oxidative stress.

Livers of aged animals did not exhibit alterations in ATP- SA; however, lithium enhanced ATP- SA in SL group in comparison with the other groups (Figure 1). The ATP-SA studies are important to

	Groups			
	C	L	SC	SL
Final body weight (g)	225 ± 10	201 ± 11.4	207.5 ± 38.6	207.5 ± 33
Food consumption (g/day)	17.6 ± 2.1	14.4 ± 3.0	14.5 ± 1.4	10.6 ± 2.1ᵃ
Energy intake (Kcal/day)	150 ± 11.9	71.3 ± 7.4ᵃ	117.26 ± 9.0ᵃᵇ	66.9 ± 6.9ᵃᶜ
Aqueous solution intake (mL/day)	27.2 ± 5.4	14.8 ± 5.2ᵃ	21.3 ± 6.4	12.2 ± 1.3ᵃᶜ
Palatability (%)	57.28 ± 7.39	25.92 ± 2.69ᵃ	42.64 ± 3.26ᵃᵇ	24.33 ± 2.53ᵃᶜ

Values were given as the mean ± standard deviation of the mean. a Statistically significant compared to the C group at p<0.05. b Statistically significant compared to the L group at p<0.05. c Statistically significant compared to the SC group at p<0.05

Table 1: Final body weight, food consumption, energy intake, aqueous solution intake and palatability in young control rats (C), young rats treated with lithium (L), aged rats (SC) and aged rats treated with lithium (SL).

	Groups			
	C	L	SC	SL
Glucose (mg/dL)	118.8 ± 9.54	150.1 ± 8.58ᵃ	76.05 ± 8.10ᵃᵇ	95.48 ± 16.83ᵇ
Triacylglycerol (mg/dL)	69.59 ± 9.57	166.91 ± 9.41ᵃ	41.54 ± 8.19ᵇ	106.97 ± 25.67ᵃᵇᶜ
Cholesterol (mg/dL)	125.63 ± 13.78	63.41 ± 9.99ᵃ	94.46 ± 9.06ᵃᵇ	109.12 ± 12.68ᵇ
VLDL-(mg/dL)	13.92 ± 1.91	33.38 ± 1.88ᵃ	8.31 ± 1.64ᵇ	19.20 ± 4.46ᵇᶜ
LDL (mg/dL)	44.73 ± 4.81	23.45 ± 8.48ᵃ	22.14 ± 8.9ᵃ	49.97 ± 11.86ᵇᶜ
HDL (mg/dL)	61.51 ± 6.12	48.26 ± 3.90	54.54 ± 9.35	34.96 ± 5.28ᵃᶜ

Values were given as the mean ± standard deviation of the mean. a Statistically significant compared to the C group at p<0.05. b Statistically significant compared to the L group at p<0.05. c Statistically significant compared to the SC group at p<0.05.

Table 2: Glucose, triacylglycerol, cholesterol, VLDL-cholesterol (VLDL), LDL-cholesterol (LDL), HDL –cholesterol (HDL) in serum of young control rats (C), young rats treated with lithium (L), aged rats (SC) and aged rats treated with lithium (SL).

	Groups			
	C	L	SC	SL
LH in liver (nmol/g tissue)	789.76 ± 111.81	574.36 ± 61.79	898.16 ± 64.48ᵇ	953.08 ± 150.68ᵇ
TAS in liver (%)	6.47 ± 0.68	9.05 ± 0.59ᵃ	6.32 ± 1.08ᵇ	6.20 ± 0.74ᵇ

Values were given as the mean ± standard deviation of the mean. a Statistically significant compared to the C group at p < 0.05. b Statistically significant compared to the L group at p<0.05. c Statistically significant compared to the SC group at p<0.05.

Table 3: Lipid hydroperoxide (LH) and total antioxidant substances (TAS) in livers of young control rats (C), young rats treated with lithium (L), aged rats (SC) and aged rats treated with lithium (SL).

analyze potential mitochondrial dysfunction and its association with oxidative stress development.

p53, Bax and Bcl2 in the liver

The liver of aged rats showed a reduction in p53 protein levels compared to the young groups (Figure 2). However, Bax protein was enhanced in the hepatic tissue of aged animals (Figure 3). The alterations in the Bax and p53 levels in the liver of aged rats were attributed to the aging effects, independent of the lithium supplementation. Lithium did not alter the liver of the young group in relation to the control group (Figure 3). Bcl 2 levels were decreased in the livers of aged animals compared to the C group. The treatment reduced Bcl2 concentration in both, aged and young livers of rats (Figure 4).

The mitochondrial dysfunction modified LH or TAS, and it could induce cell death by apoptosis. Apoptosis in hepatic tissue, represented by increased in p53 or Bax, and Bcl2 reduction ratio, could be associated with lipid profile disorders. Aged rats` livers did not present alterations in Sirt 1 in relation to the C group (Figure 5). However the lithium enhanced Sirt 1 protein in the liver (Figures 5). Sirt 1 is known as anti-aging protein, but its accumulation in the aged case indicates lower activity of this protein, and it could affect ROS enhanced or induce apoptosis in cells.

Discussion

Aging is associated with the development of metabolic disorders and liver diseases, which were triggered by the decrease of antioxidant defenses and alterations in the apoptotic process [24]. This condition promotes a progressive loss in mitochondrial function in various tissues [25]. The mitochondrial dysfunctions are responsibly by reduction in the antioxidant defenses due an increase in the production of oxidants, such as ROS [3]. However, female's rats present exhibit major mitochondrial protection when compared to male rats [15].

The choice by aged rats occurred due to decline of hepatic efficiency during aging. Aged rats presented loss of smooth-surfaced endoplasmic reticulum and therefore microsomal monooxygenases hepatics function, which could impair drugs metabolism in aged rats' livers [26]. Microsomal monooxygenases have been associated with ROS production that, on the other hands, was involved in apoptotic responses [27]. The liver is responsible by several functions, including

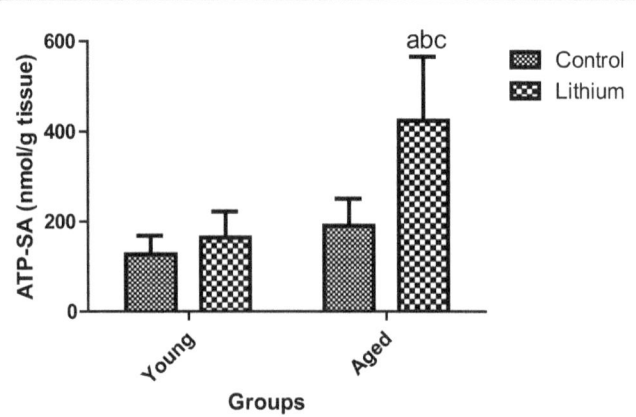

Figure 1: Increased ATP-SA in aged rats' livers treated with lithium. Values were given as the mean ± standard deviation of the mean. a Statistical analysis: two- away ANOVA. a Statistically significant compared to the C group at p<0.05. b Statistically significant compared to the L group at p<0.05. c Statistically significant compared to the SC group at p<0.05.

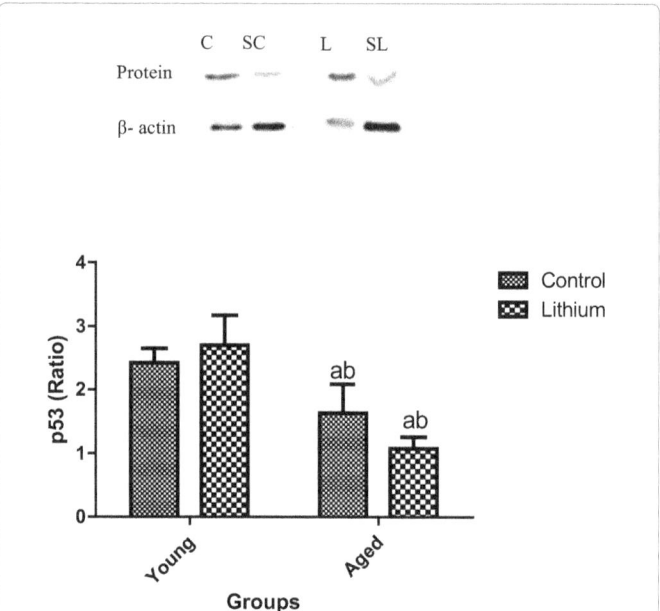

Figure 2: Reduced p53 protein ratio in aged rats' livers. Values were given as the mean ± standard deviation of the mean Statistical analysis: two- away ANOVA. a Statistically significant compared to the C group at p<0.05. b Statistically significant compared to the L group at p<0.05. c Statistically significant compared to the SC group at p<0.05.

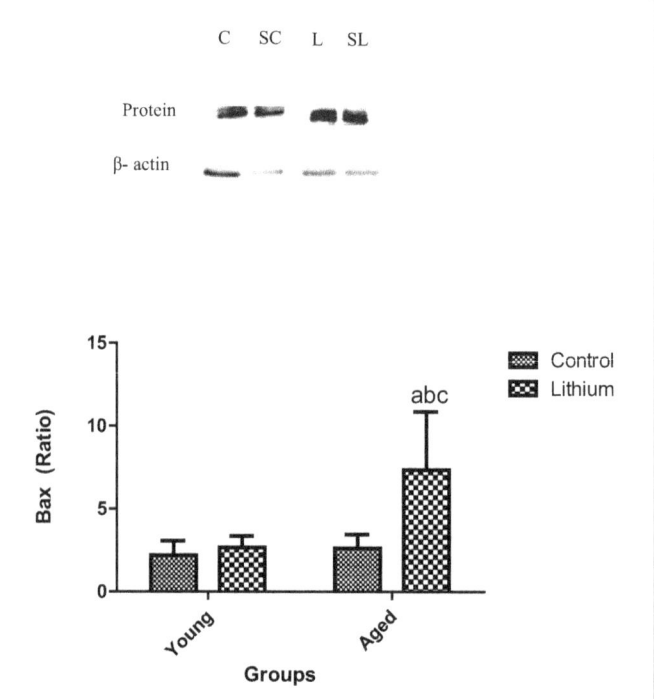

Figure 3: Increased Bax protein ratio in aged rats' livers submitted to lithium treatment. Values were given as the mean ± standard deviation of the mean Statistical analysis: two- away ANOVA. a Statistically significant compared to the C group at p<0.05. b Statistically significant compared to the L group at p<0.05. c Statistically significant compared to the SC group at p<0.05.

lipoprotein and VLDL, assembly and secretion, plasma protein synthesis, xenobiotics metabolism and more [28]. These alterations in the hepatic tissue can harm the lipid metabolism. Lithium has been

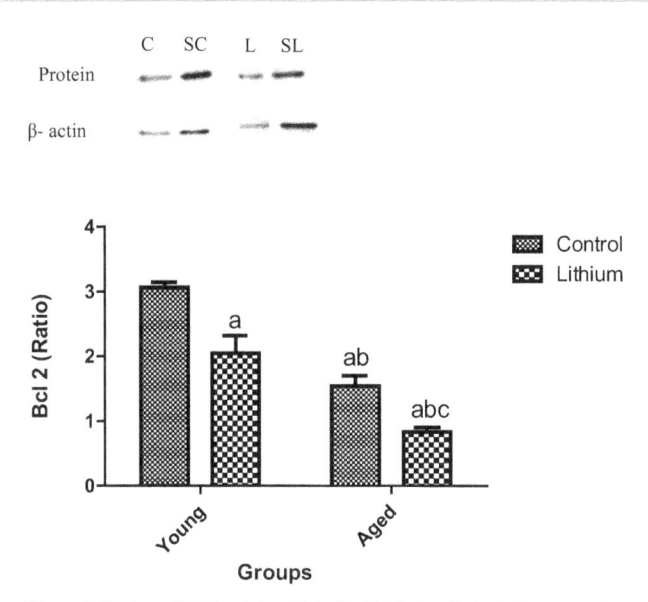

Figure 4: Reduced Bcl2 protein ratio in the liver's aged rats and young group treated with lithium. Values were given as the mean ± standard deviation of the mean Statistical analysis: two- away ANOVA. a Statistically significant compared to the C group at p<0.05. b Statistically significant compared to the L group at p<0.05. c Statistically significant compared to the SC group at p<0.05.

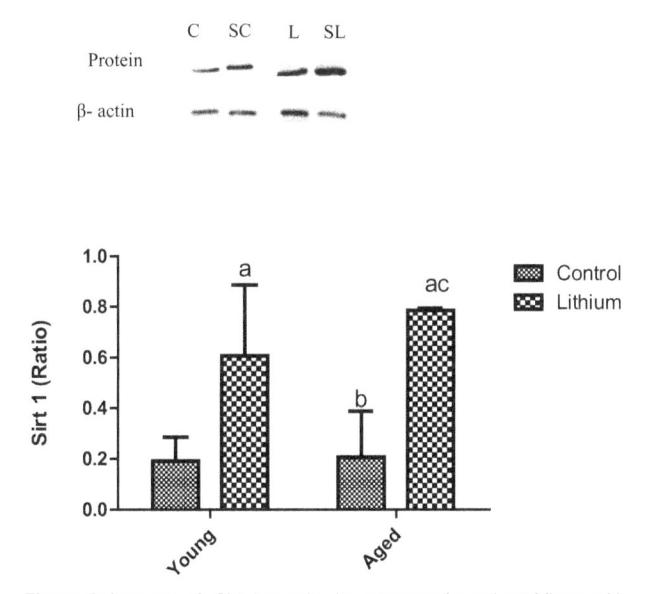

Figure 5: Increase of Sirt 1 protein in young and aged rats' livers with lithium treatment. Values were given as the mean ± standard deviation of the mean Statistical analysis: two -away ANOVA. a Statistically significant compared to the C group at p<0.05. b Statistically significant compared to the L group at p<0.05. c Statistically significant compared to the SC group at p<0.05.

emerged as a neuroprotective agent [29], but its role as a protector in aged rats' livers still has not been elucidated.

The lithium in the aged group did not promote significant differences in LH concentration; perhaps, the drug acted as an antioxidant agent [30] in the liver of the SL group. Mitochondria require oxygen to produce energy, and the deficiency or excessive generation of ROS

is associated with damage in the organelles that promote aging [31], because more oxygen is used in lipid oxidation. However, lithium could prevent excessive generation of ROS and increase LH in hepatic tissue. This fact emphasizes the increase TAS in the liver of L group, compared with the control group (Table 3); the lithium acted in the same way in the SL group. Moreover, this treatment induced the increase Sirt 1 level in the aged rats' livers involved in oxidative stress improvement (Figure 5).

It has been shown involvement of Sirt 1 protein in metabolism [32,33] by its acting in ROS reduction [34], and in the prevention of the mitochondrial damages. Sirt 1 has been determined to extend the lifespan of the cell and protect cell against injuries [35]. The raise in Sirt 1 in the liver of rats treated with lithium (L and SL), was followed by the improvement of ATP- SA only in SL group (Figures 1 and 5 respectively).

Sirt 1 has been reported to have a role in DNA repair in the aging process, blocking apoptosis cell death [36]. Nevertheless, the increasing Sirt 1 level induced by lithium was not able to prevent apoptosis in aged or young rats. This phenomenon is due to the decrease in its activity by carbonylation of this enzyme [37], altering its effect. Second Yuan et al. [38], Sirt 1 increased could cause accumulate of this protein in cell, associated with stress response during aging.

The p53 protein is known as a tumor suppressor, able to induce apoptosis by up-regulation of transcription proteins pathway [39]. However, lithium treatment did not produce p53 ratio alteration between studies groups; it could be involved in enhanced Bax ratio [40] as occurred in SL group only (Figures 2 and 3). The enhanced of Bax expression acts transactivation of this Bax in the cytosol, and induces the oligomerization of this Bax at the mitochondrial outer membrane to clearance pro-apoptotic factors [41]. In case of young rats, lithium treatment did not induce alteration of p53 and Bax ratio, but reduced Bcl 2 in a similar way to SL group (Figure 4).

The anti-apoptotic protein Bcl2 is closely associated with oxidative stress due its ability in modulates intracellular ROS concentration [42]. However, in the young rats, lithium drug acted as an antioxidant agent preventing excessive generation of ROS and apoptosis induction in young rats' livers.

The aging process can be implicated in the decline of renal function and the increase of lithium levels in blood circulation and, therefore, of the lithium elimination. These factors were responsible by increase toxicity of the drug [43], and able to induce apoptotic process development, as discussed previously. Apoptosis could be implicated in the lipid metabolism disorders presents in Table 2. Boren and Bridle [44] described the inhibition of lipogenesis enzymes and enhanced *de novo* lipid synthesis in consequences of apoptosis activation.

The treatment with lithium promoted alterations in the lipid profile of the SL group. Lithium increased TG, VLDL and LDL in the liver of SL group, compared to the SC group (Table 2). HDL, the lipoprotein responsible by reverse transport cholesterol, was reduced in this group (Table 2). The condition which TG, LDL, and VLDL increased and HDL reduced is known as dyslipidemia, a main risk factor to cardiovascular diseases development [45]; it shows higher incidence in during aging. The level of glucose was reduced in response the diminution of food consumption and energy intake after lithium administration in SL group, although the treatment did not modify animals final body weight (Tables1 and 2). This factor was related to taste aversion conditioned by lithium-induced [46], which was followed by the reduction of aqueous solution consumption, most likely due to a reduction of palatability in both, young and aged rats (Table 1). Another factor connected with the glucose reduction would be pyruvate dehydrogenase (PDH) inhibition. PDH complex act to control the balance between glucose and fatty acid substrate oxidation, with a reduction of glucose serum concentration, resulting in steatosis pathology [47], once pyruvate was used for TG formation, which is released into the blood by liver [48].

The serum of young animals submitted to lithium supplementation presented increase in glucose, TG and VLDL, and showed a reduction of total cholesterol and LDL (Table 2). The enhance of glucose level, induced by lithium in the serum of the L group, probably promoted insulin resistance [49], because this treatment may not be able to inhibit GSK3 in young animals [47]. The insulin resistance is a main disorder of diabetes pathology due ability of lower insulin response by tissues, followed by TG and VLDL enhanced in serum [50]. The TG increase was associated with a possible enhanced of non-sterified fatty acids turnover, which could occur independently of the body fat [51], explaining the absence of alterations in the L group final body (Table 1). Insulin resistance could be responsible by the increase of TG in serum due, in part by VLDL–triglyceride overproduction, secondary to increase triglyceride synthesis in the liver [51]. The higher TG concentration had been associated with large VLDL triacylglycerol-rich, which interacts with LDL. VLDL triacylglycerol -rich converts LDL in LDL-oxidized, and this fact reduced the total LDL levels [52]. Oxidized LDL are small and dense, and were not detected in method to LDL cholesterol described in this work. It was associated with a decrease of LDL and TC in young rats treated with lithium (Table 2).

In conclude, the lithium induced dyslipidemia and hyperglycemia in the young, but also acted as a possible antioxidant agent associated with Sirt 1 enhanced, to protect this tissue of damages. In the aged rats, lithium promoted dyslipidemia and could be caused cell death, however this treatment had been enhanced Sirt 1 and ATP-SA. Therefore, the supplementation with lithium may exert toxic effects in the livers of aged rats.

Acknowledgment

This article was supported by FAPESP (Fundação de Amparo à Pesquisa do Estado de São Paulo, São Paulo, Brazil).

References

1. Bartke A (2008) Insulin and aging. Cell Cycle 7: 3338-3343.

2. Hoare M, Das T, Alexander G (2010) Ageing, telomeres, senescence, and liver injury. J Hepatol 53: 950-961.

3. Lu T, Finkel T (2008) Free radicals and senescence. Exp Cell Res 314: 1918-1922.

4. HARMAN D (1956) Aging: a theory based on free radical and radiation chemistry. J Gerontol 11: 298-300.

5. Braidy N, Guillemin GJ, Mansour H, Chan-Ling T, Poljak A, et al. (2011) Age related changes in NAD+ metabolism oxidative stress and Sirt1 activity in wistar rats. PLoS One 6: e19194.

6. Novelli ELB (2005) NutriÃ§Ã £ o and healthy life. TECMED, Ribeirao Preto £ o, SÃ £ o Paulo.

7. Urano S, Sato Y, Otonari T, Makabe S, Suzuki S, et al. (1998) Aging and oxidative stress in neurodegeneration. Biofactors 7: 103-112.

8. Behl C, Moosmann B (2002) Oxidative nerve cell death in Alzheimer's disease and stroke: antioxidants as neuroprotective compounds. Biol Chem 383: 521-536.

9. Novelli EL, Souza GA, Ebaid GM, Rocha KK, Seiva FR, et al. (2010) Energy expenditure and oxygen consumption as novel biomarkers of obesity-induced cardiac disease in rats. Obesity (Silver Spring) 18: 1754-1761.

10. Diniz BS, Teixeira AL (2011) Brain-derived neurotrophic factor and Alzheimer's disease: physiopathology and beyond. Neuromolecular Med 13: 217-222.

11. Phillips ML, Travis MJ, Fagiolini A, Kupfer DJ (2008) Medication effects in neuroimaging studies of bipolar disorder. Am J Psychiatry 165: 313-320.

12. Lin D, Mok H, Yatham LN (2006) Polytherapy in bipolar disorder. CNS Drugs 20: 29-42.

13. Forlenza OV, Diniz BS, Radanovic M, Santos FS, Talib LL, et al. (2011) Disease-modifying properties of long-term lithium treatment for amnestic mild cognitive impairment: randomised controlled trial. Br J Psychiatry 198: 351-356.

14. Giles JJ, Bannigan JG (2006) Teratogenic and developmental effects of lithium. Curr Pharm Des 12: 1531-1541.

15. Borrás C, Gambini J, López-Grueso R, Pallardó FV, Viña J (2010) Direct antioxidant and protective effect of estradiol on isolated mitochondria. Biochim Biophys Acta 1802: 205-211.

16. Valdes JJ, Ramirez FM, Juarez B, Weeks OI (2010) Lithium enhances cortical mRNA expression in ovariectomized C57BL/6J mice. Acta Neurobiol Exp (Wars) 70: 288-296.

17. Rocha KK, Souza GA, Ebaid GX, Seiva FR, Cataneo AC, et al. (2009) Resveratrol toxicity: effects on risk factors for atherosclerosis and hepatic oxidative stress in standard and high-fat diets. Food Chem Toxicol 47: 1362-1367.

18. Rocha KKHR, Souza GA, Seiva FRF, Ebaid GMX, Novelli ELB (2010) Weekend ethanol consumption and high sucrose diet: resveratrol effects on energy expenditure, substrate oxidation, lipid profile, oxidative stress and hepatic energy metabolism. Pharmacology and Cell Metabolism 46: 10-16.

19. Novelli EL, Diniz YS, Galhardi CM, Ebaid GM, Rodrigues HG, et al. (2007) Anthropometrical parameters and markers of obesity in rats. Lab Anim 41: 111-119.

20. Friedewald WT, Levy RI, Fredrickson DS (1972) Estimation of the concentration of low-density lipoprotein cholesterol in plasma, without use of the preparative ultracentrifuge. Clin Chem 18: 499-502.

21. Jiang ZY, Woollard AC, Wolff SP (1991) Lipid hydroperoxide measurement by oxidation of Fe2+ in the presence of xylenol orange. Comparison with the TBA assay and an iodometric method. Lipids 26: 853-856.

22. Cheng Z, Ristow M (2013) Mitochondria and metabolic homeostasis. Antioxid Redox Signal 19: 240-242.

23. Bradford MM (1976) A rapid and sensitive method for the quantitation of microgram quantities of protein utilizing the principle of protein-dye binding. Anal Biochem 72: 248-254.

24. Lin MT, Beal MF (2006) Mitochondrial dysfunction and oxidative stress in neurodegenerative diseases. Nature 443: 787-795.

25. Rajawat YS, Hilioti Z, Bossis I (2009) Aging: central role for autophagy and the lysosomal degradative system. Ageing Res Rev 8: 199-213.

26. Schmucker DL (1998) Aging and the liver: an update. J Gerontol A Biol Sci Med Sci 53: B315-320.

27. Bhattacharyya S, Sinha K, Sil PC1 (2014) Cytochrome P450s: mechanisms and biological implications in drug metabolism and its interaction with oxidative stress. Curr Drug Metab 15: 719-742.

28. Diniz YS, Fernandes AA, Campos KE, Mani F, Ribas BO, et al. (2004) Toxicity of hypercaloric diet and monosodium glutamate: oxidative stress and metabolic shifting in hepatic tissue. Food Chem Toxicol 42: 313-319.

29. Crespo-Biel N, Camins A, Pallàs M, Canudas AM (2009) Evidence of calpain/cdk5 pathway inhibition by lithium in 3-nitropropionic acid toxicity in vivo and in vitro. Neuropharmacology 56: 422-428.

30. Machado-Vieira R, Andreazza AC, Viale CI, Zanatto V, Cereser V Jr, et al. (2007) Oxidative stress parameters in unmedicated and treated bipolar subjects during initial manic episode: a possible role for lithium antioxidant effects. Neurosci Lett 421: 33-36.

31. Wallace DC, Fan W, Procaccio V (2010) Mitochondrial energetics and therapeutics. Annu Rev Pathol 5: 297-348.

32. Kanfi Y, Naiman S, Amir G, Peshti V, Zinman G, et al. (2012) The sirtuin SIRT6 regulates lifespan in male mice. Nature 483: 218-221.

33. Houtkooper RH, Pirinen E, Auwerx J (2012) Sirtuins as regulators of metabolism and healthspan. Nat Rev Mol Cell Biol 13: 225-238.

34. Lenaz G1 (2012) Mitochondria and reactive oxygen species. Which role in physiology and pathology? Adv Exp Med Biol 942: 93-136.

35. Maiese K, Chong ZZ, Shang YC, Hou J (2011) Novel avenues of drug discovery and biomarkers for diabetes mellitus. J Clin Pharmacol 51: 128-152.

36. Audrito V, Vaisitti T, Rossi D, Gottardi D, DArena D, et al. (2011) Nicotinamide blocks proliferation and induces apoptosis of chronic lymphocytic leukemia cells through activation of the p53/miR-34a/SIRT1 tumor suppressor network. Cancer Res. 71: 4473-4483.

37. Koltai E, Szabo Z, Atalay M, Boldogh I, Naito H, et al. (2010) Exercise alters SIRT, SIRT6, NAD and NAMPT levels in skeletal muscle of aged rats. Mech Ageing Dev 131: 21-28.

38. Yuan Z, Zhang X, Sengupta N, Lane WS, Seto E (2007) SIRT1 regulates the function of the Nijmegen breakage syndrome protein. Mol Cell 27: 149-162.

39. Green DR, Kroemer G (2009) Cytoplasmic functions of the tumour suppressor p53. Nature 458: 1127-1130.

40. Miyashita T, Reed JC (1995) Tumor suppressor p53 is a direct transcriptional activator of the human bax gene. Cell 80: 293-299.

41. Chipuk JE, Kuwana T, Bouchier-Hayes L, Droin NM, Newmeyer DD, et al. (2004) Direct activation of Bax by p53 mediates mitochondrial membrane permeabilization and apoptosis. Science 303: 1010-1014.

42. Kowaltowski AJ, Cosso RG, Campos CB, Fiskum G (2002) Effect of Bcl-2 overexpression on mitochondrial structure and function. J Biol Chem 277: 42802-42807.

43. Gyulai L, Young RC (2008) New research perspectives in the treatment of bipolar disorder in older adults. Bipolar Disord 10: 659-661.

44. Boren J, Brindle KM (2012) Apoptosis-induced mitochondrial dysfunction causes cytoplasmic lipid droplet formation. Cell Death Differ 19: 1561-1570.

45. Chapman MJ, Ginsberg HN, Amarenco P, Andreotti F, Borén J, et al. (2011) Triglyceride-rich lipoproteins and high-density lipoprotein cholesterol in patients at high risk of cardiovascular disease: evidence and guidance for management. Eur Heart J 32: 1345-1361.

46. Kim KN, Kim BT, Kim YS, Lee JH, Jahng JW5 (2014) Increase of glucocorticoids is not required for the acquisition, but hinders the extinction, of lithium-induced conditioned taste aversion. Eur J Pharmacol 730: 14-19.

47. Jones HB, Reens J, Johnson E, Brocklehurst S, Slater I (2014) Myocardial steatosis and necrosis in atria and ventricles of rats givem pyruvate dehydrogenase kinase inhibitors. Toxicologic Pathology 20: 1-17.

48. Jope RS (2003) Lithium and GSK-3: one inhibitor, two inhibitory actions, multiple outcomes. Trends Pharmacol Sci 24: 441-443.

49. Henriksen EJ (2010) Dysregulation of glycogen synthase kinase-3 in skeletal muscle and the etiology of insulin resistance and type 2 diabetes. Curr Diabetes Rev 6: 285-293.

50. Choi SH, Ginsberg HN (2011) Increased very low density lipoprotein (VLDL) secretion, hepatic steatosis, and insulin resistance. Trends Endocrinol Metab 22: 353-363.

51. Mostaza JM, Vega GL, Snell P, Grundy SM (1998) Abnormal metabolism of free fatty acids in hypertriglyceridaemic men: apparent insulin resistance of adipose tissue. J Intern Med 243: 265-274.

52. Bloomgarden ZT (2004) Type 2 diabetes in the young: the evolving epidemic. Diabetes Care 27: 998-1010.

15

Nuclear Factor Erythroid 2-Related Factor 2 is Activated by Rosuvastatin via p21^{cip1} Upregulation in Endothelial Cells

Chieko Ihoriya, Minoru Satoh*, Norio Komai, Tamaki Sasaki and Naoki Kashihara

Department of Nephrology and Hypertension, Kawasaki Medical School, Kurashiki, Okayama, Japan

Abstract

Oxidative stress is a key component in the development of cardiovascular diseases and chronic kidney diseases. Statins have cardio-protective activity, and previous reports have indicated that they activate nuclear factor erythroid 2-related factor 2 (Nrf2), although their molecular mechanism is unknown. Nrf2 is an oxidative stress-responsive transcription factor with a crucial role in cellular defense against oxidative stress. We investigated the molecular mechanisms of Nrf2 activation by rosuvastatin. Nrf2 activity and Nrf2-mediated antioxidant gene expression were upregulated by rosuvastatin in human umbilical vein endothelial cells. Rosuvastatin increased Nrf2 protein levels by reducing Nrf2 degradation and upregulating the interaction between Nrf2 and p21^{Cip1}, which was inhibited by p21^{Cip1}-targeted siRNA. Rosuvastatin-mediated activation of endothelial Nrf2 provides a possible therapeutic alternative for cardiovascular diseases.

Keywords: Endothelial cell; p21^{Cip1}; Nrf2; Statin; Oxidative stress

Abbreviations: Nrf2: Nuclear Factor Erythroid 2-related Factor 2; Keap1: Kelch-like ECH-Associated Protein 1; ARE: Antioxidant Responsive Element; SOD: Superoxide Dismutase; NQO1: NAD(P)H:quinone Oxidoreductase-1; HO-1: Heme Oxygenase-1; GCLM: Glutamate-Cysteine Ligase Modulatory Subunit; Statins: 3-hydroxy-3-methyl-glutaryl-CoA reductase inhibitors; HUVECs: Human Umbilical Vein Endothelial Cells; RSV: Rosuvastatin

Introduction

The nuclear factor erythroid 2-related factor 2 (Nrf2) is an important oxidative stress-responsive transcription factor, which has a vital role in combating oxidative damage [1]. Upon activation, it becomes free from cytoplasmic sequestering and negative regulation by Kelch-like ECH-associated protein 1 (Keap1), resulting in nuclear accumulation and transactivation of a vast array of cytoprotective genes through the cognate antioxidant responsive element (ARE) [2]. Nrf2 plays a critical role in the basal activity and coordinated induction of genes encoding numerous antioxidant and phase II detoxifying enzymes, including superoxide dismutase (SOD), NAD(P)H:quinone oxidoreductase-1 (NQO1), heme oxygenase-1 (HO-1), glutamate-cysteine ligase modulatory (GCLM) subunit, and thioredoxin, among others [3,4]. Therefore, targeting the coordinated upregulation of genes coding for detoxifying proteins, antioxidants, and anti-inflammatory regulators may be a potential therapeutic strategy to protect against insults such as inflammation and oxidative stress [5]. Indeed, targeting antioxidant defenses through modulation of Nrf2 could represent a new therapeutic approach with potentially major advances over conventional therapies [6].

In many clinical trials, 3-hydroxy-3-methyl-glutaryl-CoA reductase inhibitors (statins) have shown clear benefits in cardiovascular disease beyond their lipid-lowering actions [7], as they also function as antioxidants [8]. Statins not only decrease cellular reactive oxygen species production but also enhance the antioxidant response by upregulating the expression of many antioxidants [9]. Makabe et al. reported that fluvastatin protects vascular smooth muscle cells from oxidative stress through the Nrf2-dependent antioxidant pathway [10], although the molecular mechanism is unknown. The aim of this study was to identify the molecular mechanisms of Nrf2 activation by rosuvastatin (RSV).

Materials and Methods

Cell culture and transfection

Primary human umbilical vein endothelial cells (HUVECs; Cell System, Kirkland, WA, USA) were cultured in endothelial cell basal medium-2 (Lonza, Walkersville, MD, USA) containing 5% (v/v) fetal bovine serum under humidified conditions (95% air, 5% CO_2) at 37 °C. Subconfluent cells between passages 7 and 10 were used in the experiments. These cells were divided into four groups: 5.5 mM D-Glucose (Glu) + 22 mM L-Glu (normal glucose), normal glucose + 0.1, 1.0, or 10 μM RSV (RSV), 5.5 mM D-Glu + 22 mM D-Glu (high glucose), and high glucose + RSV. RSV was provided by AstraZeneca (London, UK). The dosage of RSV for the cells was in accordance to previous studies [11,12]. The cells were incubated at 37 °C for 6 to 24 h (6 h for RNA isolation and nuclear protein preparation and 24 h for total protein preparation). Cos-7 cells (Health Protection Agency Culture Collections, Salisbury, UK) were used for the luciferase assays. Cells were cultured to 70% to 80% confluence and were transfected with 50 nmol/L p21^{Cip1}-siRNA (sc-29427; Santa Cruz Biotechnology, Dallas, TX, USA) or control-siRNA for 24 h by using Lipofectamine 2000 (Life Technology, Grand Island, NY, USA) according to the manufacturer's protocol. The extent of knockdown was assessed by western blotting.

Nrf2 reporter assay

Since transfection efficiency was low in HUVECs, we used monkey african green kidney fibroblast-like (Cos-7) cells (Health Protection Agency Culture Collections, Salisbry, UK) for the luciferase assay. Cos-7 cells were cultured with Dulbecco's Modified Eagle's

*Corresponding author: Minoru Satoh, Department of Nephrology and Hypertension, Kawasaki Medical School, 577 Matsushima, Kurashiki, Okayama 701-0192, Japan, E-mail: msatoh@med.kawasaki-m.ac.jp

Medium (Sigma-Aldrich Japan, Tokyo, Japan) containing 5% fetal bovine serum. Subconfluent cells were co-transfected with a reporter construct containing a human ARE-driven luciferase construct and a Renilla luciferase reporter as an internal control. After transfection, the cells were pretreated with RSV for 24 h. The cells were harvested, washed, homogenized, and analyzed for luciferase activity. The dual luciferase reporter assay system (Promega, Madison, WI, USA) and a luminometer (MimiLumat LB9506, Berthold Technology, Bad Wildbad, and Germany) were used to measure luciferase activity, according to the manufacturer's protocols.

mRNA stability assay

The mRNA stability of NQO1 and GCLM was determined by actinomycin D chase experiments. HUVECs were cultured under high glucose conditions for 24 h. At time 0, medium was exchanged with medium containing 1.0 μg/mL actinomycin D plus RSV or vehicle. RNA samples were prepared from RSV-treated and untreated cells in triplicate at 0, 1, 3, and 6 h. Quantitative real-time polymerase chain reaction (qPCR) of NQO1 and GCLM was performed as described below.

Cycloheximide chase assay for Nrf2 degradation/protein half-life analysis

After 24-h starvation, HUVECs were treated with 10 μM RSV for 6 h in a high glucose medium, and then harvested at 0, 15, 30, or 60 min after the addition of cycloheximide (25 μg/mL). Lysates from cycloheximide-treated cells were analyzed by western blotting.

RNA isolation and qPCR

Total RNA was extracted with TRIzol (Life Technology). Reverse transcriptase reactions were performed by using the ReverTra Ace qPCR RT Kit (Toyobo Biosciences, Osaka, Japan) for first-strand cDNA synthesis. qPCR was performed by using ABI Prism 7500 sequence-detection system (Applied Biosystems, Foster City, CA, USA). Primers and probes for TaqMan analysis were designed by Primer Express 1.5 (Applied Biosystems) by using information from the supplier based on the sequence information from GenBank or EST databases. The primers and probes used for NQO1, GCLM, and p21^{Cip1} are next: NQO1 (NM_008706) Forward, 5'- ttctctggccgattcagagt -3'; Reverse, 5'- tccagacgtttcttccatcc -3'; Probe, FAM -5'- tttacagcattggccacactccacc -3'- TAMRA. GCLM (NM_008129) Forward, 5'- caatgacccgaaagaactgc -3'; Reverse, 5'- attccctgctcttcacgat -3'; Probe, FAM-5'-attccctgctcttcacgat -3'-TAMRA. p21^{Cip1} (NM_007669) Forward, 5'-ttgcactctggtgtctgagc -3'; Reverse, 5'- tctgcgcttggagtgataga -3'; Probe, FAM -5' - aaacggaggcagaccagcctgac -3' - TAMRA. For each gene, 10 ng of cDNA was analyzed on an ABI PRISM 7500 by using the TaqMan Universal PCR Master Mix (Applied Biosystems). A standard curve was prepared from a positive control with known concentrations, and the copy numbers of 18S and the target genes were calculated. The relative ratios of target gene to 18S are shown as a bar graph. Fold change analysis was based on standardizing RNA levels by correcting for 18S levels in the sample.

Western blot analysis

Extraction of total cellular proteins and nuclear proteins was performed by using an extraction reagent (T-PER tissue protein extraction reagent, NE-PER nuclear and cytoplasmic extraction kit; Thermo Fisher Scientific, Rockford, IL, USA), according to the manufacturer's instructions. For immunoprecipitation assays, cells were lysed in radioimmunoprecipitation assay buffer (10 mM sodium phosphate, 150 mM NaCl, 1% Triton X-100, 1% sodium deoxycholate, and 0.1% sodium dodecyl sulfate SDS) in the presence of 1 mM dithiothreitol, 1 mM phenylmethanesulfonylfluoride, and a protease inhibitor cocktail (Roche Diagnostics, Indianapolis, IN, USA). For the analysis of Nrf2 expression, the proteasome inhibitor MG132 (10 μM; Sigma-Aldrich Japan) was added to the extraction buffer to avoid Nrf2 protein degradation. Cultured cells were homogenized on ice in 1.0 mL of lysis buffer containing protease inhibitors and centrifuged at 8000 g for 10 min. The protein concentration in the supernatants was determined with a Bio-Rad protein assay kit (Hercules, CA, USA). SDS-polyacrylamide gel electrophoresis was performed using cell lysates (20 μg/lane). Anti-Nrf2 (Cell Signaling Technology, Beverly, MA, USA), anti-p21^{Cip1} (Cell Signaling Technology), anti-Lamin A/C (Santa Cruz Biotechnology), anti-GAPDH (Santa Cruz Biotechnology), and anti-actin (Sigma-Aldrich Japan) antibodies were used as the primary antibodies. For immunoprecipitation assays, cell lysates were incubated with anti-p21^{Cip1} antibody and Protein A/G PLUS-Agarose (Santa Cruz Biotechnology) for overnight at 4 ℃. After washing the protein A/G agarose beads complex, proteins were extracted with SDS buffer and proceed to western-blot for Nrf2 or p21^{Cip1}. Signals were detected by using the ECL or ECL plus system (Amersham Biosciences, Piscataway, NJ, USA). The relative optical band densities were quantified by ImageJ analysis software V1.48 [13].

Statistical analyses

Data were expressed as mean ± standard error of mean (SEM). All variables were evaluated by two-tailed unpaired Student's t-test or one-way analysis of variance for comparison of multiple means. A p value < 0.05 was considered significant.

Results

RSV activates Nrf2

To determine whether RSV influences the ARE-Nrf2 pathway, we used an ARE-luciferase reporter assay in Cos-7 cells. ARE-luciferase activity was significantly higher in high glucose treated cells than in normal glucose conditions without RSV (Figure 1A). RSV increased ARE-luciferase activity under normal and high glucose conditions (Figure 1A). We then examined whether RSV increases nuclear translocation of Nrf2 protein in HUVECs. As shown in Figure 1B, rosuvastatin produced a marked increase in Nrf2 translocation into the nucleus under normal and high glucose conditions.

RSV increases Nrf2-targeted gene expression

Nrf2-targeted gene expression was evaluated by qPCR. RSV produced a dose-dependent increase in NQO1 and GCLM mRNA expression under normal and high glucose conditions (Figure 2A,2B). To examine the cause of this Nrf2-dependent induction, we assessed mRNA stability by actinomycin D chase experiments. RSV did not affect NQO1 and GCLM mRNA stability (Figure 2C, 2D).

RSV increases p21^{Cip1}-Nrf2 protein complex formation

It has been reported that p21^{Cip1} activates Nrf2 by stabilizing Nrf2 protein [14]. To elucidate the mechanisms of Nrf2 activation by RSV, we examined p21^{Cip1} expression. As shown in Figure 3A, RSV treatment produced a dose-dependent increase in p21^{Cip1} mRNA under normal and high glucose conditions. p21^{Cip1} protein expression also increased in the presence of RSV (Figure 3B). The interaction between endogenous Nrf2 and p21^{Cip1} was assessed in RSV-treated HUVECs. As shown in Figure 3C, p21^{Cip1} protein formed a complex with Nrf2.

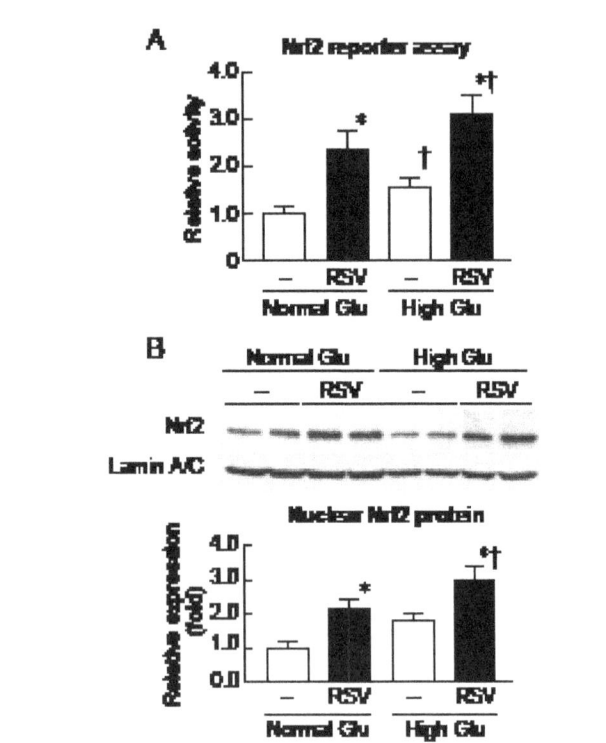

Figure 1: Nuclear factor erythroid 2-related factor 2 (Nrf2) activation by statins (A) Antioxidant response element-luciferase activity after 24 h incubation with 10 μM rosuvastatin (RSV) in Cos-7 cells in the presence of normal Glu (5.5 mM D-Glu + 22 mM L-Glu) or high Glu (5.5 mM D-Glu + 22 mM D-Glu). Data are expressed as mean ± standard error of mean (SEM). $^*p < 0.05$ vs. RSV (-), $^†p < 0.05$ as compared with normal Glu. (B) Nuclear translocation of Nrf2 following 24 h treatment with 10 μM in human umbilical vein endothelial cells (HUVECs) in the presence of normal Glu or high Glu. Data are expressed as mean ± SEM. $^*p < 0.05$ compared with RSV (-), $^†p < 0.05$ vs. normal Glu.

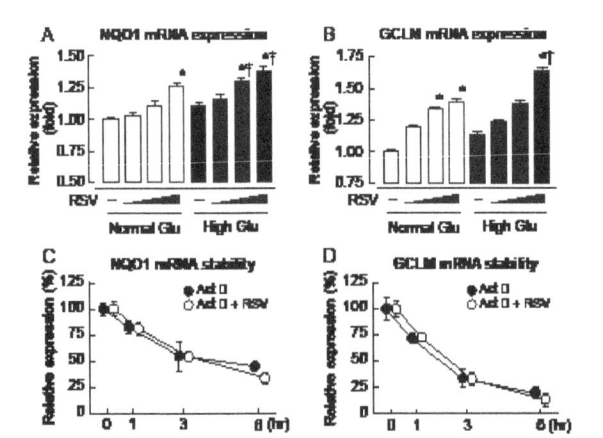

Figure 2: Nuclear factor erythroid 2-related factor 2 (Nrf2)-dependent target gene expression by rosuvastatin. NAD(P)H:quinone oxidoreductase-1 (NQO1) mRNA expression (A) and glutamate-cysteine ligase modulatory (GCLM) mRNA expression (B) after 24 h of rosuvastatin (RSV; 0.1, 1.0, 10 μM) treatment in human umbilical vein endothelial cells (HUVECs) in the presence of normal Glu (5.5 mM D-Glu + 22 mM L-Glu) or high Glu (5.5 mM D-Glu + 22 mM D-Glu). Data are expressed as mean ± standard error of mean (SEM). $^*p < 0.05$ vs. RSV (-), $^†p < 0.05$ vs. normal Glu. mRNA stability of NQO1 (C) and GCLM (D) after treatment with 10 μM RSV in the presence of normal Glu, assessed in HUVECs by using 1.0 μg/mL actinomycin D (Act D) chase assays.

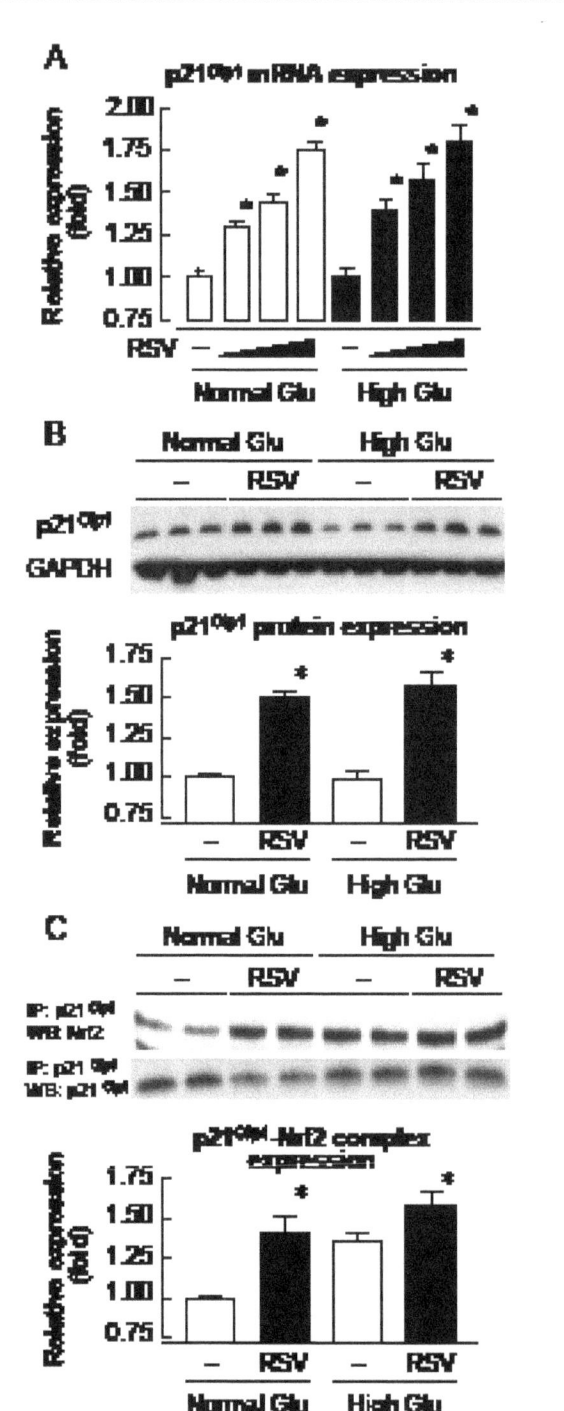

Figure 3: p21^{Cip1} expression by statins (A) p21^{Cip1} mRNA expression in human umbilical vein endothelial cells (HUVECs) after a 24 h treatment with rosuvastatin (RSV; 0.1, 1.0, 10 μM) in the presence of normal Glu (5.5 mM D-Glu + 22 mM L-Glu) or high Glu (5.5 mM D-Glu + 22 mM D-Glu). Data are expressed as the mean ± standard error of mean (SEM). $^*p < 0.05$ vs. RSV (-). (B) p21^{Cip1} protein expression in HUVECs after 24 h RSV treatment (10 μM) in the presence of normal Glu or high Glu. Data are expressed as the mean ± SEM. $^*p < 0.05$ vs. RSV (-). (C) Interaction with p21^{Cip1} and Nrf2 in HUVECs 24 h after treatment with 10 μM RSV in the presence of normal Glu or high Glu. $^*p < 0.05$ vs. RSV (-).

Furthermore, binding of endogenous p21^{Cip1} to Nrf2 was enhanced by RSV under normal and high glucose conditions.

RSV increases Nrf2 protein stability

To examine the role of p21^{Cip1} in Nrf2 activation, we examined Nrf2 protein stability in p21^{Cip1} siRNA knockdown HUVECs. p21^{Cip1} protein expression was significantly reduced by transient transfection with p21^{Cip1} siRNA versus control siRNA (Figure 4A). Nrf2 protein expression was increased by RSV in control cells but was not altered in p21^{Cip1} knockdown cells (Figure 4B). To assess the Nrf2 protein stability, a cycloheximide chase-based assay was conducted in p21^{Cip1} siRNA-transfected cells. RSV prolonged the Nrf2 half-life in control siRNA-transfected cells but did not affect the half-life of Nrf2 in p21^{Cip1} knockdown cells (Figure 4C).

Discussion

The aim of this study was to identify the molecular mechanisms of Nrf2 activation by RSV. We demonstrated that RSV activates the transcription factor Nrf2 in endothelial cells, thereby enhancing Nrf2-dependent anti-oxidant genes. To our knowledge, these findings are the first reported evidence that RSV exerts its antioxidant effect through the Nrf2/ARE pathway in endothelial cells.

We have shown that p21^{Cip1} upregulation by RSV increased Nrf2 protein levels in HUVECs. Under non-stressed conditions, Nrf2 is negatively regulated by Keap1. Nrf2 is polyubiquitinated by the Keap1-Cul3 E3 ligase, and degraded by the 26S proteasome. Some electrophiles and oxidants oxidize the cysteine thiols of Keap1 and activate Nrf2 [15]. Recent reports have indicated that p21^{Cip1} directly upregulates Nrf2 protein levels [14]. These interactions have been mapped to the DLG and ETGE motifs in Nrf2 and the KRR motif in p21^{Cip1}, which directly activates the Nrf2 pathway by competing with Keap1 for Nrf2 binding, thereby inhibiting Keap1-dependent ubiquitination of Nrf2 [14]. p21^{Cip1} regulates various cellular processes such as cell-cycle arrest, DNA replication and repair, cell differentiation, senescence, and apoptosis. We showed that RSV upregulates p21^{Cip1} expression in HUVECs, prolonging Nrf2 protein stability and activating the Nrf2/ARE pathway.

We confirmed that RSV activates the Nrf2/ARE pathway and enhances NQO1 and GCLM expression in endothelial cells. Some reports have suggested NQO1 activation is beneficial for the treatment of the metabolic syndrome by ameliorating obesity, preventing arterial smooth muscle cell proliferation, and mitigating spontaneous hypertension in animal models [16-18]. Other Nrf2-dependent antioxidants include heme oxygenase 1 (HO-1) and superoxide dismutase (SOD) [19]. Pharmacological inhibition of HO activity or deletion of the HO-1 gene worsens renal injury induced by toxic substances [20,21], ischemia reperfusion and diabetes [22]. SOD is the major antioxidant enzyme that removes superoxide, converting superoxide into hydrogen peroxide and molecular oxygen [23,24]. Thus, RSV may protect against cardiovascular diseases, including kidney diseases, through the upregulation of NQO1, HO-1, and SOD expression via Nrf2 activation.

RSV is a potent inhibitor of cholesterol biosynthesis and is used as a cholesterol-lowering drug [25]. Previous studies show that statins, including RSV, possess powerful pleiotropic effects that are independent of their effects on lipids and lipoproteins [26,27]. Recent reports have indicated that other statins also upregulate p21^{Cip1} expression [28,29], which mediates Nrf2 activation. Thus, we assume that other statins may

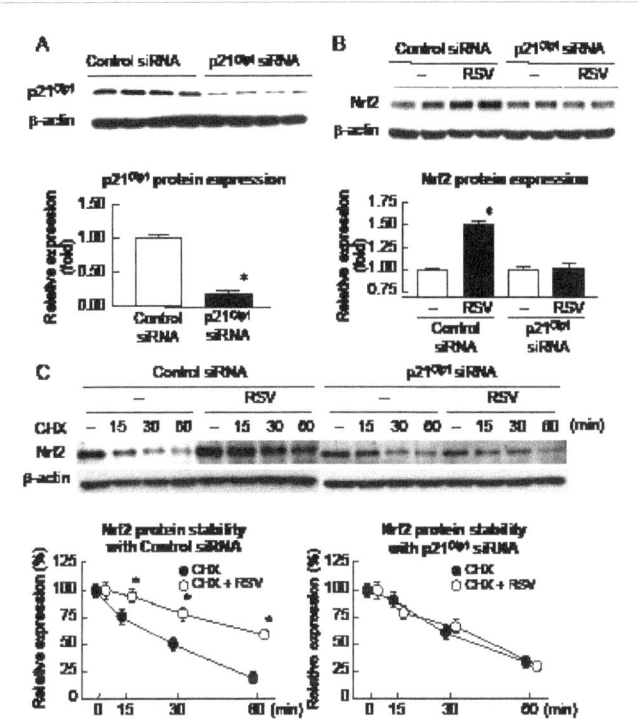

Figure 4: p21^{Cip1} enhances nuclear factor erythroid 2-related factor 2 (Nrf2) protein stability. (A) Western blot analysis of extracts from in human umbilical vein endothelial cells (HUVECs) transfected with control or p21^{Cip1} siRNA. $^*p <$ 0.05 vs. control siRNA. (B) p21^{Cip1} protein expression in HUVECS transfected with control or p21^{Cip1} siRNA following 24 h treatment with 10 μM rosuvastatin (RSV). Data are expressed as the mean ± standard error of mean (SEM). $^*p <$ 0.05 vs. RSV (-). (C) Nrf2 protein stability assessed using 25 μg/mL cycloheximide (CHX) chase-based assay. Data are expressed as the mean ± SEM. $^*p <$ 0.05 vs. RSV (-).

also activate the Nrf2/ARE pathway, contributing to their pleiotropic effects, including decreasing oxidative stress and inflammation.

In conclusion, we showed that the anti-oxidant effects of RSV include the amplification of antioxidant potential through Nrf2 activation. Numerous reports have previously described the vascular protective mechanisms of statins; however, this is the first report to suggest that statins activate Nrf2 via p21^{Cip1} upregulation. Oxidative stress is the basis of morbidity in many cardiovascular diseases, including chronic kidney disease, and statin treatment may be a useful therapeutic strategy to enhance anti-oxidative capacity.

Acknowledgement

We would like to thank Ms. Etsuko Yorimasa, Ms. Makoto Moriya, Ms. Miyuki Yokohata, Ms. Keiko Satoh, and Ms. Satomi Hanada (Kawasaki Medical School) for animal care and technical assistance. This work was supported by Grants-in-Aid for Scientific Research from the Japan Society for the Promotion of Science (No. 23591209 to N.K., No. 24390218 to N.K.), and a Research Project Grant from Kawasaki Medical School (No. 25Ki-70 to C.I.).

References

1. Gan L, Johnson JA (2014) Oxidative damage and the Nrf2-ARE pathway in neurodegenerative diseases. Biochim Biophys Acta 1842: 1208-1218.

2. Kensler TW, Wakabayashi N, Biswal S (2007) Cell survival responses to environmental stresses via the Keap1-Nrf2-ARE pathway. Annu Rev Pharmacol Toxicol 47: 89-116.

3. Kim HJ, Vaziri ND (2010) Contribution of impaired Nrf2-Keap1 pathway to oxidative stress and inflammation in chronic renal failure. Am J Physiol Renal Physiol 298: F662-671.

4. Surh YJ, Kundu JK, Na HK (2008) Nrf2 as a master redox switch in turning on the cellular signaling involved in the induction of cytoprotective genes by some chemopreventive phytochemicals. Planta Med 74: 1526-1539.

5. de Haan JB (2011) Nrf2 activators as attractive therapeutics for diabetic nephropathy. Diabetes 60: 2683-2684.

6. Jung KA, Kwak MK (2010) The Nrf2 system as a potential target for the development of indirect antioxidants. Molecules 15: 7266-7291.

7. Zhou Q, Liao JK (2010) Pleiotropic effects of statins. - Basic research and clinical perspectives. Circ J 74: 818-826.

8. Wassmann S, Laufs U, Müller K, Konkol C, Ahlbory K, et al. (2002) Cellular antioxidant effects of atorvastatin in vitro and in vivo. Arterioscler Thromb Vasc Biol 22: 300-305.

9. Haendeler J, Hoffmann J, Zeiher AM, Dimmeler S (2004) Antioxidant effects of statins via S-nitrosylation and activation of thioredoxin in endothelial cells: a novel vasculoprotective function of statins. Circulation 110: 856-861.

10. Makabe S, Takahashi Y, Watanabe H, Murakami M, Ohba T, et al. (2010) Fluvastatin protects vascular smooth muscle cells against oxidative stress through the Nrf2-dependent antioxidant pathway. Atherosclerosis 213: 377-384.

11. Marchesi M, Parolini C, Caligari S, Gilio D, Manzini S, et al. (2011) Rosuvastatin does not affect human apolipoprotein A-I expression in genetically modified mice: a clue to the disputed effect of statins on HDL. Br J Pharmacol 164: 1460-1468.

12. Pignatelli P, Carnevale R, Di Santo S, Bartimoccia S, Nocella C, et al. (2012) Rosuvastatin reduces platelet recruitment by inhibiting NADPH oxidase activation. Biochem Pharmacol 84: 1635-1642.

13. Rasband WS (1997-2014) Imagej. U S National Institutes of Health, Bethesda, Maryland, USA.

14. Chen W, Sun Z, Wang XJ, Jiang T, Huang Z, et al. (2009) Direct interaction between Nrf2 and p21(Cip1/WAF1) upregulates the Nrf2-mediated antioxidant response. Mol Cell 34: 663-673.

15. Dinkova-Kostova AT, Holtzclaw WD, Cole RN, Itoh K, Wakabayashi N, et al. (2002) Direct evidence that sulfhydryl groups of Keap1 are the sensors regulating induction of phase 2 enzymes that protect against carcinogens and oxidants. Proc Natl Acad Sci U S A 99: 11908-11913.

16. Hwang JH, Kim DW, Jo EJ, Kim YK, Jo YS, et al. (2009) Pharmacological stimulation of NADH oxidation ameliorates obesity and related phenotypes in mice. Diabetes 58: 965-974.

17. Kim SY, Jeoung NH, Oh CJ, Choi YK, Lee HJ, et al. (2009) Activation of NAD(P)H:quinone oxidoreductase 1 prevents arterial restenosis by suppressing vascular smooth muscle cell proliferation. Circ Res 104: 842-850.

18. Kim YH, Hwang JH, Noh JR, Gang GT, Tadi S, et al. (2012) Prevention of salt-induced renal injury by activation of NAD(P)H:quinone oxidoreductase , associated with NADPH oxidase. Free Radic Biol Med 52: 880-888.

19. Huang XS, Chen HP, Yu HH, Yan YF, Liao ZP, et al. (2014) Nrf2-dependent upregulation of antioxidative enzymes: a novel pathway for hypoxic preconditioning-mediated delayed cardioprotection. Mol Cell Biochem 385: 33-41.

20. Shiraishi F, Curtis LM, Truong L, Poss K, Visner GA, et al. (2000) Heme oxygenase-1 gene ablation or expression modulates cisplatin-induced renal tubular apoptosis. Am J Physiol Renal Physiol 278: F726-736.

21. Lemos FB, Ijzermans JN, Zondervan PE, Peeters AM, van den Engel S, et al. (2003) Differential expression of heme oxygenase-1 and vascular endothelial growth factor in cadaveric and living donor kidneys after ischemia-reperfusion. J Am Soc Nephrol 14: 3278-3287.

22. Ptilovanciv EO, Fernandes GS, Teixeira LC, Reis LA, Pessoa EA, et al. (2013) Heme oxygenase 1 improves glucoses metabolism and kidney histological alterations in diabetic rats. Diabetol Metab Syndr 5: 3.

23. Fridovich I (1997) Superoxide anion radical (O2-.), superoxide dismutases, and related matters. J Biol Chem 272: 18515-18517.

24. Batinic-Haberle I, Tovmasyan A, Roberts ER, Vujaskovic Z, Leong KW, et al. (2014) SOD therapeutics: latest insights into their structure-activity relationships and impact on the cellular redox-based signaling pathways. Antioxid Redox Signal 20: 2372-2415.

25. McTaggart F, Buckett L, Davidson R, Holdgate G, McCormick A, et al. (2001) Preclinical and clinical pharmacology of Rosuvastatin, a new 3-hydroxy-3-methylglutaryl coenzyme A reductase inhibitor. Am J Cardiol 87: 28B-32B.

26. Rikitake Y, Liao JK (2005) Rho GTPases, statins, and nitric oxide. Circ Res 97: 1232-1235.

27. Tanaka S, Fukumoto Y, Nochioka K, Minami T, Kudo S, et al. (2013) Statins exert the pleiotropic effects through small GTP-binding protein dissociation stimulator upregulation with a resultant Rac1 degradation. Arterioscler Thromb Vasc Biol 33: 1591-1600.

28. Li M, Liu Y, Shi H, Zhang Y, Wang G, et al. (2012) Statins inhibit pulmonary artery smooth muscle cell proliferation by upregulation of HO-1 and p21WAF1. Naunyn Schmiedebergs Arch Pharmacol 385: 961-968.

29. Klein S, Klösel J, Schierwagen R, Körner C, Granzow M, et al. (2012) Atorvastatin inhibits proliferation and apoptosis, but induces senescence in hepatic myofibroblasts and thereby attenuates hepatic fibrosis in rats. Lab Invest 92: 1440-1450.

16

Oral Intake of Krill Oil has Prophylactic and Potential Therapeutic Effects on Alcoholic Fatty Liver in Rats Fed with High-Fat Diet

Hong-ling Wang[1*], Mao-wu Guo[1], Qin Liao[1], Hui Wang[1*], Wei-juan Zhang[1*], Yun-xia Sun[1], Li Han[2*], Tomoko Tsuji[2] and Conglin Zuo[1*]

[1]Beijing Key Laboratory of Bio-products Safety Assessment, JOINN Laboratories, Beijing, China
[2]Nippon Suisan Kaisha, Ltd., Tokyo, Japan

Abstract

Aim: The objective of this study was to evaluate the prophylactic and therapeutic effects of Krill Oil on alcohol induced fatty liver in rats on high-fat diet.

Methods: Male Sprague-Dawley rats (7-8 weeks old) were gavaged with alcohol and fed with high-fat diet for six weeks to induce alcoholic fatty liver. The concentration of the alcohol formulation had a step increase to have the animal acclimated, with 8% in week 1, 12% in week 2, 20% in week 3, 30% in week 4, and 40% alcohol in the following weeks, and the dose volume was 10 ml/kg. Krill oil at daily oral dose of 10, 100 or 1000 mg/kg was given to animals along with alcohol gavage in a prophylactic experiment, or at 100 and 1000 mg/kg after six weeks of alcohol gavage in a therapeutic experiment, with or without continuing oral gavage of alcohol for four weeks. Blood samples and liver tissues were taken for triglyceride and total cholesterol assays, liver tissues were taken for microarray analysis and histopathological evaluation of hepatosteatosis at the end of the treatment.

Results: Krill Oil dose-dependently inhibited the elevation of liver triglyceride level from 17. 8% to 66.3% compared with control, and the incidence and severity of liver cytoplasmic vacuolization. In the therapeutic experiment, Krill Oil group showed an accelerated reduction of liver tissue triglyceride level and incidence and severity of liver cytoplasmic vacuolization. Krill Oil also reversed the elevated liver tissue triglyceride and the elevated incidence and severity of liver cytoplasmic vacuolization in rats which had been given alcohol for ten weeks with Krill Oil treatment initiated at the beginning of week 7.

Conclusion: Our results suggest that Krill Oil supplementation not only has prophylactic effects on alcoholic fatty liver formation, but also has potential therapeutic effects on the alcoholic fatty liver.

Keywords: Alcoholic fatty liver; Krill Oil (KO); Rat; Polyunsaturated fatty acids (PUFA); Histopathology

Introduction

Chronic and excessive alcohol consumption is a major cause of fatty liver, which is a problem in health care [1]. It is also classified as alcoholic fatty liver, an early stage of alcoholic liver disease (ALD) [2]. Over 60% heavy drinkers will develop fatty liver [3] and, if left untreated, the fatty liver will gradually aggravate and progress with high likelihood to more serious diseases, i.e. steatohepatitis, fibrosis and cirrhosis [1]. According to a WHO report [4], the deaths of about 50% of cirrhosis of the liver and about 30% of liver cancer are attributable to alcohol consumption. Fatty liver is a reversible condition where large vacuoles of triglyceride fat accumulate in liver cells via the process of steatosis at levels higher than normal, i.e. >5% of hepatocytes are steatotic. Pathogenesis of fatty liver also involves excessive calorie intake, dietary imbalance, inadequate exercise, and is associated with obesity, type 2 diabetes mellitus, coronary heart disease, hypertension, and dyslipidemia, which are all classified as non-alcoholic fatty liver [5-7].

As ambulatory patients with alcoholic fatty liver are often asymptomatic, and for most of the heavy alcohol consumption is not evitable due to physical dependency or the need of social drinking, thus the dietary supplementation becomes one of the best choices to prevent or control alcoholic fatty liver. Among which the most mentioned and reported are polyunsaturated fatty acids (PUFA). Many studies indicated that ω-3 fatty acids, the most important families of PUFA, have protective effects on fatty liver diseases [8-12]. PUFA are constituents of the animal and vegetable fats found in food. They are considered essential fatty acids, meaning that they cannot be synthesized by the human body but are vital for normal metabolism. They have to be provided from food or with an appropriate supplement [13,14]. Common sources of ω-3 PUFA include fish oils, algal oil, squid oil and some plant oils such as echium oil and flaxseed oil.

As another important source of PUFA, Krill Oil has received increasing attention in recent years for its beneficial effects on human health. Krill Oil is a mixture extracted from Antarctic krill (Euphausia superb Dana). Krill Oil contains a high proportion of ω-3 fatty acids, mainly Eicosapentaenoic Acid (EPA, C20:5) and Docosahexaenoic Acid (DHA, C22:6) which are bound to phospholipids [15, 16], in contrast to traditional ω-3 supplements such as cod liver oil and fish oil which are based on ω-3 fatty acids that bound to triglycerides. By binding with phospholipids, long-chain ω-3 fatty acids have a higher level of passage through the intestinal wall [17]. Besides ω-3 fatty acids, Krill Oil also contains many kinds of antioxidants including Vitamin E, all-trans-retinol Vitamin A, beta carotene and the carotenoid relatives, canthaxanthin and astaxanthin [17].

***Corresponding author:** Hong-ling Wang, Li Han, Beijing Key Laboratory of Bio-products Safety Assessment, JOINN Laboratories, Beijing, China, Nippon Suisan Kaisha, Ltd., Tokyo, Japan E-mail: wanghongling@joinn-lab.com

While the prophylactic effects of the Krill Oil on the non-alcoholic fatty liver had been proved in high-fat-fed mice and rats [18,19], the beneficial effects of Krill Oil on the alcoholic fatty liver are speculated but not yet demonstrated in pre-clinical studies. In this study, both prophylactic and therapeutic effects of Krill Oil on the pathogenesis of alcoholic fatty liver in rat model were investigated. The alcoholic fatty liver rat model was induced with daily alcohol gavage along with high fat diet feeding.

Materials and Methods

Chemicals and reagents

Krill Oil and Medium Chain Triglyceride (MCT) were obtained from Nippon Suisan Kaisha, Ltd., Tokyo, Japan. Alcohol (95%) was purchased from Taicang Xintai Alcohol Co. Ltd. Normal diet (ND) was purchased from Beijing Keao Xieli Diet Co. Ltd. High fat diet (HFD, fat content: 23%) was purchased from Beijing HFK Bioscience Co. Ltd. All other chemicals and solvents were of the highest grade commercially available.

Animals

Male Sprague-Dawley rats (SPF grade) were used in the whole study (Permit Numbers: ACU-11-491 and ACU12-142). Rats (160-220 g) were purchased from Vital River Laboratory Animal Technology Co. Ltd. (Beijing, China). Rats were housed in a controlled environment (temperature 22-26°C, humidity 40-70%, and 12 hour light/12 hour dark cycle) in the animal facility of JOINN Laboratories with access to food and water ad libitum unless otherwise specified. Rats were deprived of food (overnight) prior to blood sampling, and prior to terminal euthanasia. Rats were acclimated before use for the experiments.

Alcoholic Fatty Liver Model Preparation and Study Design

Fatty liver in rats was induced by alcohol gavage plus HFD feeding based on Li's method with some modifications [20]. Briefly, rats were fed with HFD plus orally administered alcohol (10 mL/kg, twice daily, at least 4 hours apart) for 6 or 10 weeks. The concentration of alcohol in the formulation increased with time along with glucose adding in the formulation to have the animal acclimated to the alcohol administration, with 8% alcohol plus 30% glucose in week 1, 12% alcohol plus 20% glucose in week 2, 20% alcohol plus 15% glucose in week 3, 30% alcohol plus 10% glucose in week 4, and 40% alcohol plus 10% glucose in following weeks.

For the prophylactic experiment, rats were randomized into six treatment groups at the initiation of alcohol gavage, and MCT or Krill Oil (diluted in MCT) was given at dose volume of 1 mL/kg via oral gavage once daily for six weeks (Figure 1). MCT, which does not contain ω-3 PUFA, was used as the vehicle control article and the diluent for Krill Oil formulation. Body weights and food consumption data were collected 3 times weekly. At the end of treatment, the rats were euthanized and necropsied. Blood samples were collected for serum triglyceride (TG) and total cholesterol (TC) analyses. Liver tissues were collected for TG and TC measurements, and for histopathological evaluation of hepatosteatosis.

For the therapeutic experiment, rats were randomized into seven groups after six-week gavage of alcohol and 10 rats from Group 2 were euthanized and necropsied on Day43 for pre-treatment data collection, then MCT or Krill Oil (diluted in MCT) was given to the remaining rats at dose volume of 1 mL/kg via oral gavage once daily through week 7 to week 10, with or without continuing oral gavage of alcohol (Figure 1). Body weights and food consumption data were collected twice weekly. At the end of treatment, the rats were euthanized and necropsied. Blood samples were collected for serum TG and TC analyses. Liver tissues were collected for TG, TC measurements, and for histopathological evaluation of hepatosteatosis.

Biochemical analyses

The serum TG, TC concentrations were measured by enzymatic methods, using GPO-PAP and COD-PAP kits (Shanghai Huashi Asia-Pacific Bio-pharmaceutical Co., Ltd). The liver TG and cholesterol were also determined using the supernatant after homogenated with PBS, individual hepatic TG and TC were quantitated enzymatically as described above.

Liver histopathology

Liver specimens from the rats were fixed in 10% neutral buffer formalin and embedded in paraffin. The specimens were sliced at 5 μm and mounted on glass slides. After staining with hematoxylin and eosin, the slides were evaluated microscopically by a veterinary pathologist. Fatty liver (cytoplasmic vacuolization) was graded according to the following grading scale [21]: slight severity (+) was recorded when cytoplasmic vacuolization was observed but was present in ≤1/3 of the hepatocytes in the section; moderate severity (++) was recorded when >1/3 and ≤2/3 of the hepatocytes in the section were affected; marked severity (+++) was recorded when >2/3 of the hepatocytes in the section were affected.

Microarray analysis

In the therapeutic experiment, liver samples from the rats were collected at necropsy and placed into RNAlater (Ambion). The samples from 3 control rats (Group 5) and 3 Krill Oil-treated rats (Group 7) were transferred to CapitalBio for Microarray analysis. Briefly, RNA was isolated from liver samples using the Ambion's kit following the manufacturer's instructions. The RNA samples were analyzed for quantity and purity by UV analysis and were evaluated for RNA integrity by gel electrophoresis. The RNA samples (≥1 μg) were used to synthesize double-stranded cDNA using the Affymetrix One-Cycle Target Labeling and Control Reagents kit. Then the cDNA was used as a template to synthesize biotin-labeled antisense cRNA using an in vitro transcription labeling kit. The cRNA was purified and fragmented according to the manual provided with the GeneChip Sample Cleanup module (Affymetrix). All GeneChip arrays (Rat Genome 230 Version 2.0 arrays) were hybridized, washed, and stained according to the Affymetrix Technical Manual. The chips were scanned using an Affymetrix GeneChip Scanner 3000 with Affymetrix® GeneChip® Command Console® Software. CEL files were imported in the R statistical package and were RMA normalized. SAM analysis was performed to identify differentially expressed genes between vehicle and Krill Oil-treated samples. The genes with q-value ≤ 5% and Fold Change ≥2 or ≤ 0.5 were identified as differentially expressed genes.

Statistical analysis

Results are expressed as means ± SD (standard deviation). Comparisons between means were performed using One-way analysis of variance (ANOVA), followed by a post-hoc LSD test. χ^2-test was used to evaluate the significances of histopathological evaluation. Differences were considered to reach statistical significance when P≤0.05. Statistical analyses were carried out with SPSS software (version 13.0 for Windows).

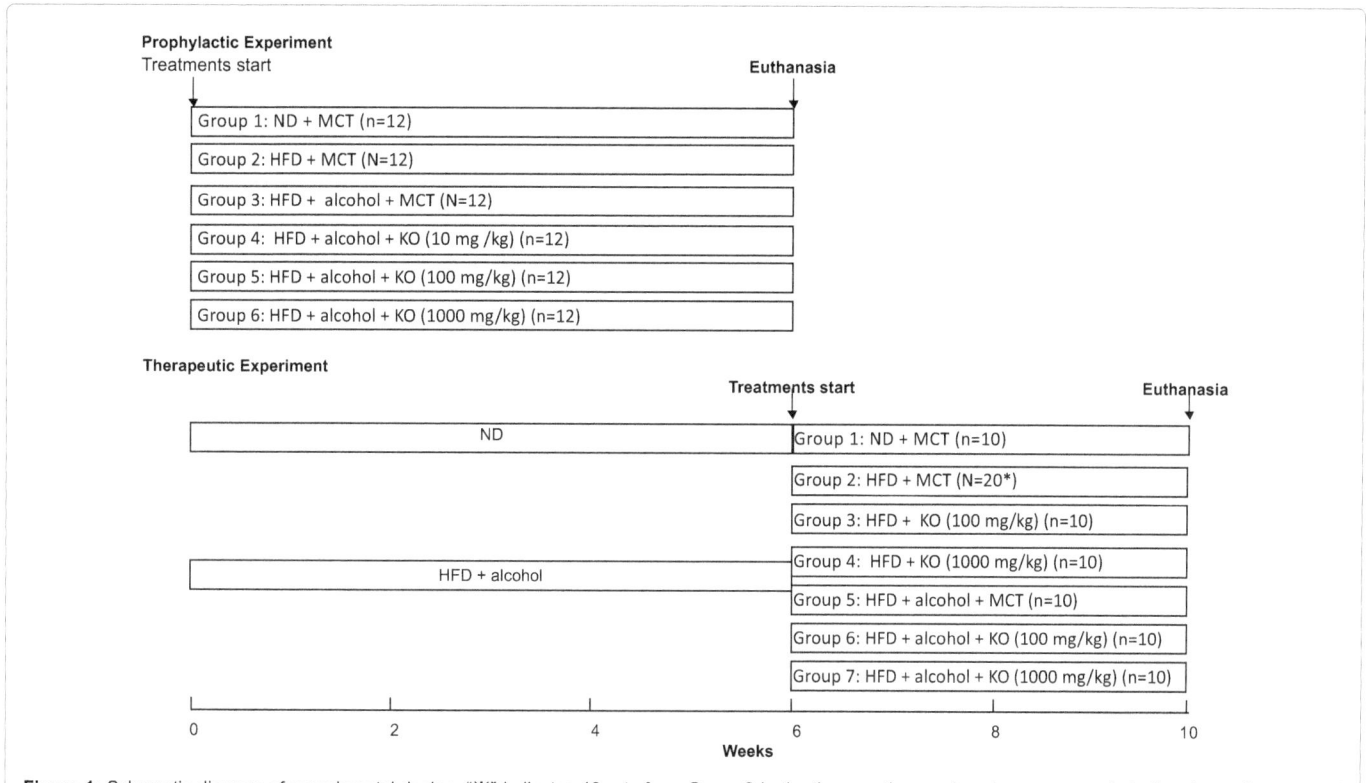

Figure 1: Schematic diagram of experimental design. "※" indicates 10 rats from Group 2 in the therapeutic experiment were necropsied after six-week gavage of alcohol on Day 43 for pre-treatment data collection.

Results

Body weight

In the prophylactic experiment, the mean body weight of ND control (ND+MCT) and HFD control (HFD+MCT) groups increased with time and there was no statistically significant difference between these two groups. The body weight of MCT control (HFD+Alcohol+MCT) group also increased with time in the initial 3 weeks. There was no apparent body weight gain in the following 2 weeks followed by body weight gain until week 6. The changes in body weight in MCT control group were considered to be related to the decrease in food consumption. After the animals acclimated to the high concentration of alcohol, the body weight gains recovered partially until week 6. By comparison with MCT control group, no apparent changes in body weight were observed in the Krill Oil treated groups (Figure 2A).

In the therapeutic experiment, similar body weight changes were observed in the initial 6 weeks for the ND control (ND+MCT) group and other groups, respectively. After alcohol treatment ended, the body weight gain in the alcohol withdrawal MCT control (HFD+Alcohol+MCT, alcohol was given for 6 weeks) group recovered to a higher level than the ND control group, and no significant differences were observed when comparing with Krill Oil treated groups. The body weight of the alcohol non-withdrawal MCT control (HFD+Alcohol+MCT, alcohol was given for 10 weeks) group increased with time during weeks 7-10 and Krill Oil treatments had no effect on body weight (Figure 2B).

Food consumption

In the prophylactic experiment, the ND control group had a consistent food consumption ranging from 22.2 to 27.7 g/rat/day, while the HFD control group had a decreased food consumption ranging from 17.8 to 21.2 g/rat/day. There was no difference between MCT control group and HFD control group in the initial 3 weeks while a marked decrease in HFD group was noted in the following 2 weeks with the lowest food consumption of 8.5 g/rat/day, and partially recovered in week 6. By comparison with MCT control group, no apparent changes in food consumption were noted in the Krill Oil treated groups except that relatively higher values were noted for 1000 mg•kg-1•d-1 Krill Oil group during D13 to D22 (Figure 3A).

In the therapeutic experiment, similar food consumption were noted in the initial 6 weeks for the ND control group and other groups, respectively. The food consumption in the alcohol withdrawal MCT control group recovered in weeks 7 to 10 while no apparent changes were noted for the alcohol non-withdrawal MCT control group, and Krill Oil treatment had no effects on food consumption compared with the model control group (Figure 3B).

Liver and serum TG and TC

In the prophylactic experiment, in comparison with ND control group, the liver TG level elevated significantly in the HFD control group, and which elevated further after alcohol exposure for six weeks, indicating an accumulation of TG in liver tissue, a characteristic sign of fatty liver. By comparison with ND control group, an elevation of liver TC was also observed in HFD control group, while no apparent further elevation was noted after alcohol exposure. Krill Oil treatment inhibited HFD and alcohol induced elevations in liver TG and TC in a dose dependent manner (Figure 4A-a; Figure 4A-b).

Unlike the changes of TG and TC noted in liver tissue, the serum TG and TC had no change either after exposure to alcohol or after treated with Krill Oil (Figure 4A-c; Figure 4A-d).

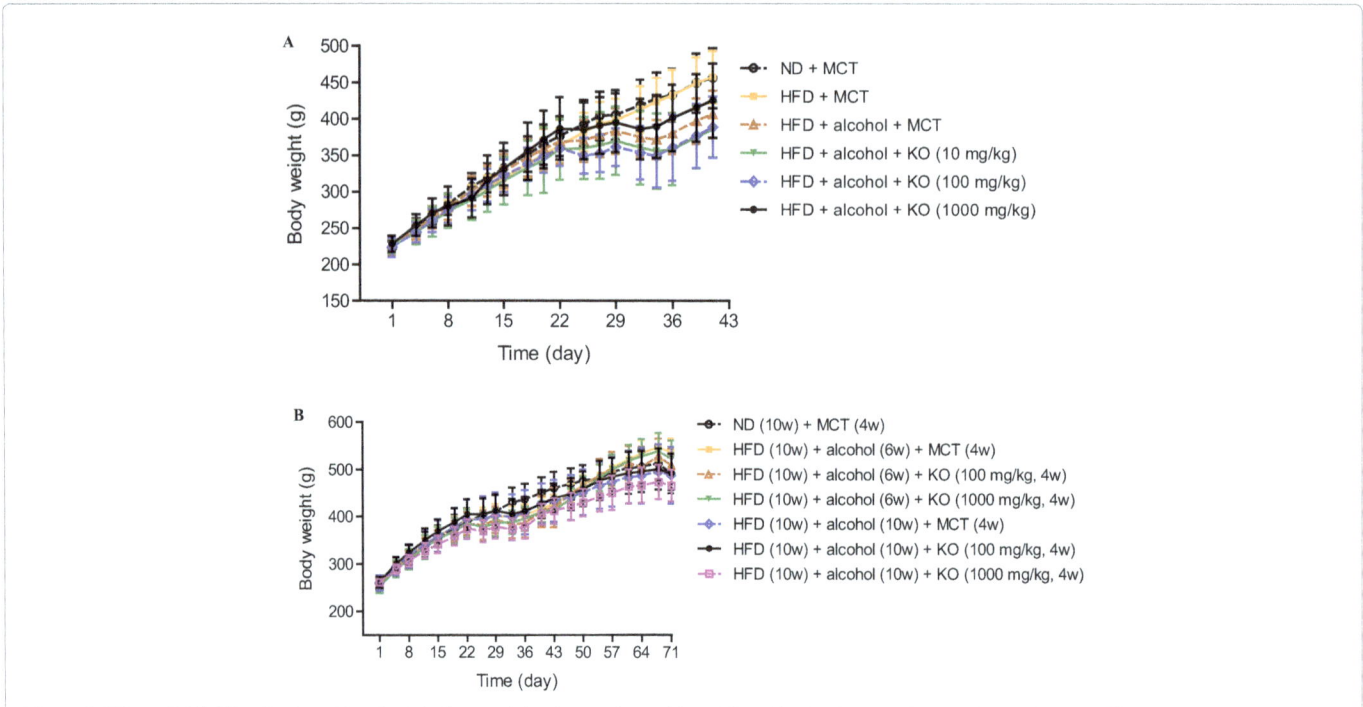

Figure 2: Effect of Krill Oil on body weight of rats in the prophylactic experiment (A, n=12) and in the therapeutic experiment (B, n=10). The results are expressed as means ± SD.

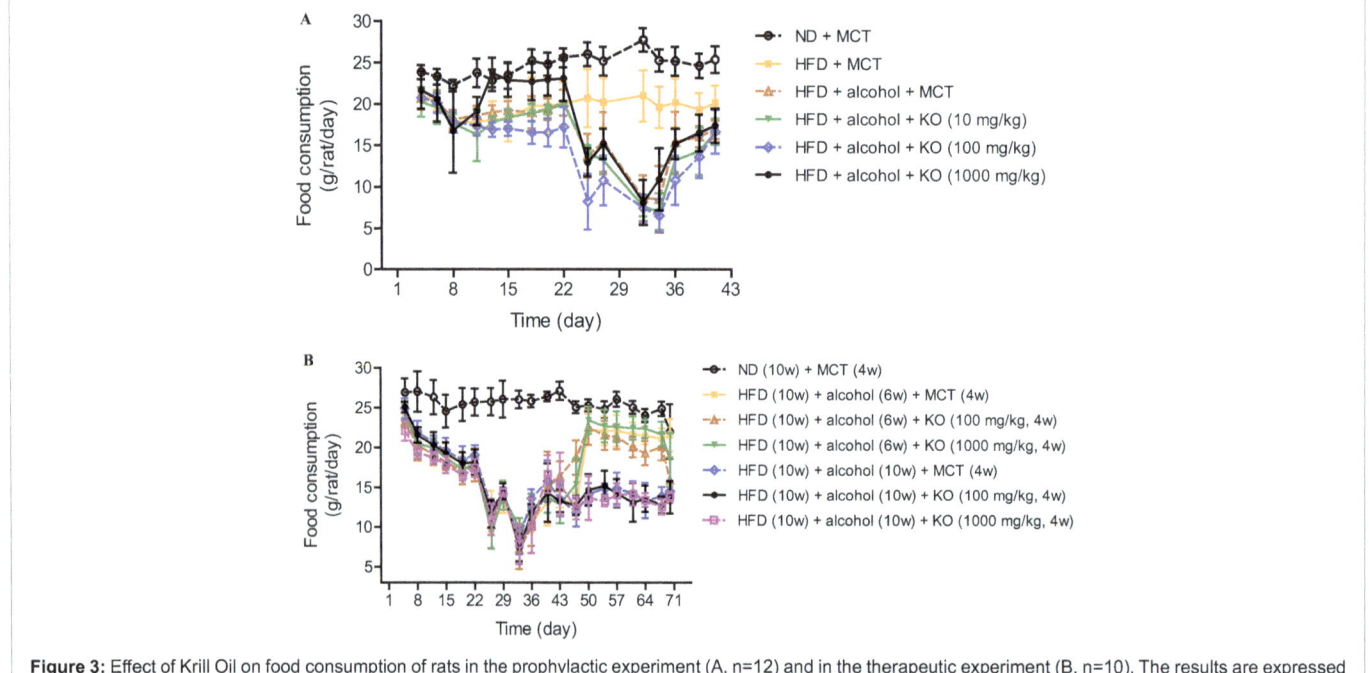

Figure 3: Effect of Krill Oil on food consumption of rats in the prophylactic experiment (A, n=12) and in the therapeutic experiment (B, n=10). The results are expressed as means ± SD.

In the therapeutic experiment, after withdrawal from alcohol exposure, the liver TG showed a spontaneous recovery. Krill Oil treatment accelerated recovery independent of doses. For the groups that continued with alcohol gavage until the end of week 10, Krill Oil treatment decreased liver TG in a dose dependent manner (Figure 4B-a). After withdrawal from alcohol gavage, the liver TC showed a slight increase in comparison with pre-treatment data, while there was no

changes in the Krill Oil treated groups. For the groups continuing with alcohol gavage until the end of week 10, no apparent change in the liver TC levels was observed in Krill Oil low-dose groups while a decrease was observed in the high-dose group (Figure 4B-b).

No change in serum TG was observed after six weeks of alcohol gavage, Serum TG was slightly increased after alcohol gavage

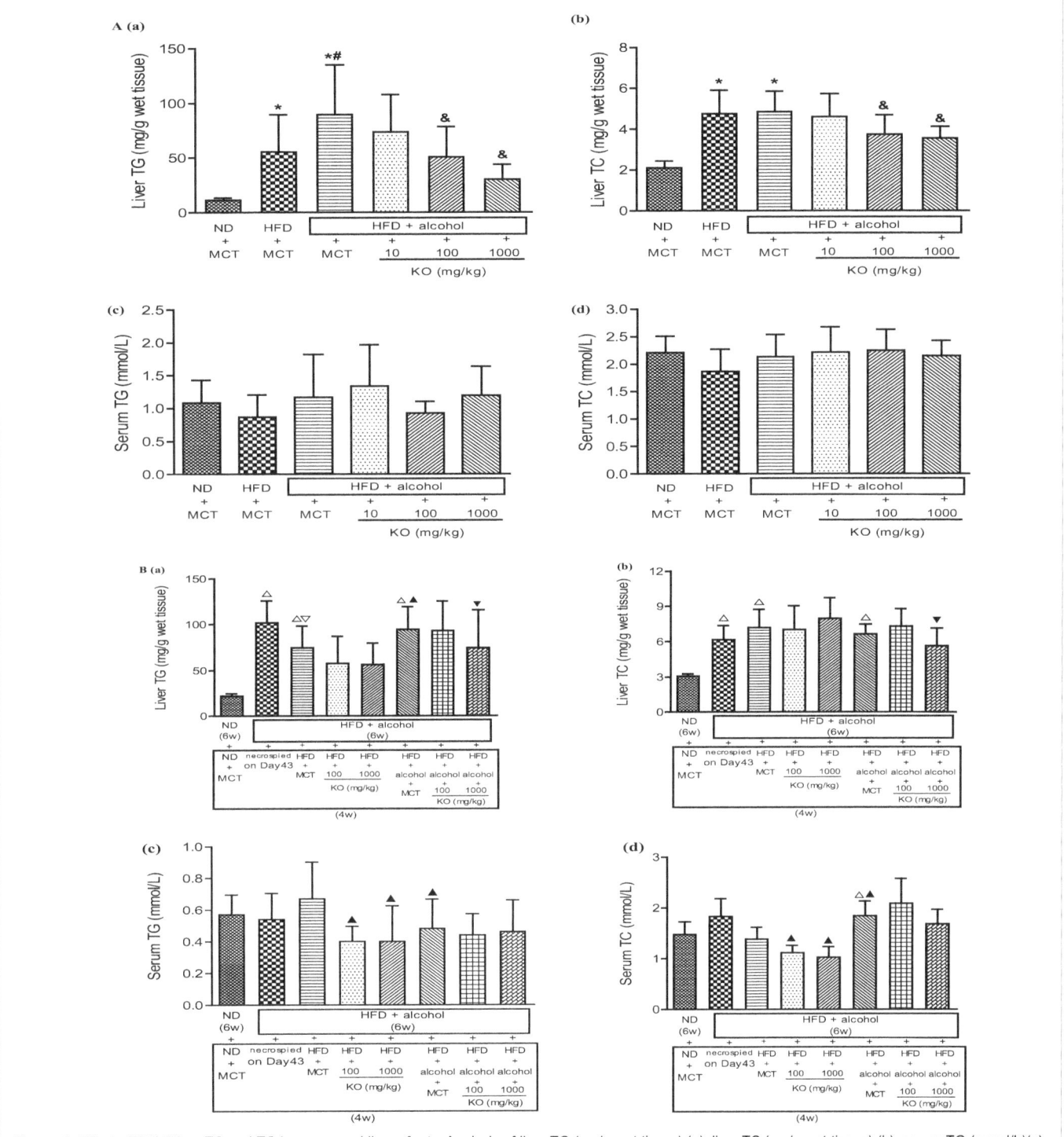

Figure 4: Effect of Krill Oil on TG and TC in serum and liver of rats. Analysis of liver TG (mg/g wet tissue) (a); liver TC (mg/g wet tissue) (b); serum TG (mmol/L)(c); serum TC (mmol/L) (d) of rats from different groups. The results are expressed as means ± SD. In the prophylactic experiment (A, n=12): *P≤0.05 vs Group 1: ND + MCT; #P≤0.05 vs Group 2: HFD + MCT; &P ≤ 0.05 vs Group 3: HFD + alcohol + MCT. In the therapeutic experiment (B, n=10): △P≤0.05 vs Group 1: ND (10w) + MCT (4w); ▽P≤0.05 vs pre-treatment data of Group 2: HFD (6w) + alcohol (6w); ▲P≤0.05 vs post-treatment data of Group 2: HFD (10w) + alcohol (6w) + MCT(4w) (alcohol withdrawal); ▼P≤0.05 vs Group 5: HFD (10w) + alcohol (10w) + MCT(4w) (alcohol non-withdrawal).

withdrawal. By comparison with the MCT control group, Krill Oil treatment (4 weeks) decreased the serum TG independent of dose. No change in serum TG level was observed after 10 weeks of alcohol gavage, and Krill Oil treatments had no effect on serum TG. The serum TC had a slight increase after six weeks of alcohol

gavage and recovered to normal value after alcohol gavage ended. Krill Oil treatments decreased serum TC. There was no further change in serum TC after ten weeks of alcohol gavage and Krill Oil treatments showed no effects on serum TC either. (Figure 4B-c; Figure 4B-d).

Liver weight and liver-to-body weight ratio

In the prophylactic experiment, by comparison with the ND control group and HFD control group, the liver to body weight ratio showed a significant increase after oral gavage of alcohol. The increased ratio was reversed by the concurrent intake of krill in a dose dependent manner (Figure 5A).

In the therapeutic experiment, after withdrawal of alcohol gavage, the liver to body weight ratio returned to normal values and there was no difference between model control group and Krill Oil treatment groups, indicating a spontaneous recovery of fatty liver and no accelerating effect was noted in Krill Oil treated groups. However, the liver to body weight ratio remained at high level when the oral gavage of alcohol continued after initiation of Krill Oil treatment. The increased ratio was reversed by oral gavage of high dose of Krill Oil (Figure 5B).

Pathology

In the prophylactic experiment, after oral gavage of alcohol for six weeks, all of the vehicle control rats showed a yellowish discoloration of the liver at necropsy. The incidence of this discoloration decreased after Krill Oil treatment in a dose dependent manner.

Moderate (++) to marked (+++) cytoplasmic vacuolization in the MCT control group were noted, alcohol treatment led to higher severity of cytoplasmic vacuolization compared with normal diet and high-fat diet control groups, indicating a successful induction of alcoholic fatty liver. Concurrent treatments with Krill Oil decreased the frequency and severity of alcohol induced cytoplasmic vacuolization in a dose-dependent manner (Figure 6A, 6C).

In the therapeutic experiment, for the alcohol withdrawal model control group, 40% rats had a liver with yellowish or whitish

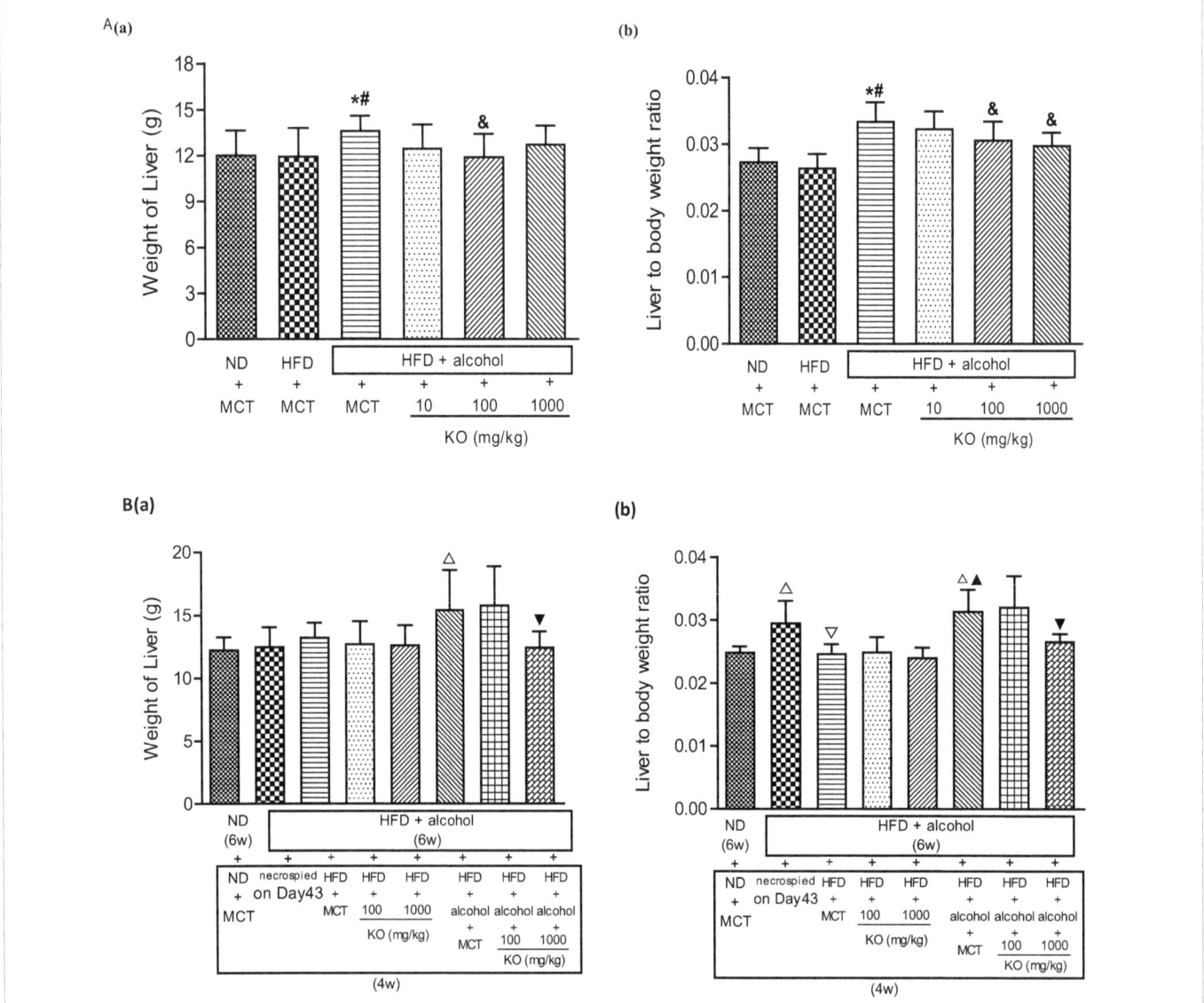

Figure 5: Effects of Krill Oil on liver weight and liver to body weight ratio of rats. Analysis of liver weight (g) (a); liver to body weight (b) of rats from different groups. The results are expressed as means ± SD. In the prophylactic experiment (A, n=12): *P≤0.05 vs Group 1: ND + MCT; #P≤0.05 vs Group 2: HFD + MCT; &P≤0.05 vs Group 3: HFD + alcohol + MCT. In the therapeutic experiment (B, n=10): △P≤0.05 vs Group 1: ND (10w) + MCT (4w); ▽P≤0.05 vs pre-treatment data of Group 2: HFD (6w) + alcohol (6w); ▲P≤0.05 vs post-treatment data of Group 2: HFD (10w) + alcohol (6w) + MCT(4w) (alcohol withdrawal); ▼P≤0.05 vs Group 5: HFD (10w) + alcohol (10w) + MCT(4w) (alcohol non-withdrawal).

Oral Intake of Krill Oil has Prophylactic and Potential Therapeutic Effects on Alcoholic Fatty Liver...

103

discoloration. No apparent changes were noted in the Krill Oil treated groups. Eight of the 10 rats in alcohol non-withdrawal model control group had liver yellowish or whitish discoloration. After treated with high-dose Krill Oil the incidence decreased to 2/10. Low-dose Krill Oil had no effects on alcohol induced discoloration.

Alcohol withdrawal vehicle control animals had fatty liver (cytoplasmic vacuolization) with 50% slight and 50% moderate. Low dose Krill Oil and high dose Krill Oil treatment improved the ratio to 70% slight and 30% moderate. All the alcohol non-withdrawal model control animals had fatty liver (cytoplasmic vacuolization) with 50% moderate and 50% marked. Krill Oil treatment did not change the overall incidence of fatty liver with 10/10 rats in both groups. However the severity of fatty liver decreased in Krill Oil treated groups with 70% moderate and 30% marked found in the low-dose group, and 30% slight, 60% moderate and 10% marked in the high-dose group (Figure 6B, 6D).

Microarray analysis

A total of 19 genes were differentially expressed after Krill Oil treatment with q-value ≤5% and Fold Change ≥2 or ≤ 0.5 (Table 2). Of these 19 genes, 1 gene was up-regulated and the other 18 genes were down-regulated. However, None of the 19 genes were directly correlated with alcohol metabolism and lipid metabolism. There are another 105 genes whose Fold Changes were ≥2 or ≤0.5 while their q-values were >5%.

Discussion

Many studies [22, 23] indicate that high-fat diet is helpful to maintain relative high blood alcohol concentration and exacerbate to induce fatty liver disease in alcoholic rats. Thus in this study, we use alcohol gavage along with feeding a high-fat diet to induce alcoholic fatty liver in Sprague-Dawley rats. Our data showed that the liver tissue TG increased from 11.42 mg/g to 48.18 mg/g after feeding high fat diet for six weeks, and the value increased further to 89.65 mg/g after alcohol exposure for six weeks. The histopathology data also showed an increased incidence and severity of liver cytoplasmic vacuolization after alcohol exposure for six weeks, indicating that the alcoholic fatty liver model was induced successfully. Concurrent supplementation of Krill Oil for six weeks inhibited the increase in liver TG and the increases in incidence and severity of liver cytoplasmic vacuolization induced by alcohol exposure, indicating Krill Oil has a prophylactic effect on fatty liver formation in this rat model. When Krill Oil was supplemented, after alcohol exposure for six weeks, i.e. after alcoholic fatty liver was already induced, the increased fatty liver related parameters either had an accelerated recovery where alcohol exposure had ended at the end of week 6, or had an attenuation when alcohol exposure continued along with Krill Oil supplementation, indicating Krill Oil had a therapeutic effect on the alcoholic fatty liver in this rat model. To find out the potential mechanisms underlying Krill Oil's effect on alcoholic fatty liver, we conducted a microarray analysis using Affymetrix GeneChip Rat Genome 230 2.0 Array. Unfortunately we did not find apparent changes at mRNA level that had a direct correlation with alcohol metabolism and lipid metabolism. Instead, the results showed most of the genes with marked changes were related to Interferon (IFN), a pluripotent cytokine in immune system modulation. The relationship between IFN and fatty liver formation has rarely been reported. Sbarbati's study showed IFN treated suckling mice had liver lipid accumulation while there is no such lipid accumulation in the control mice [24]. Wallace's data showed that PUFAs could inhibit production of IFN-γ in mice and Irons' data showed that PUFAs could impair the IFN-γ

responsiveness via diminished receptor signaling in mice [25,26]. As Krill Oil contains a high proportion of ω-3 PUFAs, its inhibitory effects on fatty liver may attribute to PUFAs' inhibitory effect on IFN signaling and subsequently inhibited fatty liver formation. Our data indicated a probable involvement of IFN in the Krill Oil's effects on fatty liver. More work needed to be done to verify this possible mechanism.

As Krill Oil contains a high proportion of ω-3 PUFAs bound to phospholipids and many kinds of antioxidants including Vitamin E, all-trans-retinol Vitamin A, canthaxanthin and astaxanthin, its inhibitory effect on alcoholic fatty liver can be attributed to PUFAs, phospholipids and astaxanthin, or any combination thereof. Song et al. showed that alcohol-DHA/AA-supplemented diet ameliorates the fatty liver induced by chronic alcohol administration in rats alcohol induced elevation in CYP2E1, nitric oxide synthase, nitrite and mitochondrial hydrogen peroxide as well as reduction in mitochondrial aldehyde dehydrogenase, ATP synthase, and 3-ketoacyl-CoA thiolase all returned to normal levels in rats fed with the alcohol-DHA/AA-supplemented diet [27].

Unlike fish oil, which is based on ω-3 fatty acids bound to triglycerides, Krill Oil's ω-3 fatty acids are bound to phospholipids [16,17]. Therefore Krill Oil contains a high proportion of phosphatidylcholine (PC). It has been reported that soybean polyenylphosphatidylcholine (PPC), a mixture of 94%-96% of polyunsaturated phosphatidylcholine, could affect the parameters in fatty liver induced by alcohol consumption. The alleviated fatty liver in the PPC-treated rats is associated with normalizing mitochondrial oxidation of palmitoyl-1-carnitine, and activities of cytochrome oxidase, serum glutamate dehydrogenase and aminotransferases which are inhibited or stimulated by alcohol exposure [28]. Aleynik's study suggests alcohol exposure induced S-adenosylmethionine (SAMe) depletion can be reversed by PPC, along with the prevention of the alcohol-induced oxidative stress. As PCs are produced in the liver via methylation of phosphatidylethanolamine by SAMe, PPC might decrease the utilization of SAMe by providing PCs, and subsequently correct GSH depletion and prevent the alcohol induced oxidative stress [29].

As for astaxanthin, Ikeuchi et al showed a reduction of high-fat diet feeding induced increases in liver weight, liver triglyceride, plasma triglyceride, and total cholesterol [30]. Bhuvaneswaria's study suggests that astaxanthin supplementation promotes insulin sensitivity and prevented liver injury by decreasing CYP2E1, myeloperoxidase, and nitro-oxidative stress and by improving the antioxidant status in them [31].

We had conducted a study to compare the prophylactic effect of Krill Oil, fish oil, soy lecithin and 1:1 mix of fish oil and soy lecithin on alcohol induced fatty liver in rats. The results indicate that Krill Oil has a prophylactic effect at dose level of 100 mg/kg, while fish oil, soy

		K-Oil	F-oil	Soy-Lec	1:1 Mix of F-O & S-L
Polar lipid (weight%)		43.4	—	64.8	32.4
Nonpolar lipid (weight%)		53.6	100	35.2	67.6
Fatty acid (%)	C14:0	11.9	5.2	—	2.6
	C16:0	21.6	7.3	29.1	18.2
	C18:0	1.3	0.7	2.5	1.6
	C18:1	17.7	8.6	12	10.3
	C18:2	1.7	1.1	50.9	26
	C18:3	1.2	0.8	5.5	3.2
	C20:5	15.2	29.3	—	14.7
	C22:6	7.7	13.1	—	6.6

Table 1: Lipid and fatty acid composition.

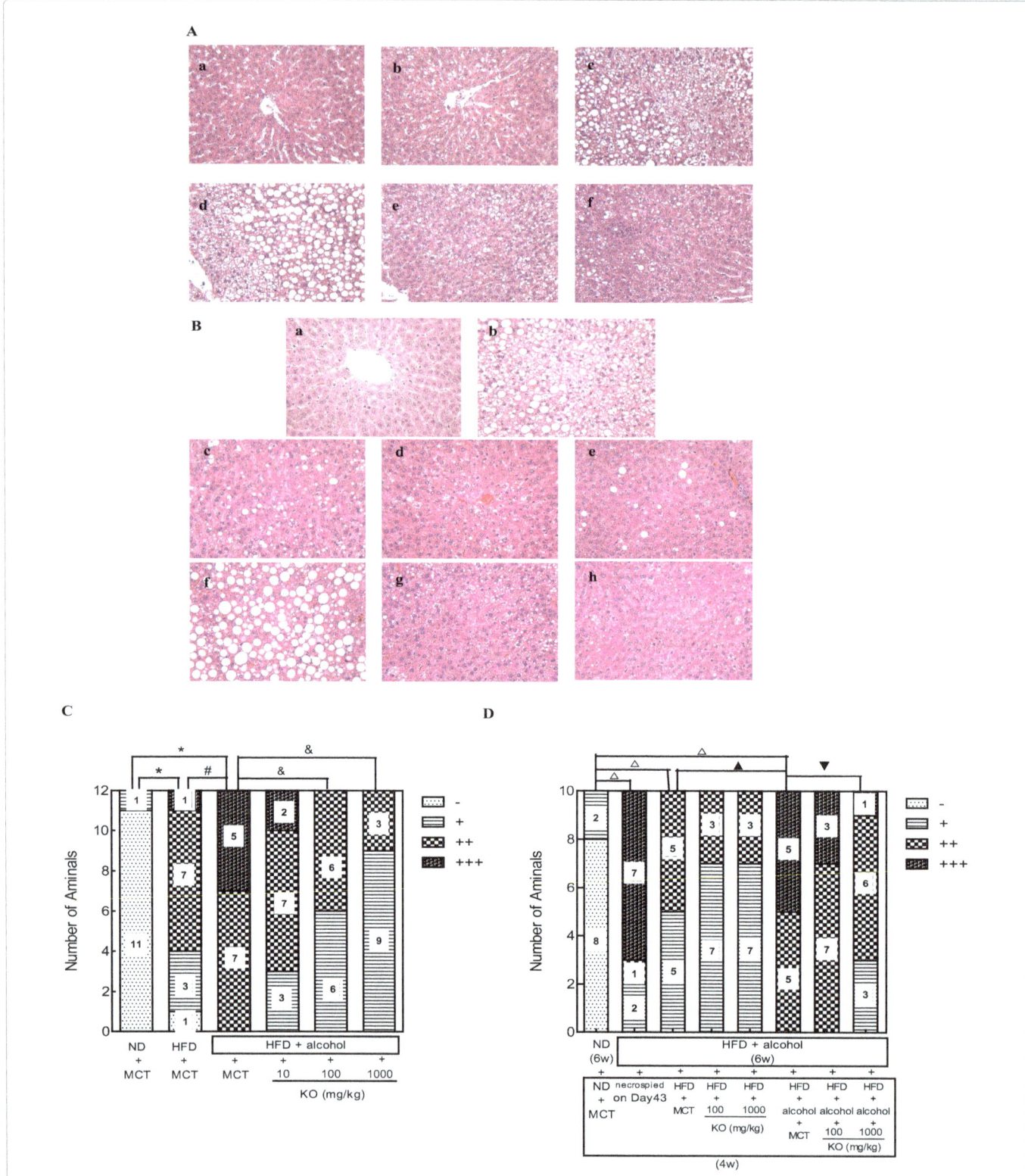

Figure 6: Effect of Krill Oil on Liver histopathology of rats. H&E × 40 objective. In the prophylactic experiment (A, n=12): (a) ND control, fatty liver (-); (b) HFD control, fatty liver (++); (c) Model control, fatty liver (+++); (d) Krill Oil 10 mg/kg, fatty liver (+++); (e) Krill Oil 100 mg/kg, fatty liver (++); (f) Krill Oil 1000 mg/kg, fatty liver (++). In the therapeutic experiment (B, n=10): (a) ND control, fatty liver (-);(b)Model control fatty liver(+++), pre-treatment; (c) Alcohol withdrawal, model control, fatty liver (++); (d) Alcohol withdrawal, Krill Oil 100 mg/kg, fatty liver (+); (e) Alcohol withdrawal, Krill Oil 1000 mg/kg, fatty liver (+); (f) Alcohol non-withdrawal, model control, fatty liver (+++); (g) Alcohol non-withdrawal, Krill Oil 100 mg/kg, fatty liver (++); (h)Alcohol non-withdrawal, Krill Oil 1000 mg/kg, fatty liver (+); (C): In the prophylactic experiment (A, n=12), *P≤0.05 vs Group 1: ND + MCT; #P≤0.05, vs post-treatment data of Group 2: HFD + MCT; &P≤0.05 vs Group 3: HFD + alcohol + MCT. (D): In the therapeutic experiment (B, n=10), ▽P≤0.05 vs pre-treatment data of Group 2: HFD (6w) + alcohol (6w); ▼P≤0.05 vs Group 5: HFD (10w) + alcohol (10w) + MCT(4w) (alcohol non-withdrawal).

Gene ID	Gene Title	Gene Symbol	Fold Change	q-value (%)
1384671_at	---	---	2.23	0.00
1387242_at	eukaryotic translation initiation factor 2-alpha kinase 2	Eif2ak2	0.49	0.00
1374337_at	---	---	0.44	0.00
1391489_at	immunity-related GTPase family, M	Irgm	0.43	0.00
1384180_at	interferon-induced protein with tetratricopeptide repeats 2	Ifit2	0.43	0.00
1379568_at	interferon-induced protein with tetratricopeptide repeats 2	Ifit2	0.41	0.00
1389034_at	ubiquitin specific peptidase 18	Usp18	0.25	0.00
1382902_at	potential ubiquitin ligase	Herc6	0.21	0.00
1370913_at	radical S-adenosyl methionine domain containing 2	Rsad2	0.21	0.00
1382314_at	interferon, alpha-inducible protein (clone IFI-15K)	G1p2	0.13	0.00
1387283_at	myxovirus (influenza virus) resistance 2	Mx2	0.13	0.00
1371970_at	family with sequence similarity 111, member A	Fam111a	0.03	0.00
1370314_at	solute carrier family 20 (phosphate transporter), member 1	Slc20a1	0.50	2.69
1373197_at	similar to Protein KIAA1404	LOC686701	0.47	3.66
1387354_at	signal transducer and activator of transcription 1	Stat1	0.46	3.66
1393044_at	cytidine monophosphate (UMP-CMP) kinase 2, mitochondrial	Cmpk2	0.44	3.66
1383564_at	interferon regulatory factor 7	Irf7	0.34	3.66
1371015_at	myxovirus (influenza virus) resistance 1	Mx1	0.30	3.66
1383075_at	cyclin D1	Ccnd1	0.34	4.65

Table 2: List of differentially expressed genes after Krill Oil treatment.

lecithin and 1:1 mix of fish oil and soy lecithin have no effects at this dose. As showed in Table 1, Krill Oil is lower in PUFA than all others. In respect of the highly unsaturated fatty acids (HUFA), a subset of PUFA which have 4 or more double bonds, Krill Oil is lower than fish oil. Krill Oil contains less polar lipid, i.e. the fatty acids which have at least one double bond, than soy lecithin. What makes Krill Oil more effective? We think that it is probably one of the characteristics of Krill Oil, i.e., the bond between PUFA with phospholipids. The supporting evidence can be found in several recently published clinical and preclinical studies. Three clinical studies showed that EPA+DHA in Krill Oil is more easily and effectively absorbed after ingestion and subsequently distributed in the blood of human subjects when compared with those in fish oil [17,32, 33]. In a study in obese Zucker rats, Krill Oil led to a significantly higher incorporation of EPA and DHA into tissue PLs than fish oil [34]. In another rat study, DHA in the form of PL had a 2-fold higher accumulation in the brain than that in the form of TG [35]. A later study in baboon neonates showed a 2.1-fold preferential incorporation and retention of dietary PL-derived arachidonic acid (AA) over TG-derived AA in the brain [36].

Based on the published data, we may attribute Krill Oil's outstanding protective effect on fatty liver to: 1) PUFAs' protective effects; 2) PC's protective effects; 3) astaxanthin's protective effects; 4) astaxanthin's antioxidative activity which makes PUFAs more stable and thus improves PUFAs' protective effects on fatty liver; 5) the bonds between PUFAs and PLs which make PUFAs more easily absorbed and thus improve PUFAs' protective effects on fatty liver.

Conclusions

Our results demonstrate that Krill Oil supplement not only has a potential prophylactic effect on alcoholic fatty liver formation, but also has a potential therapeutic effect on the already formed alcoholic fatty liver. The protective effects of Krill Oil can be attributed to its main components, i.e. ω-3polyunsaturated fatty acids, phosphatidylcholine, astaxanthin, or any combination thereof, which have been reported to have protective effects on fatty liver.

Acknowledgements

This work was supported by Nippon Suisan Kaisha, Ltd., Tokyo, Japan. The authors are solely responsible for the design and conduct of the study; collection, management, analysis, and interpretation of the data; as well as preparation of the manuscript. We would like to thank the participants who contributed their time to this project.

Authors' Contributions

HLW, LH, MWG, YXS, CLZ and TT were involved in the study design, data analysis, interpretation, and manuscript writing. Most of the experimental procedures were carried out by employees at JOINN Laboratories, Suzhou. QL was involved in the preparation of the study. The study was mainly performed by QL, WJZ and HW, who were also involved in data analysis and manuscript writing. MWG was involved in coordination of the study conduct. All authors have read and approved the final manuscript.

Competing Interests

LH is employed in Nippon Suisan Kaisha, Ltd. HLW, QL, WJZ, HW and MWG were employed at JOINN Laboratories when the study was performed.

References

1. European Association for the Study of Liver (2012) EASL clinical practical guidelines: management of alcoholic liver disease. J Hepatol 57: 399-420.

2. Marsano LS, Mendez C, Hill D, Barve S, McClain CJ (2003) Diagnosis and treatment of alcoholic liver disease and its complications. Alcohol Res Health 27: 247-256.

3. Gramenzi A, Caputo F, Biselli M, Kuria F, Loggi E, et al. (2006) Review article: alcoholic liver disease--pathophysiological aspects and risk factors. Aliment Pharmacol Ther 24: 1151-1161.

4. WHO: Global status report on alcohol and health. 2011

5. Sullivan S (2010) Implications of diet on nonalcoholic fatty liver disease. Curr Opin Gastroenterol 26: 160-164.

6. Kawano Y, Cohen DE (2013) Mechanisms of hepatic triglyceride accumulation in non-alcoholic fatty liver disease. J Gastroenterol 48: 434-441.

7. Zhang LF, Liu LS, Chu XM , Xie H, Cao LJ, et al. (2014) Combined effects of a high-fat diet and chronic valproic acid treatment on hepatic steatosis and hepatotoxicity in rats. Acta Pharmacol Sin 35: 363-372.

8. Leamy AK, Egnatchik RA, Young JD (2013) Molecular mechanisms and the role of saturated fatty acids in the progression of non-alcoholic fatty liver disease. Prog Lipid Res 52: 165-174.

9. Capanni M, Calella F, Biagini MR, Genise S, Raimondi L, et al. (2006) Prolonged n-3 polyunsaturated fatty acid supplementation ameliorates hepatic steatosis in patients with non-alcoholic fatty liver disease: a pilot study. Aliment Pharmacol Ther 23: 1143-1151.

10. Zhu FS, Liu S, Chen XM, Huang ZG, Zhang DW (2008) Effects of n-3 polyunsaturated fatty acids from seal oils on nonalcoholic fatty liver disease associated with hyperlipidemia. World J Gastroenterol 14: 6395-6400.

11. Spadaro L, Magliocco O, Spampinato D, Piro S, Oliveri C, et al. (2008) Effects of n-3 polyunsaturated fatty acids in subjects with nonalcoholic fatty liver disease. Dig Liver Dis 40: 194-199.

12. Cussons AJ, Watts GF, Mori TA, Stuckey BG (2009) Omega-3 fatty acid supplementation decreases liver fat content in polycystic ovary syndrome: a randomized controlled trial employing proton magnetic resonance spectroscopy. J Clin Endocrinol Metab 94: 3842-3848.

13. Norris AW, Spector AA (2002) Very long chain n-3 and n-6 polyunsaturated fatty acids bind strongly to liver fatty acid-binding protein. J Lipid Res 43: 646-653.

14. EL-Baz D, Salem ZA (2013) The Effect of Omega- 3 Fatty Acids on the Age Related Changes in Submandibular Salivary Glands of Albino Rats. J Am Sci 9: 149-154.

15. Winther B, Hoem N, Berge K, Reubsaet L (2011) Elucidation of phosphatidylcholine composition in krill oil extracted from Euphausia superba. Lipids 46: 25-36.

16. Schuchardt JP, Schneider I, Meyer H, Neubronner J, von Schacky C, et al. (2011) Incorporation of EPA and DHA into plasma phospholipids in response to different omega-3 fatty acid formulations--a comparative bioavailability study of fish oil vs. krill oil. Lipids Health Dis 10: 145.

17. Bunea R, El Farrah K, Deutsch L (2004) Evaluation of the effects of Neptune Krill Oil on the clinical course of hyperlipidemia. Altern Med Rev 9: 420-428.

18. Tandy S, Chung RW, Wat E, Kamili A, Berge K, et al. (2009) Dietary krill oil supplementation reduces hepatic steatosis, glycemia, and hypercholesterolemia in high-fat-fed mice. J Agric Food Chem 57: 9339-9345.

19. Ferramosca A, Conte A, Burri L, Berge K, De Nuccio F, et al. (2012) A krill oil supplemented diet suppresses hepatic steatosis in high-fat fed rats. PLoS One 7: e38797.

20. Li YG, Ji DF, Chen S, Hu GY (2008) Protective effects of sericin protein on alcohol-mediated liver damage in mice. Alcohol Alcohol 43: 246-253.

21. Zhang Y, Xie ML, Zhu LJ, Gu ZL (2007) Therapeutic effect of osthole on hyperlipidemic fatty liver in rats. Acta Pharmacol Sin 28: 398-403.

22. Fisher H, Halladay A, Ramasubramaniam N, Petrucci JC, Dagounis D, et al. (2002) Liver fat and plasma ethanol are sharply lower in rats fed ethanol in conjunction with high carbohydrate compared with high fat diets. J Nutr 132: 2732-2736.

23. Korourian S, Hakkak R, Ronis MJ, Shelnutt SR, Waldron J, et al. (1999) Diet and risk of ethanol-induced hepatotoxicity: carbohydrate-fat relationships in rats. Toxicol Sci 47: 110-117.

24. Sbarbati A, Leclercq F, Osculati F, Gresser I (1995) Interferon alpha/beta-induced abnormalities in adipocytes of suckling mice. Biol Cell 83: 163-167.

25. Wallace FA, Miles EA, Evans C, Stock TE, Yaqoob P, et al. (2001) Dietary fatty acids influence the production of Th1- but not Th2-type cytokines. J Leukoc Biol 69: 449-457.

26. Irons R, Fritsche KL (2005) Omega-3 polyunsaturated fatty acids impair in vivo interferon- gamma responsiveness via diminished receptor signaling. J Infect Dis 191: 481-486.

27. Song BJ, Moon KH, Olsson NU, Salem N Jr (2008) Prevention of alcoholic fatty liver and mitochondrial dysfunction in the rat by long-chain polyunsaturated fatty acids. J Hepatol 49: 262-273.

28. Navder KP, Baraona E, Lieber CS (1997) Polyenylphosphatidylcholine attenuates alcohol-induced fatty liver and hyperlipemia in rats. J Nutr 127: 1800-1806.

29. Aleynik SI, Lieber CS (2003) Polyenylphosphatidylcholine corrects the alcohol-induced hepatic oxidative stress by restoring s-adenosylmethionine. Alcohol Alcohol 38: 208-212.

30. Ikeuchi M, Koyama T, Takahashi J, Yazawa K (2007) Effects of astaxanthin in obese mice fed a high-fat diet. Biosci Biotechnol Biochem 71: 893-899.

31. Bhuvaneswaria S, Arunkumar E, Viswanathan P, Anuradha CV (2010) Astaxanthin restricts weight gain, promotes insulin sensitivity and curtails fatty liver disease in mice fed an obesity-promoting diet. Process Biochemistry 45: 1406- 1414.

32. Maki KC, Reeves MS, Farmer M, Griinari M, Berge K, et al. (2009) Krill oil supplementation increases plasma concentrations of eicosapentaenoic and docosahexaenoic acids in overweight and obese men and women. Nutr Res 29: 609-615.

33. Ulven SM, Kirkhus B, Lamglait A, Basu S, Elind E, et al. (2011) Metabolic effects of krill oil are essentially similar to those of fish oil but at lower dose of EPA and DHA, in healthy volunteers. Lipids 46: 37-46.

34. Batetta B, Griinari M, Carta G, Murru E, Ligresti A, et al. (2009) Endocannabinoids may mediate the ability of (n-3) fatty acids to reduce ectopic fat and inflammatory mediators in obese Zucker rats. J Nutr 139: 1495-1501.

35. Graf BA, Duchateau GS, Patterson AB, Mitchell ES, van Bruggen P, et al. (2010) Age dependent incorporation of 14C-DHA into rat brain and body tissues after dosing various 14C-DHA-esters. Prostaglandins Leukot Essent Fatty Acids 83: 89-96.

36. Wijendran V, Huang MC, Diau GY, Boehm G, Nathanielsz PW, et al. (2002) Efficacy of dietary arachidonic acid provided as triglyceride or phospholipid as substrates for brain arachidonic acid accretion in baboon neonates. Pediatr Res 51: 265-272.

17

Physical, Thermal and Spectroscopic Characterization of m-Toluic Acid: An Impact of Biofield Treatment

Mahendra Kumar Trivedi[1], Alice Branton[1], Dahryn Trivedi[1], Gopal Nayak[1], Ragini Singh[2] and Snehasis Jana[2]*

[1]Trivedi Global Inc., 10624 S Eastern Avenue Suite A-969, Henderson, NV 89052, USA
[2]Trivedi Science Research Laboratory Pvt. Ltd., Hall-A, Chinar Mega Mall, Chinar Fortune City, Hoshangabad Rd, Bhopal- 462026, Madhya Pradesh, India

Abstract

m-toluic acid (MTA) is widely used in manufacturing of dyes, pharmaceuticals, polymer stabilizers, and insect repellents. The aim of present study was to evaluate the impact of biofield treatment on physical, thermal and spectroscopic properties of MTA. MTA sample was divided into two groups that served as treated and control. The treated group received Mr. Trivedi's biofield treatment. Subsequently, the control and treated samples were evaluated using X-ray diffraction (XRD), surface area analyser, differential scanning calorimetry (DSC), thermogravimetric analysis (TGA), Fourier transform infrared (FT-IR) and ultraviolet-visible (UV-Vis) spectroscopy. XRD result showed a decrease in crystallite size in treated samples *i.e.* 42.86% in MTA along with the increase in peak intensity as compared to control. However, surface area analysis showed an increase in surface area of 107.14% in treated MTA sample as compared to control. Furthermore, DSC analysis results showed that the latent heat of fusion was considerably reduced by 40.32%, whereas, the melting temperature was increased (2.23%) in treated MTA sample as compared to control. The melting point of treated MTA was found to be 116.04°C as compared to control (113.51°C) sample. Moreover, TGA/DTG studies showed that the control sample lost 56.25% of its weight, whereas, in treated MTA, it was found 58.60%. Also, T_{max} (temperature, at which sample lost maximum of its weight) was decreased by 1.97% in treated MTA sample as compared to control. It indicates that the vaporisation temperature of treated MTA sample might decrease as compared to control. The FT-IR and UV-Vis spectra did not show any significant change in spectral properties of treated MTA sample as compared to control. These findings suggest that biofield treatment has significantly altered the physical and thermal properties of m-toluic acid, which could make them more useful as a chemical intermediate.

Keywords: Biofield treatment; m-Toluic acid; X-ray diffraction study; Surface area analysis; Differential scanning calorimetry; Thermogravimetric analysis; Fourier transform infrared spectroscopy; Ultraviolet-visible spectroscopy

Introduction

The m-toluic acid (MTA) is a benzoic acid derivative having a floral honey odour. Benzoic acid occurs naturally in many plants and its name was also derived from a plant source *i.e.* Gum benzoin. Although it is used as precursor to plasticizers, preservatives such as sodium benzoate, it also has wide application in many pharmaceutical preparations meant for treatment of fungal skin diseases, topical antiseptics, expectorants, analgesics and decongestants [1,2]. The benzoic acid derivatives are also very useful due to their bacteriostatic and fragrant properties. They are used as intermediate in the production of various pharmaceuticals having analgesic, antirheumatic and vasodilator properties [3]. MTA is used as a chemical intermediate in manufacturing of insect repellent and plastic stabilizer in the chemical industry. It is also used in the production of various chemicals like 3-carboxybenzaldehyde, 3-benzoylphenylacetic acid, 3-methylbenzophenone, and N,N-diethyl-3-methylbenzamide *etc.* [4,5]. It is **a** main component of N,N-diethyl-m-toluamide, commonly known as DEET, which is first insect repellent that can be applied to skin or clothing and provide protection against mosquitoes and other biting insects [6].

MTA is used as intermediate in various chemical reactions, hence its rate of reaction plays a crucial role. It was reported previously that any alteration in crystallite size and surface area can affect the kinetics of reaction [7]. Moreover, the rate kinetics of any chemical reaction also depends on the thermal properties of the intermediate chemical compound *i.e.* latent heat of fusion, vaporisation temperature, decomposition temperature *etc.* [8]. After considering the properties and applications of MTA, authors wanted to investigate an economically safe approach that could be beneficial to modify their physical, thermal and spectral properties.

The concept of human bioenergy has its origin thousands of years back. It is scientifically termed as the biologically produced electromagnetic and subtle energy field that provides regulatory and communication functions within the human organs [9]. It generates through internal physiological processes such as blood flow, brain and heart function, *etc.* Nowadays, many biofield therapies are in practice for their possible therapeutic potentials such as enhanced personal well-being, improved functional ability of arthritis patient, decreased pain and anxiety [10-12]. The practitioners of these therapy claim that the healers channel supraphysical energy and intentionally direct this energy towards target [13]. Thus, a human has the ability to harness the energy from environment or universe and can transmit into any living or non-living object(s). The objects always receive the energy and responding into useful way that is called biofield energy and the process is known as biofield treatment.

Mr. Trivedi's biofield treatment (The Trivedi effect®) is well known and significantly studied in different fields such as microbiology [14-16], agriculture [17,18], and biotechnology [19]. Exposure to biofield energy caused an increase in medicinal property, growth, and

*Corresponding author: Snehasis Jana, Trivedi Science Research Laboratory Pvt. Ltd., Hall-A, Chinar Mega Mall, Chinar Fortune City, Hoshangabad Rd, Bhopal- 462026, Madhya Pradesh, India, E-mail: publication@trivedisrl.com

anatomical characteristics of ashwagandha [20]. Recently, the impact of biofield treatment on atomic, crystalline and powder characteristics as well as spectroscopic characters of different materials was studied [21,22]. The biofield treatment had increased the particle size by six fold and enhanced the crystallite size by two fold in zinc powder [23]. Hence, based on the outstanding results obtained after biofield treatment on different materials and considering the pharmaceutical applications of MTA, the present study was undertaken to evaluate the impact of biofield treatment on physical, thermal and spectroscopic properties of MTA.

Materials and Methods

m-toluic acid (MTA) was procured from S D Fine Chemicals Pvt. Ltd., India. The sample was divided into two parts; one was kept as a control, while other was subjected to Mr. Trivedi's biofield treatment and coded as treated sample. The treatment sample in sealed pack was handed over to Mr. Trivedi for biofield treatment under standard laboratory conditions. Mr. Trivedi provided the treatment through his energy transmission process to the treated group without touching the sample. The biofield treated sample was returned in the similarly sealed condition for further characterization using XRD, surface area analyser, DSC, TGA, FT-IR and UV-Vis spectroscopic techniques.

X-ray diffraction (XRD) study

XRD analysis was carried out on Phillips, Holland PW 1710 X-ray diffractometer system, which had a copper anode with nickel filter. The radiation of wavelength used by the XRD system was 1.54056 Å. The data obtained were in the form of a chart of 2θ vs. intensity and a detailed table containing peak intensity counts, d value (Å), peak width (θ°), relative intensity (%) etc.

The crystallite size (G) was calculated by using formula:

$$G = k\lambda/(b\cos\theta)$$

Here, λ is the wavelength of radiation used; b is full width half maximum (FWHM) of peaks and k is the equipment constant (=0.94). However, percent change in crystallite size was calculated using the following equation:

$$\text{Percent change in crystallite size} = [(G_t - G_c)/G_c] \times 100$$

Where, G_c and G_t are crystallite size of control and treated powder samples respectively.

Surface area analysis

The surface area was measured by the Surface area analyser, Smart SORB 90 based on Brunauer–Emmett–Teller (BET). Percent changes in surface area were calculated using following equation:

$$\% \text{ change in surface area} = \frac{[S_{Treated} - S_{Control}]}{S_{Control}} \times 100$$

Where, $S_{Control}$ and $S_{Treated}$ are the surface area of control and treated samples respectively.

Differential scanning calorimetry (DSC) study

For studies related to melting temperature and latent heat of fusion of MTA, Differential Scanning Calorimeter (DSC) of Perkin Elmer/ Pyris-1, USA with a heating rate of 10°C/min under air atmosphere and flow rate of 5 ml/min was used. Melting temperature and latent heat of fusion were obtained from the DSC curve.

Percent change in latent heat of fusion was calculated using

following equations:

$$\% \text{ change in Latent heat of fusion} = \frac{[\Delta H_{Treated} - \Delta H_{Control}]}{\Delta H_{Control}} \times 100$$

Where, $\Delta H_{Control}$ and $\Delta H_{Treated}$ are the latent heat of fusion of control and treated samples, respectively. Similarly, percent change in melting point was also calculated to observe the difference in thermal properties of treated MTA sample as compared to control.

Thermogravimetric analysis/ Derivative Thermogravimetry (TGA/DTG)

Thermal stability of control and treated sample of MTA was analysed by using Mettler Toledo simultaneous Thermogravimetric analyser (TGA/DTG). The samples were heated from room temperature to 400°C with a heating rate of 5°C/min under air atmosphere. From TGA curve, onset temperature T_{onset} (temperature at which sample start losing weight) and from DTG curve, T_{max} (temperature at which sample lost its maximum weight) were recorded.

Percent change in temperature at which maximum weight loss occur in sample was calculated using following equation:

$$\% \text{ change in } T_{max} = [(T_{max, treated} - T_{max, control}) / T_{max, control}] \times 100$$

Where, $T_{max, control}$ and $T_{max, treated}$ are the temperature at which maximum weight loss occurs in control and treated sample, respectively.

Percent change in onset peak temperature was calculated using following equation:

$$\% \text{ change in onset peak temperature } T_{onset} = [(T_{onset, treated} - T_{onset, control})/ T_{onset, control}] \times 100$$

Where, $T_{onset, control}$ and $T_{onset, treated}$ are onset peak temperature in control and treated sample, respectively.

Spectroscopic studies

For determination of spectroscopic characters, the treated sample was divided into two groups i.e. T1 and T2. Both treated groups were analysed for their spectral characteristics using FT-IR and UV-Vis spectroscopy as compared to control MTA sample.

FT-IR spectroscopic characterization

FT-IR spectra were recorded on Shimadzu's Fourier transform infrared spectrometer (Japan) with the frequency range of 4000-500 cm⁻¹. The samples are prepared by grinding the dry blended powders of control and treated MTA with powdered KBr, and then compressed to form discs. The FT-IR spectroscopic analysis of MTA (control, T1 and T2) were carried out to evaluate the impact of biofield treatment at atomic and molecular level like bond strength, stability, rigidity of structure etc. [24].

UV-Vis spectroscopic analysis

The UV-Vis spectral analysis was measured using Shimadzu UV-2400 PC series spectrophotometer over a wavelength range of 200-400 nm with 1 cm quartz cell and a slit width of 2.0 nm. This analysis was performed to evaluate the effect of biofield treatment on the structural property of MTA sample. The UV-Vis spectroscopy gives the preliminary information related to the skeleton of chemical structure and possible arrangement of functional groups. With UV-Vis spectroscopy, it is possible to investigate electron transfers between orbitals or bands of atoms, ions and molecules existing in the gaseous, liquid and solid phase [24].

Results and Discussion

X-ray diffraction

X-ray diffraction study was conducted to study the crystalline nature of the control and treated sample of MTA. XRD diffractograms of control and treated samples of MTA are shown in Figure 1. The XRD diffractogram of control MTA showed an intense crystalline peak at 2θ equals to 14.00°. The single intense peak indicated the crystalline nature of MTA. However, the XRD diffractogram of treated MTA showed the crystalline peak at 2θ equals to 13.90°. The treated sample peak showed high intensity as compared to control that indicated that crystallinity of treated MTA sample increased as compared to control. It is presumed that biofield energy may be absorbed by the treated MTA molecules that may lead to formation of more symmetrical crystalline long range pattern that caused increase in intensity of peak. In addition, the crystallite size was found to be 104.211 and 59.543 nm in control and treated MTA, respectively. The crystallite size was decreased by 42.86% in treated MTA as compared to control (Figure 2). The decreased crystallite size may be due to biofield energy that can induce strain in lattice and that possibly resulted in fracturing of grains into sub grains and hence decreased crystallite size [23]. MTA is used as intermediate in synthesis of many pharmaceutical compounds hence, decrease in crystallite size may lead to fasten the rate kinetics which ultimately enhances the percentage yield of end products [8].

Surface area analysis

The surface area of control and treated samples of MTA were investigated using BET method. The control sample showed a surface area of 0.14 m^2/g however, the treated sample of MTA showed a surface area of 0.29 m^2/g. The percentage increase in surface area was 107.14% in the treated MTA sample as compared to control (Figure 2). The XRD results of treated MTA sample revealed that crystallite size decreased after biofield treatment. It could be a possible reason for increase in surface area of treated MTA sample [25]. Moreover, increase in surface area of reactant molecules fastens the rate of reaction [26]. Hence, it is hypothesized that increase in surface area of treated MTA sample can be used to increase the rate of those reactions where MTA is used as intermediate reagent.

Thermal studies

DSC analysis: DSC was used to determine ΔH and melting temperature in control and treated sample of MTA. The DSC thermograms of control and treated samples of MTA are shown in Figure 3 and the analysis results are presented in Table 1. In a solid, the amount of energy required to change the phase from solid to liquid is known as latent heat of fusion (ΔH). Further, the energy supplied during phase change *i.e.* ΔH is stored as potential energy of atoms. The

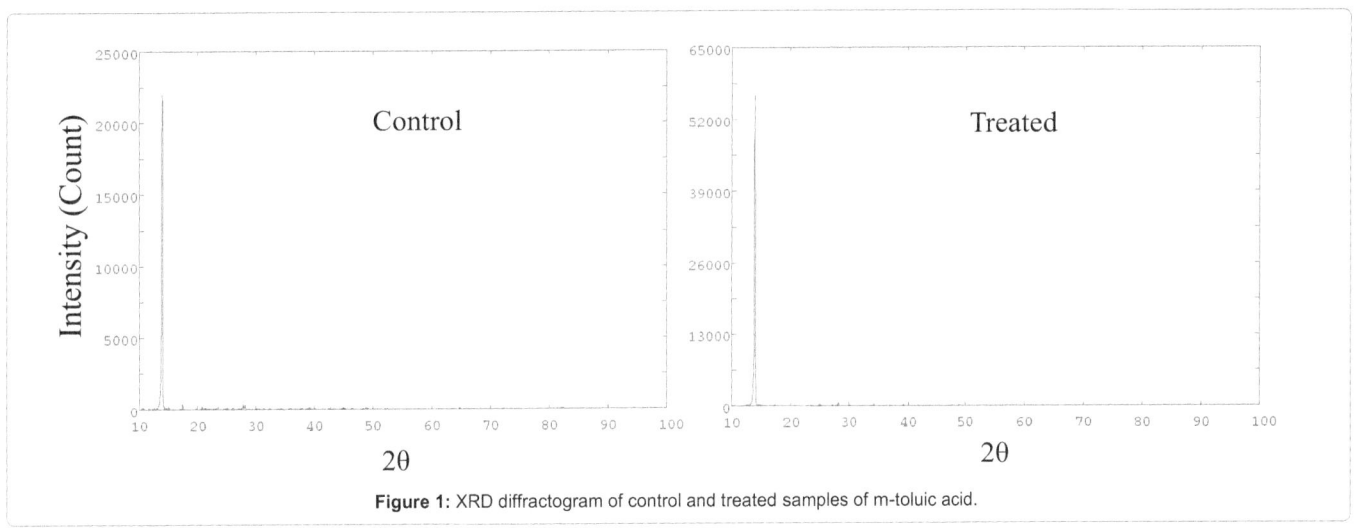

Figure 1: XRD diffractogram of control and treated samples of m-toluic acid.

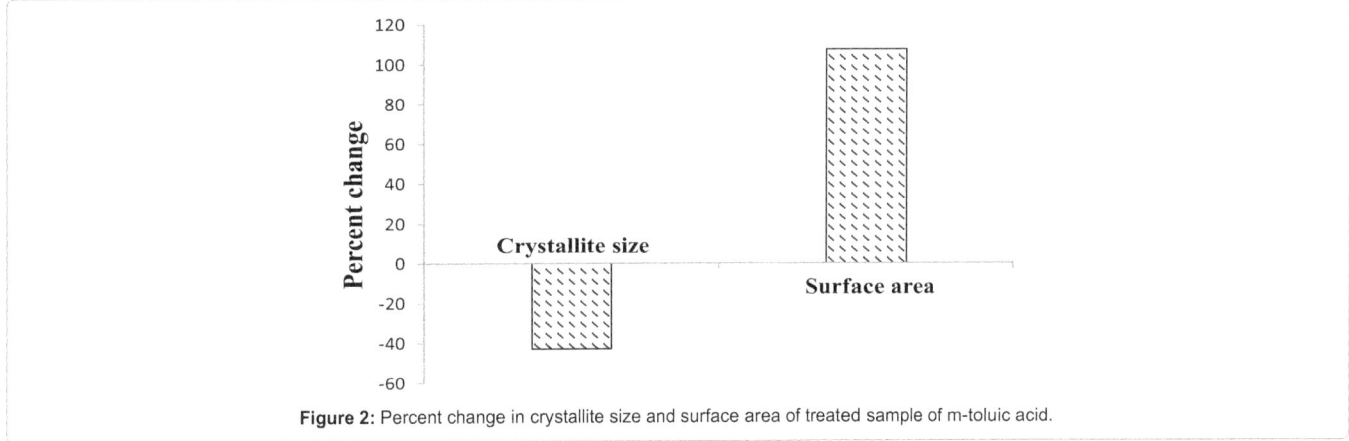

Figure 2: Percent change in crystallite size and surface area of treated sample of m-toluic acid.

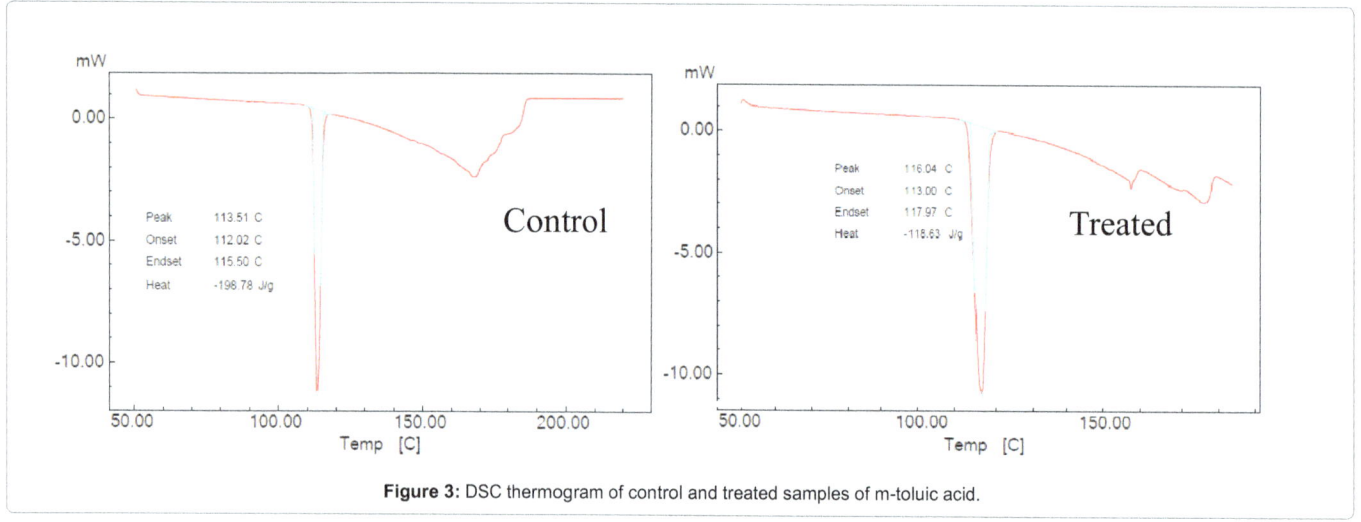

Figure 3: DSC thermogram of control and treated samples of m-toluic acid.

Parameter	Control	Treated
Latent heat of fusion ΔH (J/g)	198.78	118.63
Melting point (°C)	113.51	116.04
T_{max} (°C)	187.02	183.32
Weight loss (%)	56.25	58.60

T_{max}: temperature at which maximum weight loss occur

Table 1: Thermal analysis of control and treated sample of m-Toluic acid.

data showed that ΔH was reduced from 198.78 J/g (control) to 118.63 J/g in treated MTA. It indicates that ΔH was decreased by 40.32% in treated sample as compared to control (Figure 5). The reduction in ΔH revealed that treated MTA probably have extra internal energy in the form of potential energy as compared to control, which might be transferred through biofield treatment. This potential energy may be stored in treated MTA molecules, that could lead to lowering of ΔH in treated sample as compared to control. However, the melting temperature is related to the kinetic energy of the atoms [27]. The melting temperature of treated MTA was increased from 113.51°C (control) to 116.04°C. Thus, data suggest that melting point was increased by 2.23% as compared to control (Figure 5). Previously, our group reported that biofield treatment has altered ΔH and melting point in lead and tin powder [28]. Besides, the increase of melting point in treated MTA suggests that kinetic energy and thermal vibrations of molecules probably altered after biofield treatment. In addition, the sharpness of the endothermic peaks showed a good degree of crystallinity in control and treated sample of MTA.

TGA/DTG analysis: Thermogravimetric analysis/derivative thermogravimetry analysis (TGA/DTG) of control and biofield treated samples are summarized in Table 1. TGA thermogram (Figure 4) showed that control MTA sample started losing weight around 170°C (onset) and stopped near 212°C (end set). However, the treated MTA started losing weight near to 164°C (onset) and terminated near 209°C (end set). It indicates that onset temperature of treated MTA decreased by 3.52% as compared to control (Figure 5). Furthermore, in this process, control sample lost 56.25% and treated MTA sample lost 58.60% of its weight, which could be due to vaporisation of MTA. Besides, DTG thermogram data showed T_{max} at 187.02°C in control, whereas, it was decreased to 183.32°C in treated MTA (Table 1). It indicates that T_{max} was decreased by 1.97% in treated MTA (Figure 5). Furthermore, the reduction in T_{max} in treated MTA with respect to control sample may be correlated with increase in vaporisation

of treated MTA after biofield treatment. A possible reason for this reduction in T_{max} is that biofield energy might cause some alteration in internal energy which results into earlier vaporisation of treated MTA sample as compared to control. Moreover, it was previously reported that the state of reactant affect rate of reaction, *i.e.* gases reacts faster than solid and liquids because gases consumed less energy to separate their particles from each other [26]. Also, decrease in vaporisation temperature indicates that MTA molecules change their phase from liquid to vapour at low temperature, which may result in more frequent collision of MTA molecules with other reactants at low temperature, hence fasten the reaction rate [26]. Apart from that, it was previously reported that vapour phase reaction can be more advantageous as compared to liquid phase reaction in terms of reaction time, generation of objectionable amounts of odour and undesired by-products [29,30]. Hence, overall observations suggest that biofield treated MTA can be used to enhance the reaction kinetics and yield of the end product.

Spectroscopic studies

FT-IR analysis: FT-IR spectra of control, T1 and T2 samples of MTA are shown in Figure 6. It showed similar distribution patterns for both control and treated (T1 and T2) samples of MTA. The O-H stretching (carboxylic acid) peak was appeared at 3061-2576 cm⁻¹ in control MTA. In treated samples, O-H stretching (carboxylic acid) peak appeared in same range *i.e.* 3061-2576 cm⁻¹ in T1 and 3064-2576 cm⁻¹ in T2 sample. The peak due to C-H stretching (sp₃) was appeared at 2951, 2953 and 2951 cm⁻¹ in control, T1 and T2 sample respectively. The C=O stretching (carboxylic acid) peak was appeared at 1689 cm⁻¹ in control and 1685 cm⁻¹ in both T1 and T2 samples. The peak due to aromatic C=C stretching was appeared at 1608 cm⁻¹ in all three samples *i.e.* control, T1 and T2. Similarly C-C stretching peak (in ring) was found at 1589 cm⁻¹ in all three samples *i.e.* control, T1 and T2. O-H bending peak was found at 1417, 1415 and 1417 cm⁻¹ in control, T1 and T2 sample respectively. C-O stretching (carboxylic acid) peak was appeared at 1311 cm⁻¹ in all three samples *i.e.* control, T1 and T2. Similarly, C-OH stretching peak appeared at 1217 cm⁻¹ in all three samples *i.e.* control, T1 and T2. C-H bending (out of plane) peak was found at 931 cm⁻¹ in control and 933 cm⁻¹ in both T1 and T2 sample. The peak due to meta substituted arene was appeared at 748 cm⁻¹ in control and T1 and at 750 cm⁻¹ in T2. The FT-IR spectra were well supported by reference data [31].

The FT-IR spectroscopic study showed that no alteration was found in FT-IR spectra of treated samples (T1 and T2) as compared to

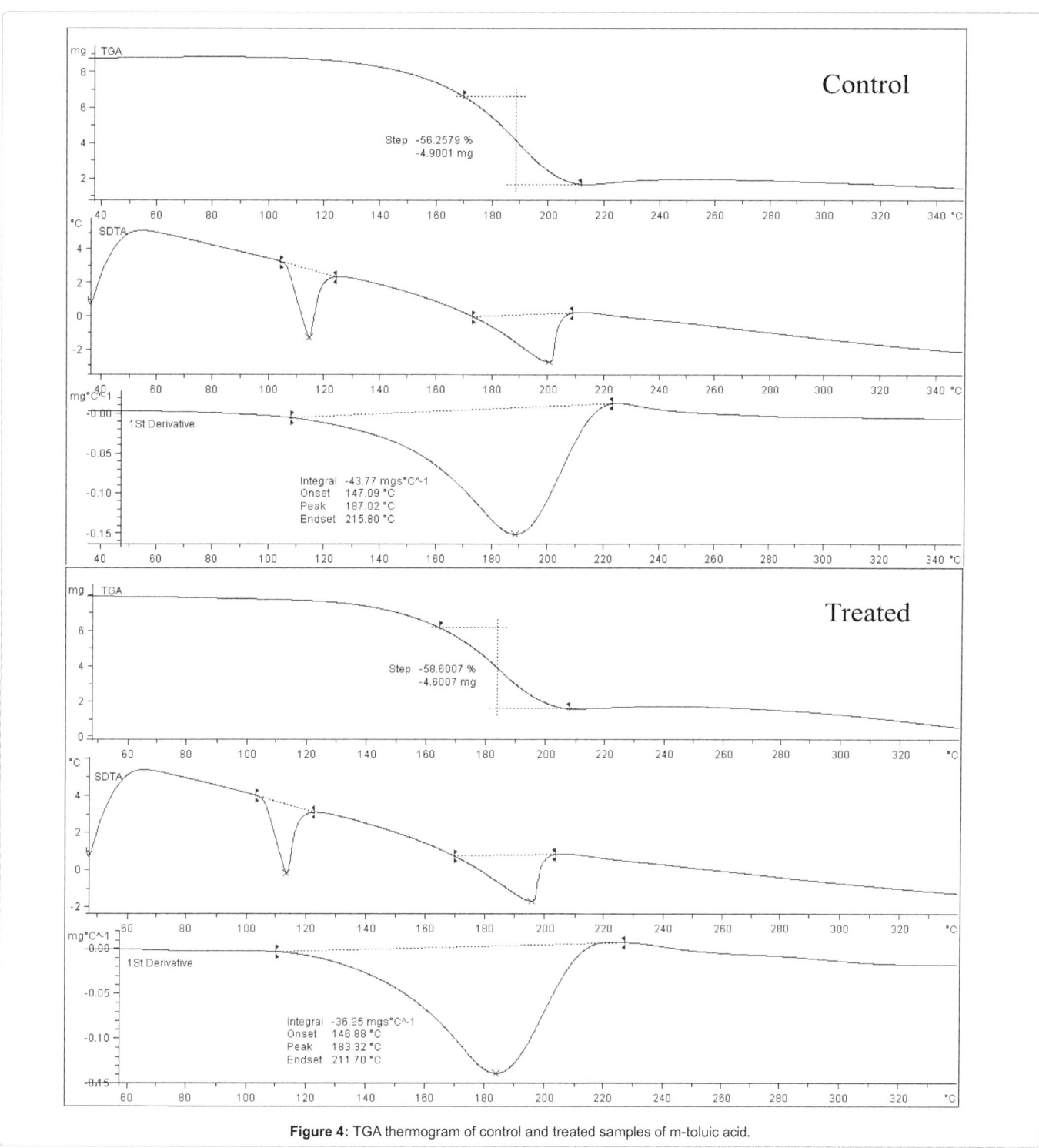

Figure 4: TGA thermogram of control and treated samples of m-toluic acid.

control. It suggests that biofield treatment did not cause any alteration in structural and bonding properties like bond strength, stability, rigidity of structure *etc*.

UV-Vis spectroscopic analysis: The UV spectra of control and treated samples (T1 and T2) of MTA are shown in Figure 7. The UV spectrum of control sample showed characteristic absorption at 204 nm which was also observed in both treated samples (T1 and T2) at 203 nm. Another absorption peak was observed at 230 nm in

control sample which was evident in T1 and T2 at 230 nm and 229 nm respectively. The spectrum of control sample showed weak absorption at 278 nm. The treated samples *i.e.* T1 and T2 also showed same kind of peak at 278 nm and 275 nm respectively. The UV spectrum of control MTA was well supported by literature data [32]. It suggests that biofield treatment could not make any alteration in chemical structure or arrangement of functional groups of treated MTA samples.

Conclusion

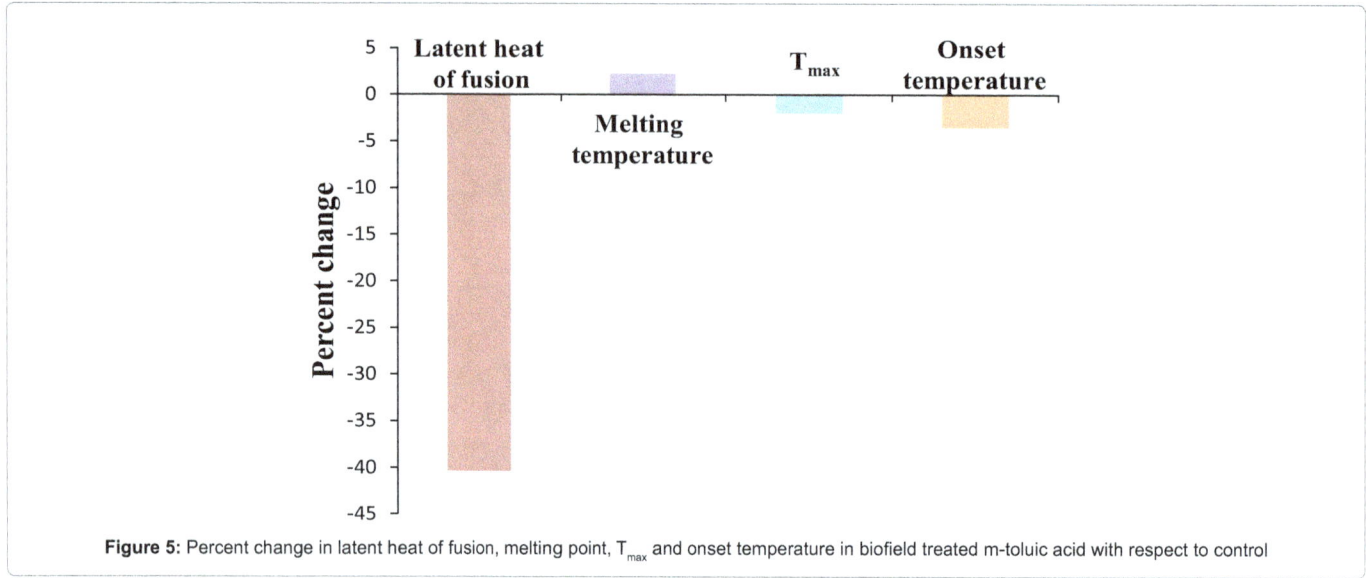

Figure 5: Percent change in latent heat of fusion, melting point, T_{max} and onset temperature in biofield treated m-toluic acid with respect to control

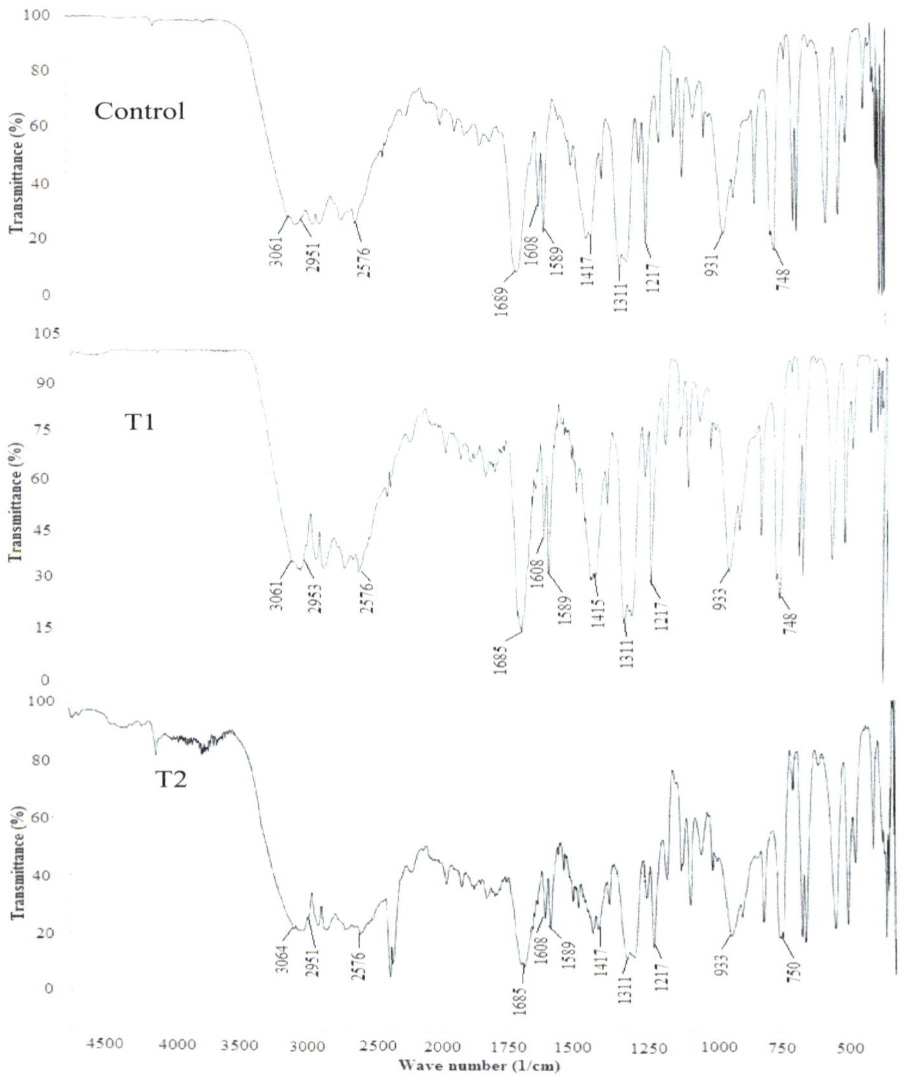

Figure 6: FT-IR spectra of control and treated samples of m-toluic acid.

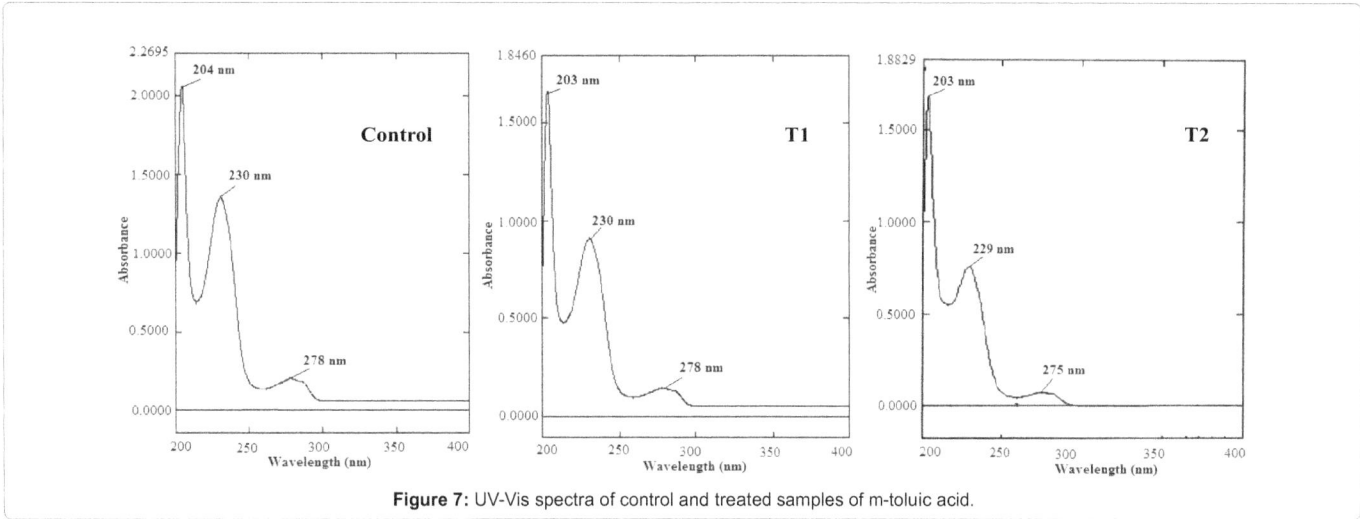

Figure 7: UV-Vis spectra of control and treated samples of m-toluic acid.

The overall study showed the influence of biofield treatment on physical and thermal properties of MTA. XRD result showed that crystallite size was decreased by 42.86% in treated MTA samples as compared to control, which might be due to fracturing of grains into sub grains caused by lattice strain produced *via* biofield energy. The surface area analysis showed an increase in surface area of 107.14% in treated MTA sample as compared to control. The reduced crystallite size and increased surface area may lead to increasing the reaction kinetics of MTA, which could make it more useful as an intermediate compound. Thermal analysis data revealed that latent heat of fusion was reduced by 40.32% in treated MTA as compared to control. TGA/DTG studies showed that T_{max} was decreased by 1.97% in treated MTA samples. On the basis of reduction in T_{max}, it is hypothesized that MTA molecules turn into vapour phase at low temperature as compared to control. Hence, molecules in vapour phase may collide more frequently with other reactants in any reaction that might enhance the rate of reaction. Therefore, it is assumed that biofield treated MTA could be more useful as an intermediate in the production of various pharmaceutical products.

Acknowledgement

The authors would like to acknowledge the whole team of Sophisticated Analytical Instrument Facility (SAIF), Nagpur, Indian Rubber Manufacturers Research Association (IRMRA), Thane and MGV Pharmacy College, Nashik for providing the instrumental facility. Authors are very grateful for the support of Trivedi Science, Trivedi Master Wellness and Trivedi Testimonials in this research work.

References

1. Wilson CO (2004) Wilson and Gisvold's textbook of organic medicinal and pharmaceutical. (11thedn), Lippincott Williams & Wilkins, Philadelphia, U.S.

2. http://www.medipharmalimited.com/whitfield_ointment.asp

3. Lillard B (1919) Practical druggist and pharmaceutical review of reviews. Lillard & Company, Michigan, U.S.

4. Knoess PH, Neeland EG (1998) A modified synthesis of the insect repellent DEET. J Chem Educ 75: 1267.

5. Bays D, Foster R (1974) Benzoylphenylacetic acids and related compounds. U.S. Patent 3828093.

6. Pavia DL, Lampman GM, Kriz GS, Engel RG (2005) Introduction to organic laboratory techniques: A small scale approach. Cengage Learning, U.S.

7. Carballo LM, Wolf EE (1978) Crystallite size effects during the catalytic oxidation of propylene on Pt/?-Al2O3. J Catal 53: 366-373.

8. Chaudhary AL, Sheppard DA, Paskevicius M, Pistidda C, Dornheim M, et al (2015) Reaction kinetic behaviour with relation to crystallite/grain size dependency in the Mg–Si–H system. Acta Mater 95: 244-253.

9. Movaffaghi Z, Farsi M (2009) Biofield therapies: biophysical basis and biological regulations? Complement Ther Clin Pract 15: 35-37.

10. Giasson M, Bouchard L (1998) Effect of therapeutic touch on the well-being of persons with terminal cancer. J Holist Nurs 16: 383-398.

11. Peck SD (1998) The efficacy of therapeutic touch for improving functional ability in elders with degenerative arthritis. Nurs Sci Q 11: 123-132.

12. Turner JG, Clark AJ, Gauthier DK, Williams M (1998) The effect of therapeutic touch on pain and anxiety in burn patients. J Adv Nurs 28: 10-20.

13. Mager J, Moore D, Bendl D, Wong B, Rachlin K, et al. (2007) Evaluating biofield treatments in a cell culture model of oxidative stress. Explore (NY) 3: 386-390.

14. Trivedi MK, Bhardwaj Y, Patil S, Shettigar H, Bulbule A (2009) Impact of an external energy on Enterococcus faecalis [ATCC-51299] in relation to antibiotic susceptibility and biochemical reactions-an experimental study. J Accord Integr Med 5: 119-130.

15. Trivedi MK, Patil S (2008) Impact of an external energy on Staphylococcus epidermis [ATCC-13518] in relation to antibiotic susceptibility and biochemical reactions-an experimental study. J Accord Integr Med 4: 230-235.

16. Trivedi MK, Patil S (2008) Impact of an external energy on Yersinia enterocolitica [ATCC-23715] in relation to antibiotic susceptibility and biochemical reactions: An experimental study. Internet J Alternat Med 6: 13.

17. Shinde V, Sances F, Patil S, Spence A (2012) Impact of biofield treatment on growth and yield of lettuce and tomato. Aust J Basic Appl Sci 6: 100-105.

18. Sances F, Flora E, Patil S, Spence A, Shinde V (2013) Impact of biofield treatment on ginseng and organic blueberry yield. Agrivita J Agric Sci 35: 22-29.

19. Patil SA, Nayak GB, Barve SS, Tembe RP, Khan RR (2012) Impact of biofield treatment on growth and anatomical characteristics of Pogostemon cablin (Benth.). Biotechnology 11: 154-162.

20. Altekar N, Nayak G (2015) Effect of biofield treatment on plant growth and adaptation. J Environ Health Sci 1: 1-9.

21. Dabhade VV, Tallapragada RR, Trivedi MK (2009) Effect of external energy on atomic, crystalline and powder characteristics of antimony and bismuth powders. Bull Mater Sci 32: 471-479.

22. Trivedi MK, Nayak G, Patil S, Tallapragada RM, Latiyal O, et al. (2015) Studies of the atomic and crystalline characteristics of ceramic oxide nano powders after bio field treatment. Ind Eng Manage 4: 161.

23. Trivedi MK, Tallapragada RR (2008) A transcendental to changing metal powder characteristics. Met Powder Rep 63: 22-28.

24. Pavia DL, Lampman GM, Kriz GS (2001) Introduction to spectroscopy. (3rdedn), Thomson Learning, Singapore.

25. Okada K, Nagashima T, Kameshima Y, Yasumori A, Tsukada T (2002) Relationship between formation conditions, properties, and crystallite size of boehmite. J Colloid Interface Sci 253: 308-314.

26. Espenson JH (1995) Chemical kinetics and reaction mechanisms. (2ndedn) Mcgraw-Hill, U.S.

27. Moore J (2010) Chemistry: The molecular science. (4thedn), Brooks Cole, Belmont, U.S.

28. Trivedi MK, Patil S, Tallapragada RM (2013) Effect of biofield treatment on the physical and thermal characteristics of silicon, tin and lead powders. J Material Sci Eng 2: 125.

29. Morrell CE, Beach LK (1948) Oxidation of aromatic compounds. U.S. Patent 2443832.

30. Hull EH (1979) Production of N,N-di(ethyl)-meta-toluamide from meta-toluic acid by liquid phase catalytic reaction with diethylamine. U.S. Patent 4133833.

31. Cutler HG (1999) Biologically active natural products: Agrochemicals. CRC Press, U.S.

32. Lang L (1969) Absorption spectra in the ultraviolet and visible region. Akademiai Kiado Publishers Budapest 10: 115-400.

18

Phytochemical Analysis of Wild and *In vitro* Raised Plants of *Rheum* Species using HPLC

Tabin S[1]*, Gupta RC[1], Kamili AN[2] and Bansal G[3]

[1]*Department of Botany, Punjabi University Patiala, Punjab, India*
[2]*Centre of Research for Development, University of Kashmir, Srinagar, India*
[3]*Department of Pharmaceutical Sciences and Drug Research, Punjabi University Patiala, Punjab, India*

Abstract

The plants are micro-biosynthetic factories for variety of compounds which are their secondary metabolites. These mainly include alkaloids, glycosides, flavonoids, volatile oils, saponins, etc. The medicinal properties are attributed to the specific bioactive compound or combination of phytochemicals. In present study, Phytochemical analysis of two *Rheum* species namely, *Rheum spiciforme* and *Rheum webbianum* was carried out using different plant parts from wild populations and also from tissue culture raised plants derived from these wild populations. Anthraquinone derivatives including emodin, aloe-emodin and rhein was quantified in analysed plant parts using HPLC method and a comparative analysis was done. The analyzed samples showed presence of various alkaloids, carbohydrates, proteins and tannins. Furthermore, *Rheum* spp. are shown to contain emodin, aloe-emodin and rhein as main active principles. Among the various populations of *R. spiciforme* maximum yield of aloe-emodin and Rhein was detected in Chakwali population while maximum amount of emodin was found in Dahi nala. Similarly, in *R. webbianum* maximum yield of aloe-emodin and rhein was detected in Panzila top population while maximum amount of emodin was found in Tangsti population. The different regenerants from tissue cultured plants showed very low yield of these active compounds as compared to wild populations in both the species. The reported contents of different phytochemicals can be useful in determination of best chemotypes which will be significant for the future use of these chemotypes in pharmaceutical industries (Graphical Abstract).

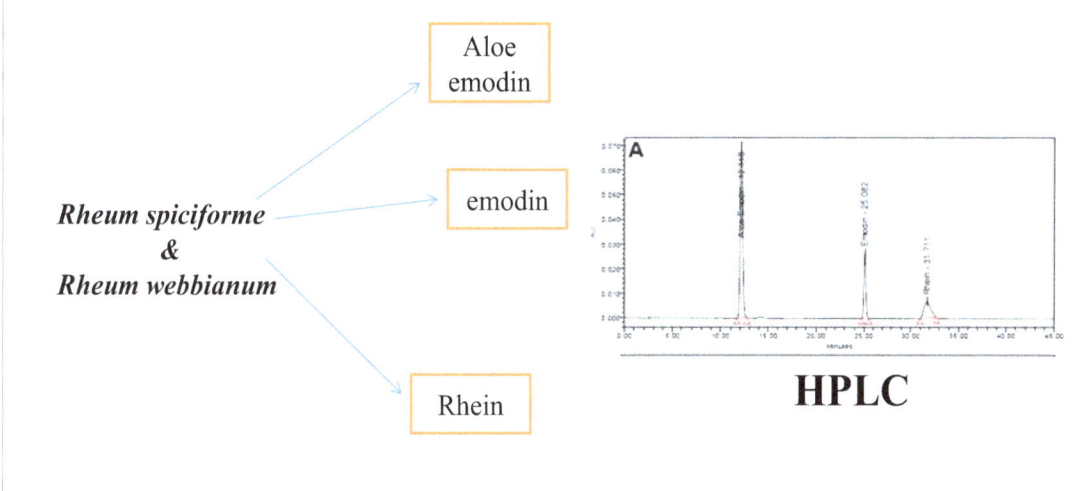

Keywords: *Rheum*; HPLC; Aloe-emodin; Anthraquinones; Phytochemicals; Anticancer; Antioxidant compounds

Introduction

Rheum species, commonly called rhubarb, are included in endangered plants list and are under great threat. It has been listed as vulnerable by various agencies like IUCN, UNEP and WWF particularly from Kashmir Himalaya [1]. *Rheum* has sixty species all over the world and mostly famous for its medicinal value, as recent studies have proved rhubarb as one of the anticancer plant. *Rheum* includes perennial, stout herbs, mainly distributed in the temperate and sub- tropical regions of world chiefly in Asian countries viz. India, Nepal, Bhutan, China, Pakistan, Korea, Turkey, Russia and Tibet. Many compounds used in today's medicine have a complex structure, and synthesizing these bioactive compounds chemically at a low price is not easy [2]. The age old traditional values attached with the various forest types and the varieties of forest products (i.e.,

medicinal plants) have gained tremendous importance in the present century [3]. In china, *Rheum* plant is worshipped as it cures so many diseases and it is called as Dahuang in China. The *Rheum* plant is an eatable plant. It can be taken as a food ad it can be also cooked. Its juicy stalks are eaten raw and its leaves are cooked as a vegetable. In India it is found in Western Himalaya, and Northern Himalaya. In

*Corresponding author: Shagoon Tabin, Department of Botany, Punjabi University Patiala, Punjab-147002, India, E-mail: shagoonkhan@gmail.com

Kashmir it is found in all in over the Kashmir Himalaya which includes regions of Ladakh, Guerz, Anantnag and Baramulla districts. *R. webbianum* is used in treatment of indigestion, abdominal disorders, boils, wounds and flactuaence [4]. It is also helpful in managing cancers [5]. *R. emodi* is puragative, stomachache, astringent, tonic and effective in curing skin diseases [6,7] it is an antioxidant [8] and [9] cytotoxic in nature [10], Kinase II inhibitory [11], anti-viral [12] and nephroprotective [13]. Moreover, it is used as textile dyeing [14], anti-microbial, anti-tumor, anti-inflammatory [15] used in cosmetics ad as food colorant [16], live stimulant, purgative, anticholesterololeamic, antitumor, antiseptic, tonic, and, antiparlinson [17]. Hypatoprotective principles that can prevent and treat liver damage [18], blocks the binding of SARS-CoV S proein to ACE2 and infectivity of S protein pseudotyped retrovirus to vero E6 cells [19], Antidiabetic, similar to insulin [20], Nephroroprotective properties [21] anticancer, anti-oxidant [22,23]. *R. spiciforme* is also an adulterant and also used also in the treatment of boils, wounds, rheumatic pain. Roots are frequently used for the treatment of bone fractures, backache and joints pain [24]. Chromatography is one of the fast emerging tools by which the quality control and fingerprint of herbs can be assessed accurately. Using this technique, the identification of various chemical markers of the herbal drugs can be easily done and it also helps to identify the specific herb in combination of other herbs. Popularity of HPLC for analysis of herbal drugs is due to its economic, rapid and simultaneous screening of large number of herbal samples in less time. The main active ingredients of the *Rheum* species are a series of anthraquinones, dianthrones, glycosides and tannins. The anthraquinone derivatives including emodin, aloe-emodin, rhein, physcion, chrysophanol and their glucosides are the accepted important active principles. Rhaponticin, a distyrene derivative, only exists in non-quality (inferior-grade) rhubarb. In quality rhubarb and most exported rhubarbs, the content of rhaponticin is not detected. Like all such substances, rhein is a cathartic. Rhein is commonly found as a glycoside such as rhein-8-glucoside or glucorhein. Rhein was first isolated in Yu et al. [25]. Originally the rhubarb plant which contains rhein was used as a laxative. It was believed that rhein along with other anthraquinone glycosides imparted this activity. Rhein has been reevaluated as an antibacterial agent against *Staphylococcus aureus* [26]. Present study was aimed to find out the anthraquinones from the two *Rheum spp.* for which three standards were used i.e., aloe emodin, emodin and rhein.

Materials and Methods

The roots and rhizomes of *R. webbianum* and *R. spiciforme* were kept in brown paper bags dried under room temperature. The *in vitro* explants i.e., leaves, roots and callus [27] of these species were also dried in room temperature in paper bags. The dried roots and rhizomes of all these species were grinded in pestle and mortar to powder form for making methanol (HPLC grade) extracts. The glassware and methanol (HPLC grade) was procured from commercial suppliers. Triple distilled water was used in the laboratory for different steps.

Extraction of plant material

The powdered roots and rhizomes of each sample (30 g) were charged in a soxhlet apparatus and extracted with 500 ml of HPLC methanol on water bath. The extraction was continued for one week. The extract was concentrated and dried on rotary evaporator under reduced pressure. The resultant semisolid, sticky extract of each sample was stored at 4°C till further analysis. Each extract was subjected to phytochemical screening to detect the different types of constituents present in it. We used Dragendorff's test for alkaloids, Fehling

solutions test for carbohydrates, Millions test for proteins and amino acids, Salkowski reaction for steroids, Shinoda test for Flavonoids, Keller-Killiani test for glycosides, $FeCl_3$ test for tannins and phenolic compounds and Sudan Reagent test for Fats and oils.

HPLC analysis

The chromatographic analysis was carried out on a Waters HPLC system comprising binary pumps (515), auto injector (2707) and PDA detector (2998), controlled by Empower Pro software. Each standard marker (rhein, emodin, aloe-emodin) and extract (1 g extract dissolved in 5 ml methanol) was chromatographed on a C_{18} column (250 mm × 4.6 mm; Sunfire) with gradient elution by using methanol (mobile phase A) and 2% acetic acid (mobile phase B) at a flow rate of 0.5 ml/min. The column was maintained at a temperature of 30°C. The injection volume was fixed at 10 µl and LC-UV chromatographs were extracted at 254 nm. The gradient program for elution is given in Table 1. Purity of each marker peak in LC-UV chromatogram of each sample was ascertained by PDA analysis.

For quantification of the three markers (aloe-emodin, rhein & emodin), a standard solution containing these three markers (1 µg/ml) in methanol was prepared and analysed (n=6) using the optimized HPLC methanol. Peak area of each marker (mean ± SD) was determined, and it was used to calculate the content of markers in samples of *Rheum* collected from different sources. For sample analyses, each extract obtained after recovery of the solvent was dissolved in 150 ml of methanol. This extract solution was analysed by the HPLC method and contents of markers were calculated as follows:

Content of markers in (µg/30 g) = $(A_S/A_T) \times 1 \times 150$

Where, A_S = peak area of marker in standard solution A_T = peak area of marker in extract solution 1= concentration of marker in standard solution in 150 µg/ml = dilution factor.

Results

Rheum webbianum

The phytochemical screening of extracts of *R. webbianum* showed that the amino acids were absent in the samples of Panzila Top, Khardungla and Tangsti, whereas glycosides were absent in the samples of Khardungla and Tangsti. It was also observed that all types of phytoconstituents were present in each of the *in vitro* explants also (Table 1).

HPLC analysis

The contents of aloe-emodin, emodin and rhein in various samples of *R. webbianum* were found to be in the range of 67.5-4500, 255-2385 and 0.4-1143 µg/30 g of the plant material, respectively (Table 2). The LC-UV chromatograms of extracts of different samples of *R. webbianum* along with *in vitro* explants are shown in Figure 1. The roots showed the presence of anthraquinones i.e., aloe-emodin, emodin and rhein in all the observed samples. The maximum content of aloe-emodin and rhein was found in Panzila Top sample, whereas maximum content of emodin was found in Tangsti sample (Table 2 and Figure 2). Of these, Panzila Top, populations (2n=22), whereas all other populations are tetraploid (2n=44). The amount of aloe emodin and rhein is found to be very high in diploid cytotype, compared with all the populations of tetraploid cytotypes. However, the amount of emodin is more than two populations and less than other two populations. The leaves, roots and callus of *in vitro* explants were also analysed for anthraquinones content (Table 2 and Figure 2). The maximum content of the markers of aloe-emodin and rhein was found in *in vitro* callus, while the maximum content of emodin was found in *in vitro* leaves (Table 2, Figure 2).

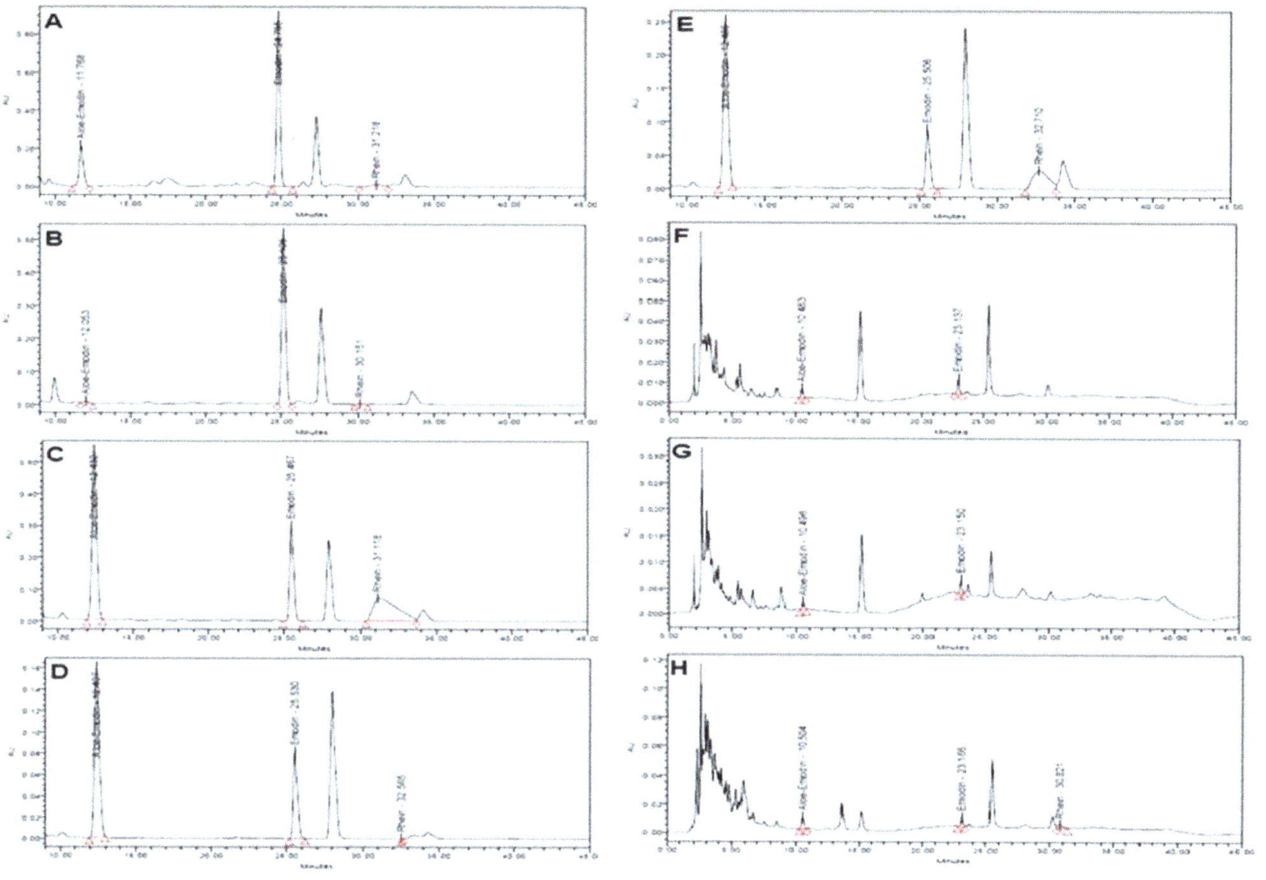

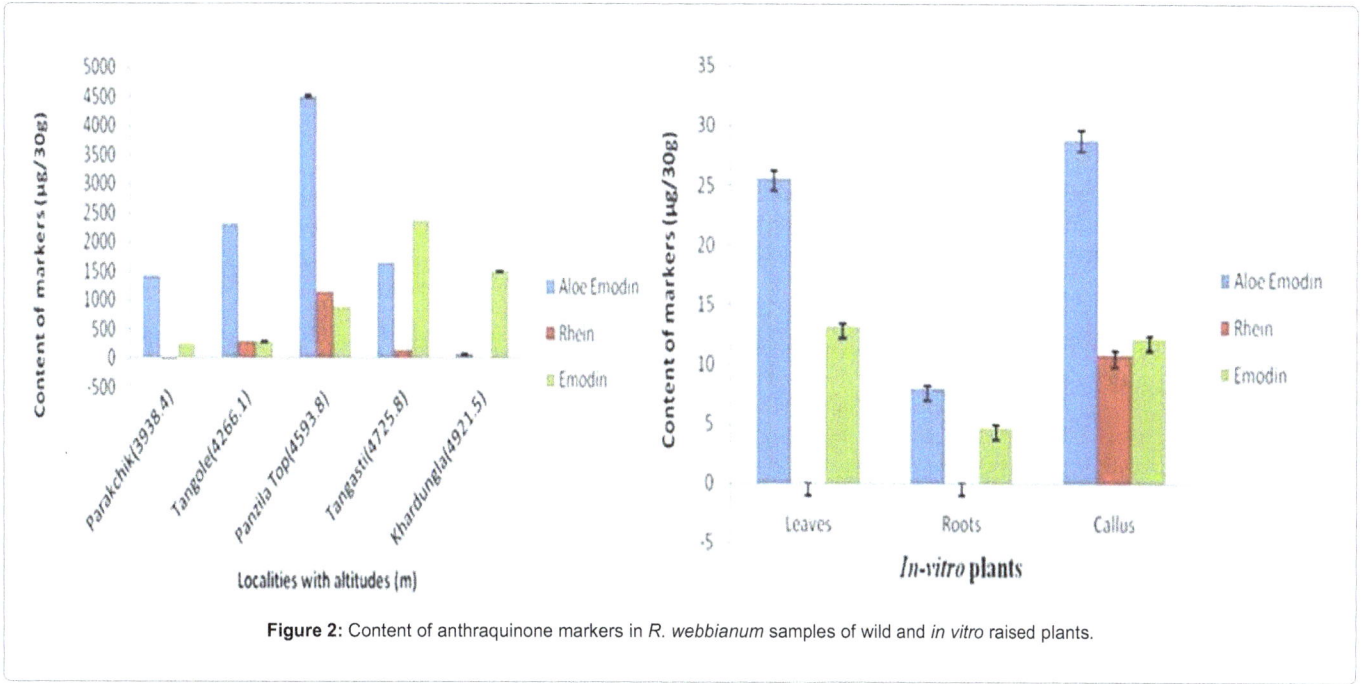

Figure 1: (A-H): LC-UV chromatographs of *R. webbianum* samples collected from Tangsti (A), Khardungla (B), Pazila top (C), Parakhchik (D), Tangole (E), *In vitro* leaves (F), *In vitro* roots (G), *In vitro* callus (H).

Figure 2: Content of anthraquinone markers in *R. webbianum* samples of wild and *in vitro* raised plants.

Samples	Alkaloids	Carbohydrates	proteins	Amino acids	Steroids	Flavonoids	Glycosides	Tannins and phenols	Fats and oils
Panzila top (4x)	+	+	+	−	+	+	+	+	+
Tangole (4x)	+	+	+	+	+	+	+	+	+
Parakhchik (2x)	+	+	+	+	+	+	+	+	+
Tangtsi (4x)	+	+	+	−	+	+	−	+	+
Khardungla (4x)	+	+	+	−	+	+	−	+	+
Roots (in-vitro)	+	+	+	+	+	+	+	+	+
Leaves (in-vitro)	+	+	+	+	+	+	+	+	+
Callus(in-vitro)	+	+	+	+	+	+	+	+	+

(+): Present; (-): Absent

Table 1: Estimation of different compounds from methanolic extracts of *R. webbianum*.

Samples	Altitude (m)	Content (µg/30 g of samples)		
		Aloe-emodin	Emodin	Rhein
Khardungla (4x)	4921.5	67.5 ± 0.8	1500.0 ± 9.3	5.7 ± 0.1
Tangsti (4x)	4725.8	1650 ± 10.4	2385 ± 18.6	130.5 ± 1.7
Panzila top (2x)	4593.8	4500 ± 29.2	885 ± 9.5	1143.0 ± 12.7
Tangole (4x)	4266.1	2130 ± 16.7	279.0 ± 3.1	282.0 ± 3.7
Parakachik (4x)	3938.4	1410.0 ± 12.3	255.0 ± 3.6	0.4 ± 0.01
Leaves (in vitro raised)	-	15.3 ± 0.7	13.2 ± 0.2	ND
Roots (in vitro raised)	-	7.95 ± 0.3	4.65 ± 0.2	ND
Callus (in vitro raised)	-	48 ± 0.8	12.15 ± 0.2	10.8 ± 0.3

ND: Not Detected

Table 2: Content of different active constituents in various samples of wild *R. webbianum* populations and in regenerants of *in vitro* raised plants.

Rheum spiciforme

Phytochemical screening: The extracts along with the *in vitro* explants of *R. spiciforme* were screened for phytochemical tests, and it was observed that all the compounds i.e., amino acids, steroids, glycosides, etc., were present in all the samples (Table 3).

HPLC analysis: The sharp and symmetrical peaks were observed for all the three marker anthraquinones i.e., aloe-emodin, emodin and rhein in all the samples of *R. spiciforme* (Figure 3 and Table 3). The maximum content of aloe-emodin (3409.5 µg/30 g) and rhein (531.4 µg/30 g) was found in Chakwali, whereas, maximum content of emodin (915.0 µg/30 g) was found in Dahi Nala. The different parts of *in vitro* explant i.e., leaves, roots and callus were also analysed for markers. The maximum content of aloe-emodin and emodin was found in *in vitro* callus whereas rhein was absent in all the three explants (Table 4 and Figure 4).

Discussion

Plants are rich source of effective and safe medicines due to presence of different bioactive molecules such as alkaloids, flavonoids, glycosides, tannins, phenolic compounds, etc. [28,29]. *Rheum* is a well-known medicinal plant having anti-cancer and anti-oxidant activities. Anthraquinone is the major class of phytochemicals, which is responsible for its pharmacological activities. These constituents are mainly present in roots and rhizomes. The main members of anthraquinone class include aloe-emodin, emodin, chrysaphanol, physcion and rhein, which are proved as anticancer agents [30]. Anthocyanins and flavonols are also found in *Rheum* [31,32]. In the present study, three anthraquinones were analysed i.e., aloe-emodin, rhein and emodin. Aloe-emodin (1,8-Dihydroxy-3-(hydroxymethyl)-

9,10-anthraquinone) has been reported to exhibit anticancer activity on neuroectodermal tumors, lung squamous cell carcinoma and hepatoma cells [33]. Emodin (1,3,8-trihydroxy-6-methylanthraquinone) is an active constituent of many herbal laxatives. It has been used for the treatment of inflammatory diseases such as peptic ulcers and as a laxative, and others such as skin burns, gallstone, hepatitis, inflammation and osteomyelitis, etc. [34]. Rhein (1,8-dihydroxy-3-carboxyl anthraquinone) is also known as cassic acid, is a substance in the anthraquinone group obtained from rhubarb. Rhein is a cathartic and is commonly found as a glycoside such as rhein-8-glucoside or glucorhein. Rhein was first isolated [25]. Originally the rhubarb plant which contains rhein was used as a laxative. It was believed that rhein along with other anthraquinone glycosides imparted this activity. Rhein has been reevaluated as an antibacterial agent against *Staphylococcus aureus* in 2008 [26].

In the present study, the two species of *Rheum* i.e., *R. webbianum* and *R. spiciforme* were screened for the presence of different phytoconstituents. These were collected from the different parts of Kashmir (India) at different altitudes and were also grown *in vitro*. There were total 17 samples, including the *in vitro* explants of each species from which the anthraquinones were derived. In case of *R. webbianum*, amino acids were absent in the sample collected from Panzila Top, Khardungla and Tangsti. Glycosides were absent in Khardungla and Tangsti samples. All these compounds were also present in *in vitro* explants. Raashid [35] has also reported the similar phytochemical behavior for *R. webbianum*. All these constituents i.e.,

Altitudes	Alkaloids	Carbohydrates	proteins	Amino acids	Steroids	Flavonoids	Glycosides	Tannins and phenols	Fats & oils
Dawar Hills	+	+	+	+	+	+	+	+	+
Satni Mountain	+	+	+	+	+	+	+	+	+
Tragbal	+	+	+	+	+	+	+	+	+
Dahinala	+	+	+	+	+	+	+	+	+
Chakwali	+	+	+	+	+	+	+	+	+
Habakhatoon Mountain	+	+	+	+	+	+	+	+	+
Roots (in-vitro)	+	+	+	+	+	+	+	+	+
Leaves (in-vitro)	+	+	+	+	+	+	+	+	+
Callus (in-vitro)	+	+	+	+	+	+	+	+	+

(+): Present, (-): Absent

Table 3: Estimation of different compounds from methanolic extracts of *R. spiciforme*.

Collection Area	Altitude (m)	Content (µg/30 g of samples)		
		Aloe emodin	Emodin	Rhein
Dawar Hills	4419.6	996 ± 12.6	189.0 ± 2.7	279.1 ± 4.1
Chakwali	4684.8	3409.5 ± 28.4	538.5 ± 7.6	531.4 ± 8.3
Dahi Nala	3810.0	3102.0 ± 32.6	915.0 ± 16.6	384.2 ± 5.6
Satni Mountain	3962.4	2124.0 ± 19.4	376.5 ± 5.2	301.5 ± 5.0
Habbakhatoon Mountain	4756.8	2856.0 ± 31.7	622.5 ± 8.9	421.5 ± 6.4
Tragbal	3352.8	2887.5 ± 40.2	505.5 ± 7.6	478.5 ± 7.2
Leaves (in vitro raised)	-	7.95 ± 0.5	3 ± 0.5	ND
Roots (in vitro raised)	-	31.5 ± 0.3	15 ± 0.1	ND
Callus (in vitro raised)	-	31.35 ± 0.3	22.5 ± 0.3	ND

ND: Not Detected

Table 4: Content of different active constituents in various samples of wild *R. spiciforme* populations and in regenerants of *in vitro* raised plants.

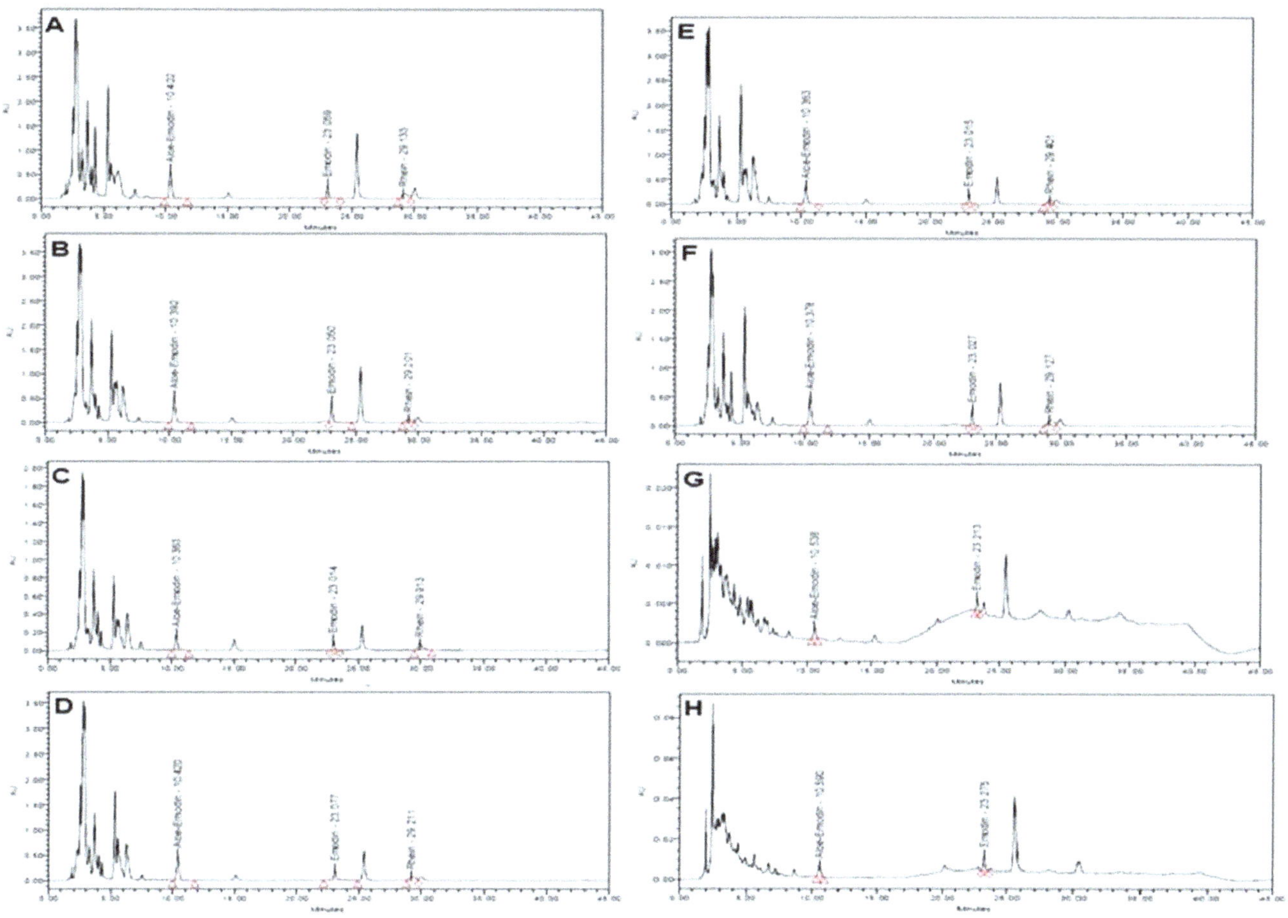

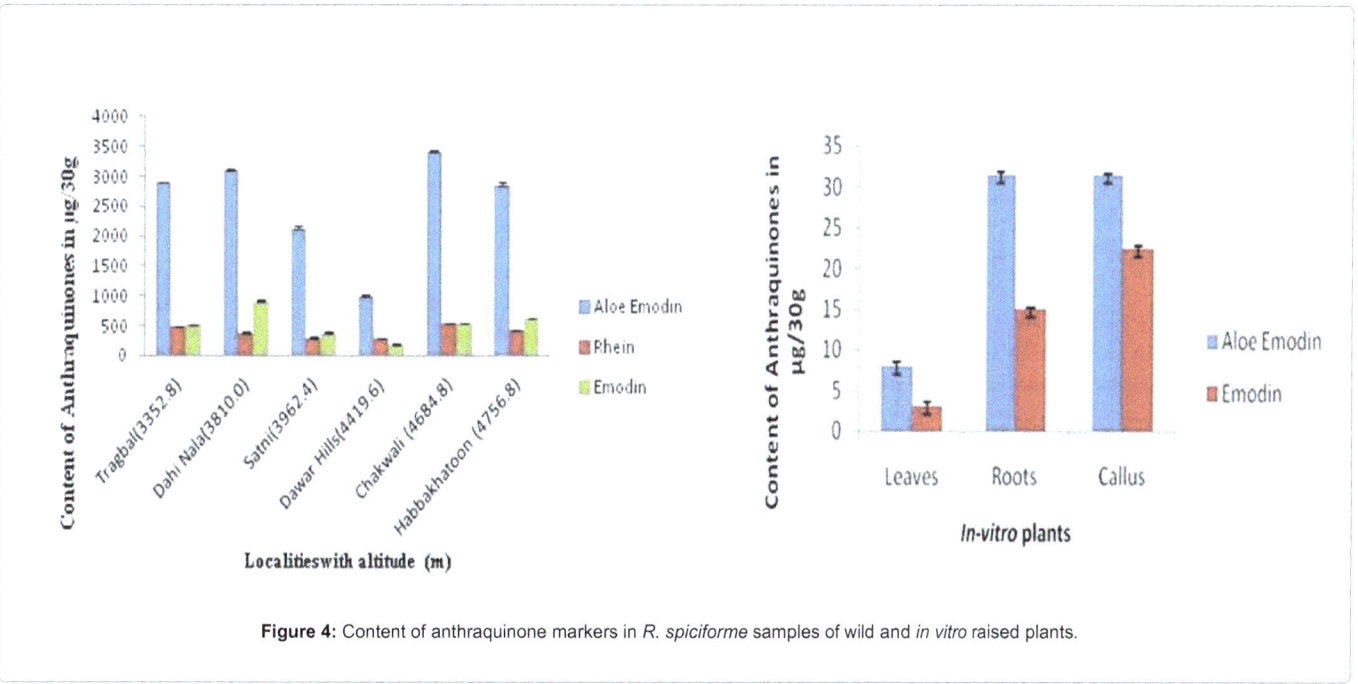

Figure 3: (A-I): LC-UV chromatographs of *R. spiciforme* samples collected from (A) Chakwali, (B) Dahinala, (C) Dawar hills, (D) Habba Khatoon mountain, (E) Satni mountain, (F) Tragbal, (G) *In vitro* leaves, (H) *In vitro* roots, (I) *In vitro* callus.

Figure 4: Content of anthraquinone markers in *R. spiciforme* samples of wild and *in vitro* raised plants.

alkaloids, proteins, flavonoids, carbohydrates, amino acids, steroids, glycosides, tannins and phenols, fats and oils were also present in all the samples of *R. spiciforme*, as well as in the *in vitro* raised explants. These results indicate that there is no uniform effect of altitude on the presence of phytochemicals in any of the two species. In present studies, the glycosides were screened in roots of *Rheum* species and also from *in vitro* explants (roots, callus and leaves). All samples of *R. webbianum* were also analyzed for the content of these three markers. All the three markers were present in all samples of *R. webbianum*. The maximum content of aloe-emodin (4500 μm/30 g) and rhein (1143 μm/30 g) was found in sample collected from Panzila Top whereas maximum content of emodin (2385 μm/30 g) was found in Tangsti sample. Rhein was also present in all these samples. In the case of *in vitro* explants, the maximum content of aloe-emodin (48 μm/30 g) was found in *in vitro* callus, the maximum content of emodin (13 μm/30 g) was found in *in vitro* leaves, rhein was absent in *in vitro* roots and leaves, whereas rhein (10 μm/30 g) was only present in *in vitro* callus. The amount of these anthraquinones and their derivatives has also been studied in many other species of *Rheum* such as *R. tanguticum* [36]. *R. officinale* [37], *R. palmatum* [38] and *R. ribes* [39] etc. (Supplementary Table S1).

The nine samples of *R. spiciforme* were also analyzed through HPLC for the quantification of the markers. All of these markers were present in each sample of *R. spiciforme*. The maximum content of aloe-emodin (3409 μm/30 g) was found in Chakwali, whereas, maximum content of emodin (915 μm/30 g) was found in Dahi Nala sample. The maximum content of rhein (531 μm/30 g) was also found in Chakwali. It was also observed that rhein was present in all the samples of *R. spiciforme*, whereas it was absent in some of the samples of *R. emodi*. In case of *in vitro* explants, it was noted that the maximum content of aloe-emodin (31.35 μm/30 g) and emodin (22 μm/30 g) was found in *in vitro* callus whereas rhein was absent in all these three explants.

It was observed that maximum aloe-emodin, emodin and rhein were found in *R. webbianum* as compared to *R. spiciforme*. The maximum content of aloe-emodin and rhein of the *in vitro* explants was also found in *R. webbianum*, whereas rhein was absent in explants (*in vitro*) of *R. spiciforme*. Only maximum content of emodin was found in *in vitro* explants of *R. spiciforme*.

Present study is the first report on *R. spiciforme* from India for phytochemical screening as no previous work was done in India and it was also observed that the *R. webbianum* contains highest content of these three anthraquinones and it was also observed that in *R. webbianum has* the amount of active compounds present in tetraploid plants was less than diploid plant. Similarly, the amount of active principle is reported to be more in the diploid than polyploids by some other workers [40-42]. Generally the amount of these active principles are found to be more in polyploids as compared to diploids [43,44].

It was observed in the present study, that the amount of these compounds show great variation, to check the variation we must go for authenticated plants and must explore extensively area to know the best chemotype plant. The value of contents must be varying due to genetic diversity and/or ecological factors, so we must mark out the best genotype growing in specific type of environment which is having the maximum amount of these active principles, only then we can have the standardized drug with specific amount of the active principles. Also, the amount of these active principles is known to vary with the age of plants, so we must study the amount of these active principles in the cultivated plants at different stages of age. The tissue cultured plants show less amount of active principles as compared to wild grown plants which might be due to the young age of tissue cultured plants as they

were hardly 4-5 months old whereas the wild plants were very old, as the amount of active principles increase with increase in age of plants, so the age differences between tissue cultured and wild grown plants might showed the variation in content of active principles. Correlation in amount of secondary metabolite with altitude has been reported in *R. emodi* [7,45-46]. Prasad and Purohit [7] reported the concentration of active constituents and calorific value of *R. emodi* and *R. nobile* in Sikkim Himalaya. In their study, high calorific values was recorded in *R. nobile* in comparison to *R. emodi,* and active constituents of both the plant species were found to decrease in low-altitudes conserved plants compared to the wild plants. But in the present study, it was found that no co-relation between altitude and content of markers was found. This lack of correlation may be attributed to the other factors such as age of the plant and magnitude of exposure of the plant to sunlight also affects concentration of markers in the plants.

Conclusion

Phytochemical screening showed the presence of amino acids, alkaloids, flavonoids, steroids, fats and oils, tannins and phenols, carbohydrates and glycosides in different samples of *Rheum* species. In some samples of *R. emodi*, amino acids, steroids and glycosides were absent. In R. *webbianum*, constituents like alkaloids, proteins, steroids, etc., were also present. Only amino acids and glycosides were absent in two of the samples, whereas all the compounds were present in *in vitro* explants of *R. webbianum*. In *R. spiciforme*, all constituents i.e., alkaloids, proteins, flavonoids, carbohydrates, amino acids, steroids, glycosides, tannins and phenols, fats and oils were also present in all the samples as well as in samples of *in vitro* explants. These species of *Rheum* were also screened to quantify the anthraquinone markers (aloe-emodin, emodin and rhein). The methanolic extracts were analysed to determine the content of aloe-emodin, emodin and rhein by HPLC method. All the three anthraquinones i.e., aloe-emodin, emodin and rhein were present in *R. webbianum*, but in case of *in vitro* explants of *R. webbianum*, rhein was present only in callus. The highest amount of aloe emodin (4500/30 g), emodin (1500.0/30 g) and rhein (1143.0/30 g) was observed in Panzila Top, Khardungla and Panzila Top samples respectively. In *R. spiciforme* highest content of aloe-emodin (3409.5/30 g) and rhein (531.4/30 g) was found in Chakwali samples, while highest content of emodin (915.0/30 g) was present in the samples of Dahi Nala. Rhein was absent in all *in vitro* explants of this species. Among all the three species, the maximum contents of aloe-emodin, emodin and rhein were found in samples of *R. webbianum* and amongst the *in vitro* explants, the maximum content of aloe-emodin and rhein was found in *R. webbianum* and that of emodin was observed in *R. spiciforme*. The observation of present study showed that *R. webbianum* is most abundant and rich in contents of active compounds. The results of present study can be efficiently utilized in future research programmes for the selection of elite material and for devising the utilization strategies for best chemotypes.

Author's Contributions

All authors equally participated in designing experiments analysis and interpretation of data. All authors read and approved the final manuscript.

Acknowledgement

This study was supported by DST, GoI, New Delhi funded women entrepreneurship project, the assistance of which is highly acknowledged.

References

1. Kabir Dar A, Siddiqui MAA, Wahid-ul H, Lone AH, Manzoor N, et al. (2015) Threat Status of Rheum emodi - A Study in Selected Cis-Himalayan Regions of Kashmir Valley Jammu & Kashmir India. Med Aromat Plants 4: 183.

2. Shimomura K, Yoshimatsu K, Jaziri M, Ishimaru K (1997) Traditional medicinal plant genetic resources and biotechnology applications. In: Watanabe K and Pehu ERG (eds.) Plant Biotechnology and Plant Genetic Resources for Sustainability and Productivity, RG Landes Company and Academic Press Inc., Austin, Texas, pp: 209-225.

3. Stein R (2004) Alternative remedies gaining popularity-Majority in U. S. Try some form, survey finds. The Washington Post.

4. Chaurasia OP, Ballabh B (2009) Medicinal Plants of cold desert Ladakh used in treatment of stomach disorders. Indian J Traditional Knowled 82: 185-192.

5. Srinivas G, Babykutty S, Sathiadevan PP, Srinivas P (2007) Molecular mechanism of emodin action: transition from laxative ingredient to an antitumor agent. Med Res Rev 27: 591-608.

6. Kapoor LD (1990) Handbook of Ayurvedic Medicinal Plants, CRC Press, Boca Raton, FL and London, pp: 487.

7. Prasad P, Purohit MC (2001) Altitude acclimatization and concentration of active constituents and calorific value of two medicinal plant species Rheum emodi and R. nobile (Rhubarb) in Sikkim Himalaya. Current Science 80: 734-736.

8. Yen GC, Duh PD, Chuang DY (2000) Antioxidant activity of anthraquinones and anthrone. Food Chemistry 70: 437-441.

9. Cai YZ, Sun M, Xing J, Corke H (2004) Antioxidant phenolic constituents in roots of Rheum officinale and Rubia cordifolia: structure- radical scavenging activity relationships. J Agric Food Chem 52: 7884-7890.

10. Kubo I, Murai Y, Soediro I, Soeetarno S, Sastrodihardjo S (1992) Cytotoxic anthraquinones from Rheum palmatum. Phytochemistry 31: 1063-1065.

11. Yim H, Lee YH, Lee CH, Lee SK (1999) Emodin, an anthraquinone derivative isolated from the rhizomes of Rheum palmatum, selectively inhibits the activity of casein II as a competitive inhibitor. Planta Med 65: 9-13.

12. Semple SJ, Pyke SM, Reynolds GD, Flower RL (2001) In vitro antiviral activity of the anthraquinone chrysophanic acid against poliovirus. Antiviral Research 49: 169-178.

13. Kala CP (2002) Indigenous knowledge of Bhotiya tribal community on wool dyeing and its present status in the Garhwal Himalaya, India. Current Sci 83: 814-817.

14. Anonymous (1972) The Wealth of India Publication and Information Directorate (CSIR), New Delhi. Vol-IX.

15. Malik S, Kumar R, Vats SK, Bhushan S, Sharma M, et al. (2009) Regeneration in Rheum emodi Wall: A step towards conservation of an endangered medicinal plant species. Engineer Life Sci 9: 130-134.

16. Kong LD, Cheng CH, Tan RX (2004) Inhibition of MAO A and B by some plant-derived alkaloids, phenols and anthraquinones. J Ethnopharmacol 91: 351-355.

17. Akhtar MS, Amin M, Ahmad M, Alamgeer A (2009) Hepatoprotective effect of Rheum emodi roots (Revand chini) and Akseer-e-Jigar against Paracetamol-induced hepatotoxicity in rats. Ethnobotanical Leaflets 13: 310- 315.

18. Ho TY, Wu SL, Chen JC, Li CC, Hsiang CY (2007) Emodin blocks the SARS coronavirus spike protein and angiotensin-converting enzyme 2 interaction. Antiviral Res 74: 92-101.

19. Radhika R, Kumari DK, Sudarsanam D (2010) Anti-diabetic activity of R. emodi in Alloxan induced diabetic rats. Internat J Pharmaceut Sci Res 1: 296-300.

20. Alam MM, Javed K, Jafri MA (2005) Effect of Rheum emodi (Revand Hindi) on renal functions in rats. J Ethnopharmacol 96: 121-125.

21. Rajkumar V, Guha G, Kumar RA (2010) Antioxidant and anti-cancer potentials of Rheum emodi rhizome extracts. Evidence-based Complementary and Alternative Medicine, pp: 1-9.

22. Kuo PL, Lin TC, Lin CC (2002) The antiproliferative activity of aloe-emodin is through p53-dependent and p21-dependent apoptotic pathway in human hepatoma cell lines. Life Sci 71: 1879-1892.

23. Ganie AH, Tali BA, Khuroo AA, Nawchoo IA, Rather AM (2014) Rheum spiciforme Royle (Polygonaceae): A new record to the flora of Kashmir Valley, India. National Academy Science Letters 37: 561-565.

24. Hesse O (1895) The chemistry of Rhubarb. Pharmaceutical J 55: 325-327.

25. Yu L, Xiang H, Fan J, Wang D, Yang F, et al. (2008) Global transcriptional response of Staphylococcus aureus to rhein, a natural plant product. J Biotechnol 135: 304-308.

26. Tabin S, Gupta RC, Kamili AN (2014) In vitro micro propagation of Rheum explants supplemented with various types of growth hormones. IOSR-JAVS 7: 97-100.

27. Edeoga HO, Okwu DE, Mbaebie BO (2005) Phytochemical constituents of some Nigerian medicinal plants. African J Biotechnology 4: 685-688.

28. Meena AK, Bansal P, Kumar S (2009) Plants-herbal wealth as a potential source of ayurvedic drugs. Asian Journal of Traditional Medicines 4: 152-170.

29. Krenn L, Pradhan R, Presser A, Reznicek G, Kopp B (2004) Anthrone C-glucosides from Rheum emodi. Chem Pharm Bull (Tokyo) 52: 391-393.

30. Hertog MG, Hollman PC (1996) Potential health effects of the dietary flavonol quercetin. Eur J Clin Nutr 50: 63-71.

31. Wang LS, Stoner GD (2008) Anthocyanins and their role in cancer prevention. Cancer Lett 269: 281-290.

32. Lee HZ (2001) Protein kinase C involvement in aloe-emodin- and emodin-induced apoptosis in lung carcinoma cell. Br J Pharmacol 134: 1093-1103.

33. Tsai JC, Tsai S, Chang WC (2004) Effect of ethanol extracts of three Chinese medicinal plants with laxative properties on ion transport of the rat intestinal epithelia. Biological Pharmaceutical Bulletin 27: 162-165.

34. Rashid S, Kaloo ZA, Singh S, Bashir I (2014) Callus induction and shoot regeneration from rhizome explants of Rheum webbianum Royle-a threatened medicinal plant growing in Kashmir Himalaya. J Scientific Innovative Res 3: 515-518.

35. Gao XY, Jiang Y, Lu J, Tu PF (2009) One single standard substance for the determination of multiple anthraquinone derivatives in rhubarb using high-performance liquid chromatography-diode array detection. J Chromatography A 1216: 2118-2123.

36. Zheng-xiang XIA, Zhong-yan T, Rui A, Chen Y, Yi-zhu Z, et al. (2012) A new anthraquinone glycoside from the root of Rheum officinale Baill. Acta Pharmaceutica Sinica 47: 1183-1186.

37. Zhao LC, Liang J, Li W, Cheng KM, Xia X, et al. (2011) The use of response surface methodology to optimize the ultrasound-assisted extraction of five anthraquinones from Rheum palmatum L. Molecules 16: 5928-5937.

38. Abdulla KK, Taha EM, Rahim SM (2014) Phenolic profile, antioxidant, and antibacterial effects of ethanol and aqueous extracts of Rheum ribes L. roots. Der Pharma Chemica, 6: 201-205.

39. Eliasova A, Repcak M, Pastirova A (2004) Quantitative changes of secondary metabolites of Matricaria chamomilla by abiotic stress. Zeitschrift fur Naturforschung Teil C Biochemie Biophysik Biologie Virlogie 59: 543-548.

40. Sharma N (2012) Cytomorphological diversity and chemical characterization of selected anti-diabetic medicinal plants from North India. A Ph. D. Thesis. Department of Botany, Punjabi University, Patiala.

41. Goyal H (2013) Cytogenetical and chemical characterization of some selected North Indian medicinal Composits. A Ph. D. Thesis. Department of Botany, Punjabi University, Patiala.

42. Berkov S (2001) Size and alkaloid content of seeds in induced aututetraploids of Datura innoxia, Datura stramonium and Hyoscyamus niger. Pharmaceutical Biology 39: 329-331.

43. Svehlikova V, Repcak M (2008) Variation of apigenin quantity in diploid and tetraploid Chamomilla recutita (L.) Rauschert. Plant Biology 2: 403-407.

44. Pandith SA, Hussain A, Bhat WW, Dhar N, Qazi AK, et al. (2014). Evaluation of anthraquinones from Himalayan rhubarb (Rheum emodi Wall. ex Meissn.) as antiproliferative agents. South African J Botany 95: 1-8.

45. Farroq U (2013) Evaluation of cytomorphological diversity in the members of Monochlamydeae from Kashmir. PhD thesis, Punjabi University, Patiala, Punjab, India.

46. Carey DB, Wink M (1994) Elevational variation of quinolizidine alkaloid contents in a lupine (Lupinus argenteus) of the Rocky Mountains. J Chem Ecol 20: 849-857.

19

Regulated Intramembrane Proteolysis of the Colony-Stimulating Factor 1 Receptor during Macrophage Activation

Spencer Swarts, Theresa Carlson and Peter van der Geer*

Department of Chemistry and Biochemistry, San Diego State University, San Diego, CA, USA

Introduction

The colony-stimulating factor (CSF-1) receptor is a protein-tyrosine kinase expressed on monocytes and macrophages. Binding of CSF-1 to its receptor results in receptor dimerization, cross-phosphorylation, and recruitment of cellular signaling proteins. More recently, we discovered that the CSF-1 receptor is subject to regulated intramembrane proteolysis or RIPping. RIPping involves ectodomain shedding and release of the cytoplasmic region into the interior of the cell. It is carried out by tumor necrosis factor α-converting enzyme (TACE) and γ-secretase, following the encounter of macrophages with molecules that are derived from microbial pathogens. CSF-1 receptor RIPping is likely to play a role in macrophage activation in response to microbial infection.

The CSF-1 receptor uses tyrosine phosphorylation sites to recruit and activate cellular signaling proteins. CSF-1 is a cytokine that acts as a key regulator for growth, survival, differentiation, and activation of monocytes, macrophages, and other cell types [1,2]. It acts by binding to a receptor that is present on the surface of a variety of cell types, including primitive multipotent hematopoietic stem cells, B cells, neurons, placental trophoblasts, osteoclasts, monocytes and macrophages [3]. The CSF-1 receptor is a protein-tyrosine kinase, composed of an extracellular ligand-binding region, a transmembrane region, and a cytoplasmic region [4-6]. The cytoplasmic portion of the receptor is divided into a juxta membrane region, a kinase domain that is separated into two parts by a kinase insert, and a carboxy-terminal tail [2]. It is well established that ligand binding results in receptor dimerization and autophosphorylation on a number of tyrosine residues (Figure 1). Phosphorylation at tyrosine 807 in the activation loop increases kinase activity [7]. Additional phosphorylation sites have been characterized as binding sites for intracellular signaling proteins (Figure 1). These signaling proteins are activated directly or indirectly as a consequence of their interaction with the receptor and they relay information along intracellular signal transduction pathways [1,2]. Thus, like other receptor protein-tyrosine kinases, the CSF-1 receptor uses phosphotyrosine-containing protein-binding sites to recruit cytoplasmic signaling proteins. Upon binding to the receptor, these proteins activate signal transduction pathways that cause the biochemical changes that make it possible for the cell to respond to the presence of CSF-1.

Regulated intramembrane proteolysis

Regulated intramembrane proteolysis is a process that involves two cleavage events and that results in the release of the cytoplasmic region of an integral membrane protein into the interior of the cell [8]. Proteins that are present on the cell surface as well as proteins present in intracellular membranes have been shown to undergo RIPping [8]. Cell surface proteins are first cleaved in their extracellular region within 5-20 residues of the plasma membrane. This first cleavage event, which is usually regulated, results in release of the extracellular domain and the production of an integral membrane protein with a very short section extending from surface the cell and a longer cytoplasmic region that contains one or more functional domains. This cleavage product,

in turn, is recognized by a second protease, resulting in cleavage within the transmembrane region, followed by release of a soluble protein product into the cytoplasm. Following its release from the membrane this protein can travel to other locations within the cell to carry out a particular function [8,9].

RIPping was first observed in the context of sterol-regulated gene transcription. During this process, the expression of proteins that participate in the uptake or biosynthesis of cholesterol is turned on in response to the absence of sterols [10]. Regulation of sterol sensitive gene transcription is mediated by sterol-regulatory element binding proteins or SREBPs. SREBPs are produced as integral membrane protein precursors that are localized in the endoplasmic reticulum in the presence of cholesterol. These precursor proteins are composed of an amino-terminal region that can function as a transcription factor and that project into the cytoplasm, a transmembrane region, a short loop projecting into the lumen of the endoplasmic reticulum, a second transmembrane region, and a regulatory region that is present in the cytoplasm [11]. In the absence of sterols, these proteins move from the endoplasmic reticulum to the Golgi apparatus where they are proteolytically cleaved, resulting in the release of their amino-terminal transcription factors [12]. Maturation of the SREBP precursor proteins involves two distinct cleavage events. The precursor protein is first cleaved within its luminal loop by the site 1 protease [13]. The amino-terminal half is subsequently recognized and cleaved within its transmembrane region by the site 2 protease [14]. This results in the release of the mature SREBP into the cytosol, followed by its translocation into the nucleus. Like many transcription factors, SREBPs are short lived; they are poly-ubiquitinated and degraded in the proteasome [15]. We recently discovered that the CSF-1 receptor is processed in a similar fashion during macrophage activation [16-20].

Regulated intramembrane proteolysis of the CSF-1 receptor

We followed up experiments showing that treatment of macrophages with 12-O-tetradecanoylphorbol-13-acetate (TPA), an activator of protein kinase C, or lipopolysaccharides (LPS), a component of bacterial cell walls caused the disappearance of CSF-1 receptors from the cell surface [21,22]. To investigate the dynamics of this process, P388D1 macrophages were incubated with TPA for various amounts of time before the cells were lysed and analyzed

---

*Corresponding author: Peter van der Geer, Department of Chemistry and Biochemistry, San Diego State University, San Diego, CA, USA
E-mail: pvanderg@mail.sdsu.edu

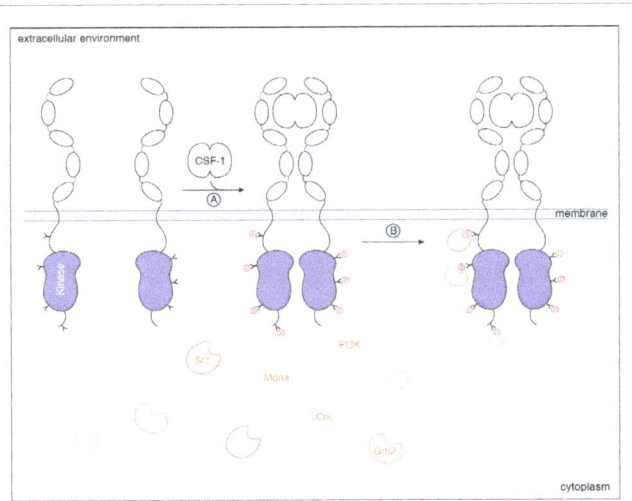

Figure 1: *The CSF-1 receptor uses tyrosine phosphorylation sites to recruit and activate cellular signaling proteins.* The CSF-1 receptor is a protein-tyrosine kinase expressed on the cell surface of a variety of cells. It contains an extracellular ligand binding domain (light purple) and a cytoplasmic kinase domain (dark purple). CSF-1 (yellow) is a dimer that contains two receptor-binding sites. Binding of CSF-1 to its receptor results in receptor dimerization (arrow A) making it possible for receptors to phosphorylate each other on tyrosine residues (tyrosine residues are indicated with the letter Y and phosphate groups are shown as an encircled p). A number of autophosphorylation sites have been identified in the CSF-1 receptor, including tyrosines 559, 697, 706, 721, 807 and 973 [42-46]. Phosphorylation on tyrosine 807 contributes to activation of the catalytic domain [7,47]. Other tyrosine phosphorylation sites act as binding sites for Src-homology domain-containing signaling proteins (red and orange globular structures in the cytoplasm). Upon autophosphorylation of the receptor, these proteins move from the cytoplasm to their docking sites on the receptor (arrow B). Cytoplasmic proteins known to bind to the activated CSF-1 receptor include: the protein-tyrosine kinase Src, growth factor receptor binding protein 2 (Grb2), signal transducer and activator of transcription 1 and 3 (STAT 1 and 3), phosphatidyl-inositol 3-kinase, the monocytic adaptor protein Mona, phospholipase Cγ, and the ubiquitin protein ligase c-Cbl [42,45,46,48-52]. Upon binding to the receptor, these proteins are activated resulting in the relay of information along cellular signal transduction cascades.

for the presence of CSF-1 receptors by immunoblotting. Following addition of TPA it takes 5 to 10 minutes before receptors start to disappear. Receptor downregulation reaches maximal levels after 1.5 hours [23]. As receptors disappear, a 55 kDa protein that represents the carboxy-terminal half of the receptor emerges [23]. Separation of the cells into particulate and soluble fractions showed that the formation of this CSF-1 receptor fragment involves two steps. First, the receptor is cleaved amino-terminally to the membrane, resulting in the formation of a 55 kDa membrane-associated fragment (Figure 2). The membrane-bound cleavage product is often referred to as the carboxy-terminal fragment or CTF. The CSF-1 receptor CTF is cleaved again, resulting in the release of a slightly smaller fragment into the cytoplasm (Figure 2). This soluble product is often referred to as the intracellular domain or ICD. The first cleavage can be blocked using inhibitors of TACE, a metalloprotease composed of an extracellular catalytic domain, a single transmembrane domain and a short cytoplasmic tail [21,24]. The second cleavage can be blocked using pharmacological inhibitors of γ-secretase or dominant interfering mutants [23].

γ-Secretase is a complex of several integral membrane proteins that cleaves proteins within their transmembrane region [25]. γ-Secretase has been implicated in the production of Aβ, which is a major constituent of amyloid plagues, and the onset of Alzheimer's

disease [25]. Our results suggest that the CSF-1 receptor is cleaved in its extracellular region by TACE, followed by cleavage in the transmembrane region by γ-secretase.

Identification of the TACE and γ-secretase cleavage sites in the CSF-1 receptor

While we had good evidence showing that the CSF-1 receptor undergoes proteolytic processing, the exact location of the cleavage sites has remained unknown. Identification of the cleavage sites involves purification of the cleavage products followed by amino-terminal sequencing. To facilitate purification, we engineered CSF-1 receptors containing several affinity tags at their carboxy-terminus. Tagged receptors were stably expressed in 293A cells, cells were stimulated to initiate receptor processing, and cleavage products were purified using affinity chromatography [26]. The TPA-inducible TACE cleavage site was identified following pretreatment of cells with the γ-secretase inhibitor, L-685,458, for 1 hour, followed by stimulation with TPA for 20 minutes. The γ-secretase inhibitor was included to prevent the second cleavage. Edman degradation yielded the following amino-terminal sequence, SKQLPDES, indicating that the receptor is cleaved 12 amino acid residues before the start of the transmembrane domain (Figure 3). The γ-secretase cleavage site was identified from cells that were stimulated for 20 minutes with TPA in the presence of H_2O_2; H_2O_2 was included because in our experiments it appears to inhibit degradation of the soluble product in the proteasome [27]. Amino-terminal sequencing yielded a major and a minor sequence, LLLYKYKQKP and YKYKQKP respectively, thus identifying a major and minor cleavage site within the transmembrane region (Figure 3). Identification of the cleavage sites will provide insight into substrate recognition by both TACE and γ-secretase. Analysis of cleavage site mutants will help elucidate the role of CSF-1 receptor RIPping in macrophage activation.

Nuclear localization of the CSF-1 receptor ICD

In most cases studied, RIPping results in the transient appearance of cleavage products that move to the nucleus where they regulate gene expression, followed by their degradation in the proteasome. For example, the Notch ICD transiently translocates to the nucleus where it interacts with members of the CSL family of transcription factors before it is degraded [28,29]. Because the cytoplasmic cleavage products are usually unstable, it has remained difficult to document their presence in the nucleus. Immunofluorescence data suggested that the CSF-1 receptor ICD, following its release from the plasma membrane, localizes in part to the nucleus [23]. The interpretation of these experiments is complicated by the fact that the CSF-1 receptor ICD becomes ubiquitinated followed by its degradation in the proteasome [23,27]. To further investigate the localization of the ICD following its release from the membrane, we have generated an amino-terminally tagged version of the cleavage product. Preliminary data suggest that this protein may be present in the nucleus. Together these observations suggest that the CSF-1 receptor ICD travels to the nucleus where it may be involved in regulation of gene transcription. It remains unclear, however, exactly how the CSF-1 receptor ICD is marked for translocation to the nucleus. Because a well-recognized nuclear localization signal is absent from the ICD, we propose that the ICD associates with an unidentified binding partner, which directs the ICD towards the nucleus. Alternatively, it is possible that the ICD contains an unusual nuclear localization signal. Expression of stable ICD mutants, which are currently being constructed, would make it possible to initiate a more thorough investigation of the localization of the ICD, following its release into the cytoplasm.

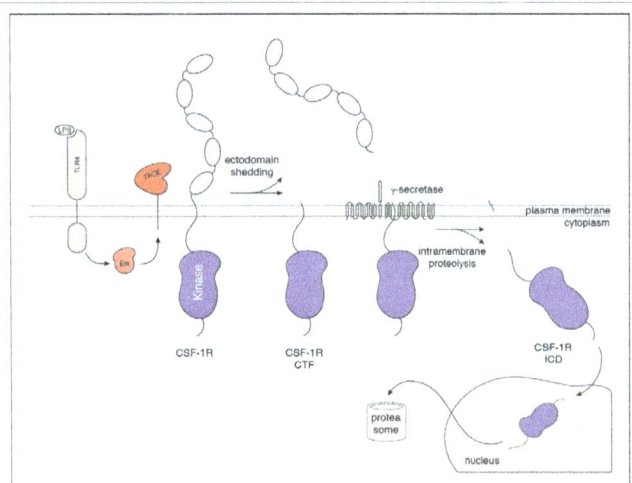

Figure 2: *Regulated intramembrane proteolysis of the CSF-1 receptor following the interaction of macrophages with pathogen-derived molecules.* Pathogen-derived molecules are recognized by dedicated families of receptors on the surface of macrophages. For example, LPS binds to Toll-like receptor 4 (TLR4). TLR4 activates various intracellular kinases, including Erk-1 and Erk-2 [40,41]. This leads to activation of TACE, a protease with a short cytoplasmic region and an extracellular catalytic domain [53]. TACE cleaves the CSF-1 receptor (CSF-1R) at a site 12 residues amino-terminal to the transmembrane region. This results in the release of most of the ligand-binding region into the extracellular environment (ectodomain shedding) leaving behind a protein with a very short extracellular region. This product is often referred to as the carboxy-terminal fragment or CTF. The CTF is cleaved by γ-secretase within its transmembrane region resulting in the release of the intracellular domain or ICD into the cytoplasm [53]. The ICD can be detected in the nucleus where it may be involved in the regulation of gene transcription. It is short lived and is degraded in the proteasome.

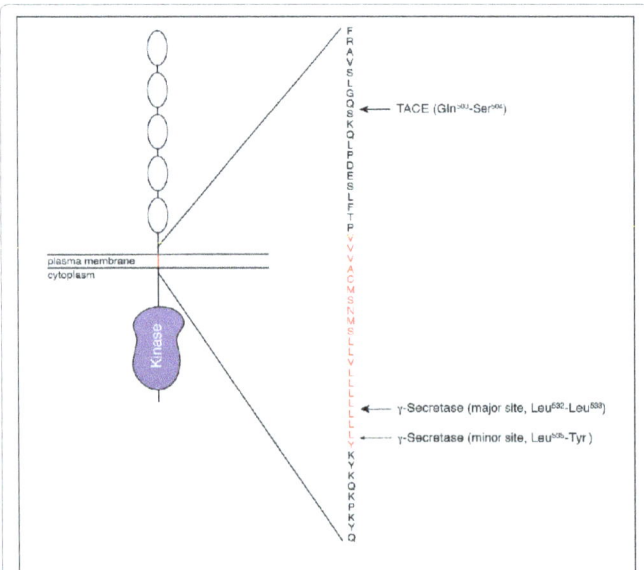

Figure 3: *Location of the TACE and γ-secretase cleavage sites in the CSF-1 receptor.* The sites were identified by automated Edman degradation following purification of the cleavage products [26].

CSF-1 receptor RIPping during the immune response

A successful response against microbial infections depends on the interplay between the innate and the adaptive immune systems [30,31]. The innate immune system recognizes the invader as foreign, based on

the presence of pathogen-associated molecular patterns, such as LPS or double stranded RNA [32]. It initiates the anti-microbial response and helps to recruit and activate the adaptive immune system. The adaptive immune system generates responses against specific antigens associated with the intruder and solicits the help of the innate immune system to terminate the infection [33]. Macrophages, which are found in most tissues, form the first line of defense by recognizing invading microorganisms using pattern recognition receptors, initiating the anti-microbial response, and alerting the rest of the immune system by producing proinflammatory cytokines, including IL-1β, IL-6 and TNF [30]. Toll-like receptors (TLRs) are one of several families of pattern recognition receptors that are expressed on macrophages [34,35]. They recognize molecules that are associated specifically with microorganisms, including lipopolysaccharide, a major component of gram-negative bacterial cell walls (which binds to TLR4), bacterial lipoproteins (TLR2), double-stranded RNA (TLR3), and CpG islands in bacterial DNA (TLR9) [36-39]. Upon ligand binding, TLRs recruit death domain-containing adaptor proteins that relay information along signal transduction cascades, which leads to the activation of the stress activated protein kinases p38 and JNK, Tank-binding kinase 1, an IκB kinase, and the extracellular signal regulated kinases Erk-1 and Erk-2, ultimately resulting in macrophage activation [40,41].

Interestingly, we observed that LPS induces RIPping of the CSF-1 receptor in a dose and time dependent manner [21]. Other Toll-like receptor ligands such as Lipid A, Lipoteichoic acid, poly I: poly C, and bacterial DNA also stimulated proteolytic processing of the CSF-1 receptor [21]. These observations lend support to the idea that CSF-1 receptor RIPping and release of the ICD from the plasma membrane into the cytoplasm plays a role in macrophage activation during the response to a microbial infection. While this remains to be proven, it seems likely that the CSF-1 receptor ICD moves to the nucleus to contribute to the activation of pro-inflammatory gene transcription.

Acknowledgement

This work was supported in part by the California Metabolic Research Foundation.

References

1. Mouchemore KA, Pixley FJ (2012) CSF-1 signaling in macrophages: pleiotrophy through phosphotyrosine-based signaling pathways. Crit Rev Clin Lab Sci 49: 49-61.

2. Pixley FJ, Stanley ER (2004) CSF-1 regulation of the wandering macrophage: complexity in action. Trends Cell Biol 14: 628-638.

3. Dai XM, Ryan GR, Hapel AJ, Dominguez MG, Russell RG, et al. (2002) Targeted disruption of the mouse colony-stimulating factor 1 receptor gene results in osteopetrosis, mononuclear phagocyte deficiency, increased primitive progenitor cell frequencies, and reproductive defects. Blood 99: 111-120.

4. Coussens L, Van Beveren C, Smith D, Chen E, Mitchell RL, et al. (1986) Structural alteration of viral homologue of receptor proto-oncogene fms at carboxyl terminus. Nature 320: 277-280.

5. Rothwell VM, Rohrschneider LR (1987) Murine c-fms cDNA: cloning, sequence analysis and retroviral expression. Oncogene Res 1: 311-324.

6. Sherr CJ, Rettenmier CW, Sacca R, Roussel MF, Look AT, et al. (1985) The c-fms proto-oncogene product is related to the receptor for the mononuclear phagocyte growth factor, CSF-1. Cell 41: 665-676.

7. van der Geer P, Hunter T (1991) Tyrosine 706 and 807 phosphorylation site mutants in the murine colony-stimulating factor-1 receptor are unaffected in their ability to bind or phosphorylate phosphatidylinositol-3 kinase but show differential defects in their ability to induce early response gene transcription. Mol Cell Biol 11: 4698-4709.

8. Brown MS, Ye J, Rawson RB, Goldstein JL (2000) Regulated intramembrane proteolysis: a control mechanism conserved from bacteria to humans. Cell 100: 391-398.

9. Urban S, Freeman M (2002) Intramembrane proteolysis controls diverse signalling pathways throughout evolution. Curr Opin Genet Dev 12: 512-518.

10. Goldstein JL, Brown MS (1990) Regulation of the mevalonate pathway. Nature 343: 425-430.

11. Wang X, Sato R, Brown MS, Hua X, Goldstein JL (1994) SREBP- a membrane-bound transcription factor released by sterol-regulated proteolysis. Cell 77: 53-62.

12. DeBose-Boyd RA, Brown MS, Li WP, Nohturfft A, Goldstein JL, et al. (1999) Transport-dependent proteolysis of SREBP: relocation of site-1 protease from Golgi to ER obviates the need for SREBP transport to Golgi. Cell 99: 703-712.

13. Sakai J, Rawson RB, Espenshade PJ, Cheng D, Seegmiller AC, et al. (1998) Molecular identification of the sterol-regulated luminal protease that cleaves SREBPs and controls lipid composition of animal cells. Mol Cell 2: 505-514.

14. Rawson RB, Zelenski NG, Nijhawan D, Ye J, Sakai J, et al. (1997) Complementation cloning of S2P, a gene encoding a putative metalloprotease required for intramembrane cleavage of SREBPs. Mol Cell 1: 47-57.

15. Sundqvist A, Bengoechea-Alonso MT, Ye X, Lukiyanchuk V, Jin J, et al. (2005) Control of lipid metabolism by phosphorylation-dependent degradation of the SREBP family of transcription factors by SCF(Fbw7). Cell Metab 1: 379-391.

16. Palsson-McDermott EM, O'Neill LA (2004) Signal transduction by the lipopolysaccharide receptor, Toll-like receptor-4. Immunology 113: 153-162.

17. Downing JR, Roussel MF, Sherr CJ (1989) Ligand and protein kinase C downmodulate the colony-stimulating factor 1 receptor by independent mechanisms. Mol Cell Biol 9: 2890-2896.

18. Baccarini M, Dello Sbarba P, Buscher D, Bartocci A, Stanley ER (1992) IFN-gamma/lipopolysaccharide activation of macrophages is associated with protein kinase C-dependent down-modulation of the colony-stimulating factor-1 receptor. J Immunol 149: 2656-2661.

19. Chen BD, Lin HS, Hsu S (1983) Lipopolysaccharide inhibits the binding of colony-stimulating factor (CSF-1) to murine peritoneal exudate macrophages. J Immunol 130: 2256-2260.

20. Chen BD, Lin HS, Hsu S (1983) Tumor-promoting phorbol esters inhibit the binding of colony-stimulating factor (CSF-1) to murine peritoneal exudate macrophages. J Cell Physiol 116: 207-212.

21. Glenn G, van der Geer P (2008) Toll-like receptors stimulate regulated intramembrane proteolysis of the CSF-1 receptor through Erk activation. FEBS Lett 582: 911-915.

22. Wilhelmsen K, Copp J, Glenn G, Hoffman RC, Tucker P, et al. (2004) Purification and identification of protein-tyrosine kinase-binding proteins using synthetic phosphopeptides as affinity reagents. Mol Cell Proteomics 3: 887-895.

23. Wilhelmsen K, P van der Geer (2004) Phorbol 12-myristate 13-acetate- induced release of the colony-stimulating factor 1 receptor cytoplasmic domain into the cytosol involves two separate cleavage events. Mol Cell Biol 24: 454-464.

24. Rovida E, Paccagnini A, Del Rosso M, Peschon J, Dello Sbarba P (2001) TNF-alpha-converting enzyme cleaves the macrophage colony-stimulating factor receptor in macrophages undergoing activation. J Immunol 166: 1583-1589.

25. Selkoe DJ, Wolfe MS (2007) Presenilin: running with scissors in the membrane. Cell 131: 215-221.

26. Vahidi A, Glenn G, van der Geer P (2014) Identification and mutagenesis of the TACE and Î³-secretase cleavage sites in the colony-stimulating factor 1 receptor. Biochem Biophys Res Commun 450: 782-787.

27. Glenn G, van der Geer P (2007) CSF-1 and TPA stimulate independent pathways leading to lysosomal degradation or regulated intramembrane proteolysis of the CSF-1 receptor. FEBS Lett 581: 5377-5381.

28. Kopan R (2012) Notch signaling. Cold Spring Harb Perspect Biol 4.

29. Kopan R (1999) All good things must come to an end: how is Notch signaling turned off? Sci STKE 1999: PE1.

30. Medzhitov R, Janeway C Jr (2000) Innate immunity. N Engl J Med 343: 338-344.

31. Medzhitov R (2007) Recognition of microorganisms and activation of the immune response. Nature 449: 819-826.

32. Janeway CA Jr (1989) Approaching the asymptote? Evolution and revolution in immunology. Cold Spring Harb Symp Quant Biol 54: 1-13.

33. Schatz DG, Oettinger MA, Schlissel MS (1992) V(D)J recombination: molecular biology and regulation. Annu Rev Immunol 10: 359-383.

34. Medzhitov R, Janeway C Jr (2000) The Toll receptor family and microbial recognition. Trends Microbiol 8: 452-456.

35. Medzhitov R, Preston-Hurlburt P, Janeway CA Jr (1997) A human homologue of the Drosophila Toll protein signals activation of adaptive immunity. Nature 388: 394-397.

36. Alexopoulou L, Holt AC, Medzhitov R, Flavell RA (2001) Recognition of double-stranded RNA and activation of NF-kappaB by Toll-like receptor 3. Nature 413: 732-738.

37. Hemmi H, Takeuchi O, Kawai T, Kaisho T, Sato S, et al. (2000) A Toll-like receptor recognizes bacterial DNA. Nature 408: 740-745.

38. Poltorak A, He X, Smirnova I, Liu MY, Van Huffel C, et al. (1998) Defective LPS signaling in C3H/HeJ and C57BL/10ScCr mice: mutations in Tlr4 gene. Science 282: 2085-2088.

39. Schwandner R, Dziarski R, Wesche H, Rothe M, Kirschning CJ (1999) Peptidoglycan- and lipoteichoic acid-induced cell activation is mediated by toll-like receptor 2. J Biol Chem 274: 17406-17409.

40. Aderem A, Ulevitch RJ (2000) Toll-like receptors in the induction of the innate immune response. Nature 406: 782-787.

41. Banerjee A, Gerondakis S (2007) Coordinating TLR-activated signaling pathways in cells of the immune system. Immunol Cell Biol 85: 420-424.

42. Reedijk M, Liu X, van der Geer P, Letwin K, Waterfield MD, et al. (1992) Tyr721 regulates specific binding of the CSF-1 receptor kinase insert to PI 3'-kinase SH2 domains: a model for SH2-mediated receptor-target interactions. EMBO J 11: 1365-1372.

43. Tapley P, Kazlauskas A, Cooper JA, Rohrschneider LR (1990) Macrophage colony-stimulating factor-induced tyrosine phosphorylation of c-fms proteins expressed in FDC-P1 and BALB/c 3T3 cells. Mol Cell Biol 10: 2528-2538.

44. van der Geer P, T Hunter (1990) Identification of tyrosine 706 in the kinase insert as the major colony- stimulating factor 1 (CSF-1)-stimulated autophosphorylation site in the CSF-1 receptor in a murine macrophage cell line. Mol Cell Biol 10: 2991-3002.

45. van der Geer P, Hunter T (1993) Mutation of Tyr697, a GRB2-binding site, and Tyr72 a PI 3-kinase binding site, abrogates signal transduction by the murine CSF-1 receptor expressed in Rat-2 fibroblasts. EMBO J 12: 5161-5172.

46. Wilhelmsen K, Burkhalter S, van der Geer P (2002) C-Cbl binds the CSF-1 receptor at tyrosine 973, a novel phosphorylation site in the receptor's carboxy-terminus. Oncogene 21: 1079-1089.

47. Roussel MF, Shurtleff SA, Downing JR, CJ Sherr (1990) A point mutation at tyrosine-809 in the human colony-stimulating factor 1 receptor impairs mitogenesis without abrogating tyrosine kinase activity, association with phosphatidylinositol 3-kinase, or induction of c-fos and junB genes. Proc Natl Acad Sci USA 87: 6738-6742.

48. Alonso G, Koegl M, Mazurenko N, Courtneidge SA (1995) Sequence requirements for binding of Src family tyrosine kinases to activated growth factor receptors. J Biol Chem 270: 9840-9848.

49. Novak U, Nice E, Hamilton JA, Paradiso L (1996) Requirement for Y706 of the murine (or Y708 of the human) CSF-1 receptor for STAT1 activation in response to CSF-1. Oncogene 13: 2607-2613.

50. Lioubin MN, Myles GM, Carlberg K, Bowtell D, Rohrschneider LR (1994) Shc, Grb2, Sos and a 150-kilodalton tyrosine-phosphorylated protein form complexes with Fms in hematopoietic cells. Mol Cell Biol 14: 5682-5691.

51. Bourette RP, Arnaud S, Myles GM, Blanchet JP, Rohrschneider LR, et al. (1998) Mona, a novel hematopoietic-specific adaptor interacting with the macrophage colony-stimulating factor receptor, is implicated in monocyte/macrophage development. EMBO J 17: 7273-7281.

52. Bourette RP Myles GM, Choi JL, Rohrschneider LR (1997) Sequential activation of phoshatidylinositol 3-kinase and phospholipase C-gamma2 by the M-CSF receptor is necessary for differentiation signaling. EMBO J 16: 5880-5893.

53. Black RA (2002) Tumor necrosis factor-alpha converting enzyme. Int J Biochem Cell Biol 34: 1-5.

20

Role of Copper and Selenium in Reproductive Biology

Pal A*

Department of Biochemistry, PGIMER, Chandigarh 160012, India

Abstract

Among the indispensable trace elements required for normal physiological growth and development of the body; Copper (Cu) and Selenium (Se) have a paramount significance in human reproduction. Male testosterone levels have been suggested to play a role in the severity of Cu deficiency. In females, estrogen causes increase in plasma Cu levels by inducing ceruloplasmin and alteration of hepatic subcellular distribution of Cu. Thus, changes in Cu levels due to estrogen are thought to protect Cu-deficient females against mortality.

During pubertal maturation, the Se content of male gonads increases and it is localized in the mitochondrial capsule protein of the mid-piece. In females, infertility and abortion aberrations are caused due to Se deficiency.

Keywords: Copper; Selenium; Human reproduction

Introduction

Trace elements [Copper (Cu), Selenium (Se), Zinc (Zn), Iron (Fe), Molybdenum (Mo), Manganese (Mn), Cobalt (Co), Chromium (Cr), and Iodine (I)], inorganic substances that are vital for sustaining life, are required in minute amounts every day (generally less than 100 mg/day [1,2]. Trace element homeostasis is important for optimal health, enzymatic reactions, immune function, respiration, gene transcription, and cell proliferation, nervous and reproductive system. Various diseases that include genetic disorders [3,4], cancer [5], diabetes [6], neurodegenerative diseases [7,8] and reproductive abnormalities [2] are associated with aberrant trace element homeostasis. Accumulating evidences intensely indicate that loss of trace element homeostasis have a profound effect on reproductive system of animals, including humans. Among the outlined trace elements, Zn, Cu, and Se have an imposing role in human reproduction. Contrary to Zn and Cu which are metals, Se is non-metal with diverse biological effects which are mediated through Se containing proteins (seleno-proteins) that are present in all three domains of life. All seleno-proteins contain at least one selenocysteine, a Se containing amino acid. Most of the seleno-proteins serve as oxidoreductases [9-13]. Cu and Se are redox active elements due to presence of unpaired electrons which allow their participation in redox reactions involving mostly one electron loss (oxidation) or gain (reduction). On the other hand, Zn has no unpaired electrons when in the Zn^{2+} state, preventing its participation in redox reactions. However, this redox activity of Cu and Se results in formation of highly damaging free hydroxyl radicals, which subsequently causes oxidative stress, unless homeostasis is tightly regulated. In biological systems Zn, Cu and Se are mostly bound to proteins, forming metalloproteins. In biological system Zn, Cu and Se accomplish pivotal roles to maintain optimum health. Apart from Cu and Se, other trace elements are the focus of several recent comprehensive reviews/books and will not be considered further [1,2,14-17]. The remainder of this chapter will instead focus on essentiality, and clinical and biochemical spectrum conditions pertaining to Cu and Se (Table 1) in human reproductive system.

Copper

Cu is the third-most abundant transition metal in the body [22] and a vital trace metal that plays a fundamental role in the biochemistry of all living organisms; affecting enzyme activity, both as a cofactor and as an integral component of many metalloenzymes [23]. The average intake of Cu by human adults varies from 0.6 to 1.6 mg/d. In human body Cu is found in relatively high amounts: a healthy 70 kg adult contains about 110 mg of Cu, approximately 10 mg in liver, 8.8 mg in brain and 6 mg in blood [24,25]. Duodenum is the primary site of Cu absorption. The biological functions of redox active Cu includes electron-transfer catalysis by means of its two accessible oxidation states: Cu^+ (cuprous) and Cu^{2+} (cupric) [26]. Cu is involved in many aspects of metabolism, including mitochondrial oxidative phosphorylation, neurotransmitter synthesis and function, pigment formation, connective tissue biosynthesis, and Fe metabolism [27] (Table 1). Biliary excretion is the main route of Cu excretion from the body. Due to immaturity of biliary excretion system and high proficiency of Cu absorption, neonates are more susceptible to Cu poisoning [28]. Cu homeostasis in the body is securely synchronized as it is an important component of numerous metalloenzymes and metalloproteins, and perturbations in Cu levels are known to underlie the pathoetiology of wide spectrum of diseases including reproductive, hemopoietic, nervous, skeletal, cardiovascular integumentary, and immune systems [1].

Wilson's disease, an autosomal recessive disorder, is caused by mutations in ATP7B gene in which Cu accumulates in liver and secondarily in other organs. Grossly elevated hepatic Cu content, augmented urinary Cu excretion and decreased serum ceruloplasmin levels are good indicators of the Wilson's disease [29-32]. Cu poisoning manifestations include nausea, epigastric pain, vomiting, diarrhea, intravascular hemolysis, and severe Cu toxicity may also cause death. Indian childhood cirrhosis and idiopathic Cu toxicity are the other examples of Cu toxicity associated diseases in humans [33]. Strikingly, accumulating evidences suggest that increased Cu levels in brain due to chronic Cu toxicity can result in cognition waning in rats [34,35].

On the other hand, Menkes disease, X-chromosome linked human disorder characterized by progressive neurological impairment, peculiar hair and death in infancy, is associated with abnormal Cu metabolism. Cu deficiency results from alteration in Cu transport, the entrapment of Cu in intestinal and kidney cells or vascular endothelial cells in the blood-brain barrier (BBB). The Menkes disease patients

***Corresponding author:** Amit Pal, Department of Biochemistry, P.G.I.M.E.R., Chandigarh, 160012, India, E-mail: maximus1134@gmail.com; apal1134@gmail.com

Cu dependent enzymes/proteins	Selenoproteins
Monoamine oxidase	Glutathione peroxidases (GPx 1-6)
Ceruloplasmin	Thioredoxin reductase (TR 1-3)
Cytochrome c oxidase	Cytochrome c oxidase
Lysyl oxidase	Selenoprotein P
Diamine oxidase	Selenoprotein W
Dopamine β-hydroxylase	Selenophosphate synthetase
Hephaestin	15 kDa selenoprotein
Glycosylphosphatidylinositol- anchored ceruloplasmin	Selenoprotein H, I, K, M, N, O, R, S, T, V
β-amyloid precursor protein	
Glucose regulated protein 78	
peptidylglycine α-amidating- mono-oxygenase	
Prion protein	
Cu-Zn superoxide dismutase	
Tyrosinase	
Metallothionein	
Blood-clotting factors V and VIII	
Transcuprein	
Albumin	
Angiogenin	

Source: [17-21]

Table 1: Copper and selenium dependent enzymes/proteins.

have low hepatic Cu and plasma ceruloplasmin levels. The disorder is a result of a mutation on the X-chromosome close to band q-13 and Menkes disease gene (ATP7A) has been shown to be expressed in intestinal epithelial cells [36,37]. Generally, anemia and leukopenia are related to Cu deficiency. In addition to Wilson's and Menkes disease, other diseased conditions like albinism, Down's syndrome [38], cytochrome-coxidase deficiency [39] and Cutis-laxa [40] also lead to fluctuations in Cu metabolism.

Role of copper in reproductive system:

Effect of copper on male reproduction: Male rats fed with low Cu diets exhibited decreased Cu levels in testis [41]. Anemia, heart hypertrophy and death in male rat (castrated or not) are also caused by Cu deficiency. Testosterone level in the male has been suggested to play a role in the severity of Cu deficiency. The presence of testosterone could influence male rats to the toxic effects of Cu deficiency. There is an observed 50% reduction in testosterone levels in castrated male, and this testosterone reduction significantly improved the anemia induced by Cu deficiency and increased the survival of rats by two weeks compared to non-castrated males, thus it improved the severity of the Cu deficiency. However, the protection was only temporary [42].

Copper deficiency in female reproduction and pregnancy: As opposed to Cu-deficient male rats, Cu-deficient female rats are protected against mortality due to Cu deficiency [43]. Endogenous estrogens are suggested to play a role in the protection against Cu-deficient state, as evidences indicate that estrogens alter the hepatic subcellular distribution of Cu, and induce the synthesis of ceruloplasmin thereby increasing the plasma Cu levels [44-46]. Notwithstanding, even ovariectomized females, where plasma estrogen is reduced by 48%, are protected against the severity of Cu deficiency. Thus, ovariectomized or intact female rats are not susceptible to severe Cu deficiency [47-52].

Cu, required for various enzymes/proteins involved in normal central nervous system (CNS) functioning, also affect norepinephrine and dopamine levels in the CNS by synthesis and/or release of neurotransmitters [8,53-56]. Thus, females taking oral contraceptives

are at higher risk of acquiring physiological and behavioral changes due to altered amine metabolism in brain [57]. There is an increased pressure on indispensable metal homeostasis of the pregnant female towards the completion of fetus development at the end of gestation [58]. Despite the fact that liver has the highest Cu concentration compared to other organs of the body; Cu is not significantly withdrawn from maternal storage tissues such as liver during pregnancy. Increased intestinal absorption of Cu and food consumption is responsible for transient augmentation in plasma Cu level observed during mid-pregnancy [59,60]. Infants completely dependent upon parenteral nutrition, without supplementation of Cu, develop hypochromic normocytic anemia, neutropenia and skeletal abnormalities in association with profound hypocupremia 14~ and these abnormalities responded well to oral Cu supplementation [2]. Hypomyelination is also reported in pups of Cu-deficient rat dams [53].

Selenium

Se is of fundamental prominence to human health. Owing to comprehensive study by Schwarz and Foltz, Se was proved as an indispensable nutrient necessary for both normal growth and reproduction in animals [61]. Se is a crucial component of several major metabolic pathways, including antioxidant defense function, thyroid hormone metabolism, and immune system. Se, an important trace element, deficiency is involved in heart disease and increased cancer risk. Keshan disease in humans is caused due to Se deficiency. Se toxicity, characterized by loss of hair and changes in ectodermal appendages, has also been reported in humans [62]. Se is as a cofactor of glutathione peroxidase which confers protection to cell from free radicals [18,63-68]. Se is a component of the unusual amino acids selenomethionine and selenocysteine. Se plays a key role in the physiological functioning of the thyroid gland which produces thyroid hormone (TH) and in every cell that uses TH, by participating as a cofactor for three iodothyronine deiodinases (Table 1). The iodothyronine deiodinases are the subfamily of deiodinase enzymes that use Se [21,69-71,18]. There are widespread variances in Se dietary intake across different populations, depending on the soil Se content and thus the Se content in foodstuffs and inter-individual dietary habits. So, Se enters the food chain through plants. Dietary Se is absorbed in the small intestine and incorporated into proteins by yet unknown complex mechanisms. According to WHO, 40 μg and 30 μg Se/day is sufficient to meet normal requirements of adult male and female, respectively [72].

Effect of Selenium on male reproduction: Low fertility and poor growth are associated with consumption of Se-deficient in farm animals [73]. During pubertal maturation in males, there is a significant increase in Se content of male gonads [74,75]. In addition to this, oligospermia, increase in abnormal spermatozoa, and a decline in the ratio of motile to immotile spermatozoa also been reported in Se-deficient rats. Increased fragility and decreased stability of the mitochondrial sheath causes disorganization of the mitochondrial sheath of the mid-piece. Se is localized in the mitochondrial capsule protein [(MCP), cysteine- and proline-rich selenoprotein)] of the mid-piece [76-80].

Testosterone secretion is affected by Se deficiency as its deficiency causes changes in the LH receptors of Leydig cells [74,75]. Pituitary gland, the bulbourethral and prostate glands, and the caput and corpus epididymis have shown the highest Se retentions [75,81]. Numerous studies have demonstrated the protecting effect of Se against Cd-induced toxicity [82]. Se also inhibits DNA, RNA and protein synthesis. Prostate cancer is caused due to high level of Cd in the prostate [83,84] and Se at non-toxic levels could help in the inhibition of the growth of cancerous cells (Table 2) [85]. A recent study has shown that dietary

Sex	Manifestations	References
Male	Testosterone biosynthesis	[87]
	Formation and normal development of spermatozoa	[88]
	Gluthathione peroxidase-4 shields developing- sperm cells from oxidative DNA damage	[89,90]
	Increased dietary Se intake increases male fertility, improved sperm quality, sperm motility, sperm count	[90-94]
Female	Low serum Se associated with miscarriage in pregnancy	[95,96]
	Probably linked with preeclampsia	[97]
	Lower Se concentration linked with preterm labor	[98]
	Decreased serum Se and glutathione peroxidase associated with obstetric cholestasis	
	Decrease in maternal plasma Se concentration connected to gestational diabetes mellitus	

Source: [18,21,66]

Table 2: Effects of selenium dyshomeostasis on human reproductive system.

Se of roosters can affect apoptosis of germ cells and cell cycle-related genes in the testis during spermatogenesis [86].

Selenium deficiency, female reproduction, pregnancy and lactation: Among the major outcomes resulting from Se deficiency in females are infertility, abortion and retained placenta. In addition to this, the offspring born from Se-deficient mother suffer from muscular weakness [61,99,100]. Se requirement of lactating and pregnant mothers is increased which can be explained on the basis of Se transport to the fetus via the placenta as well as to the infant via the breast milk [101,102]. It's worth noting here that Se level in human milk is robustly affected by maternal Se intake and status [103]. Molecular sieve chromatography have revealed that majority of the Se in human milk is protein-bound [104]. Infants and young children Se requirements are high because of their rapid growth (Table 2). Se deficiency may lead to miscarriages, gestational complications as well as damage to the nervous and immune systems of the fetus. During the early stage of pregnancy, low concentration of Se in serum, has been associated with low birth weight of child at birth [105].

References

1. Prasad AS (1982) Clinical, biochemical, and nutritional aspects of trace elements. Publisher: A.R. Liss, Vol 6: Current topics in nutrition and disease.

2. Bedwal RS, Bahuguna A (1994) Zinc, copper and selenium in reproduction. Experientia 50: 626-640.

3. Turski ML, Thiele DJ (2009) New roles for copper metabolism in cell proliferation, signaling, and disease. J Biol Chem 284: 717-721.

4. Prasad AS, Oberleas D (1976) Trace Elements in Human Health and Disease: Zinc and copper. Academic Press

5. Lichten LA, Cousins RJ (2009) Mammalian zinc transporters: Nutritional and physiologic regulation. Annu Rev Nutr 29: 153-176.

6. Jansen J, Karges W, Rink L (2009) Zinc and diabetes--clinical links and molecular mechanisms. J Nutr Biochem 20: 399-417.

7. Vonk WI, Klomp LW (2008) Role of transition metals in the pathogenesis of amyotrophic lateral sclerosis. Biochem Soc Trans 36: 1322-1328.

8. Desai V, Kaler SG (2008) Role of copper in human neurological disorders. Am J Clin Nutr 88: 855S-8S.

9. Labunskyy VM, Hatfield DL, Gladyshev VN (2014) Selenoproteins: Molecular pathways and physiological roles. Physiol Rev 94: 739-777.

10. Hatfield DL, Tsuji PA, Carlson BA, Gladyshev VN (2014) Selenium and selenocysteine: roles in cancer, health, and development. Trends Biochem Sci 39: 112-120.

11. Roman M, Jitaru P, Barbante C (2014) Selenium biochemistry and its role for human health. Metallomics 6: 25-54.

12. Weeks BS, Hanna MS, Cooperstein D (2012) Dietary selenium and selenoprotein function. Med Sci Monit 18: RA127-132.

13. Combs GF Jr (2015) Biomarkers of selenium status. Nutrients 7: 2209-2236.

14. Nath R (2000) Health and Disease Role of Micronutrients and Trace Elements: Recent Advances in the Assessment of Micronutrients and Trace Elements Deficiency in Humans. A.P.H Publishing

15. Rennert OM, Chan WY (1984) Metabolism of Trace Metals in Man: Developmental aspects. CRC Press

16. Brown SS, Kodama Y, Pure IUo, Chemistry A (1987) Toxicology of Metals: Clinical and Experimental Research : Proceedings of the VIth UOEH International Symposium and IIIrd COMPTOX, Held in Kitakyushu, Japan, 27-31 July 1986. Ellis Horwood Limited

17. Fraga CG (2005) Relevance, essentiality and toxicity of trace elements in human health. Mol Aspects Med 26: 235-244.

18. Brown KM, Arthur JR (2001) Selenium, selenoproteins and human health: a review. Public Health Nutr 4: 593-599.

19. Tapiero H, Tew KD (2003) Trace elements in human physiology and pathology: zinc and metallothioneins. Biomed Pharmacother 57: 399-411.

20. Tapiero H, Townsend DM, Tew KD (2003) Trace elements in human physiology and pathology. Copper. Biomed Pharmacother 57: 386-398.

21. Mistry HD, Broughton Pipkin F, Redman CW, Poston L (2012) Selenium in reproductive health. Am J Obstet Gynecol 206: 21-30.

22. Gaggelli E, Kozlowski H, Valensin D, Valensin G (2006) Copper homeostasis and neurodegenerative disorders (Alzheimer's, prion, and Parkinson's diseases and amyotrophic lateral sclerosis). Chem Rev 106: 1995-2044.

23. Uauy R, Olivares M, Gonzalez M (1998) Essentiality of copper in humans. Am J Clin Nutr 67: 952S-959S.

24. de Romaña DL, Olivares M, Uauy R, Araya M (2011) Risks and benefits of copper in light of new insights of copper homeostasis. J Trace Elem Med Biol 25: 3-13.

25. Linder MC, Hazegh-Azam M (1996) Copper biochemistry and molecular biology. Am J Clin Nutr 63: 797S-811S.

26. Georgopoulos PG, Roy A, Yonone-Lioy MJ, Opiekun RE, Lioy PJ (2001) Environmental copper: its dynamics and human exposure issues. J Toxicol Environ Health B Crit Rev 4: 341-394.

27. Madsen E, Gitlin JD (2007) Copper and iron disorders of the brain. Annu Rev Neurosci 30: 317-337.

28. Pandit A, Bhave S (1996) Present interpretation of the role of copper in Indian childhood cirrhosis. Am J Clin Nutr 63: 830S-835S.

29. European Association for Study of Liver (2012) EASL Clinical Practice Guidelines: Wilson's disease. J Hepatol 56: 671-685.

30. Gouider-Khouja N (2009) Wilson's disease. Parkinsonism Relat Disord 15 Suppl 3: S126-129.

31. Rosencrantz R, Schilsky M (2011) Wilson disease: pathogenesis and clinical considerations in diagnosis and treatment. Semin Liver Dis 31: 245-259.

32. Prasad R, Kaur G, Walia BN (1998) A critical evaluation of copper metabolism in Indian Wilson's disease children with special reference to their phenotypes and relatives. Biol Trace Elem Res 65: 153-165.

33. Prasad R, Kaur G, Nath R, Walia BN (1996) Molecular basis of pathophysiology of Indian childhood cirrhosis: role of nuclear copper accumulation in liver. Mol Cell Biochem 156: 25-30.

34. Pal A, Badyal RK, Vasishta RK, Attri SV, Thapa BR, et al. (2013) Biochemical, histological, and memory impairment effects of chronic copper toxicity: A model for non-Wilsonian brain copper toxicosis in Wistar rat. Biol Trace Elem Res 153: 257-268.

35. Pal A, Vasishta Rk, Prasad R (2013) Hepatic and hippocampus iron status is not altered in response to increased serum ceruloplasmin and serum "free" copper in Wistar rat model for non-Wilsonian brain copper toxicosis. Biol Trace Elem Res 154: 403-411.

36. Kaler SG (2011) ATP7A-related copper transport diseases-emerging concepts and future trends. Nat Rev Neurol 7: 15-29.

37. Kaler SG, Holmes CS, Goldstein DS, Tang J, Godwin SC, et al. (2008) Neonatal diagnosis and treatment of Menkes disease. N Engl J Med 358: 605-614.

38. Brooksbank BW, Balázs R (1983) Superoxide dismutase and lipo-peroxidation in Down's syndrome fetal brain. Lancet 1: 881-882.

39. Williams RB, Davies NT, McDonald I (1977) The effects of pregnancy and lactation on copper and zinc retention in the rat. Br J Nutr 38: 407-416.

40. Byers PH, Siegel RC, Holbrook KA, Narayanan AS, Bornstein P, et al. (1980) X-linked cutis laxa: defective cross-link formation in collagen due to decreased lysyl oxidase activity. N Engl J Med 303: 61-65.

41. Keen CL, Reinstein NH, Goudey-Lefevre J, Lefevre M, Lönnerdal B, et al. (1985) Effect of dietary copper and zinc levels on tissue copper, zinc, and iron in male rats. Biol Trace Elem Res 8: 123-136.

42. Fields M, Lewis CG, Beal T, Scholfield D, Patterson K, et al. (1987) Sexual differences in the expression of copper deficiency in rats. Proc Soc Exp Biol Med 186: 183-187.

43. Fields M, Lewis C, Scholfield DJ, Powell AS, Rose AJ, et al. (1986) Female rats are protected against the fructose induced mortality of copper deficiency. Proc Soc Exp Biol Med 183: 145-149.

44. Carruthers ME, Hobbs CB, Warren RL (1966) Raised serum copper and caeruloplasmin levels in subjects taking oral contraceptives. J Clin Pathol 19: 498-500.

45. Russanov E, Banskalieva V, Ljutakova S (1981) Influence of sex hormones on the subcellular distribution of copper in sheep liver. Res Vet Sci 30: 223-225.

46. Saylor WW, Downer JV (1986) Copper and zinc distribution in the liver and oviduct of estrogen- and testosterone-treated hens (Gallus domesticus). Nutrition Research 6:181-190.

47. Evans GW, Cornatzer NF, Cornatzer WE (1970) Mechanism for hormone-induced alterations in serum ceruloplasmin. Am J Physiol 218: 613-615.

48. Sorenson JRJ, Association ICR (1982) Inflammatory diseases and copper: the metabolic and therapeutic roles of copper and other essential metalloelements in humans. Humana Press.

49. Mehta SW, Eikum R (1989) Effect of estrogen on serum and tissue levels of copper and zinc. Adv Exp Med Biol 258: 155-162.

50. Meyer BJ, Meyer AC, Horwitt MK (1958) Factors influencing serum copper and ceruloplasmin oxidative activity in the rat. Am J Physiol 194: 581-584.

51. Vir SC, Love AH (1981) Zinc and copper nutriture of women taking oral contraceptive agents. Am J Clin Nutr 34: 1479-1483.

52. Yunice AA, Lindeman RD (1975) Effect of estrogen-progestogen administration on tissue cation concentrations in the rat. Endocrinology 97: 1263-1269.

53. Prohaska JR (1990) Development of copper deficiency in neonatal mice. J Nutr Biochem 1: 415-419.

54. Gaier ED, Eipper BA, Mains RE (2013) Copper signaling in the mammalian nervous system: synaptic effects. J Neurosci Res 91: 2-19.

55. Lutsenko S, Bhattacharjee A, Hubbard AL (2010) Copper handling machinery of the brain. Metallomics 2: 596-608.

56. Tiffany-Castiglioni E, Hong S, Qian Y (2011) Copper handling by astrocytes: Insights into neurodegenerative diseases. Int J Dev Neurosci 29: 811-818.

57. Feller DJ, O'Dell BL (1980) Dopamine and norepinephrine in discrete areas of the copper-deficient rat brain. J Neurochem 34: 1259-1263.

58. Hall GA, Howell JM (1969) The effect of copper deficiency on reproduction in the female rat. Br J Nutr 23: 41-45.

59. Gohary ME, Cavazos LF, Manning JP (1962) Effects of testosterone on histochemical reactions of epithelium of hamster ductus epididymidis and seminal vesicle. The Anatomical Record 144: 229-237.

60. Masters DG, Keen CL, Lönnerdal B, Hurley LS (1983) Zinc deficiency teratogenicity: the protective role of maternal tissue catabolism. J Nutr 113: 905-912.

61. Schwarz K, Foltz CM (1999) Selenium as an integral part of factor 3 against dietary necrotic liver degeneration. 1951. Nutrition 15: 255.

62. Yang GQ, Wang SZ, Zhou RH, Sun SZ (1983) Endemic selenium intoxication of humans in China. Am J Clin Nutr 37: 872-881.

63. Burk RF, Hill KE, Motley AK (2003) Selenoprotein metabolism and function: evidence for more than one function for selenoprotein P. J Nutr 133: 1517S-20S.

64. Zachara BA (1992) Mammalian selenoproteins. J Trace Elem Electrolytes Health Dis 6: 137-151.

65. Holben DH, Smith AM (1999) The diverse role of selenium within selenoproteins: A review. J Am Diet Assoc 99: 836-843.

66. Allan CB, Lacourciere GM, Stadtman TC (1999) Responsiveness of selenoproteins to dietary selenium. Annu Rev Nutr 19: 1-16.

67. [No authors listed] (1987) Incorporation of selenium into glutathione peroxidase. Nutr Rev 45: 344-345.

68. Zhu Z, Kimura M, Itokawa Y (1993) Effect of selenium and protein deficiency on selenium and glutathione peroxidase in rats. Biol Trace Elem Res 36: 15-23.

69. Drutel A, Archambeaud F, Caron P (2013) Selenium and the thyroid gland: more good news for clinicians. Clin Endocrinol (Oxf) 78: 155-164.

70. Darras VM, Van Herck SL (2012) Iodothyronine deiodinase structure and function: from ascidians to humans. J Endocrinol 215: 189-206.

71. Orozco A, Valverde-R C, Olvera A, García-G C (2012) Iodothyronine deiodinases: A functional and evolutionary perspective. J Endocrinol 215: 207-219.

72. Levander OA, Whanger PD (1996) Deliberations and evaluations of the approaches, endpoints and paradigms for selenium and iodine dietary recommendations. J Nutr 126: 2427S-2434S.

73. Hartfiel W, Bahners N (1988) Selenium deficiency in the Federal Republic of Germany. Biol Trace Elem Res 15: 1-12.

74. Behne D, Höfer T, von Berswordt-Wallrabe R, Elger W (1982) Selenium in the testis of the rat: studies on its regulation and its importance for the organism. J Nutr 112: 1682-1687.

75. Behne D, Duk M, Elger W (1986) Selenium content and glutathione peroxidase activity in the testis of the maturing rat. J Nutr 116: 1442-1447.

76. Maiorino M, Roveri A, Benazzi L, Bosello V, Mauri P, et al. (2005) Functional interaction of phospholipid hydro peroxide glutathione peroxidase with sperm mitochondrion-associated cysteine-rich protein discloses the adjacent cysteine motif as a new substrate of the selenoperoxidase. J Biol Chem 280: 38395-38402.

77. Wu AS, Oldfield JE, Shull LR, Cheeke PR (1979) Specific effect of selenium deficiency on rat sperm. Biol Reprod 20: 793-798.

78. Sánchez-Gutiérrez M, García-Montalvo EA, Izquierdo-Vega JA, Del Razo LM (2008) Effect of dietary selenium deficiency on the in vitro fertilizing ability of mice spermatozoa. Cell Biol Toxicol 24: 321-329.

79. Noblanc A, Kocer A, Chabory E, Vernet P, Saez F, et al. (2011) Glutathione peroxidases at work on epididymal spermatozoa: an example of the dual effect of reactive oxygen species on mammalian male fertilizing ability. J Androl 32: 641-650.

80. Wu SH, Oldfield JE, Whanger PD, Weswig PH (1973) Effect of selenium, vitamin E, and antioxidants on testicular function in rats. Biol Reprod 8: 625-629.

81. Burk RF, Brown DG, Seely RJ, Scaief CC 3rd (1972) Influence of dietary and injected selenium on whole-blody retention, route of excretion, and tissue retention of 75SeO3 2- in the rat. J Nutr 102: 1049-1055.

82. Olsson U (1986) Selenium deficiency and detoxication functions in the rat: short-term effects of cadmium. Drug Nutr Interact 4: 309-319.

83. Bako G, Smith ES, Hanson J, Dewar R (1982) The geographical distribution of high cadmium concentrations in the environment and prostate cancer in Alberta. Can J Public Health 73: 92-94.

84. Webber MM, Perez-Ripoll EA, James GT (1985) Inhibitory effects of selenium on the growth of DU-145 human prostate carcinoma cells in vitro. Biochem Biophys Res Commun 130: 603-609.

85. Combs GF Jr, Clark LC (1985) Can dietary selenium modify cancer risk? Nutr Rev 43: 325-331.

86. Song R, Yao X, Shi L, Ren Y, Zhao H (2015) Effects of dietary selenium on apoptosis of germ cells in the testis during spermatogenesis in roosters. Theriogenology 84: 583-588.

87. Behne D, Weiler H, Kyriakopoulos A (1996) Effects of selenium deficiency on testicular morphology and function in rats. J Reprod Fertil 106: 291-297.

88. Flohé L (2007) Selenium in mammalian spermiogenesis. Biol Chem 388: 987-995.

89. Ursini F, Heim S, Kiess M, Maiorino M, Roveri A, et al. (1999) Dual function of the selenoprotein PHGPx during sperm maturation. Science 285: 1393-1396.

90. Safarinejad MR, Safarinejad S (2009) Efficacy of selenium and/or N-acetyl-cysteine for improving semen parameters in infertile men: a double-blind, placebo controlled, randomized study. J Urol 181: 741-751.

91. Irvine DS (1996) Glutathione as a treatment for male infertility. Rev Reprod 1: 6-12.

92. Bleau G, Lemarbre J, Faucher G, Roberts KD, Chapdelaine A (1984) Semen selenium and human fertility. Fertil Steril 42: 890-894.

93. Scott R, MacPherson A, Yates RW, Hussain B, Dixon J (1998) The effect of oral selenium supplementation on human sperm motility. Br J Urol 82: 76-80.

94. Keskes-Ammar L, Feki-Chakroun N, Rebai T, Sahnoun Z, Ghozzi H, et al. (2003) Sperm oxidative stress and the effect of an oral vitamin E and selenium supplement on semen quality in infertile men. Arch Androl 49: 83-94.

95. Barrington JW, Lindsay P, James D, Smith S, Roberts A (1996) Selenium deficiency and miscarriage: A possible link? Br J Obstet Gynaecol 103: 130-132.

96. Koçak I, Aksoy E, Ustün C (1999) Recurrent spontaneous abortion and selenium deficiency. Int J Gynaecol Obstet 65: 79-80.

97. Hesketh J (2008) Nutrigenomics and selenium: gene expression patterns, physiological targets, and genetics. Annu Rev Nutr 28: 157-177.

98. Rayman MP, Wijnen H, Vader H, Kooistra L, Pop V (2011) Maternal selenium status during early gestation and risk for preterm birth. CMAJ 183: 549-555.

99. Shamberger RJ (1983) Biochemistry of Selenium. Plenum Press.

100. Westermarck T, Raunu P, Kirjarinta M, Lappalainen L (1977) Selenium content of whole blood and serum in adults and children of different ages from different parts of Finland. Acta Pharmacol Toxicol (Copenh) 40: 465-475.

101. Higashi A, Tamari H, Kuroki Y, Matsuda I (1983) Longitudinal changes in selenium content of breast milk. Acta Paediatr Scand 72: 433-436.

102. Smith AM, Picciano MF, Milner JA (1982) Selenium intakes and status of human milk and formula fed infants. Am J Clin Nutr 35: 521-526.

103. Kumpulainen J, Salmenperä L, Siimes MA, Koivistoinen P, Perheentupa J (1985) Selenium status of exclusively breast-fed infants as influenced by maternal organic or inorganic selenium supplementation. Am J Clin Nutr 42: 829-835.

104. Milner JA, Sherman L, Picciano MF (1987) Distribution of selenium in human milk. Am J Clin Nutr 45: 617-624.

105. PieczyÅ ska J, Grajeta H (2015) The role of selenium in human conception and pregnancy. J Trace Elem Med Biol 29: 31-38.

21

Sequential Responses of Bacteria to Noxious Agents (Antibiotics) Leading to Accumulation of Mutations and Permanent Resistance

Ana Martins[1,2,3], Gabriella Spengler[2], Joseph Molnar[2] and Leonard Amaral[1,2,4]*

[1]*Grupo de Micobacterias, UEI Microbiology, Medical Microbiology and Parasitology Unidade de (UPMM), Instituto de Medicina Tropical and Higiene, Universidade Nova de Lisboa, Portugal*
[2]*Institute of Medical Microbiology and Immunobiology, Faculty of Medicine, University of Szeged, Hungary*
[3]*Institute of Pharmacognosy, Faculty of Pharmacy, University of Szeged, Hungary*
[4]*Grupo de Micobacterias, UEI Microbiology, Centro de Malaria and Outras doenças Tropicais (CMDT), Instituto de Medicina Tropical and Higiene, Universidade Nova de Lisboa, Portugal*

Abstract

Bacteria have the capacity, as all living cells, to escape harm from a noxious agent by extruding the agent before it reaches its target and harms to the cell. This initial response is intrinsic and involves plasma membrane bound efflux pumps which have the capacity to recognise and extrude a large variety of structurally unrelated molecules. When the concentration of the agent is progressively increased, the number of efflux pumps is also progressively increased as a consequence of over-expression of genes that regulate and code for the synthesis of these pumps. Often, when the bacterium is transferred to drug free medium, the number of pump units returns to baseline levels. However, when the concentration of agent is maintained over a prolonged period of time, mutations in genes that code for essential proteins which are usual targets of antibiotics, begin to accumulate and the expression of genes that code for the efflux pumps decreases, oftentimes reaching wild type levels.

When the patient is treated with an antibiotic over a prolonged period of time and initial therapy is ineffective, the bacterium most likely escapes via its own intrinsic efflux pump system and with time, it is expected that the number of efflux pump units progressively increase rendering the clinical isolate resistant to the given antibiotic. The amount of energy needed to maintain a high level of efflux pump activity is great and at the expense of other activities that are needed for survival and replication. When this point is reached, and following the second law of thermodynamics, the bacterium goes through changes to survive at low energy costs (for example: switches its mutator gene and a number of predicted mutations of essential proteins take place). These changes render the bacterium permanently resistant to given antibiotics, the need for efflux is no longer and the number of efflux pump units returns to baseline levels. This review will discuss the structure, genetic regulation, physiology of efflux pumps and the means by which a clinical isolate can be characterized for the components that contribute to its resistance during therapy, namely, evaluation of efflux pump activity versus mutations. The ability of a laboratory to perform these evaluations will go a long way toward the selection of effective antibiotic therapy on a real-basis.

Keywords: Bacteria; Mycobacterium; Efflux pumps; Control; Genetic regulation; Biophysics; Physiology; Inhibitors of efflux pumps; Role of efflux pumps in infection; Role of efflux pumps in quorum sensing

Introduction

Bacteria have multiple ways to survive the presence of noxious agents in their environment whether that environment is in the wild (toxic agents produced by competing bacteria and other microorganisms [1], toxic agents introduced by human populations [2]) or the human body (antibiotics [3], natural immune defences of the host [4], etc). Concerning the environment of the bacterially infected host, bacteria have the capacity to escape the activity of antibiotics if and when therapy is ineffective due to the presence of mutations that render the antibiotic intended target immune to the antibiotic [5], or to the secretion of enzymes by the given bacteria that destroy the activity of a given antibiotic (examples-lactamases [6]), or to poorly delivered therapy which favours the selection of spontaneous mutations rendering the antibiotic ineffective [7] and induces responses that are transient until the antibiotic is no longer present [8]. Among the transient responses are down-regulation of porins (channels through the bacterial envelope of Gram-negative bacteria which mediate the passage of hydrophilic agents into the cell [9]), induction of two-component regulon systems which render the bacterium relatively immune to many noxious agents [10], and up-regulation of efflux pumps [11]. It is the intent of this mini-review to primarily discuss the structure, function, control and genetic regulation of efflux pumps of pathogenic bacteria and the role that efflux pumps play in rendering the infective bacterium including

mycobacteria, intrinsically resistant, transiently resistant and multi-drug resistant (MDR) and their interaction with other mechanisms that supplement induced drug resistance such as the two-component regulon systems, quorum sensing and activation of a mutator system that as of this writing remains to be proven. In addition, assays, which can at this time be adopted for the evaluation and quantification of efflux pumps of a clinical isolate, will be presented and discussed.

The Structure of the Efflux Pump of Gram-Negative Bacterium

Efflux pumps are proteins that are present in the cell envelope of

*Corresponding author: Leonard Amaral, M.D., Ph.D., Grupo de Micobacterias, UEI Microbiology, Institute of Tropical Medicine and Higiene, Universidade Nova de Lisboa, Rua Junqueira 100, 1349-008 Lisbon, Portugal
E-mail: lamaral@ihmt.unl.pt

all bacteria, are firmly attached to the bacterial plasma membrane and traverse the cell envelope such that a conduit from the plasma membrane to the surface of the cell makes it possible for the extrusion of noxious agents from the cytoplasm and periplasm. Because the efflux pumps of the Gram-negative *E. coli* have been very much studied and their structure, genetic regulation and control, physiological activity, energy sources for their function, interaction with other drug resistant mechanisms, means by which their function can be reduced or obviated and the means by which they can be evaluated when over-expressed in a given Gram-negative isolate are confirmed, we will restrict our discussion to the AcrAB-TolC the main efflux pump of this bacterial pathogen.

Structure of the Main Efflux Pump of *E. coli*

E. coli has a wide variety of efflux pumps that may at one time or another extrude a given noxious agent [12]. The main efflux pump of *E. coli* is the AcrAB-TolC pump, which belongs to the genetic family of transporters termed "resistant nodulation division" (RND). This pump has a trimer structure that consists of two fusion proteins coded by the *acrA* gene that anchor the pump to the plasma membrane of the cell and may mechanically assist the pump [13,14] in the translocation of a recognised noxious agent that is bound to the transporter component of the pump to the external environment. The second component of the efflux pump trimer is the transporter AcrB that is coded by the *acrB* gene and which has the capacity to recognise and bind noxious agent that are structurally unrelated [15-19]. The means by this recognition takes place is not yet understood. The third component is TolC, which is a barrel like structure that forms a contiguous channel with the AcrB transporter affording the conduit of the noxious agent to the surface of the cell [20-22]. Although the structures of the AcrA fusion [17], the AcrB transporter [19] and TolC [23, 24] are fully known, the actual position and structure within the cell envelope remains elusive. Nevertheless, a schematic figure of the AcrAB-TolC efflux pump of *E. coli* is presented by figure 1 modified from that of Pos [17]. Briefly, a noxious agent that has traversed the outer membrane to the periplasm or the cytoplasmic side of the plasma membrane, enters the transporter, is bound and extruded to the outside of the cell via the conduit TolC

channel. The process is dependent on energy, which has been commonly accepted as coming from the proton motive force of the cell [8,25]. This concept has been challenged recently and modified within the context of what takes place for the maintenance of the proton motive force (PMF) when the pH of the environment is low or high and the source of protons that supply the energy for the pump [11,25,26].

Energy Source for the Function of the Acrab-Tolc Efflux Pump of *E. coli*

The PMF is derived from the differential concentration of protons at opposite sides of a unit membrane as defined by Mitchell's chemiosmotic hypothesis [27]. The generation of protons results from metabolic activity of the cell and the transfer of these protons to the surface of the plasma membrane cause a relative difference between the concentrations of protons on the surface being much greater than that on the cytoplasmic (medial) side of the plasma membrane. This concentration difference results in an electrochemical gradient termed as the PMF. When certain activities of the cell, such as transport mediated by an RND efflux pump, take place, the movement of these protons to the periplasm makes it possible for the pump to extrude the substrate bound to the AcrB component of the transporter. However, this theory has been modified from results that examined the effect of pH on the source of energy required for the activity of the pump [28-30]. Briefly, whereas at pH 5.5 or below, metabolic energy is not required for the extrusion of an AcrAB-TolC substrate such as ethidium bromide, at pH of 6.5 to 7.0, efflux is totally dependent upon a metabolic source of energy (glucose, glycolytic intermediates etc. [31]). Because the main contributor to the PMF is the activity of ATP synthase [32,33], and at low pH, it favours the synthesis of ATP whereas at high pH it favours the hydrolysis of ATP, at low pH protons are not generated by the synthase and the source of protons needed for the function of the pump must lie elsewhere. Mitchell's theory, when applied to the PMF of bacteria, would result in the movement of protons into the vast ocean milieu that would soon eliminate the differential difference between the two concentrations of protons, and hence, the PMF would collapse [28] The modification of Mitchell's chemiosmotic theory involves the now known fact that the protons generated by metabolic

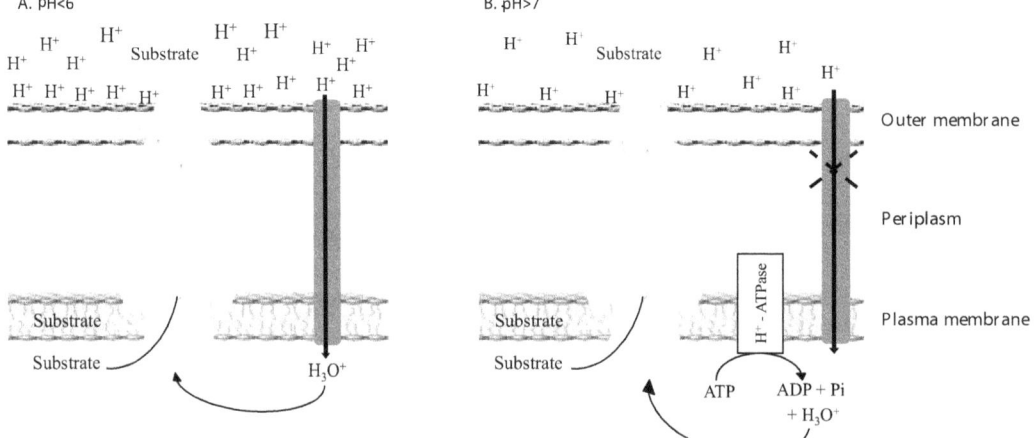

Figure 1: At pH lower than 6, the concentration of hydronium ions at the surface of the cell is considerably higher than that in the milieu. This drives the hydronium ions toward the cytoplasmic side of the plasma membrane (inner membrane) via porins. The hydronium ions then pass through the transporter and reduce internal pH causing the release of the bound substrate. The peristaltic action of the fusion proteins promotes the passage of water and the substrate is carried out to the surface. The energy required for the conformational change in the fusion proteins that generate the peristaltic action as described by Pos et al. is provided by metabolism.

At pH above 7, the primary source of hydronium ions which are to pass through the transporter and promote the release of the substrate from the transporter, results from the activity of the ATP synthase.

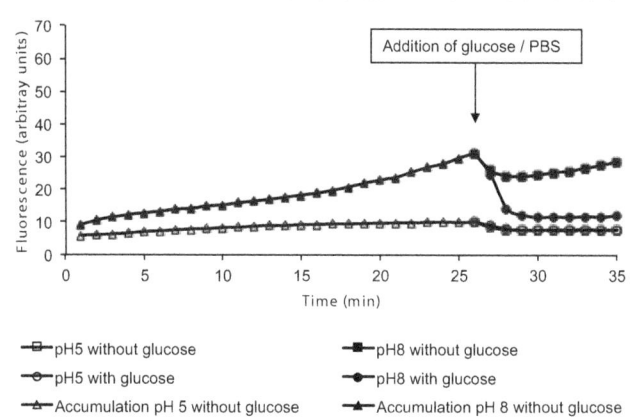

Figure 2 – Efflux of EB by the strain *E. coli* AG100.

activity are distributed over the surface of the cell and bound to the lipopolysaccharide layer of the outer cell membrane and to basic amino acids of various proteins adsorbed to the surface of the cell [30]. These bound protons (hydronium ions) produce a pH at the surface of the cell that is two to three pH units lower than that of the bulk milieu [29,30]. Consequently, when the pH of the environment is low and there is a need for protons, the bound hydronium ions are mobilised to the periplasm through porin channels that normally permit the movement of water into the cell [34]. In the absence of metabolic energy, at low pH, the attraction of hydronium ions to the surface of the cell contributes to the PMF. At high pH, the attraction of hydronium ions will be considerably lower, hence the need for metabolic energy as a source of protons that may passively reach the surface of the cell via the efflux pump channel itself and contribute to the PMF [25,26]. Significant to this theory is the recent observation that at high pH the dissociation of a substrate from the AcrB transporter is very slow or not at all whereas at low pH the dissociation constant is very high [35]. Therefore, the movement of hydronium ions through the efflux pump reduces the pH and the AcrB bound substrate is released and carried to the surface by the movement of water [25,26] mechanically assisted by the peristaltic action of fusion proteins AcrA [13,14]. The facts presented above also explain why the PMF of a bacterium is maintained in very acidic and very basic media [36-40]. Figure 1 depicts the events related to the anticipated sources of hydronium ions (protons) needed for the activity of the AcrAB-TolC efflux pump at low and high pH.

Experiments that Support the Theory Presented for the Sources of Energy that Contribute to the PMF and the Effectiveness of Efflux Pump Activity

The effect of pH on efflux has been studied and, as an example, figure 2 demonstrates the effect of low pH (5.5) and the need for metabolic energy when the pH is high (pH 8.0) on the real time efflux of the universal substrate ethidium bromide (EB) by *E. coli* [41]. Similar studies had also been done for *Salmonella enterica* serovar Typhimurium [26,42], *Enterobacter aerogenes* [43], *Enterococcus feacalis* [44] and *Straphylococcus aereus* [45]. As noted by this figure, at low pH metabolic energy is not needed whereas at high pH metabolic energy (glucose) is an absolute requirement for efflux of EB. Other sources of metabolic energy can replace the need for glucose at high pH [42]. The method for real time as well as other methods for the evaluation of efflux pump activity will be fully described in later sections of this review.

In Vitro Responses of Bacteria to Prolonged Exposure to Antibiotics and the Inducement of Efflux Pump Genes

The genetic regulation of the AcrAB efflux pump involves the

activation of stress genes *sox* and *rob* sequentially followed by the activation of local regulators *mar A* and *marB*, *acrA* (codes for fusion protein A) and *acrB* (codes for transporter B). Prolonged exposure to increasing concentration of given antibiotics results in the increased resistance to the antibiotic as well as to other unrelated antibiotics (mdr). Exposure of *E. coli* to increasing concentrations of tetracycline increases the MIC of the agent [12,46], as well as increases the activity of genes that regulate and code for efflux pump components of the efflux pump AcrAB of *E. coli* (Table 1 [12,46]). The transfer of the bacterium to drug free medium or medium containing an inhibitor of the pump results in the restoration of the MIC as well as the genes that regulate and code for the efflux pump components. However, if the efflux pump is over-expressed and then the organism is placed in medium containing the last concentration of the antibiotic used to induce efflux pump expression, and serially transferred to this constant concentration, with time, the MIC to tetracycline continues to increase whereas the activity of the gene that codes for the AcrB transporter returns to baseline levels (Table 1) [47]. The cause for the progressive increase of resistance to tetracycline as well as to the main antibiotic targets of beta lactams, 30S ribosomes and gyrase [47] is due to the accumulation of mutations with prolonged exposure to a constant concentration of a given antibiotic. This development of an MDR phenotype is predicated on the initial response to the antibiotic, which is the increased activity of genes that regulate and code for the AcrAB-TolC efflux pump. In other words, the increased expression of the efflux pump system makes it possible for the generation and accumulation of mutations in the essential proteins of the organism. It also explains why a constant dose of an antibiotic for a prolonged period of time yields a clinical isolate for which the MIC of the given antibiotic may increase to 10, 50 or even 100 fold over that for the wild type strain.

Inducement of an efflux pump system of *Mycobacterium tuberculosis* by exposure to increasing concentrations of isoniazid (INH) has also been shown [48,49]. Moreover, as noted for *E. coli* prolonged exposure to a constant concentration of INH will at first be accompanied with increase in the expression of genes *mmpL7*, *p55*, *efpA*, *mmr*, *Rv1258c* and *Rv2459* that code for the main efflux pumps of the organism followed by mutations in essential genes [49].

Genes	AG100$_{TET}$ [12,46]	AG100$_{TET10}$ [47]
acrF	↑↑	↑
acrA	↑↑↑	n.a.
acrB	↑↑↑	↑
acrR	↑↑	n.a.
marR	↑↑	n.a.
marA	↑↑↑	↑
marB	↑↑	n.a.
tolC	↑↑	n.a.
micF	↑↑↑	n.a.
ompF	↑	n.a.
ompX	↑↑↑	↑
soxS	↑	↑
rob	↑	↑

Table 1: Changes in the expression of genes that code for or regulate the expression of AcrAB efflux pump. Table represents the relative quantity of gene mRNA compared with the parental strain AG100 not adapted to tetracycline (TET). ↑↑↑-increase over 6 times; ↑↑-increase over 2 times; ↑-slight increase till 2 times; →-same level of expression; n.a.: data not available. AG100$_{TET}$ refers to the strains after increasing concentrations of TET [12,46]. AG100$_{TET10}$ refers to the strain AG100$_{TET}$ after serial passages at 10 ug/mL of TET [47].

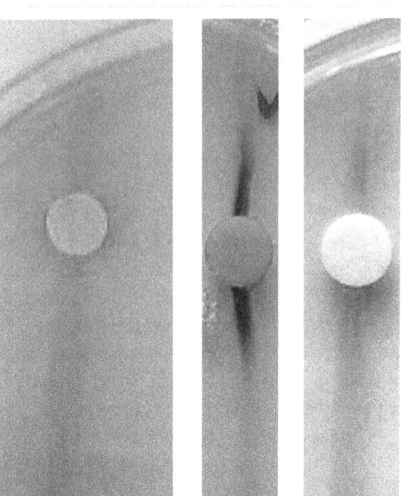

Figure 3: The effect of a trifluoromethyl ketone (TF) on the response of CV026 to the QS signal acylated hydroxyl lactone (AHL). **A**: Control disk with TFK MM4 (20 µg) alone (no colour). **B**: Control disk impregnated with QS signal pure acylated hydroxyl lactone (AHL) (10 ng) alone (deep purple coloration indicates response by the responding bacterium that is obviated by the TFK MM4 compound) [52].

Similar results have been obtained with Gram-positive bacteria [45].

The Role of the Efflux Pump in quorum sensing

Communication between bacteria of the same strain or species and between species contributes to their survival [50-52]. The secretion of signals that invoke a specific response from the responder is termed Quorum sensing (QS). When it takes place between strains of the same species, communication is directed towards the reduction of population growth and hence, reducing the possibility of exceeding the nutritional support of the environment [53, 54]. Other signals involve the secretion of bioactive molecules that inhibit the replication of a competing population species [55] or even kill (biocidins) [56] or promote a swarming effect that recruits members of the same species to migrate to a specific location [57,58]. Other responses involving "community action" are also invoked and these result in secretion of materials that will protect the bacterium from external danger. These materials, termed biofilm, encase the bacteria at distances from each other and within the matrix of this biofilm are channels used for further communication [59-61]. Biofilms are produced in the wild to maintain the bacterial population *in situ* (for example: surface of rocks) [31] and are also produced at sites of the human colonised by infecting bacteria [62]. There is a relationship between efflux pumps (EP), QS and biofilm secretion, which has come to the forefront only recently [13]. In this case, the absence of the main efflux pump of a Gram-negative bacterium inhibits the secretion of biofilm suggesting that the efflux pump provides the means by which the synthesised biofilm is extruded much as is the case for the extrusion of toxic products produced by the metabolic processes of the bacterium [63]. These aspects suggest that efflux pumps perform other roles than simply extruding noxious agents that have penetrated the cell envelope. To this extent the question of whether efflux pumps have a role in the secretion of QS signals has been indirectly shown by the demonstration that agents which inhibit the PMF of a Gram-negative bacterium not only inhibit the activity of an efflux pump but also inhibit responses from a bacterium to which the QS signal is directed [52,64]. As shown by figure 3, agents such as trifluoromethyl ketones (TKFs) that inhibit the PMF of bacteria [52], and their efflux pump system also inhibit the response to a QS signal

[52]. Other inhibitors of the PMF such as phenothiazines that also inhibit efflux pumps of bacteria have also been shown to inhibit the responses to QS signals.

Other studies will more closely examine the relationship between the efflux pump and secretion of QS signals since the inhibition of the latter is considered to be of great significance for the prevention of biofilm secretion, as well as other secretions that promote tissue damage to the infected host.

The Role of Efflux Pumps and the Two Component Regulon of *Salmonella*

The neutrophil does not readily kill phagocytosed *Salmonella* once it is entrapped by the lysosome [10]. The reason for this is due to the inducement of the pmrA/pmrB two component regulon by the acidic pH of the phagolysosome that results in rendering the organism practically resistant to almost everything [10]. The pmrA/pmrB regulon is activated by pH [10] and functions as follows: Activation of the *pmrb* gene produces a product pmrB, which undergoes self-phosphorylation. The phophorylated pmrB acts as a kinase and transfers the phosphate to pmrA which activates a series of nine genes that result in the synthesis of Lipid A that is introduced into the nascent polysaccharide (LPS) layer of the outer membrane of the organism [10]. Because this increased LPS renders the organism immune to the action of lysosomal hydrolases and prevents the penetration of antibiotics [10]; a systemic infection that results from the invasion of the organism into the peritoneal cavity is accompanied by high mortality. Clinical isolates of *Salmonella* from peritoneal infections or extracted from the phagolysosomes of the neutrophil have over-expressed efflux pumps. These over-expressed efflux pumps result from the activation of the gene *pmrd* by the pmrA protein and the product of *pmrd*, pmrD, directly activates *ramA*, the global regulator of the AcrAB efflux pump of the organism [10]. Over-expression of the AcrAB-TolC efflux pump contributes to the difficulties associated with the therapy of a salmonella infection of the colon [26]. Although an inhibition of the efflux pump system of the strain whose pmrA/pmrB two-component regulon has been induced will not contribute much to therapy of a *Salmonella* peritoneal infection. The salmonella strain that eventually colonises the colon is expected to have its efflux pump over-expressed as it passes through the stomach (pH as low as 3 or less) as a consequence of the activation of its induced pmrD product. Moreover, when the organism reaches the colon, it is already prepared to extrude the toxic bile salts present [23,41]. Consequently, inhibition of the AcrAB-TolC efflux pump of colon-colonising *Salmonella* by non-toxic agents known to inhibit the

Genes	0.5h	1h	4h	8h	16h
soxS	→	↑↑	↑	→	→
rob	↑	↑	↑	→	↑
ramA	↑	↑	↑↑↑	↑↑	↑
marA	→	→	↑↑	↑	→
acrB	→	↑	↑	↑↑↑	↑↑
pmrA	↑	↑	↑	↑↑	↑
pmrB	→	↑	↑↑	↑	↑

Table 2: Activity of genes that regulate and code for the AcrAB efflux pump of *Salmonella*. During the first 8 h, the organism was not growing, but genes evolved in the expression of the AcrB transporter were sequentially activated: first *soxS*, whose expression was elevated after 1h of culture; followed by *ramA*, *marA* and *pmrB* (4 h culture). After 8 h of culture, *ramA* decreased its activity, *marA* returned to baseline activity, *acrB* was maximally increased in activity and *pmrA* was now active. By the end of the 16 h culture, only *acrB* activity remained elevated. Table represents the relative quantity of gene mRNA compared with the untreated *Salmonella* strain: ↑↑↑-increase over 15 times; ↑↑-increase from 5 to 15 times; ↑-increase till 5 times; →-same level of expression.

pump may effectively treat a *Salmonella* infection of the colon when used in combination with antibiotics.

The response of salmonella to chlorpromazine (CPZ) and thioridazine (TZ) has resulted in the understanding that the MIC determined 16 h later does not fully characterise the response of the organism. As an example, during the first 8 hours of exposure to various concentrations of CPZ, the organism does not grow, demonstrating susceptibility to the agent. However, following this period, the organism grows at the same rate as the drug free control culture [65]. The same result is obtained with TZ [42]. Obviously, the events after the initial period of 8 hours, an adaptive response must have taken place. As evident from the data presented by table 2, the genes that regulate and code for efflux pumps of *Salmonella* are sequentially expressed during the first 8 hours of culture [42]. By the end of 16 hrs, the MIC of TZ is over 200 mg/L and the expression of efflux pumps has returned to almost normal baseline levels [42]. Nevertheless, the activity of the efflux pump after 24 h of exposure is not sufficient to permit the organism to survive a sub-inhibitory concentration. Survival appears to involve huge changes in the appearance of the cell envelope as well as the protein composition extracted from this envelope [65]. These studies show how well equipped *Salmonella* is for dealing with high concentrations of a noxious agent in its environment suggesting that in all probability, the dangers posed by food-borne infections of *Salmonella* will be with us for a long time.

Methods for Assessing Efflux Pump Activity and Evaluation of Compounds for Activity against the Efflux Pump System of Bacteria

We have developed a number of methods that can easily be adapted to the daily routine of a general bacteriology laboratory. Among the simplest to use is the EB (ethidium bromide) agar method that requires no instrumentation and its preparation evaluation of results is performed with material that is universally present in these laboratories.

The EB Agar Method for Characterising the Presence of an Over-Expressed Pump System of a Clinical Isolate

The fluorochrome EB is a universal efflux pump substrate [66] which when added to agar in increasing concentrations will identify the highest concentration that a clinical bacterial isolate can readily extrude. This concentration is readily noted by the presence of pink fluorescence associated with the colonies present on the surface of the cell [67-69]. The higher the concentration of EB that produces

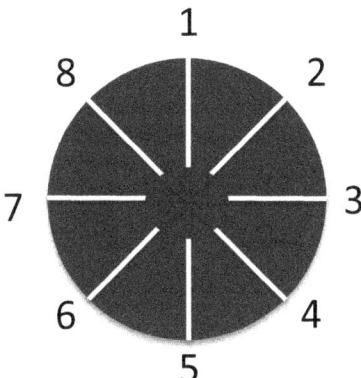

Figure 4: Schematic representation of the EB or AO plates. Cells are swabbed in the plate in lines that start nearly the center (without touching each other) to the outer part of the agar.

fluorescence of the colony as compared to that of a wild type reference control of the same species, the more active is the efflux pump system of the clinical isolate. The method is simple, reproducible and can readily be phased into a bacteriological laboratory. No special skills or laboratory equipment other than a short/long wave hand held UV light, is needed. For a more effective evaluation, a UV box will do the trick. The method and its variations have been fully described [67-69]. Figure 4 shows a schematic presentation of a common EB plate, which can be used for evaluation of as many as 8 to 12 strains at the same time. Characterisation of the clinical isolate in a quantitative manner is also possible and the reader is encouraged to adapt this part of the method [69]. For those situations where the use of EB is controlled or prohibited, a replacement method has been developed using acridine orange as the efflux pump substrate [70].

The Automated Real-Time Assessment of an Efflux Pump System of a Clinical Bacterial Isolate

Assessment of efflux pump activity conducted by the automated EB method has been completely described [72]. This method affords a real-time estimation of accumulation of EB and its efflux. Briefly, bacterial strains are cultured in a suitable medium until they reach an optical density at 600nm of 0.6 and centrifuged. The pellets are washed twice with saline buffer, the OD at 600 adjusted again to 0.6 in glucose-free saline buffers at pH 7 (or other according to the objective of the experiment). Because metabolic energy is required for efflux of EB, the absence of glucose ensures sufficient accumulation of the agent. The final concentration of EB for all experiments is to be determined empirically for each bacterial species (note concentration of EB varies from 0.5 mg/L for enterococci and may be as high as 3 mg/L for salmonella). At concentrations of EB that exceed the ability of the cell to extrude the agent, the level of intracellular agent rapidly increases and results in its intercalation between the nucleic bases of DNA. EB when bound to DNA is no longer available for extrusion [71]. The tubes are rapidly transferred to a Corbett 3000 thermo cycler (Qiagen, Doncaster, Australia) programmed with cycles of 1 min at a constant temperature of 37°C. Accumulation of EB in each tube is followed on a real-time basis by assessment of fluorescence emitted. Excitation and emission wavelengths are 535 nm and 585 nm, respectively. Whereas the medium containing as much as 4.0 mg/L of EB does not appreciably fluoresce, as the concentration of EB builds up in the periplasm of the Gram-negative bacterium, the instrument readily detects fluorescence.

For controls that demonstrate the accumulation of EB that results from a concentration of EB that exceeds the cell's ability to extrude, varying concentrations of carbonyl cyanide m-chlorophenylhydrazone (CCCP) and Phe-Arg-naphthylamide (PAβN) can be used as described [71]. The methods for determination of efflux, physiological parameters that affect efflux and evaluation of compounds for activity against the efflux pump of mycobacteria have been fully described [72]. The data presented by figure 2 present raw data directly from the Corbette 3000 instrument used.

Concluding Remarks and Perspectives

The response of bacteria to a noxious agent such an antibiotic initially involves intrinsic efflux pumps, which can be over-expressed as the concentration of the agent increases. When the concentration of the agent is then maintained, efflux pumps continue to be over-expressed and mutations in essential genes take place, supposedly by activation of a master mutator gene. Soon thereafter the level of efflux pump activity returns to baseline level. The sequence of these processes has been confirmed for mycobacteria and other bacterial species. Moreover, as is the case for all matter in the universe, conservation of energy goes from a high to a lower level (second law of thermodynamics), and bacteria are no exception. Therefore, because the maintenance of high efflux activity extols a high-energy cost, mutations that render essential proteins immune from antibiotic actions provide a more energy efficient response that can be maintained indefinitely. However, if the environment is purged of the noxious agent, the bacteria that contain mutations in essential genes cannot compete and within a few serial passages in drug free medium with their wild type relatives, they cease to exist [41].

It is the consensus of the pharmacologically oriented microbiologists that with the use of non-toxic modulators of efflux pump activity in combination with antibiotics, to which the initial strain is resistant, will render the organism fully susceptible to the antibiotic. This consensus must be qualified to "provide of course that the initial resistance was due entirely to efflux pump activity". However, if mutations have taken place, even if efflux is still evident, this form of combinational therapy will probably fail. Because therapy of some infections is prolonged to as long as one month (example Lyme disease) and even years (therapy of an MDR TB infection), in all probability, the clinical bacterial isolate will express some efflux and mutations. Consequently, the ability to determine the contributions made by efflux and mutations for the antibiotic resistance of the clinical isolate may prove useful for the selection of appropriate therapy. The methods presented in this review are directed at this potential need and should be considered for introduction into general bacteriology laboratories.

Acknowledgments

Martins A is supported by SFRH/BPD/81118/2011 from Fundação para a Ciência e a Tecnologia, Portugal.

GS was supported by TÁMOP-4.2.1/B-09/1/KONV-2010-0005-Creating the Center of Excellence at the University of Szeged supported by the European Union and co-financed by the European Regional Fund and TÁMOP-4.2.2/B-10/1-2010-0012 project: "Broadening the knowledge base and supporting the long term professional sustainability of the Research University Center of Excellence at the University of Szeged by ensuring the rising generation of excellent scientists" European Union grant.

The authors acknowledge the support of the Szeged Cancer Foundation.

References

1. Nagarajan M, Maruthanayagam V, Sundararaman M (2012) A review of pharmacological and toxicological potentials of marine cyanobacterial metabolites. J Appl Toxicol 32: 153-185.

2. Schreiber F, Szewzyk U (2008) Environmentally relevant concentrations of pharmaceuticals influence the initial adhesion of bacteria. Aquat Toxicol 87: 227-233.

3. Gauzit R, Lakhdari M (2012) Generic antibiotic drugs: is effectiveness guaranteed? Med Mal Infect 42: 141-148.

4. Leung DT, Chowdhury F, Calderwood SB, Qadri F, Ryan ET (2012) Immune responses to cholera in children. Expert Rev Anti Infect Ther 10: 435-444.

5. Wu W, Yang Y, Sun G (2012) Recent Insights into Antibiotic Resistance in Helicobacter pylori Eradication. Gastroenterol Res Pract 2012: 723183.

6. Akova M, Daikos GL, Tzouvelekis L, Carmeli Y (2012) Interventional strategies and current clinical experience with carbapenemase-producing Gram-negative bacteria. Clin Microbiol Infect 18: 439-448.

7. Zhang Y, Yew WW (2009) Mechanisms of drug resistance in Mycobacterium tuberculosis. Int J Tuberc Lung Dis 13: 1320-1330.

8. Nienhuis WA, Stienstra Y, Abass KM, Tuah W, Thompson WA, et al. (2012) Paradoxical responses after start of antimicrobial treatment in Mycobacterium ulcerans infection. Clin Infect Dis 54: 519-526.

9. Davin-Regli A, Bolla JM, James CE, Lavigne JP, Chevalier J, et al. (2008) Membrane permeability and regulation of drug "influx and efflux" in enterobacterial pathogens. Curr Drug Targets 9: 750-759.

10. Gunn JS (2008) The Salmonella PmrAB regulon: lipopolysaccharide modifications, antimicrobial peptide resistance and more. Trends Microbiol 16: 284-290.

11. Amaral L, Martins A, Spengler G, Martins M, Rodrigues L, et al. (2012) Structure, Genetic Regulation, Physiology and Function of the AcrAB–TolC Efflux Pump of Escherichia coli and Salmonella. Antimicrobial Drug Discovery 44-61.

12. Viveiros M, Jesus A, Brito M, Leandro C, Martins M, et al. (2005) Inducement and reversal of tetracycline resistance in Escherichia coli K-12 and expression of proton gradient-dependent multidrug efflux pump genes. Antimicrob Agents Chemother 49: 3578-3582.

13. Seeger MA, Diederichs K, Eicher T, Brandstätter L, Schiefner A, et al. (2008) The AcrB efflux pump: conformational cycling and peristalsis lead to multidrug resistance. Curr Drug Targets 9: 729-749.

14. Pos KM (2009) Drug transport mechanism of the AcrB efflux pump. Biochim Biophys Acta 1794: 782-793.

15. Elkins CA, Nikaido H (2003) 3D structure of AcrB: the archetypal multidrug efflux transporter of Escherichia coli likely captures substrates from periplasm. Drug Resist Updat 6: 9-13.

16. Yu EW, McDermott G, Zgurskaya HI, Nikaido H, Koshland DE Jr (2003) Structural basis of multiple drug-binding capacity of the AcrB multidrug efflux pump. Science 300: 976-980.

17. Pietras Z, Bavro VN, Furnham N, Pellegrini-Calace M, Milner-White EJ, et al. (2008) Structure and mechanism of drug efflux machinery in Gram negative bacteria. Curr Drug Targets 9: 719-728.

18. Vargiu AV, Collu F, Schulz R, Pos KM, Zacharias M, et al. (2011) Effect of the F610A mutation on substrate extrusion in the AcrB transporter: explanation and rationale by molecular dynamics simulations. J Am Chem Soc 133: 10704-10707.

19. Eicher T, Brandstätter L, Pos KM (2009) Structural and functional aspects of the multidrug efflux pump AcrB. Biol Chem 390: 693-699.

20. Routh MD, Zalucki Y, Su CC, Zhang Q, Shafer WM, et al. (2011) Efflux pumps of the resistance-nodulation-division family: a perspective of their structure, function, and regulation in gram-negative bacteria. Adv Enzymol Relat Areas Mol Biol 77: 109-146.

21. Misra R, Bavro VN (2009) Assembly and transport mechanism of tripartite drug efflux systems. Biochim Biophys Acta 1794: 817-825.

22. Pagès JM, Amaral L (2009) Mechanisms of drug efflux and strategies to combat them: challenging the efflux pump of Gram-negative bacteria. Biochim Biophys Acta 1794: 826-833.

23. Nikaido H (2011) Structure and mechanism of RND-type multidrug efflux pumps. Adv Enzymol Relat Areas Mol Biol 77: 1-60.

24. Murakami S (2008) Multidrug efflux transporter, AcrB--the pumping mechanism. Curr Opin Struct Biol 18: 459-465.

25. Amaral L, Fanning S, Pagès JM (2011) Efflux pumps of gram-negative bacteria: genetic responses to stress and the modulation of their activity by pH, inhibitors, and phenothiazines. Adv Enzymol Relat Areas Mol Biol 77: 61-108.

26. Amaral L, Cerca P, Spengler G, Machado L, Martins A, et al. (2011) Ethidium bromide efflux by Salmonella: modulation by metabolic energy, pH, ions and phenothiazines. Int J Antimicrob Agents 38: 140-145.

27. Mitchell P (1961) Coupling of phosphorylation to electron and hydrogen transfer by a chemi-osmotic type of mechanism. Nature 191: 144-148.

28. Mulkidjanian AY (2006) Proton in the well and through the desolvation barrier. Biochim Biophys Acta 1757: 415-427.

29. Mulkidjanian AY, Heberle J, Cherepanov DA (2006) Protons @ interfaces: implications for biological energy conversion. Biochim Biophys Acta 1757: 913-930.

30. Mulkidjanian AY, Cherepanov DA, Heberle J, Junge W (2005) Proton transfer dynamics at membrane/water interface and mechanism of biological energy conversion. Biochemistry (Mosc) 70: 251-256.

31. Spengler G, Martins A, Schelz Z, Rodrigues L, Aagaard L, et al. (2009) Characterization of intrinsic efflux activity of Enterococcus faecalis ATCC29212 by a semi-automated ethidium bromide method. In Vivo 23: 81-87.

32. Hurdle JG, O'Neill AJ, Chopra I, Lee RE (2011) Targeting bacterial membrane function: an underexploited mechanism for treating persistent infections. Nat Rev Microbiol 9: 62-75.

33. Feniouk BA, Yoshida M (2008) Regulatory mechanisms of proton-translocating F(O)F (1)-ATP synthase. Results Probl Cell Differ 45: 279-308.

34. Lavigne JP, Sotto A, Nicolas-Chanoine MH, Bouziges N, Bourg G, et al. (2012) Membrane permeability, a pivotal function involved in antibiotic resistance and virulence in Enterobacter aerogenes clinical isolates. Clin Microbiol Infect 18: 539-545.

35. Su CC, Yu EW (2007) Ligand-transporter interaction in the AcrB multidrug efflux pump determined by fluorescence polarization assay. FEBS Lett 581: 4972-4976.

36. Lee K, Lee HG, Pi K, Choi YJ (2008) The effect of low pH on protein expression by the probiotic bacterium *Lactobacillus reuteri*. Proteomics 8: 1624-1630.

37. Tseng CP, Tsau JL, Montville TJ (1991) Bioenergetic consequences of catabolic shifts by *Lactobacillus plantarum* in response to shifts in environmental oxygen and pH in chemostat cultures. J Bacteriol 173: 4411-4416.

38. Hamilton IR (1990) Maintenance of proton motive force by *Streptococcus mutans* and *Streptococcus sobrinus* during growth in continuous culture. Oral Microbiol Immunol 5: 280-287.

39. Setty OH, Hendler RW, Shrager RI (1983) Simultaneous measurements of proton motive force, delta pH, membrane potential, and H+/O ratios in intact Escherichia coli. Biophys J 43: 371-381.

40. Kashket ER (1981) Proton motive force in growing Streptococcus lactis and Staphylococcus aureus cells under aerobic and anaerobic conditions. J Bacteriol 146: 369-376.

41. Martins A, Spengler G, Rodrigues L, Viveiros M, Ramos J, et al. (2009) pH Modulation of Efflux Pump Activity of Multi-Drug Resistant *E. coli*: Protection During its Passage and Eventual Colonization of the Colon. PLoS One 4: e6656.

42. Spengler G, Rodrigues L, Martins A, Martins M, McCusker M, et al. (2012) Genetic response of Salmonella enterica serotype Enteritidis to thioridazine rendering the organism resistant to the agent. Int J Antimicrob Agents 39: 16-21.

43. Martins A, Spengler G, Martins M, Rodrigues L, Viveiros M, et al. (2010) Physiological characterisation of the efflux pump system of antibiotic-susceptible and multidrug-resistant Enterobacter aerogenes. Int J Antimicrob Agents 36: 313-318.

44. Spengler G, Martins A, Schelz Z, Rodrigues L, Aagaard L, et al. (2009) Characterization of intrinsic efflux activity of Enterococcus faecalis ATCC29212 by a semi-automated ethidium bromide method. In Vivo 23: 81-87.

45. Costa SS, Ntokou E, Martins A, Viveiros M, Pouranas S, et al. (2010) Identification of the plasmid encoded qacA efflux pump gene in the methicillin-resistant Staphylococcus aureus (MRSA) strain HPV107, a representative of the MRSA Iberian clone. Int J Antimicrob Agents 36: 557-561.

46. Viveiros M, Dupont M, Rodrigues L, Couto I, Davin-Regli A, et al. (2007) Antibiotic stress, genetic response and altered permeability of E. coli. PLoS One 2: e365.

47. Martins A, Iversen C, Rodrigues L, Spengler G, Ramos J, et al. (2009) An AcrAB-mediated multidrug-resistant phenotype is maintained following restoration of wild-type activities by efflux pump genes and their regulators. Int J Antimicrob Agents 34: 602-604.

48. Viveiros M, Portugal I, Bettencourt R, Victor TC, Jordaan AM, et al. (2002) Isoniazid-induced transient high-level resistance in Mycobacterium tuberculosis. Antimicrob Agents Chemother 46: 2804-2810.

49. Machado D, Couto I, Perdigão J, Rodrigues L, Portugal I, et al. (2012) Contribution of efflux to the emergence of isoniazid and multidrug resistance in Mycobacterium tuberculosis. PLoS One 7: e34538.

50. Szabó MA, Varga GZ, Hohmann J, Schelz Z, Szegedi E, et al. (2010) Inhibition of quorum-sensing signals by essential oils. Phytother Res 24: 782-786.

51. Varga ZG, Szabo MA, Hohmann J, Schelz Z, Szegedi E, et al. (2011) Effect of phenothiazines and related compounds on quorum sensing regulated functions. Lett Drug Discovery Design 8: 133-137.

52. Varga ZG, Armada A, Cerca P, Amaral L, Mior Ahmad Subki MA, et al. (2012) Inhibition of quorum sensing and efflux pump system by trifluoromethyl ketone proton pump inhibitors. In Vivo 26: 277-285.

53. Guillier L, Stahl V, Hezard B, Notz E, Briandet R (2008) Modelling the competitive growth between Listeria monocytogenes and biofilm microflora of smear cheese wooden shelves. Int J Food Microbiol 128: 51-57.

54. Komitopoulou E, Bainton NJ, Adams MR (2004) Premature Salmonella Typhimurium growth inhibition in competition with other Gram-negative organisms is redox potential regulated via RpoS induction. J Appl Microbiol 97: 964-972.

55. Yoon H, Klinzing G, Blanch HW (1977) Competition for mixed substrates by microbial populations. Biotechnol Bioeng 19: 1193-1210.

56. Stewart CR, Burnside DM, Cianciotto NP (2011) The surfactant of Legionella pneumophila Is secreted in a TolC-dependent manner and is antagonistic toward other Legionella species. J Bacteriol 193: 5971-5984.

57. Venturi V, Bertani I, Kerényi A, Netotea S, Pongor S (2010) Co-swarming and local collapse: quorum sensing conveys resilience to bacterial communities by localizing cheater mutants in Pseudomonas aeruginosa. PLoS One 5: e9998.

58. Netotea S, Bertani I, Steindler L, Kerényi A, Venturi V, et al. (2009) A simple model for the early events of quorum sensing in Pseudomonas aeruginosa: modeling bacterial swarming as the movement of an "activation zone". Biol Direct 4: 6.

59. Lazar V (2011) Quorum sensing in biofilms--how to destroy the bacterial citadels or their cohesion/power? Anaerobe 17: 280-285.

60. Lazar, Chifiriuc MC (2010) Architecture and physiology of microbial biofilms. Roum Arch Microbiol Immunol 69: 95-107.

61. Bjarnsholt T, Tolker-Nielsen T, Høiby N, Givskov M (2010) Interference of Pseudomonas aeruginosa signalling and biofilm formation for infection control. Expert Rev Mol Med 12: e11.

62. Lear G, Anderson MJ, Smith JP, Boxen K, Lewis GD (2008) Spatial and temporal heterogeneity of the bacterial communities in stream epilithic biofilms. FEMS Microbiol Ecol 65: 463-473.

63. Piddock LJ (2006) Multidrug-resistance efflux pumps - not just for resistance. Nat Rev Microbiol 4: 629-636.

64. Amaral L, Molnar J (2012) Inhibitors of efflux pumps of Gram-negative bacteria inhibits Quorum Sensing. Open Journal of Pharmacology 2: 2.

65. Amaral L, Kristiansen JE, Frolund Thomsen V, Markovich B (2000) The effects of chlorpromazine on the outer cell wall of Salmonella typhimurium in ensuring resistance to the drug. Int J Antimicrob Agents 14: 225-229.

66. Viveiros M, Martins A, Paixão L, Rodrigues L, Martins M, et al. (2008) Demonstration of intrinsic efflux activity of Escherichia coli K-12 AG100 by an automated ethidium bromide method. Int J Antimicrob Agents 31: 458-462.

67. Martins M, Santos B, Martins A, Viveiros M, Couto I, et al. (2006) An instrument-free method for the demonstration of efflux pump activity of bacteria. In Vivo 20: 657-664.

68. Martins M, Couto I, Viveiros M, Amaral L (2010) Identification of efflux-mediated multi-drug resistance in bacterial clinical isolates by two simple methods. Methods Mol Biol 642: 143-157.

69. Martins M, Viveiros M, Couto I, Costa SS, Pacheco T, et al. (2011) Identification of efflux pump-mediated multidrug-resistant bacteria by the ethidium bromide-agar cartwheel method. In Vivo 25: 171-178.

70. Martins A, Amaral L (2012) Screening for efflux pump systems of bacteria by the new acridine orange agar method. In Vivo 26: 203-206.

71. Viveiros M, Rodrigues L, Martins M, Couto I, Spengler G, et al. (2010) Evaluation of efflux activity of bacteria by a semi-automated fluorometric system. Methods Mol Biol 642: 159-172.

72. Rodrigues L, Machado D, Couto I, Amaral L, Viveiros M (2012) Contribution of efflux activity to isoniazid resistance in the *Mycobacterium tuberculosis* complex. Infect Genet Evol 12: 695-700.

22

Sodium, Potassium, Calcium and Copper Levels in Seminal Plasma are Associated with Sperm Quality in Fertile and Infertile Men

Abdul-Wahab R Hamad[1*], Hala I Al-Daghistani[2], Walid D Shquirat[2], Muna Abdel-Dayem[3] and Mohammad Al-Swaifi[3]

[1]Department of Medical Allied Sciences, Zarka University College, Al-Balqa Applied University, Zarka13115, Jordan
[2]Department of Medical Allied Sciences; Al-Salt College for Humanitarian Sciences, Al-Balqa Applied University, Al-Salt 19117, Jordan
[3]Medical Al-Hussein City Hospital, Amman 11855, Jordan

Abstract

Concentrations of Sodium (Na), Potassium (K), Calcium (Ca) and Copper (Cu) in the semen of infertile male with and without varicocele in relation to serum steroid hormones, spermato¬zoa quality were evaluated. The study group comprised of 300 males, 102(34%) with varicocele, 123(41%) without varicocele, and 75(25%) fertile control groups which were randomly selected. Seminal analysis was performed (including volume, sperm count, motility, viscosity, viability and morphology) with biochemical measurements of fructose and mixed agglutination reaction (MAR) for ASA. Atomic absorption was used to estimate the level of Cu, and flame photometer for Na, K and Ca in seminal plasma. Serum levels of progesterone and testosterone were estimated using a competitive chemoluminescent enzyme immunoassay.

A significant difference in sperm viscosity, sluggish and immotile sperms, progesterone was appeared among infertile males with and without varicocele in comparison to fertile groups. Despite the significant decreases of semen K and Ca among infertile male (with and without varicocele) in comparison with fertile ($p<0.05$), the mean Na and Cu concentrations were none significantly between groups. Potassium concentration was highly significant with abnormal testosterone level ($p=0.001$) and Cu concentration was highly significant with abnormal progesterone level ($p=0.001$). Furthermore, calcium level was significantly increased ($p=0.001$) with sluggish and immotile sperms, sperm account, fructose and ASA among normal and abnormal cases. Cu level appeared to be decreased in fertile male compared to infertile male with and without varicocele. Yet, the proportion of abnormality in fructose and % ASA is increased with increasing Cu levels in seminal plasma, whereas low level of Cu showed a negative effect on seminal fluid volume, morphology and sperm count. It is suggested that seminal plasma K and Cu exert particular effects on steroid hormone and semen quality. However, measurement of seminal plasma trace elements may serve as an accurate parameter to evaluate male fertility since they are correlated with the disturbance of semen parameters especially sperm motility, volume, count and viability.

Keywords: Sodium; Potassium; Calcium; Copper; Steroid hormone

Introduction

World health organization defined infertility as failure of conceiving a child for at least 12 month of unprotected intercourse [1]. Infertility has been shown to have a high prevalence worldwide (affects one in six). It has been reported that male factor infertility plays a role in approximately 30-55% of infertile couples [2]. However, despite advances in diagnostic methods in the field of andrology, there remains a significant subset of these sub fertile men who are classified as having unexplained male infertility. Male infertility has multiple causes and the commonest single defined cause is sperm dysfunction [2]. Despite the problem in assessing the prevalence of infertility in developing countries, between 8-12% of couples around the world have difficulty conceiving a child at some point in their lives.

The etiologies of male infertility include gene mutations, aneuploidies, infectious diseases, ejaculatory duct occlusion, varcocele, radiation, chemotherapy and erectile dysfunction [3].

Infertility is complex and has many causes and consequences depending on the gender, sexual abnormalities, and environmental factors [4]. Human semen contains high concentrations of trace elements like calcium (Ca), magnesium (Mg), copper (Cu), selenium (Se), and zinc (Zn) in bound and free (ionic) forms. These trace elements play very vital role in affecting various parameters of semen [5].

There are some studies which demonstrate the significance of trace elements in male fertility. Zinc was found to have high levels in semen from mammals, and zinc has been found to be critical to spermatogenesis [6].

Increased levels of metal ions in blood plasma [7] or semen [8] appear to be significantly and positively correlated with male infertility [9]. Spermatogenesis in mammals requires the action of a number of peptide and steroid hormones (sex hormones), each of which plays an important role in normal functioning of the seminiferous epithelium. Sex hormones are not critical only for regulation of male germ cell development, but also for proliferation and function of the somatic cell types required for proper development of the testis [9]. Among the most common somatic cells that are affected by sex hormones are the interstitial steroidogenic leydig cells, whose primary function appears to be production of testosterone [10]. The sertoli cells, whose direct contact with proliferating and differentiating germ cells within the seminiferous tubules makes them essential for providing both

*Corresponding author: Abdul-Wahab R Hamad, Department of Medical Allied Sciences, Zarka University College, Al-Balqa Applied University, Zarka 13115, Jordan, E-mail: wahabhamad2004@yahoo.com

physical and nutritional support for spermatogenesis [11]. FSH and LH are secreted by the anterior pituitary and act directly on the testes to stimulate somatic cell function in support of spermatogenesis [12]. LH is known to act on leydig cells to produce testosterone while FSH acts on sertoli cells to promote spermatogenesis [13].

Seminal plasma is very important for sperm metabolism, function, survival, and transport in the female genital tract. Cations such as Na, K, Ca, and P in the seminal plasma establish osmotic balance, while essential trace elements are components of many important enzymes. Thus, biochemical evaluation of seminal plasma is an important criterion for assessing fertility and diagnosing male reproductive disorders [14-16].

Abnormal levels of Ca, Na, K, Zn, and Cu in seminal plasma have been reported to be correlated with infertility in humans. Ca is the trigger for the acrosome reaction in mammalian spermatozoa and there is substantial evidence that Ca is differentially involved in sperm motility, depending on the stage of sperm maturation. However, Magnus et al. [17] reported no association between ionized calcium concentrations and the proportion of spermatozoa displaying progressive movement. Prien et al. [18] compared sperm motility, velocity and progressive movement with total and ionized calcium. The ions present in the semen help in stimulating the motility and glycolysis. The addition of potassium to semen extenders has been shown to improve motility of stallion Padilla et al. [19] and human sperm Karow et al. [20] but Rossato et al. [21] found no correlation between the ionic composition and the osmolarity of human seminal plasma.

Intracellular concentrations of potassium are higher than those of seminal plasma, and therefore potassium levels are linked to sperm concentration. In ram, increasing potassium levels are negatively correlated to progressive motility, while the reverse is true for sodium and chloride Abdel-Rahman et al. [22]. In ram ejaculates, intracellular calcium and magnesium concentrations were higher than in seminal plasma as opposed to phosphate levels. Furthermore, lower values of progressive motility has been reported to be correlated to increasing levels of calcium and decreasing magnesium and phosphate concentrations levels Abdel-Rahman et al. [22].

Copper is an important element for numerous metalloenzymes and metalloproteins that are involved in energy or antioxidant metabolism. However, in its ionic form

(Cu^{+2}) and at high level, this trace element rapidly becomes toxic to a variety of cells, including human spermatozoa [23]. It has been identified that Cu is highly toxic for sperm [24]. *In vitro* studies, it has been demonstrated the effect of Cu in intrauterine devices preventing conception [25]. The present study was designed to evaluate seminal plasma levels of copper, sodium, potassium and calcium and to correlate their concentrations with various semen parameters among fertile and infertile male subjects.

Materials and Methods

Study groups

Two hundred and twenty-five infertile males including 102 (34%) patient with varicocele and 123 (41%) without varicocele which were recruited in this study. Their mean ages were 31.3 ± 5.2 and 32.3 ± 5.9 years, respectively. Men were attending the infertility department at Medical Hussein City Hospital in Jordan with complete medical and clinical histories. Patients married and infertile (with their fertile female partner) which were for at least more than one year of unproductive

intercourse. A questionnaire survey collected data regarding patient occupation, marital status, infertility history and other data. Patients with a history of trace metals exposure or who resided in areas known to have heavy metals contamination, smokers, and alcoholic consumers were excluded from this study. Varicocele was diagnosed after physical examination, duplex, and Color Doppler Ultrasonography. All cases of varicocele were classified as grade I (palpable distension detected only during a valsalva manoeuvre) [25]. Control group was randomly selected from other outpatient clinics of the same hospital and consists of 75 (25%) fertile married males with mean age of 33.36 ± 6.27 years. They are clinically asymptomatic males without varicocele and normal seminal fluids. Informed consent was obtained from all study cases.

Seminal Fluid Samples

Semen specimens were collected through masturbation after 3 days abstinence. Each patient provided at least two samples within one month. Samples were incubated for 30 min at 37°C for liquefaction. A routine semen analysis was performed upon liquefaction according to WHO to measure volume, pH, sperm concentration, motility, viscosity, viability and morphology (WHO, 2010). The remaining semen sample was centrifuged at 1000 ×g for 10 min; the seminal plasma was separated for three equal parts and stored at -70°C until further analyses. Morphology was determined after incubation of the sample with trypsin for 10 minutes at 25°C according to the methylene blue eosin staining procedure, feathering, and fixation by flame. At least 100 cells were examined at a final magnification of 1000x. Viscosity of the liquefied sample was estimated by introducing a glass rod into the sample and observing the thread that forms on withdrawal of the rod. Threads obtained from normal samples should not exceed 2 cm in length [26]. Motility was expressed as a percentage of motile spermatozoa and their mean velocity. The conventional analysis is recommended in which a fixed volume of semen is delivered onto a clean glass slide and covered with a mm cover slip (WHO, 2010). The preparation is then examined at a magnification of 400xs. The microscopic field is scanned systematically, and the motility of each spermatozoon encountered is graded a, b, c, or d. At least 100 spermatozoa are classified in this way. The presence of 50% or more with forward progression (categories a and b) or 25% or more with rapid progression (category a) within 60 minutes of ejaculation were considered as normal results. The results were averaged for the two samples, and a single value was used for each parameter. Sperm motility was calculated by multiplying sperm concentration x10^6/ml) and semen volume (ml).

Trace elements determination

Determination of Cupper (Cu) concentration was carried out according to a method of using Atomic absorption spectrophotometer (AA 6650 Shimadzu, Japan). While, the determination of Sodium (Na), Potassium (K) and Calicium (Ca) concentrations were analyzed by using Flame photometer (Microprocessor Scientific International, India).

Frozen semen samples were liquefied at room temperature and digested in covered beakers in a fume cupboard with a 1:1 solution of highly purified HNO_3 under moderate heating conditions (85°C). All laboratory ware used was previously treated with 10% nitric acid for 48 hours and copiously rinsed with distilled-deionized water to eliminate possible traces of metals. Semen samples were diluted 1:50 for Cu, Na, K, and Ca determination. Concentrations were determined by comparison with standard curves covering different concentration ranges. Aqueous standards for plotting calibration graphs were obtained by serial dilution of stock solutions containing 1000 pg/mL of the analyte as nitrates. Blanks were prepared in a similar fashion as samples.

Mixed Anti-globulin Reaction (MAR) Test

The MAR test is performed by mixing fresh, untreated semen with sheep blood cells (SRBs) coated with human IgG. A monospecific antihuman-IgG antiserum is added to this mixture, which was mixed and read within 10 minutes. Positive and negative control samples were run along with each experiment. The formation of mixed agglutinates between sRBC and motile spermatozoa proves the presence of IgG antibodies on the sperms. Immunologic infertility is suspected when 10%-90% of the motile spermatozoa attached to the RBCs [27].

Determination of seminal fluid fructose

The method is adopted from that of Seliwanoff. The principle depends upon the presence of fructose (ketoses), which forms a pink color when heated, with resorcinol in the presence of hydrochloric acid (ARCOMEX, Fructose. S.F). Intensity of the red complex is proportional to the fructose concentration and measured photometrically at 490 nm [28]. Normal fructose level in the seminal plasma is 120-500 g/dl.

Hormone estimation

Serum levels of progesterone and testosterone were estimated by a competitive chemoluminescent enzyme immunoassay using IMMULITE 2000 Progesterone and IMMULITE 2000. Total Testosterone which was utilized specific antibody-coated polystyrene beads as a solid phase [29,30]. Samples were incubated with alkaline phosphatase-labeled regent and the bound label was then quantified using a specific chemoluminescent substrate. Light emission was detected by photomultiplier tube, and the results were calculated for each sample. The normal ranges for progesterone is 0.27-0.9 ng/ml and for testosterone 262-1593 ng/dl.

Statistical analysis

The collected data was entered to statistical Package for Social Sciences (SPSS) version 19. The descriptive statistics using frequency and percentage was used to describe the study variables. The continuous variables within the database were converted to rank cases using four ranks. The ranking was used as a procedure to make possible to test two discrete variable using non-parametric statistics. Kruskal-Wallis test was used to test the effect of independent variables.

Results

Serum and seminal plasma obtained from 300 men including infertile with varicocele, infertile without varicocele, and fertile control males. Their ages varied from 25 to 47 years, thus covering the entire span of the reproductive years. Seminal fluid and serum samples were investigated for the possible relations between trace metals (Cu, Na, K and Ca), seminal fluid parameters, fructose levels, autoimmunity to sperm antigen and steroid hormones.

Seminal fluid parameters

The criteria for normozoospermia was a concentration of ≥ 20×10(6)/ml, with grade a motility in 25% or grade a and b motility in 50% of spermatozoa, normal morphology in at least 30% of the spermatozoa, viability >75% of the total sperms, and semen volume >2 ml. The mean values for normal sperm count(x10⁶), viability(%), progressive motility (x10⁶), and normal morphology(%) were 96 ± 78.0, 84 ± 82.4, and 60 ± 80.0; 6 ± 4.9, 6 ± 5.9, and 9 ± 12.0; 6 ± 4.9, 15 ± 14.7, and 9 ± 12.0; 3±2.4, 0±0, and 3 ± 4 for infertile without varicocele,

infertile with varicocele, and fertile males, respectively (Table 1).

The proportion with sperm viability (>75%), was 117(95.1%), 96(94.1%), and 66(88.0%); asthenospermia (progressive motility >50%) was 117(95.1%), 87(85.3%), and 66(88.0%); oligospermia (sperm density <20×10⁶/mL) was 36(48.8%), 39(88.2%), and 18(24%); azospermia (no sperm in the ejaculate) was 21(17.1%), 6(5.9%), and 0(0%), and teratospermia (morphology <30%) was 120(97.6%), 102(100%), and 72(96%) for infertile without varicocele, with varicocele, and fertile male, respectively. Analyzing of seminal fluid samples revealed significant differences in sperm viscosity, sluggish motility, and immotility (P<0.05).

Seminal fructose concentration was estimated among our study groups. The mean ranges of fructose in the seminal plasma was 102-1040, 35-671, and 113-909 mg/dl in infertile males without varicocele, with varicocele, and fertile, respectively. No significant differences in the level of seminal fructose among infertile and fertile males were recorded. MAR test was used to detect sperm autoantibodies in the seminal plasma. ASA was present in 30(24.4%) infertile male without varicocele, 30(29.4%) infertile with varicocele, and in 18 (24%) fertile males. These results showed no significant differences.

Progesterone and testosterone in the serum

The mean ranges values for serum testosterone and progesterone were: (140-1342), (173-903), and (42-788) ng/dl for testosterone, while (0.15-0.86), (0.15-1.10), and (0.09-0.89) ng/ml for progesterone in males with varicocele, without varicocele, and fertile males, respectively (Table 1). However, no significant differences appeared in testosterone concentration between infertile and fertile group. Progesterone level was found to be significant among infertile and fertile cases.

Trace elements concentration in the seminal fluid

The mean concentration of Na, K, Ca and Cu in the seminal fluid among infertile male without varicocele was 1541, 777, 125 and 1.9 µg/ml as compared to 1375, 764, 115 and 2.0 µg/ml for infertile with varicocele and 1703, 883, 150 and 1.7 µg/ml for fertile male (Table 2 and Figure 1). This decreases in K and Ca among infertile as compared to fertile males appeared significant (0.001, 0.04 respectively). However, Na and Cu showed a non-significant difference among infertile without varicocele, infertile with varicocele and fertile males.

Trace elements and steroid hormones

The concentration of trace elements measured in the seminal plasma and their relation to hormones in the serum are presented in Table 3. The mean Cu was highly significantly (p=0.001) among cases of normal and abnormal increases in progesterone and testosterone concentration. While Na, K, Ca showed a non-significant in cases with normal and abnormal progesterone levels.

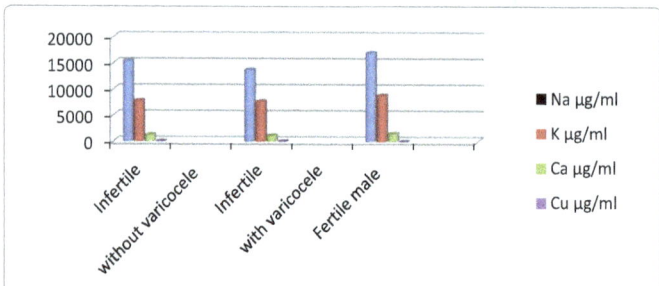

Figure 1: Comparison between trace elements concentration among study groups

Seminal fluid parameters		Infertile without varicocele Mean ±SD	Infertile with varicocele Mean ±SD	Fertile male Mean ±SD	Count (% of total)	P- value
Sperm count (x10⁶)	Normal	96(78.0%)	84(82.4%)	60(80.0%)	240(80%)	NS
	Abnormal	27(22.0%)	18(17.6%)	15(20.0%)	60(20%)	
Viability (%)	Normal	6(4.9%)	6(5.9%)	9(12.0%)	21(7%)	NS
	Abnormal	117(95.1%)	96(94.1%)	66(88.0%)	279(93%)	
Viscosity(cm)	Normal	102(82.9%)	81(79.4%)	60(80.0%)	243(81%)	0.05
	Abnormal	21(17.0%)	21(20.6%)	15(20.0%)	57(19.0%)	
Sperm morphology (%)	Normal	3(2.4%)	0(0%)	3(4%)	6(2%)	NS
	Abnormal	120(97.6%)	102(100%)	72(96%)	294(98%)	
Progressive Motility (a+b) (%)	Existed	6(4.9%)	15(14.7%)	9(12%)	30(10%)	NS
	Not existed	117(95.1%)	87(85.3%)	66(88%)	270(90%)	
Sluggish motility(c) (%)	Existed	99(80.5%)	90(88.2%)	75(100%)	264(88%)	0.001
	Not existed	24(19.5%)	12(11.8%)	0(0%)	36(12.0%)	
Immotile (d) (%)	Existed	105(85.4%)	96(94.1%)	75(100%)	276(92.%)	0.001
	Not existed	18(14.6%)	6(5.9%)	0(0%)	24(8%)	
Fructose Concentration (g/dl)	Normal	114(92.7%)	78(76.5%)	69(92%)	261(87%)	NS
	Abnormal	9(7.3%)	24(23.5%)	6(8%)	39(13%)	
Antisperm antibody(%)	Absent	93(75.6%)	72(70.6%)	57(76.0%)	222(74%)	NS
	Present	30(24.4%)	30(29.4%)	18(24%)	78(26.0%)	
Testosterone ng/dl	Normal	93(75.6%)	78(76.5%)	57(76%)	228(76%)	NS
	Abnormal	30(24.4%)	24(23.5%)	18(24%)	72(24%)	
Progesterone ng/dl	Normal	63(51.2%)	45(44.1%)	48(64%)	135(45%)	0.03
	Abnormal	60(48.8%)	57(55.9%)	27(36%)	165(55%)	

Table 1: A comparison between Sperm parameters, fructose level, and steroid hormones among infertile males with varicocele, without varicocele, and fertile.

Infertility status	Na µg/ml means ±SD	K µg/ml means ±SD	Ca µg/ml means ±SD	Cu µg/ml means ±SD
Infertile without varicocele	1541.6 ±665.8	776.8± 379.7	124.8±114.15	1.88±1.623
Infertile with varicocele	1374.9±626.5	764.1±484.1	115.4±90.02	1.961±2.054
Fertile male	1703.4±853.5	883.5±464.3	150.39±118.71	1.73±1.83
P value	**NS**	**0.001**	**0.04**	**NS**

Table 2: Trace elements concentration among infertile and fertile males

		Na µg/ml Mean ±SD	K µg/ml Mean± SD	Ca µg/ml Mean± SD	Cu µg/ml Mean± SD
Testosterone ng/dl	Abnormal	1648.7(811.3%)	837.5(400.1%)	137.7(101.5%)	1.72(1.86%)
	Normal	1486.4(677.4%)	787.1(452.2%)	124.9(110.4%)	1.92(1.81%)
	Total	1525.4(713.8%)	799.1(440.1%)	128.0(108.3%)	1.87(1.82%)
	P- value	NS	0.001	NS	NS
Progesterone ng/dl	Abnormal	1458.8(670.4%)	467.9(410.1%)	125.2(106.5%)	1.46(1.34%)
	Normal	1606.7(758.2%)	841.0(472.5%)	131.4(110.7%)	2.36(2.18%)
	Total	1525.4(713.8%)	799.1(440.1%)	128.0(108.3%)	1.87(1.82%)
	P- value	NS	NS	NS	0.001

Note: Normal value for testosterone= 262-1593 ng/dl, progesterone= 0.27- 0.9 ng/dl, and fructose= 120-500 g/dl

Table 3: Means of Na, K, Ca, and Cu concentrations in relation to progesterone and testosterone concentration in the serum of the study groups

Trace elements and seminal fluid parameters

Semen parameters were divided into two groups (normal and abnormal), according to the WHO recommended reference values (WHO, 2010) and the level of Na, K, Ca, and Cu were compared between these two groups using rank sum tests (Table 4). The mean concentrations of Na and K was increases significantly (p=0.05-0.001) in cases with viability, motility, sluggish and immotile sperms. However, Ca and Cu was slightly increase in cases with abnormal viability, motility, sperm count (p<0.05). No significant correlation was observed between Na, K, and Ca and fructose seminal fluid parameter. On the other hand, there were significant differences (p<0.05) in Cu concentrations between men with normal and abnormal

sperm fructose. Mean serum Cu level in cases with abnormal sperm viability, volume, fructose and ASA was 1.93, 1.81, 2.22 and 1.99 µg/ml compared to 1.09, 1.88, 1.82 and 1.53 µg/ml in cases with normal values, respectively (p<0.05).

Discussion

Male factor infertility has been estimated to account for approximately 50% of all problems with fertility. These problems either interfere with the sperm production process or disrupt their motility after production. Population-based studies are needed to investigate the trends in male reproductive disorders and to explore environmental factors influencing male reproductive health. Patients with and without varicocele tend to have a statistically different semen parameters as compared with fertile regarding sperm viscosity, sluggish and immotile sperms, in addition to progesterone level (p=0.05, 0.001, 0.001, and 0.05, respectively). These results are in accordance with previous studies that demonstrated the detrimental effect of varicocele on sperm quality [26-28]. However, they revealed the association of varicocele with the stress sperm pattern in the form of increased number of abnormal forms, decreased progressive motility and sperm density. In addition, a significant differences was reported in the level of progesterone mainly cases with varicocele group which explained their importance as an infertility determinant among varicocele-related infertility. In addition, viscosity of ejaculate was reported to occur more frequently among infertile couples than in fertile [29]. The importance of semen viscosity lies in the fact that the spermatozoa are tangled in the mucoid mass in the semen and prevented from migrating into the cervical tract to ascend the site of fertilization [30]. Several conditions, such as concentrations of prostate-specific antigen, zinc, calcium, and activity of neutral α-glucosidase in seminal plasma, were found to be correlated with abnormal semen viscosity [31,32].

Some trace amounts of metals are essential for physiological homeostasis; it is well known that excessive or insufficient concentrations of these elements will induce toxicity and deficiency symptoms. The result of other studies showed significance differences of seminal plasma copper concentration between infertile and fertile males, while in recent study there was no significant correlation between seminal plasma copper concentration and infertility.

In the present study the trace elements (Cu, Ca, K and Na) in the seminal plasma of infertile men were investigated and compared to fertile. Semen from infertile male with and without varicocele appeared to contain a significant low concentration of K and Ca (p=0.001, 0.04, respectively) compared to fertile males, while, Cu and Na levels were not.

Although, the role of copper in male reproductive capacity appears to be largely unknown, but this metal appears to be involved in spermatozoa motility and it may also act at the pituitary receptors which control the release of LH [23,33,34] demonstrated a weak but significant positive correlation between blood copper concentrations and sperm motility. The recent study was not in agreement with above both studies.

This study showed that the seminal plasma calcium level was significantly lower in the infertile men compared to the fertile controls (p<0.05). Wong et al. [23] in his study in Netherland reported similar findings of low Ca in the seminal plasma of infertile men which accounts for hypomotility. This has demonstrated the importance of calcium in sperm physiology, including motility [5] metabolism [35], acrosome reaction and fertilization [36]. It is known that calcium is required to initiate the acrosome reaction with its attendant release of enzymes and membrane alterations needed for successful egg-sperm interaction. This accounts for the significantly higher seminal plasma calcium level in normospermic compared to the oligospermic, azoospermic and

		Na µg/ml Mean ±SD	K µg/ml Mean± SD	Ca µg/ml Mean± SD	Cu µg/ml Mean± SD
Viability (%)	Abnormal	1546(721.8%)	808.0(441.8%)	130.5(107.2%)	1.93(1.85%)
	Normal	1245(534.2%)	681.4(407.9%)	94.31(119.3%)	1.09(1.12%)
	P-value	NS	0.01	0.001	0.003
Volume (ml)	Abnormal	1592(834.3%)	823.85(366.9%)	159.5(123.1%)	1.81(2.09%)
	Normal	1508(681.3%)	792.9(457.1%)	122.6(103.8%)	1.88(1.75%)
	P-value	0.002	0.01	0.05	NS
Progressive motility (%)	Not existed	1555(723.8%)	814.6(446.8%)	134.8(110.3%)	1.90(1.85%)
	existed	1255(556.8%)	659.5(350.2%)	66.69(63.83%)	1.59(1.57%)
	P-value	0.01	0.008	0.008	NS
Sperm morphology (%)	Abnormal	1835(483.8%)	991.7(110.7%)	107.1(110.3%)	1.85(1.82%)
	Normal	1328(689.7%)	731.5(343.8%)	150.9(68.45%)	2.66(2.34%)
	P-value	0.001	0.02	0.02	NS
Sluggish motility (%)	Not existed	1271(584.2%)	674.1(265.1%)	69.02(79.35%)	2.29(2.21%)
	Existed	1559(723.8%)	816.3(456.6%)	136.1(109.3%)	1.81(1.76%)
	P –value	NS	NS	0.001	NS
Immotile sperm (%)	Not existed	1269(632.9%)	648.1(253.5%)	74.55(91.98%)	2.37(1.79%)
	Existed	1547(717.1%)	812.2(450.6%)	132.69(108.4%)	1.83(±1.82%)
	P-value	NS	NS	0.001	NS
Count x10⁶/ml	Abnormal	1486(666.6%)	826.1(411.4%)	142.6(1167%)	2.03(1.90%)
	Normal	1550(743.2%)	781.9(457.8%)	118.6(101.7%)	1.772(1.77%)
	P-value	0.03	NS	0.03	NS
Fructose	Abnormal	1415(638.2%)	649.9(374.4%)	125.3(93.18%)	2.22(2.12%)
	Normal	1541(724.1%)	821.4(445.4%)	128.4(110.5%)	1.82(1.77%)
	P- value	NS	NS	NS	0.05
ASA(%)	Negative	1525(690.5%)	794.0(43.2%)	121.7(109.1%)	1.99(1.87%)
	Positive	1524(781.1%)	813.6(433.8%)	145.9(104.6%)	1.53(1.64%)
	P –value	NS	NS	NS	0.006

Table 4: Means of Na, K, Ca, and Cu concentrations in relation to sperm count, volume, viability, motility, fructose, leukocyte and the presence of sperm autoantibody.

asthenoligospermic subjects. Calcium is also necessary for maximum motility of sperm cells.

Semen volume, morphology and motility showed a significant difference between normal and abnormal with Ca, Na and K but non-significant with Cu indicating that the higher the volume of semen the more will be the concentration of Ca, Na and K in the seminal fluid. This finding agrees with the observation of Kanwal et al. [37] who reported that Ca related to semen volume in bull. Abdel-Rahman et al. [22] also reported a positive correlation between K and semen volume. In the same vein, Na and K showed a positive and significant correlation with sperm motility. This signifies that the progressive active movement of spermatozoa may be improved or increased with higher concentration of Na, Na and K in the seminal fluid of the bucks. This is in contrary to the report by Kaya et al. [38] who observed a negative correlation between sperm motility and Na and K concentrations in ram. However, a positive but non-significant correlation of r = 0.17 has been reported by Kanwal et al. [37] between K and sperm motility in bull. Intracellular calcium (Ca) is essential for the sperm motility, metabolism and acrosomal reaction [39]. Potassium and sodium are also present in high concentrations in the seminal plasma that have the great role in acrosomal reactions [40].

Examinations of the seminal plasma suggest that the concentrations of all elements were within the physiological limits and comparable to the results of other authors [41-43], their concentrations were significantly (p<0.001) higher in the infertile group compared to other groups. As we found no data available to compare and discuss our detected statistical differences, we assume that unlike the blood plasma, the seminal plasma does not have a proper filtration system and therefore acts as an accumulator of any organic or inorganic substance. At the same time, lower concentrations of chemical elements in the sperm cells prove that spermatozoa lack a typical cytoplasm as a source of potential binding molecules for the minerals. Nonetheless, we have to be aware of the fact that the content of chemical elements within spermatozoa may vary and is highly dependent on the concentration of the sperm cell within the ejaculate. The results of this study may give an indication about the involvement of trace elements as an important etiological role in the pathogenicity of unexplained infertility and therapeutic intervention with these elements supplement in a suitable formula may be beneficial and might give a promise in this respect.

References

1. La Vignera S, Vicari E, Condorelli RA, D'Agata R, Calogero AE (2011) Male accessory gland infection and sperm parameters (review). Int J Androl 34: e330-347.

2. Hamada AJ, Esteves SC, Agarwal A (2013) A comprehensive review of genetics and genetic testing in azoospermia. Clinics (Sao Paulo) 68 Suppl 1: 39-60.

3. Ollero M, Gil-Guzman E, Lopez MC, Sharma RK, Agarwal A, et al. (2001) Characterization of subsets of human spermatozoa at different stages of maturation: implications in the diagnosis and treatment of male infertility. Hum Reprod 16: 1912-1921.

4. Burtis CA, Ashwood ER, Bruns DE (2006) In Tietz Textbook of Clinical Chemistry and Molecular Diagnostics pp: 2079-2152.

5. Sørensen MB, Bergdahl IA, Hjøllund NH, Bonde JP, Stoltenberg M, et al. (1999) Zinc, magnesium and calcium in human seminal fluid: relations to other semen parameters and fertility. Mol Hum Reprod 5: 331-337.

6. Shquirat WD, Daghistani HIA, Hamad AWR, Dayem MA, Swaifi MA (2013) Zinc, Manganese, and Magnesium in seminal fluid and their relationship to male infertility in Jordan. International Journal of Pharmacy and Medical Sciences 3: 1-10.

7. Umeyama T, Ishikawa H, Takeshima H, Yoshii S, Koiso K (1986) A comparative study of seminal trace elements in fertile and infertile men. Fertil Steril 46: 494-499.

8. Irvine DS (1996) Glutathione as a treatment for male infertility. Rev Reprod 1: 6-12.

9. Gutteridge JM (1986) Antioxidant properties of the proteins caeruloplasmin, albumin and transferrin. A study of their activity in serum and synovial fluid from patients with rheumatoid arthritis. Biochim Biophys Acta 869: 119-127.

10. Mclachan RI, O'Donnell L, Meachen SJ, Stanton PG, de Krester DM, et al. (2002) Identification of specific sites of hormonal regulation in spermatogenesis in rats, monkeys and man. Recent Prog Horm Res 57: 149-179.

11. Mendis-Handagama SM (1997) Luteinizing hormone on Leydig cell structure and function. Histol Histopathol 12: 869-882.

12. Pierce JG, Parsons TF (1981) Glycoprotein hormones: structure and function. Annu Rev Biochem 50: 465-495.

13. Griswold MD (1998) The central role of Sertoli cells in spermatogenesis. Semin Cell Dev Biol 9: 411-416.

14. Barrier Battut I, Delajarraud H, Legrand E, Buyas JF, Fieni F, et al. (2002) Calcium, magnesium, copper and zinc in seminal plasma of fertile stallions and their relationship with semen freezability. Theriogenology 58: 229-232.

15. Massányi P, Toman R, Trandzik J, Nad P, Skalická M, et al. (2004) Concentration of copper, zinc, iron, cadmium, lead and nickel in bull, ram, boar, stallion and fox semen. Trace Elements and Electrolytes 21: 45-49.

16. Massányi P, Trandzik J, Nad P, Koréneková B, Skalická M, et al. (2004) Concentration of copper, iron, zinc, cadmium, lead, and nickel in bull and ram semen and relation to the occurrence of pathological spermatozoa. J Environ Sci Health A Tox Hazard Subst Environ Eng 39: 3005-3014.

17. Magnus O, Abyholm T, Kofstad J, Purvis K (1990) Ionized calcium in human male and female reproductive fluids: relationships to sperm motility. Hum Reprod 5: 94-98.

18. Prien SD, Lox CD, Messer RH, DeLeon FD (1990) Seminal concentssrations of total and ionized calcium from men with normal and decreased motility. Fertil Steril 54: 171-172.

19. Padilla AW, Foote RH (1991) Extender and centrifugation effects on the motility patterns of slow-cooled stallion spermatozoa. J Anim Sci 69: 3308-3313.

20. Karow AM, Gilbert WB, Black JB (1992) Effects of temperature, potassium concentration, and sugar on human spermatozoa motility: a cell preservation model from reproductive medicine. Cryobiology 29: 250-254.

21. Rossato M, Balercia G, Lucarelli G, Foresta C, Mantero F (2002) Role of seminal osmolarity in the reduction of human sperm motility. Int J Androl 25: 230-235.

22. Abdel-Rahman HA1, El-Belely MS, Al-Qarawi AA, El-Mougy SA (2000) The relationship between semen quality and mineral composition of semen in various ram breeds. Small Rumin Res 38: 45-49.

23. Wong WY, Flik G, Groenen PM, Swinkels DW, Thomas CM, et al. (2001) The impact of calcium, magnesium, zinc, and copper in blood and seminal plasma on semen parameters in men. Reprod Toxicol 15: 131-136.

24. Skandhan KP (1992) Review on copper in male reproduction and contraception. Rev Fr Gynecol Obstet 87: 594-598.

25. Roblero L, Guadarrama A, Lopez T, Zegers-Hochschild F (1996) Effect of copper ion on the motility, viability, acrosome reaction and fertilizing capacity of human spermatozoa in vitro. Reprod Fertil Dev 8: 871-874.

26. Zini A (2002) Varicocele: Evaluation and treatment. J Sex Reprod Med 2:119-24.

27. Pasqualotto FF1, Lucon AM, de Góes PM, Sobreiro BP, Hallak J, et al. (2005) Semen profile, testicular volume, and hormonal levels in infertile patients with varicoceles compared with fertile men with and without varicoceles. Fertil Steril 83: 74-77.

28. Al-Daghistani HI, Hamad AW, Abdel-Dayem M, Al-Swaifi M, Abu Zaid M (2010) Evaluation of Serum Testosterone, Progesterone, Seminal Antisperm Antibody, and Fructose Levels among Jordanian Males with a History of Infertility. Biochem Res Int.

29. ELzanaty S, Malm J, Giwercman A (2004) Visco-elasticity of seminal fluid in relation to the epididymal and accessory sex gland function and its impact on sperm motility. Int J Androl 27: 94-100.

30. Gopalkrishnan K, Padwal V, Balaiah D (2000) Does seminal fluid viscosity influence sperm chromatin integrity? Arch Androl 45: 99-103.

31. Mendeluk G, González Flecha FL, Castello PR, Bregni C (2000) Factors involved in the biochemical etiology of human seminal plasma hyperviscosity. J Androl 21: 262-267.

32. Andrade-Rocha FT (2005) Physical analysis of ejaculate to evaluate the secretory activity of the seminal vesicles and prostate. Clin Chem Lab Med 43: 1203-1210.

33. Slivkova J, Popelkova M, Massanyi P, Toporcerova S, Stawarz R, et al. (2009) Concentration of trace elements in human semen and relation to spermatozoa quality. J Environ Sci Health A Tox Hazard Subst Environ Eng 44: 370-375.

34. Jockenhövel F, Bals-Pratsch M, Bertram HP, Nieschlag E (1990) Seminal lead and copper in fertile and infertile men. Andrologia 22: 503-511.

35. Peterson RN, Freund M (1976) Relationship between motility and the transport and binding of divalent captions to the plasma membrane of human spermatozoa. Fertil Steril 27: 1301-1307.

36. Yanagimachi, R (1981) Mechanisms of Fertilization in Mammals. Fertilization and Embryonic Development In vitro, Plenum Press, New York, pp: 88-182.

37. Kanwal MR, Rehman NU, Ahmad N, Samad HA, Zia-ur-rehman, et al. (2000) Bulk Cations and Trace Elements in the Nili-Ravi Buffalo and Crossbred Cow Bull Semen. International Journal of Agriculture and Biology 2: 302-305.

38. Kaya A, Aksoy M, Tekeli T (2002) Influence of ejaculation frequency on sperm characteristics, ionic composition and enzymatic activity of seminal plasma in rams. Small Ruminant Research 44: 153-158.

39. Aitken RJ, Clarkson JS, Fishel S (1989) Generation of reactive oxygen species, lipid peroxidation, and human sperm function. Biol Reprod 41: 183-197.

40. Vickram AS, Ramesh PM, Sridharan TB (2012) Effect of various biomolecules for normal functioning of human sperm for fertilization:A Review. Int J Pharm Pharm Sci 4: 18-24.

41. Eghbali M, Alavi-Shoushtari SM, Asri Rezaii S (2008) Effects of copper and superoxide dismutase content of seminal plasma on buffalo semen characteristics, Pak J Biol Sci 11: 1964-1968.

42. Gur S, Demirci E (2000) Effect of calcium, magnesium, sodium and potassium levels in seminal plasma of holstein bulls on spermatological characters. Turk J Vet Anim Sci 24: 275-281.

43. Çevik M, Tuncer PB, Tasdemir U, Ozgurtas T (2007) Comparison of spermatological characteristics and biochemical seminal plasma parameters of normozoospermic and oligoasthenozoospermic bulls of two breeds. Turk J Vet Anim Sci 31: 381-387.

23

State of Art: Review of Theoretical Study of GSK-3 β and a New Neural Networks QSAR Studies for the Design of New Inhibitors using 2D-Descriptors

García I[1] and Prado-Prado F[2*]

[1]*Department of Organic Chemistry, University of Vigo, 36200, Spain*
[2]*Biomedical Sciences Department, Health Sciences Division, University of Quintana Roo, 77039, Mexico*

Abstract

Alzheimer's disease (AD) is characterized by several pathologies, as this disease involves neuropathological lesions in the brain. Indeed, a wealth of evidence suggests that β-amyloid is central to the pathophysiology of AD and is likely to play an early role in this intractable neurodegenerative disorder. AD is the most prevalent form of dementia, and current indications show that twenty-nine million people live with AD worldwide, a figure expected to rise exponentially over the coming decades. Clearly, blocking disease progression or, in the best-case scenario, preventing AD altogether would be of benefit in both social and economic terms. However, current AD therapies are merely palliative and only temporarily slow cognitive decline, and treatments that address the underlying pathologic mechanisms of AD are completely lacking. While familial AD (FAD) is caused by autosomal dominant mutations in either amyloid precursor protein (APP) or the presenilin (PS1, PS2) genes. First, we have reviewed 2D QSAR, 3D QSAR, CoMFA, CoMSIA and docking for GSK-3α and GSK-3β with different compounds to find out their structural requirements. Next, we develop a QSAR for GSK-3β, because is one of the most important enzymes that intervenes in neuropathological disease such as Alzheimer. QSAR could play an important role in studying these GSK-3 inhibitors. For this reason we developed QSAR models for GSK-3β, LDA, ANNs and CT from more than 40000 cases with more than 2400 different molecules inhibitors of GSK-3β obtained from ChEMBL database server; in total we used more than 45000 different molecules to develop the QSAR models. We used 237 molecular descriptors calculated with DRAGON software. The model correctly classified 1310 out of 1643 active compounds (79.7%) and 24823 out of 26156 non-active compounds (94.9%) in the training series. The overall training performance was 94.0%. Validation of the model was carried out using an external predicting series. In this series the model classified correctly 757 out of 940 (80.5%) active compounds and 14 166 out of 14 937 non-active compounds (94.8%). The overall predictability performance was 94.0%. In this work, we propose five types of non Linear ANN and we show that it is another alternative model to the already existing ones in the literature, such as LDA. The best model obtained was RBF 166:166-402-1:1 which had an overall training performance of 94.2%. All this can help to design new inhibitors of GSK-3β. The present work reports the attempts to calculate within a unified framework probabilities of GSK-3β inhibitors against different molecules found in the literature.

Keywords: GSK-3β; QSAR; Artificial neural network; Linear neural network; Linear discriminant analysis

Introduction

Glycogen synthase kinase-3 (GSK-3) has two isoforms, GSK-3α and GSK-3β, [1] and they are serine/threonine kinases involved in numerous cellular processes and diverse diseases as Alzheimer disease, cancer, and diabetes. GSK-3α and GSK-3β have been shown to be present in mammals and the latter is specifically expressed in the central nervous system [2,3]. In particular, GSK-3β is well known to play critical roles in oxidative stress-induced neurodegenerative diseases such as Alzheimer′s disease (AD) [2,4]. Despite intensive investigation into the physiological roles of GSK-3 isoforms, the basis for their differential activities remains unresolved. A more comprehensive understanding of the mechanistic basis for GSK-3 isoform-specific functions could lead to the development of isoform-specific inhibitors [5]. GSK-3β knock-out mice die *in utero* [6], whereas GSK-3α knock-out mice are viable and display improved glucose tolerance in response to glucose load and elevated hepatic glycogen storage and insulin sensitivity [7,8].

Alzheimer′s disease [9] is a serious and degenerative disorder that causes a gradual loss of neurons, and in spite of the efforts realized by the big pharmaceutical companies of the world, the origin of this pathology is still not very clear. β-amyloid (Aβ) is an important protein implicated in the pathogenesis of AD, but the mechanism by which it causes neurotoxicity is still unknown [10,11]. In particular, there are few literature reports to study the direct link between the pathological hyperphosphorylation of tau protein, a microtubule-

associated protein, and the formation of neurofibrillary tangles (NFT) [12]. The last decades had marked a very significant era of AD research. During this period, the nature of amyloid plaques and NTFs, the two histopathological hallmarks of AD, had been elucidated. Recent research efforts have led to several hypotheses to explain AD. Amyloid β toxicity is believed to play a primary role in the development of AD [13]. GSK-3β activity may increase with aging [14], which is consistent with the fact that aging is the most important risk factor for AD. Both *in vitro* and *in vivo* studies have demonstrated that inhibition of GSK-3β, can reverse hyperphosphorylation of tau and prevent behavioral impairments in mice [15-20]. These studies make GSK-3β inhibition very attractive as a therapeutic target for AD [21].

In the last years, a number of publications have been published suggesting GSK-3 as a target for the treatment of AD. There are two isoforms of GSK-3, GSK-3α and GSK-3β, both sharing a high homology

*Corresponding author: Prado-Prado F, Biomedical Sciences Department, Health Sciences Division, University of Quintana Roo, 77039, Chetumal, Mexico, E-mail: fenol1@hotmail.com

at their catalytic site, but the α form possesses an extended N-terminus with respect to the β form [22,23]. The phosphorylation of proteins by GSK-3 is an important link in neural function [24-26]. There are two characteristic neuropathological hallmarks of AD, Neurofibrillary Tangles (NFT's) and an increased production of amyloid beta (Aβ) peptides, where NFT's are composed of highly phosphorylated forms of the microtubule-associated protein tau [27] and studies have shown that GSK-3 is one of the main *in vivo* players of phosphorylation of tau protein [28]. It has been reported that Lithium, a GSK-3 inhibitor, blocks production of Aβ peptides by interfering with APP cleavage at γ-secretase step, where the target for Lithium is GSK-3α [22,29]. Phiel et al. [29] showed that selective reduction in concentration of the α isoform led to a decrease in the concentration of Aβ40 and Aβ42, primary constituents of amyloid plaques in AD. Thus, inhibition of GSK-3α could potentially provide dual therapy against AD, preventing the buildup of amyloid plaques and of neurofibrillary tangles [29-31].

GSK-3β is a serine/threonine kinase and is thought to be a key factor for aberrant tau phosphorylation [32]. Activated GSK-3β coexists with progression of NFT's and neurodegeneration in the AD brain [33-35]. A conditional GSK-3β overexpressing transgenic mouse exhibits persistent tau hyperphosphorylation, pretangle-like somatodendritic localization of tau, neuronal death in hippocampus and cognitive deficits [36,37]. These studies suggest that GSK-3β is associated with AD progression, and GSK-3β inhibition is expected to be a promising therapeutic approach for AD.

In this sense, quantitative structure-activity relationships (QSAR) could play an important role in studying these β and γ-secretase inhibitors. QSAR models are necessary in order to guide the β and γ-secretase inhibitors.

On the other hand, QSAR models can be used to explore the relationships between the structural spaces of compounds as inhibitors for specific enzymes, such as MAO inhibitors [38], HIV-1 integrase inhibitors [39], and/or protease inhibitors [40] or tyrosinase inhibitors [41-43]. In fact, almost all QSAR techniques are based on the use of molecular descriptors, which are numerical series that codify useful chemical information and enable correlations between statistical and biological properties [44,45]. Recently, the field has moved from small molecules to proteins and other systems. For instance, González-Díaz et al. have discussed the use of these methods but only from the point of view of proteins [46]. Later, some groups have published different papers in one special issue on QSAR but they have been also restricted to the field of protein and proteomics [47-53]. In other recent issue, guest-edited by González-Díaz [54] a series of papers have been published, devoted to QSAR/QSPR techniques for low-molecular-weight drugs [54-63]. Most recently, Prado-Prado et al. [64] have published a mt-QSAR for anti-parasitic drugs. This year we have published another issue [65] focused on QSAR/QSPR models and a graph theory used to approach Drug ADMET processes and Metabolomics [66-73]. Last, one of the most recent issues published has discussed the applications of QSAR in Pharmaceutical Design [74-83].

The functions of GSK-3 and its implication in various human diseases have triggered an active search for potent and selective GSK-3 inhibitors [12] in the last years. QSARs can be used as predictive tools for the development of molecules [84,85]. The QSAR approach involves the development of models that relate the structure of drugs with their biological activity against different targets [86,87]. Furthermore, there are multiple chemometric approaches that can, in principle, be selected for this step. Multiple linear regression (MLR), LDA, partial least squares (PLS) and different kinds of artificial neural networks

can be used to relate molecular structure (represented by molecular descriptors) with biological properties. The ANNs are particularly useful in QSAR studies in which the linear models fit poorly due to high data complexity; an example was the work of Prado-Prado et al. in which four types of non-ANN were developed to calculate within an unified framework probabilities of antiparasitic action of drugs against different parasite species [64,88,89]. There are several different kinds of ANN and these include multilayer perceptron (MLP), radial basis functions (RBF) and PNNs; the latter ANN is a variant of RBF systems. In particular, PNN is a type of neural network that uses a kernel-based approximation to form an estimate of the probability density functions of classes in a classification problem [90]. In the present work, we have reviewed previous works based on 2D-QSAR, 3D-QSAR, CoMFA, CoMSIA and docking techniques, which studied different compounds to find out the structural requirements. Last, in this review, we developed quantitative structure-activity relationships (QSAR) models for GSK-3β, linear discriminant analysis (LDA) [91] and linear artificial neural networks (ANNs) from more than 40000 cases with more than 24000 different inhibitors of GSK-3β obtained from ChEMBL database http://www.ebi.ac.uk/chembldb/index.php/target/browser/classification [92,93]; in total we used more than 45000 different cases to develop the QSAR models. In addition, we did a study of different fragments that exist in the molecules of the database in order to see which fragments had more influence in the activity, and which fragments interact more with the protein. As there are very studies with GSK-3β that can be found in the literature the design of new inhibitors of this enzyme is very important for study of the neurodegenerative diseases [94,95]. The topics reviewed, discussed, and/or reported in this paper are:

1. Studies of GSK-3α inhibitors

1.1. 2D-QSAR for 3-anilino-4-phenylmaleimides

1.2. 3D-QSAR and docking of 3-anilino-4-phenylmaleimides

1.3. QSAR studies of Some GSK-3α Inhibitory pyrimidines

2. Studies of GSK-3β inhibitors

2.1. Design, synthesis and structure-activity relationships of 1,3,4-oxadiazole derivatives

2.2. Linear/Nonlinear Regression Methods for Prediction of Glycogen Synthase Kinase-3β Inhibitory Activities

2.3. Molecular modeling, docking and 3D-QSAR studies for maleimides

2.4. Molecular Docking and biological testing of new GSK-3β inhibitors

2.5. 3D-QSAR Modeling of Paullones

2.6. Modeling of Binding Mode of Benzo[*e*]isoindole-1,3-diones

3. QSAR studies of GSK-3β

3.1. Theoretical study of GSK-3β: Neural Networks QSAR studies

Studies of GSK-3α Inhibitors

2D-QSAR for 3-anilino-4-phenylmaleimides

Sivaprakasam et al. [31] reported in their study a 2D-QSAR exploration of the physicochemical (hydrophobic, electronic, and steric) and structural requirements among 3-anilino-4-phenylmaleimides toward GSK-3α binding. Using Fujita-Ban and Hansch QSAR analyses, electronic and steric interactions at the 4-phenyl ring and hydrophobic interactions at the 3-anilino ring were shown to be crucial. Hansch-type QSAR was still widely used in the lead optimization stage of synthetic and other projects.

Fujita-Ban analysis of 3-anilino-4-phenylmaleimides revealed that certain structural features such as Cl, OCH$_3$, and NO2 mono substitution at any position around the 4-phenyl ring were favorable for GSK-3α inhibition. Substituents at the 3-anilino ring such as 3-Cl, 4-Cl, 5-Cl, 3-COOH, 4-OH, and 4-SCH$_3$ were positively and 3-OH was negatively correlated with GSK-3α inhibitory activity.

Through Hansch QSAR analyses, they found that the GSK-3α inhibitory activity was enhanced by: 1. Electron-withdrawing, bulky *ortho* substituents at 4-phenyl ring; 2. 4-chloro substitution around anilino ring; 3. 3-anilino rather than 3-N-methylanilino derivatives; 4. Hydrophobic *meta* substituents on the anilino ring. Overall, QSAR models 13a and 14a suggested electronic and steric effects at the 4-phenyl ring and hydrophobic effects at the 3-anilino or 3-N-methylanilino ring were crucial. Their 2D-model (Figure 1) illustrated these effects which are essential for binding the maleimides to the GSK-3α enzyme. Their analysis provided key information regarding ligand–target interactions which they believed would help medicinal chemists to design more potent GSK-3α inhibitors.

3D-QSAR and docking of 3-anilino-4-phenylmaleimides

3D-QSAR analyses were reported in this article [96], using CoMFA and CoMSIA and molecular docking studies on 3-anilino-4-phenylmaleimides as GSK-3α inhibitors, in order to better understand the mechanism of action and structure-activity relationship of these compounds. The comparison of the active site residues of GSK-3α showed that all the key amino acids involved in polar interactions with the maleimides for the β isoform were the same in the α isoform, except for Asp133 in the β isoform, which was replaced by Glu196 in the α isoform. The authors prepared a homology model for GSK-3α and showed that the change from Asp to Glu should not affect maleimide binding significantly. Their best CoMFA model contained steric and electrostatic fields and had $n = 56$, $q^2 = 0.844$, $r^2 = 0.942$, $SEE = 0.104$, $F = 162.49$ and $r^2_{pred} = 0.779$ for five components. CoMFA electrostatic contours revealed that increased negative charge at the *meta* position of the 4-phenyl ring was favorable for the activity. They found that electron withdrawing groups at the *meta* and *para* positions around the anilino ring were important for enhancing activity.

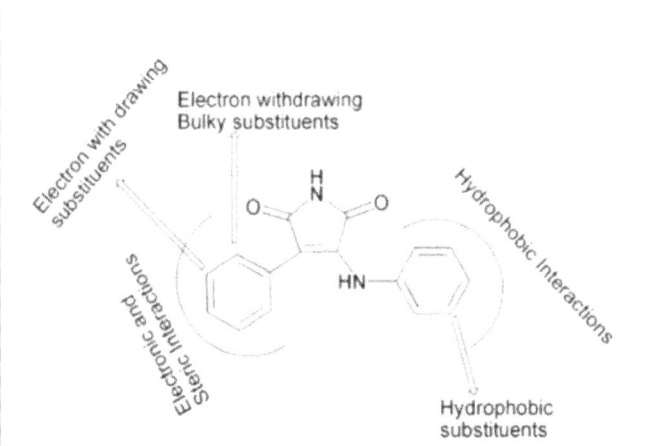

Figure 1: Proposed model based on 2D-QSAR analyses showing the nature of interactions and substitution requirements for effective binding of 3-anilino-4-phenylmaleimides with the GSK-3α isoform.

Electron-withdrawing bulky *ortho* substituents on the 4-phenyl ring were conducive to GSK-3α inhibition. CoMSIA model showed the importance of hydrogen bond donor groups on these ligands for enhanced activity. The best CoMSIA model (S + E + D) had $n = 56$, $q^2 = 0.833$, $r^2 = 0.932$, $SEE = 0.113$, $F = 111.67$ and $r^2_{pred} = 0.803$ for six components. Comparatively, 3-N-methylanilino derivatives were less active than 3-anilino derivatives.

Docking studies revealed the binding poses of three subclasses of these ligands, namely anilino, N-methylanilino and indoline derivatives, within the active site of the β isoform, and helped to explain the difference in their inhibitory activity.

QSAR studies of some GSK-3α inhibitory pyrimidines

Jamloky et al. studied in this paper [22] a series of pyrimidines which was performed to gain structural insight into the binding mode of the molecules to the GSK-3α. The molecular modeling studies were performed using CS Chem. Office 2001 molecular modeling software version 6.0. MOPAC module was used to minimize the energy and calculate the descriptors. The thermodynamic and steric features of the pyrimidines were highly correlated with GSK-3α inhibitory activity. The positive coefficient of PMI-Y in the model suggested that the presence of bulky substituents positioned towards the Y-axis of the molecule would enhance the GSK-3α inhibitory activity. The observation supports the hypothesis that the presence of the bulky substituents like bromine with inherent hydrophobic character may be involved in the nonspecific interaction with the ATP binding site. The results of the study suggested that the introduction of bulky groups at C-5 position of the hydrophobic interaction with the ATP binding site of the enzyme may be attributed to the strain exerted by the two adjacent phenyl rings on the planar pyrazolo (3,4-*b*) pyridine ring, thereby partly disrupting the hydrogen bonding interaction between nitrogen in the pyrazolo group and the complementary group in the enzyme.

Studies of GSK-3β Inhibitors

Design, synthesis and structure-activity relationships of 1,3,4-oxadiazole derivatives

Saitoh et al. [97] reported design, synthesis and structure–activity relationships of a novel series of oxadiazole derivatives as GSK-3β inhibitors. Among these inhibitors, compound 20x showed highly selective and potent GSK-3β inhibitory activity *in vitro* and its binding mode was determined by obtaining the X-ray co-crystal structure of 20x (Figure 2) and GSK-3β (Figure 3). The hydrogen bonding interaction of the benzimidazole core with the hinge region and the oxadiazole with Asp200 were observed. Additionally, the interaction of 4-methoxyphenyl group with Arg141 was also observed.

Linear/nonlinear regression methods for prediction of glycogen synthase Kinase-3β inhibitory activities

Freitas et al. [98] applied linear/nonlinear regression methods as multiple linear regression (MLR), artificial neural network (ANN), and support vector machines (SVM) with a series of glycogen synthase kinase-3β (GSK-3β) inhibitors using calculated Dragon descriptors. Few variables were selected from a pool of calculated Dragon descriptors through three different feature selection methods, namely genetic algorithm (GA), successive projections algorithm (SPA), and fuzzy rough set ant colony optimization (fuzzy rough set ACO). The fuzzy rough set ACO/SVM-based model gave the best estimation/prediction results, demonstrating the nonlinear nature of this analysis

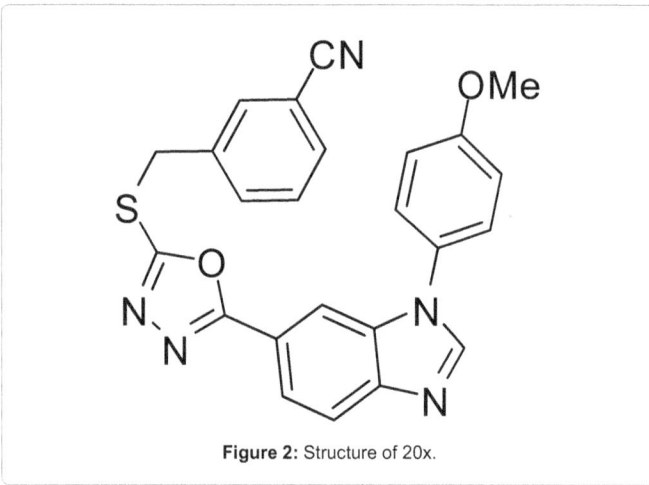

Figure 2: Structure of 20x.

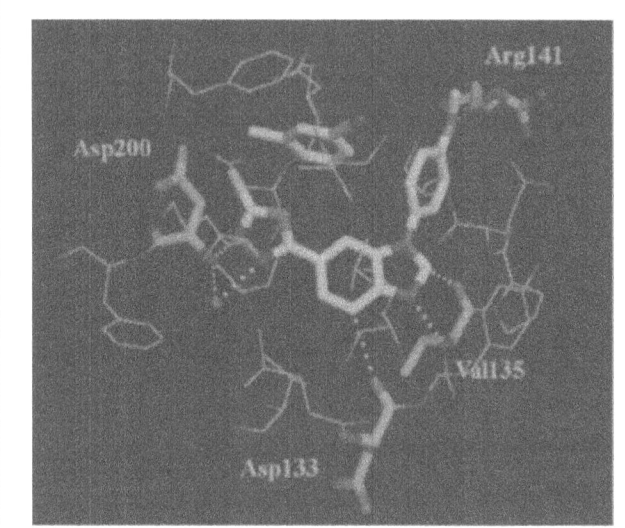

Figure 3: X-ray co-crystal structure of 1 in complex with GSK-3β.

and suggesting fuzzy rough set ACO, introduced in chemistry for the first time, as an improved variable selection method in QSAR for the class of GSK-3β inhibitors. MLR yielded QSAR models only reasonably predictable, with r^2 ranging from 0.77 to 0.81 and r^2_{test} of 0.67 to 0.76, ANN and specially SVM were capable of estimating and predicting biological activities very accurately.

Molecular modeling, docking and 3D-QSAR studies for maleimides

Hwan-Kim et al. [99] carried out molecular modeling and docking studies with three-dimensional quantitative structure relationships (3D-QSAR) to determine the correct binding mode of glycogen synthase kinase 3β (GSK-3β) inhibitors. For the 3D-QSAR (CoMFA and CoMSIA), they used 51 substituted benzofuran-3-yl-(indol-3-yl) maleimides. Two binding modes of the inhibitors to the binding site of GSK-3β were analyzed. The binding mode 1 yielded better 3D-QSAR correlations using both CoMFA and CoMSIA methodologies. The three-component CoMFA model from the steric and electrostatic fields for the experimentally determined pIC$_{50}$ values had the following statistics: $R^2(cv) = 0.386$ and $SE(cv) = 0.854$ for the cross-validation, and

$R^2 = 0.811$ and $SE = 0.474$ for the fitted correlation. $F_{(3.47)} = 67.034$, and probability of $R^2 = 0$ (3.47) = 0.000. The binding mode suggested by the results of this study was consistent with the preliminary results of X-ray crystal structures of inhibitor-bound GSK-3β. The 3D-QSAR models were used for the estimation of the inhibitory potency of two additional compounds.

Molecular docking and biological testing of new GSK-3β inhibitors

Lavrovskii et al. [100] used a series of new heteroaryl-substituted oxadiazole-5-carboxamide inhibitors of GSK-3β. Molecular docking was used for the rational selection of synthesized compounds for the subsequent biological testing. It was established that the inhibitory activity of the synthesized compounds strongly depends on the character of substituents in the phenyl ring and the nature of terminal heterocyclic fragments. The most active compounds inhibit GSK-3β at IC$_{50}$ in the micro molar range and could be considered as potential drug candidates.

3D-QSAR modeling of paullones

Osolodkin et al. [101] carried out a 3D-QSAR study which suggested ways of modification of the molecule to increase its physiological activity. A comparative molecular field analysis (CoMFA) [7] and a comparative molecular similarity indices analysis (CoMSIA) [8] are among the most widely used 3D-QSAR methods. The energy of Van der Waals and electrostatic interactions of a probe atom (with the charge +1) with molecules of the training set (CoMFA) or the electrostatic, Van der Waals, hydrophobic, and donor/acceptor similarity indices (CoMSIA) were used as descriptors. The equation for activity prediction was derived using the partial least squares (PLS) method. The advantages of the methods were the ability of graphic representation of PLS model coefficients and the fact that they allowed the user to suggest substitutions affecting activity and/or selectivity of the molecules. The authors built a new 3D-QSAR model for GSK-3β inhibition by paullones by means of the CoMFA method. This model can be used as a guide for designing new paullone GSK-3β inhibitors.

Modeling of binding mode of Benzo[e]isoindole-1,3-diones

Yang et al. [102] synthesized benzo[e]isoindole-1,3-dione derivatives and the effects on GSK-3β activity and zebrafish embryo growth were evaluated. A series of derivatives showed obvious inhibitory activity against GSK-3β. The most potent inhibitor, 7,8-dimethoxy-5-methylbenzo[e]isoindole-1,3-dione, showed nanomolar IC$_{50}$ and obvious phenotype on zebrafish embryo growth associated with the inhibition of GSK-3β at low micro molar concentration. The interaction mode between this compound and GSK-3β was characterized by computational modeling. To rationalize the structure-activity relationships of these compounds, the binding modes of the most potent inhibitors 8a and 8b (Figure 4) were modeled using docking simulations. Compounds 8a and 8b were docked into the ATP binding site of GSK-3β, and the binding modes of the lowest energy were analyzed. Compounds 8a and 8b fit the ATP pocket of GSK-3β well. The maleimide motif of type II formed a pair of hydrogen bonds with the hinge region (Glu133 and Val135) of GSK-3β, similar to the binding mode of other known maleimides GSK-3β inhibitors. The two methoxy oxygen atoms formed another two hydrogen bonds with the positively charged Lys85. The methyl group of the methoxy at C-8 position docked to the small back cleft of GSK-3β. This binding mode explicitly explained the important role of the two methoxy groups at C-7 and C-8 positions. Another result was the 4-ethyl group of 8b

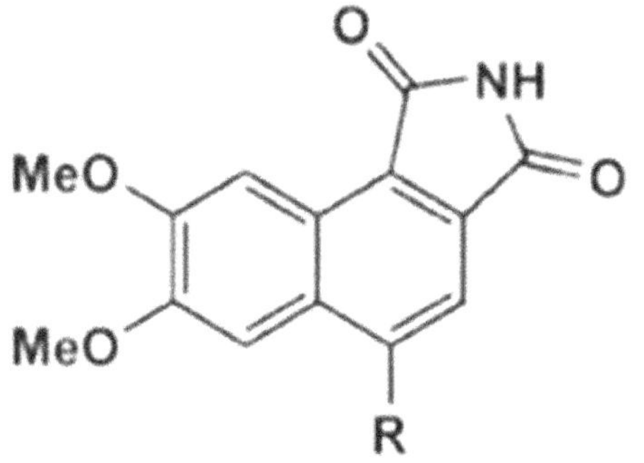

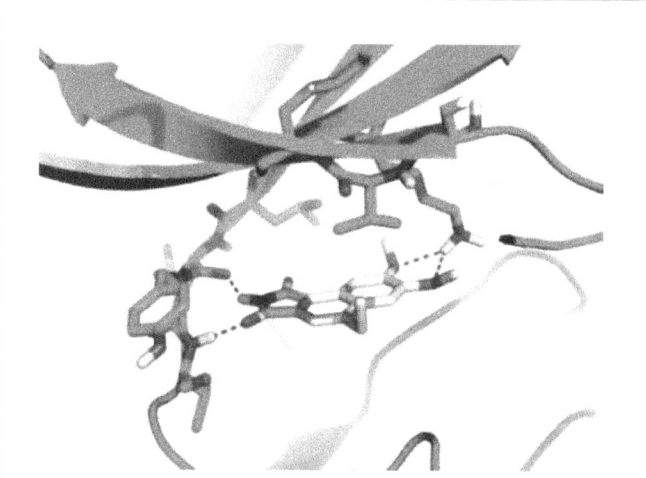

Figure 4: Structure of 8a and 8b.

docks to the minor hydrophobic pocket made up of Ile62 and Val70 in front of the ATP binding site of GSK-3β (Figure 5), which contributed to its higher binding affinity compared to 8a. The docking results also provided a template to understand the structure-activity relationships of other compounds.

QSAR Studies of GSK-3β

Theoretical study of GSK-3β: Neural Networks QSAR studies for the design of new inhibitors using 2D-descriptors

Alzheimer´s disease [9] is a serious and degenerative disorder that causes a gradual loss of neurons, and in spite of the efforts realized by the big pharmaceutical companies of the world, the origin of this pathology is still not very clear. β-amyloid (Aβ) is an important protein implicated in the pathogenesis of AD, but the mechanism by which it causes neurotoxicity is still unknown [10,11]. In particular, there are few literatures report to study the direct link between the pathological hyperphosphorylation of tau protein, a microtubule-associated protein, and the formation of neurofibrillary tangles (NFT) [12]. The last decades had marked a very significant era of AD research. During this period, the nature of amyloid plaques and NTFs, the two histopathological hallmarks of AD, had been elucidated. Recent research efforts have led to several hypotheses to explain AD. Amyloid β toxicity is believed to play a primary role in the development of AD [13]. GSK-3β activity may increase with aging [14], which is consistent with the fact that aging is the most important risk factor for AD. Both *in vitro* and *in vivo* studies have demonstrated that inhibition of GSK-3β, can reverse hyperphosphorylation of tau and prevent behavioral impairments in mice [15-20]. These studies make GSK-3β inhibition very attractive as a therapeutic target for AD [21].

We developed quantitative structure-activity relationships (QSAR) models for GSK-3β, linear discriminant analysis (LDA) [91] and linear artificial neural networks (ANNs) from more than 40000 cases with more than 24000 different molecules inhibitors of GSK-3β obtained from ChEMBL database http://www.ebi.ac.uk/chembldb/index.php/target/browser/classification [92,93]; in total we used more than 45000 different molecules to develop the QSAR models. In addition, we did a study of different fragments that exist in the molecules of the database

in order to see which fragments had more influence in the activity, and which fragments interact more with the protein. As there many studies with GSK-3β that can be found in the literature the design of new inhibitors of this enzyme is very important for the study of neurodegenerative diseases [94,95].

Methods

Linear classifier

A database from ChEMBL database [92] containing assayed GSK-3β inhibitors was used (Table SM from the Supplementary Material). The DRAGON software 4.0 [14] was utilized here and provides 1664 descriptors classified as zero- (0D) one- (1D), two- (2D) and three-dimensional (3D) descriptors depending on the fact they are computed from the chemical formula, substructure list representation, molecular graph or geometrical representation of the molecule, respectively [103]. In this work, we calculated the following descriptors: 2D autocorrelations, Burden eigenvalues, topological charge indices, eigenvalue-based indices, functional group counts, atoms-centred fragments, charge descriptors and molecular properties. The QSAR model was constructed with the multivariate regression technique, the LDA, employing the Forward stepwise method for the selection of variables. All statistical analyses and data exploration were carried out in STATISTICA 6.0 [104]. In the actual work, the independent data test is used by splitting the data randomly in a training series used for a model construction and a cross-validation (CV) one. The general formula of the QSAR classification function is the following:

$$GSKI - 3\beta_{score} = \sum W_m \cdot {}^m 2D_i + W_0 \qquad (1)$$

where GSKI-3β$_{score}$ is the continuous and dimensionless score value for the GSKI-3β/non-GSKI-3β classification that gives relatively higher values to molecules with more probability to act as GSKI-3β, ${}^m2D_i$ are the $2Ds$ of type m, W_m is the coefficient (weights) of these indices in the QSAR model and W_0 is the independent term.

The reported statistical parameters of the QSAR model are the following: N, χ^2, F, and p-level as well as Sensitivity, Specificity, and Accuracy for both training and CV [104]. N is the number of molecules used to train the model, λ is Wilks statistic parameter, χ^2 is Chi-square and p-level is the probability of error.

Figure 5: Docked binding modes of compounds 8b in the ATP binding site of GSK-3β.

Nonlinear classifiers

We processed our data with different ANNs using the STATISTICA 6.0 software [104] looking for a better model to predict activity against GSK-3β. Five types of ANNs were used, namely, Probabilistic Neural Network (PNN), Radial Basis Function (RBF) [105], Three Layers Perceptron (MLP-3), and Four Layer Perceptron (MLP-4) and Linear (LNN). The profile of a ANN is: Ni:I-H1-H2-O:No. It means that we have inputs variables (Ni), neurons in the input layer (I), neurons in the first hidden layer (H1), in the second hidden layer (H2), neuron in the output layer (O) and output variable (No).

We can used a very simple type of ANN called Linear Neural Network (RBF) to fit this discriminant function. The model deals with the classification of a compound set with or without affinity on different receptors. A dummy variable Affinity Class (AC) was used as input to codify the affinity. This variable indicates either high (AC = 1) or low (AC = 0) affinity of the drug by the receptor. $S(DTP)_{pred}$ or DTP affinity predicted score is the output of the model and it is a continuous dimensionless score that sorts compounds from low to high affinity to the target coinciding DTPs with higher values of $S(DTP)_{pred}$ and nDTPs with lowest values. In equation (6), b represents the coefficients of the RBF classification function, determined by the ANN module of the STATISTICA 6.0 software package [104]. We used Forward Stepwise algorithm for a variable selection.

Let be $^k\chi(G)$ drugs molecular descriptors and $^k\xi(R)$ receptor or drug target descriptors for different drugs (d) with different receptor; we can attempt to develop a simple linear classifier of mt-QSAR type with the general formula:

$$S(DTP)_{pred} = \sum_{k=0}^{5} b_i(G_k) \cdot {}^k\chi(G) + b_0 \qquad (2)$$

We assessed the quality of models with different statistical parameters like Specificity (Equation 2), Sensitivity (Equation 3), Accuracy (Equation 4) and ROC curve (Receiver Operating Characteristic curve) which is a graphical plot of the sensitivity, or true positives, vs. (1−specificity), or false positives,

$$specificity = \frac{NTN}{NTN + NFP} \qquad (3)$$

$$sensitivity = \frac{NTP}{NTP + NFN} \qquad (4)$$

$$accuracy = \frac{NTP + NTN}{NTP + FN + FP + TN} \qquad (5)$$

where NTN means number of true negatives, NFP is number of false positives, NTP is number of true positives, NFN is number of false negatives, FN is false negatives, FP is false positives and TN is true negatives.

The data set used in this article was obtained from ChEMBL database [92,93]. It has more than 56000 cases and more than 24000 different compounds inhibitors of GSK-3β. In total we used more than 45000 different molecules to develop the QSAR models obtained in ChEMBL. This is a database of bioactive drug-like small molecules, it contains 2-D structures, calculated properties (e.g. logP, Molecular Weight, Lipinski Parameters, etc.) and abstracted bioactivities (e.g. binding constants, pharmacology and ADMET data). ChEMBL

normalises the bioactivities into a uniform set of end-points and units where possible, and also tags the links between a molecular target and a published assay with a set of varying confidence levels. The data is abstracted and curated from the primary scientific literature, and covers a significant fraction of the structure activity relationship (SAR) and discovery of modern drugs. The codes and activity for all compounds as well as the references used to collect them are depicted in Table SM of the supplementary material file.

Results and Discussion

LDA

In this paper we obtained a LDA study with Equation 6, and we can observe that eighteen variables entry inside equation:

$$GSK1-3\beta_{score} = -18.1 \cdot D1 + 18.9 \cdot D2 + 0.7 \cdot D3 + 22.0 \cdot D4 - 37.7 \cdot D5 + 11.7 \cdot D6 + 6.6 \cdot D7 - 8.5 \cdot D8 - 20.9 \cdot D9 + 5.4 \cdot D10 +$$
$$+ 7.2 \cdot D11 - 2.4 \cdot D12 + 1.2 \cdot D13 + 14.3 \cdot D14 - 14.6 \cdot D15 - 10.8 \cdot D16 + 12.4 \cdot D17 + 20.1 \cdot D18 - 9.4 \cdot D19 + 13.6 \cdot D20 + 8.8 \cdot D21 +$$
$$+ 14.1 \cdot D22 - 168.3 \cdot D23 - 122.8 \cdot D24 - 2.8 \cdot D25 + 0.1 \cdot D26 - 0.7 \cdot D27 - 86.4 \qquad (6)$$
$$N = 45,299 \qquad \lambda = 0.64 \qquad \chi^2 = 12201.95 \qquad p-level < 0.001$$

In Table 1, we show the code names of descriptors used in the equation 6. The nomenclature used in the descriptors of the equation is the same as establishing the Dragon software, where N is the number of compounds used for training, λ is the Wilks statistic parameter, χ^2 is the Chi-square and p is the level of error. The model correctly classified 1310 out of 1643 active compounds (79.7%) and 24823 out of 26156 non-active compounds (94.9%) in the training series. The overall training performance was 94.0%. Validation of the model was carried out using an external predicting series. In this series the model classified correctly 757 out of 940 (80.5%) compounds and 14166 out of 14937 non-active compounds (94.8%). The overall predictability performance was 94.0% (Table 2).

ANN models

The ANN models are non-linear models useful to predict the biological activity of a large datasets of molecules. This technique is an alternative to linear methods such as LDA [106,107]. Figure 6 depicts the networks maps for some of the ANN models. In general, at least one ANN of every types tested was statically significant. However, one must note that the profiles of each network indicate that these are highly nonlinear and complicated models [108-110].

In Figure 7, we depict the ROC-curve [111,112] for RBF tested. Notably, almost model presented and an area under curve higher than 0.5 (the value for a random classifier). The vitality of this type of procedures developing ANN-QSAR models has been demonstrated before [113]; see, for instance, the work of Fernandez and Caballero [114]. The same is true about the ANNs tested, where is illustrated ROC-curves of ANN RBF with an area higher than 0.99. To show how important is this result, we compared the present model with other model used to address the same problem. We processed our data with ANNs looking for a better model. In general, the ANN RBF tested was statically significant [107].

The network found was RBF and it showed training performance higher than 94.2%. The summary of results is showed in Table 2. After direct inspection of the results reported in Table 2 for ANN methods, we can conclude that a complex ANN method is a good method to predict the activity. We compare different types of networks to obtain a better model; Table 2 shows the classification matrix of the different networks. RBF 166:166-402-1:1 was taken as the main network because it presented a wider range of variables, 166 inputs in the first layer and 166 neurons in second layer, and two sets of cases (Training and Validation). Another tested networks found were LNN 233:233-1:1 and

Definition	Name Descriptor
D1	ATS1m
D2	ATS2m
D3	ATS8m
D4	ATS3v
D5	ATS3e
D6	MATS3m
D7	MATS4m
D8	MATS3e
D9	MATS2p
D10	GATS1v
D11	GATS4v
D12	GATS1e
D13	GATS7e
D14	GATS3p
D15	BELm4
D16	BELm5
D17	BELv2
D18	BEHe1
D19	BEHe8
D20	BELe5
D21	BELe8
D22	BELp4
D23	JGI4
D24	JGI7
D25	Ui
D26	AMR
D27	MLOGP

Table 1: Code names of the different molecular descriptor used in the equation 6.

Model	Train			Stat.		Validation	
profile	Active	Non-Active	%	Par.	%	Active	Non-Active
	1310	333	79.9	Sn	80.5	757	183
LDA	1333	24823	94.9	Sp	94.8	771	14166
			94.0	Ac	94.0		
RBF	1552	100	94.0	Sn	94.3	889	53
166:166-402-1:1	1572	25613	94.2	Sp	94.1	909	14611
			94.0	Ac	94.2		

Table 2: Comparison of LDA and ANN classification model.

LNN 232:232-1:1 presented low accuracy and PNN 233:233-20619-2-2:1 had a very low percentage of DTPs leading to possible errors in the model although its accuracy was very good, (Table 1). We depict the ROC-curve for RBF 166:166-402-1:1 to show how reliable was the network model developed, (Figure 7).

Conclusion

The functions of GSK-3 and its implication in various human diseases have triggered an active search for potent and selective GSK-3 inhibitors. Nowadays, theoretical studies such as QSAR models have become a very useful tool in this context to substantially reduce time and resources consuming experiments. In this work we developed a new LDA model using the Dragon descriptors, with a large data base using about 20000 different drugs obtained from the ChEMBL server. We conclude that a large database gives a much more precise model; the use of tools such as ChEMBL database enables us to develop

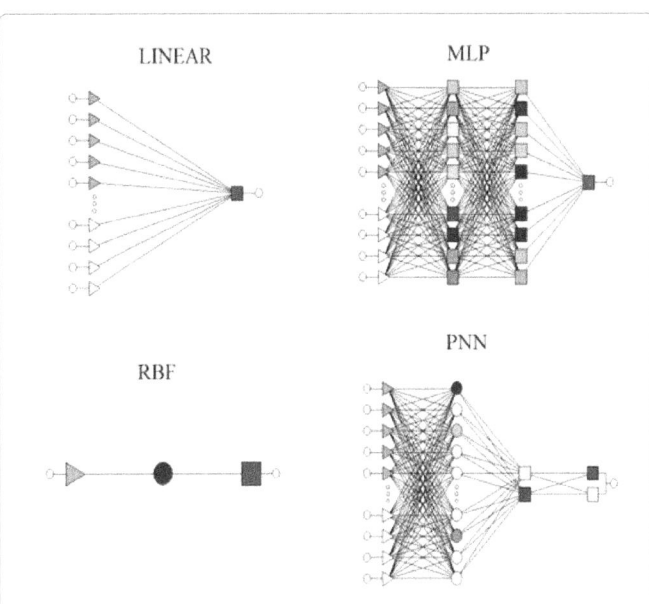

Figure 6: Depicts the networks maps for some of the ANN models used in this manuscript.

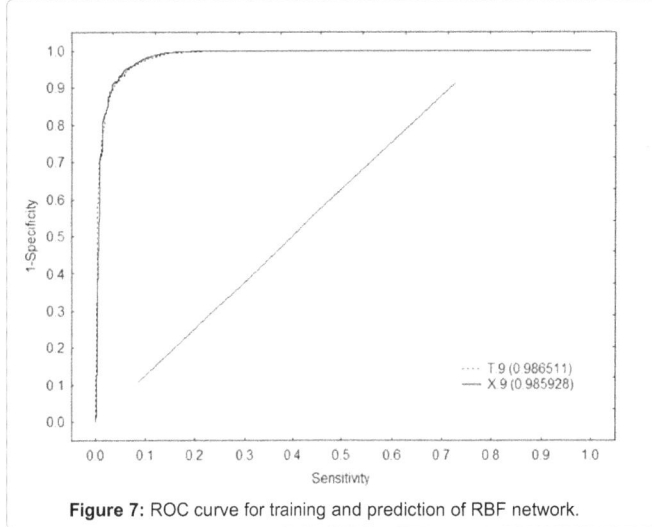

Figure 7: ROC curve for training and prediction of RBF network.

models with large data bases, and this helps us to make the results more reliable. To improve the model we developed non-linear models and compared them to LDA. We proposed non-linear models, and for the first time, we proposed ANN models based on Dragon Descriptors series of GSK-3β, and we concluded that they are alternative methods to study the activity of different families of molecules compared with other methods found in the literature.

Acknowledgments

The authors thank the sponsorship DCS-UQROO PIFI (P/PIFI-2012-23MSU0140Z-09 DCS) and FJPP thanks sponsorshipsfor a research position at the University of Quintana Roo from the project.

References

1. Woodgett JR (1990) Molecular cloning and expression of glycogen synthase kinase-3/factor A. EMBO J 9: 2431-2438.

2. Cai F, Wang F, Lin FK, Liu C, Ma LQ, et al. (2008) Redox modulation of long-term potentiation in the hippocampus via regulation of the glycogen synthase kinase-3beta pathway. Free Radic Biol Med 45: 964-970.

3. Woodgett JR (1991) cDNA cloning and properties of glycogen synthase kinase-3. Methods Enzymol 200: 564-577.

4. Maiese K, Chong ZZ (2004) Insights into oxidative stress and potential novel therapeutic targets for Alzheimer disease. Restor Neurol Neurosci 22: 87-104.

5. Buescher JL, Phiel CJ (2010) A noncatalytic domain of glycogen synthase kinase-3 (GSK-3) is essential for activity. J Biol Chem 285: 7957-7963.

6. Hoeflich KP, Luo J, Rubie EA, Tsao MS, Jin O, et al. (2000) Requirement for glycogen synthase kinase-3beta in cell survival and NF-kappaB activation. Nature 406: 86-90.

7. Hooper C, Killick R, Lovestone S (2008) The GSK3 hypothesis of Alzheimer's disease. J Neurochem 104: 1433-1439.

8. MacAulay K, Doble BW, Patel S, Hansotia T, Sinclair EM, et al. (2007) Glycogen synthase kinase 3alpha-specific regulation of murine hepatic glycogen metabolism. Cell Metab 6: 329-337.

9. Olson RE (2000) Secretase inhibitors as therapeutics for Alzheimer's disease. Annu Rep Med Chem 35: 31-40.

10. Deguchi K (2006) Insights into oxidative stress and potential novel therapeutic targets for Alzheimer disease. J Cereb Blood Flow Metab 26: 1263-1273.

11. Stabenfeldt SE, García AJ, LaPlaca MC (2006) Thermoreversible laminin-functionalized hydrogel for neural tissue engineering. J Biomed Mater Res A 77: 718-725.

12. Huang J, Chen YJ, Bian WH, Yu J, Zhao YW, et al. (2010) Unilateral amyloid-beta25-35 injection into the rat amygdala increases the expressions of aberrant tau phosphorylation kinases. Chin Med J (Engl) 123: 1311-1314.

13. Hardy J, Selkoe DJ (2002) The amyloid hypothesis of Alzheimer's disease: progress and problems on the road to therapeutics. Science 297: 353-356.

14. Wen Y, Planel E, Herman M, Figueroa HY, Wang L, et al. (2008) Interplay between cyclin-dependent kinase 5 and glycogen synthase kinase 3 beta mediated by neuregulin signaling leads to differential effects on tau phosphorylation and amyloid precursor protein processing. J Neurosci 28: 2624-2632.

15. Pérez M, Hernández F, Lim F, Díaz-Nido J, Avila J (2003) Chronic lithium treatment decreases mutant tau protein aggregation in a transgenic mouse model. J Alzheimers Dis 5: 301-308.

16. Engel T, Goñi-Oliver P, Lucas JJ, Avila J, Hernández F (2006) Chronic lithium administration to FTDP-17 tau and GSK-3beta overexpressing mice prevents tau hyperphosphorylation and neurofibrillary tangle formation, but pre-formed neurofibrillary tangles do not revert. J Neurochem 99: 1445-1455.

17. Engel T, Hernández F, Avila J, Lucas JJ (2006) Full reversal of Alzheimer's disease-like phenotype in a mouse model with conditional overexpression of glycogen synthase kinase-3. J Neurosci 26: 5083-5090.

18. Le Corre S, Klafki HW, Plesnila N, Hübinger G, Obermeier A, et al. (2006) An inhibitor of tau hyperphosphorylation prevents severe motor impairments in tau transgenic mice. Proc Natl Acad Sci U S A 103: 9673-9678.

19. Nakashima H, Ishihara T, Suguimoto P, Yokota O, Oshima E, et al. (2005) Chronic lithium treatment decreases tau lesions by promoting ubiquitination in a mouse model of tauopathies. Acta Neuropathol 110: 547-556.

20. Noble W, Planel E, Zehr C, Olm V, Meyerson J, et al. (2005) Inhibition of glycogen synthase kinase-3 by lithium correlates with reduced tauopathy and degeneration in vivo. Proc Natl Acad Sci U S A 102: 6990-6995.

21. Gong CX, Iqbal K (2008) Hyperphosphorylation of microtubule-associated protein tau: a promising therapeutic target for Alzheimer disease. Curr Med Chem 15: 2321-2328.

22. Jamloki A, Karthikeyan C, Sharma SK, Hari Narayana Murthy NS, et al. (2006) QSAR Studies on Some GSK-3a Inhibitory 6-aryl-pyrazolo-(3,4-b) pyrimidines. Asian Journal of Biochemistry 1: 236-243.

23. Ali A, Hoeflich KP, Woodgett JR (2001) Glycogen synthase kinase-3: properties, functions, and regulation. Chem Rev 101: 2527-2540.

24. Martinez A, Castro A, Dorronsoro I, Alonso M (2002) Glycogen synthase kinase 3 (GSK-3) inhibitors as new promising drugs for diabetes, neurodegeneration, cancer, and inflammation. Med Res Rev 22: 373-384.

25. Martinez A, Alonso M, Castro A, Pérez C, Moreno FJ (2002) First non-ATP competitive glycogen synthase kinase 3 beta (GSK-3beta) inhibitors: thiadiazolidinones (TDZD) as potential drugs for the treatment of Alzheimer's disease. J Med Chem 45: 1292-1299.

26. Eldar-Finkelman H (2002) Glycogen synthase kinase 3: an emerging therapeutic target. Trends Mol Med 8: 126-132.

27. Lee VM, Goedert M, Trojanowski JQ (2001) Neurodegenerative tauopathies. Annu Rev Neurosci 24: 1121-1159.

28. Flaherty DB, Soria JP, Tomasiewicz HG, Wood JG (2000) Phosphorylation of human tau protein by microtubule-associated kinases: GSK3beta and cdk5 are key participants. J Neurosci Res 62: 463-472.

29. Phiel CJ, Wilson CA, Lee VM, Klein PS (2003) GSK-3alpha regulates production of Alzheimer's disease amyloid-beta peptides. Nature 423: 435-439.

30. Bhat RV, Budd Haeberlein SL, Avila J (2004) Glycogen synthase kinase 3: a drug target for CNS therapies. J Neurochem 89: 1313-1317.

31. Sivaprakasam P, Xie A, Doerksen RJ (2006) Probing the physicochemical and structural requirements for glycogen synthase kinase-3alpha inhibition: 2D-QSAR for 3-anilino-4-phenylmaleimides. Bioorg Med Chem 14: 8210-8218.

32. Ishiguro K, Takamatsu M, Tomizawa K, Omori A, Takahashi M, et al. (1992) Tau protein kinase I converts normal tau protein into A68-like component of paired helical filaments. J Biol Chem 267: 10897-10901.

33. Pei JJ, Tanaka T, Tung YC, Braak E, Iqbal K, et al. (1997) Distribution, levels, and activity of glycogen synthase kinase-3 in the Alzheimer disease brain. J Neuropathol Exp Neurol 56: 70-78.

34. Pei JJ, Braak E, Braak H, Grundke-Iqbal I, Iqbal K, et al. (1999) Distribution of active glycogen synthase kinase 3beta (GSK-3beta) in brains staged for Alzheimer disease neurofibrillary changes. J Neuropathol Exp Neurol 58: 1010-1019.

35. Baum L, Hansen L, Masliah E, Saitoh T (1996) Glycogen synthase kinase 3 alteration in Alzheimer disease is related to neurofibrillary tangle formation. Mol Chem Neuropathol 29: 253-261.

36. Lucas JJ, Hernández F, Gómez-Ramos P, Morán MA, Hen R, et al. (2001) Decreased nuclear beta-catenin, tau hyperphosphorylation and neurodegeneration in GSK-3beta conditional transgenic mice. EMBO J 20: 27-39.

37. Hernández F, Borrell J, Guaza C, Avila J, Lucas JJ (2002) Spatial learning deficit in transgenic mice that conditionally over-express GSK-3beta in the brain but do not form tau filaments. J Neurochem 83: 1529-1533.

38. Santana L, Uriarte E, González-Díaz H, Zagotto G, Soto-Otero R, et al. (2006) A QSAR model for in silico screening of MAO-A inhibitors. Prediction, synthesis, and biological assay of novel coumarins. J Med Chem 49: 1149-1156.

39. Marrero-Ponce Y (2004) Linear indices of the "molecular pseudograph's atom adjacency matrix": definition, significance-interpretation, and application to QSAR analysis of flavone derivatives as HIV-1 integrase inhibitors. J Chem Inf Comput Sci 44: 2010-2026.

40. Vilar S, Santana L, Uriarte E (2006) Probabilistic neural network model for the in silico evaluation of anti-HIV activity and mechanism of action. J Med Chem 49: 1118-1124.

41. Marrero-Ponce Y, Khan MT, Casañola Martín GM, Ather A, Sultankhodzhaev MN, et al. (2007) Prediction of tyrosinase inhibition activity using atom-based bilinear indices. Chem Med Chem 2: 449-478.

42. Casanola Martin, Marrero Ponce Y, Khan MT, Ather A, Sultan S, et al. (2007) TOMOCOMD-CARDD descriptors-based virtual screening of tyrosinase inhibitors: evaluation of different classification model combinations using bond-based linear indices. Bio Org Med Chem 15: 1483-1503.

43. Casañola-Martín GM, Marrero-Ponce Y, Khan MT, Ather A, Khan KM, et al. (2007) Dragon method for finding novel tyrosinase inhibitors: Biosilico identification and experimental in vitro assays. Eur J Med Chem 42: 1370-1381.

44. Núñez MB, Maguna FP, Okulik NB, Castro EA (2004) QSAR modeling of the MAO inhibitory activity of xanthones derivatives. Bioorg Med Chem Lett 14: 5611-5617.

45. Todeschini R, Consonni V (2000) Handbook of Molecular Descriptors. Wiley VCH.

46. González-Díaz H, González-Díaz Y, Santana L, Ubeira FM, Uriarte E (2008) Proteomics, networks and connectivity indices. Proteomics 8: 750-778.

47. Zhao CJ, Dai QY (2009) [Recent advances in study of antinociceptive conotoxins]. Yao Xue Xue Bao 44: 561-565.

48. Jacob RB, McDougal OM (2010) The M-superfamily of conotoxins: a review. Cell Mol Life Sci 67: 17-27.

49. Giuliani A, Di Paola L, Setola R (2009) Proteins as Networks: A Mesoscopic Approach Using Haemoglobin Molecule as Case Study. Curr Proteomics 6: 235-245.

50. Vilar S, González-Díaz H, Santana L, Uriarte E (2009) A network-QSAR model for prediction of genetic-component biomarkers in human colorectal cancer. J Theor Biol 261: 449-458.

51. Concu R, Dea-Ayuela MA, Perez-Montoto LG, Prado-Prado FJ, Uriarte E, et al. (2009) 3D entropy and moments prediction of enzyme classes and experimental-theoretic study of peptide fingerprints in Leishmania parasites. Biochim Biophys Acta 1794: 1784-1794.

52. Torrens F, Castellano G (2009) Topological Charge-Transfer Indices: From Small Molecules to Proteins. Curr Proteomics 6: 204-213.

53. Vázquez JM, Vanessa A, Seoane JA, Freire A, Serantes JA, et al. (2009) Star Graphs of Protein Sequences and Proteome Mass Spectra in Cancer Prediction. Curr Proteomics 6: 275-288.

54. González-Díaz H (2008) Quantitative studies on Structure-Activity and Structure-Property Relationships (QSAR/QSPR). Curr Top Med Chem 8: 1554.

55. Ivanciuc O (2008) Weka machine learning for predicting the phospholipidosis inducing potential. Curr Top Med Chem 8: 1691-1709.

56. González-Díaz H, Prado-Prado F, Ubeira FM (2008) Predicting antimicrobial drugs and targets with the March-Inside approach. Curr Top Med Chem 8: 1676-1690.

57. Duardo-Sánchez A, Patlewicz G, López-Díaz A (2008) Current topics on software use in medicinal chemistry: intellectual property, taxes, and regulatory issues. Curr Top Med Chem 8: 1666-1675.

58. Wang JF, Wei DQ, Chou KC (2008) Drug candidates from traditional chinese medicines. Curr Top Med Chem 8: 1656-1665.

59. Helguera AM, Combes RD, González MP, Cordeiro MN (2008) Applications of 2D descriptors in drug design: a Dragon tale. Curr Top Med Chem 8: 1628-1655.

60. González MP, Terán C, Saíz-Urra L, Teijeira M (2008) Variable selection methods in QSAR: an overview. Curr Top Med Chem 8: 1606-1627.

61. Caballero J, Fernandez M (2008) Artificial neural networks from MATLAB in medicinal chemistry. Bayesian-regularized genetic neural networks (BRGNN): application to the prediction of the antagonistic activity against human platelet thrombin receptor (PAR-1). Curr Top Med Chem 8: 1580-1605.

62. Wang JF, Wei DQ, Chou KC (2008) Pharmacogenomics and personalized use of drugs. Curr Top Med Chem 8: 1573-1579.

63. Vilar S, Cozza G, Moro S (2008) Medicinal chemistry and the molecular operating environment (MOE): application of QSAR and molecular docking to drug discovery. Curr Top Med Chem 8: 1555-1572.

64. Prado-Prado FJ, García-Mera X, González-Díaz H (2010) Multi-target spectral moment QSAR versus ANN for antiparasitic drugs against different parasite species. Bioorg Med Chem 18: 2225-2231.

65. González-Díaz H (2010) Network topological indices, drug metabolism, and distribution. Curr Drug Metab 11: 283-284.

66. Khan MT (2010) Predictions of the ADMET properties of candidate drug molecules utilizing different QSAR/QSPR modelling approaches. Curr Drug Metab 11: 285-295.

67. Mrabet Y, Semmar N (2010) Mathematical methods to analysis of topology, functional variability and evolution of metabolic systems based on different decomposition concepts. Curr Drug Metab 11: 315-341.

68. Martínez-Romero M, Vázquez-Naya JM, Rabuñal JR, Pita-Fernández S, Macenlle R, et al. (2010) Artificial intelligence techniques for colorectal cancer drug metabolism: ontology and complex network. Curr Drug Metab 11: 347-368.

69. Zhong WZ, Zhan J, Kang P, Yamazaki S (2010) Gender specific drug metabolism of PF-02341066 in rats--role of sulfoconjugation. Curr Drug Metab 11: 296-306.

70. Wang JF, Chou KC (2010) Molecular modeling of cytochrome P450 and drug metabolism. Curr Drug Metab 11: 342-346.

71. González-Díaz H, Duardo-Sanchez A, Ubeira FM, Prado-Prado F, Pérez-Montoto LG, et al. (2010) Review of MARCH-INSIDE & complex networks prediction of drugs: ADMET, anti-parasite activity, metabolizing enzymes and cardiotoxicity proteome biomarkers. Curr Drug Metab 11: 379-406.

72. García I, Diop YF, Gómez G (2010) QSAR & complex network study of the HMGR inhibitors structural diversity. Curr Drug Metab 11: 307-314.

73. Chou KC (2010) Graphic rule for drug metabolism systems. Curr Drug Metab 11: 369-378.

74. Concu R, Podda G, Ubeira FM, González-Díaz H (2010) Review of QSAR models for enzyme classes of drug targets: Theoretical background and applications in parasites, hosts, and other organisms. Curr Pharm Des 16: 2710-2723.

75. Estrada E, Molina E, Nodarse D, Uriarte E (2010) Structural contributions of substrates to their binding to P-Glycoprotein. A TOPS-MODE approach. Curr Pharm Des 16: 2676-2709.

76. García I, Fall Y, Gómez G (2010) QSAR, docking, and CoMFA studies of GSK3 inhibitors. Curr Pharm Des 16: 2666-2675.

77. González-Díaz H (2010) QSAR and complex networks in pharmaceutical design, microbiology, parasitology, toxicology, cancer, and neurosciences. Curr Pharm Des 16: 2598-2600.

78. Gonzalez-Diaz H, Romaris F, Duardo-Sanchez A, Pérez-Montoto LG, Prado-Prado F, et al. (2010) Predicting drugs and proteins in parasite infections with topological indices of complex networks: theoretical backgrounds, aplications, and legal issues. Current Pharmaceutical Design 16: 2737-2764.

79. Marrero-Ponce Y (2010) Ligand-Based Computer-Aided Discovery of Tyrosinase Inhibitors. Applications of the Tomocomd-Cardd Method to the Elucidation of New Compounds. Current Pharmaceutical Design 16: 2601-2624.

80. Munteanu CR, Fernández-Blanco E, Seoane JA, Izquierdo-Novo P, Rodríguez-Fernández JA, et al. (2010) Drug discovery and design for complex diseases through QSAR computational methods. Curr Pharm Des 16: 2640-2655.

81. Roy K, Ghosh G (2010) Exploring QSARs with Extended Topochemical Atom (ETA) indices for modeling chemical and drug toxicity. Curr Pharm Des 16: 2625-2639.

82. Speck-Planche A, Scotti MT, de Paulo-Emerenciano V (2010) Current pharmaceutical design of antituberculosis drugs: future perspectives. Current Pharmaceutical Design 16: 2656-2665.

83. Vázquez-Naya JM, Martínez-Romero M, Porto-Pazos AB, Novoa F, Valladares-Ayerbes M, et al. (2010) Ontologies of drug discovery and design for neurology, cardiology and oncology. Curr Pharm Des 16: 2724-2736.

84. Chou KC (2004) Structural bioinformatics and its impact to biomedical science. Curr Med Chem 11: 2105-2134.

85. Chou KC, Wei DQ, Du QS, Sirois S, Zhong WZ (2006) Progress in computational approach to drug development against SARS. Curr Med Chem 13: 3263-3270.

86. Prado-Prado FJ, González-Díaz H, de la Vega OM, Ubeira FM, Chou KC, et al. (2008) Unified QSAR Approach to antimicrobials. Part 3: first multi-tasking QSAR model for input-coded prediction, structural back-projection, and complex networks clustering of antiprotozoal compounds. Bioorg Med Chem 16: 5871-5880.

87. Prado-Prado FJ, Martinez de la Vega O, Uriarte E, Ubeira FM, Chou KC, et al. (2009) Unified QSAR approach to antimicrobials. 4. Multi-target QSAR modeling and comparative multi-distance study of the giant components of antiviral drug-drug complex networks. Bioorg Med Chem 17: 569-575.

88. Vanyúr R, Héberger K, Jakus J (2003) Prediction of anti-HIV-1 activity of a series of tetrapyrrole molecules. J Chem Inf Comput Sci 43: 1829-1836.

89. Vilar S, Santana L, Uriarte E (2006) Probabilistic neural network model for the in silico evaluation of anti-HIV activity and mechanism of action. J Med Chem 49: 1118-1124.

90. Mosier PD, Jurs PC (2002) QSAR/QSPR studies using probabilistic neural networks and generalized regression neural networks. J Chem Inf Comput Sci 42: 1460-1470.

91. Prado-Prado FJ, Borges F, Perez-Montoto LG, González-Díaz H (2009) Multi-

target spectral moment: QSAR for antifungal drugs vs. different fungi species. Eur J Med Chem 44: 4051-4056.

92. Overington J (2009) ChEMBL. An interview with John Overington, team leader, chemogenomics at the European Bioinformatics Institute Outstation of the European Molecular Biology Laboratory (EMBL-EBI). Interview by Wendy A. Warr. J Comput Aided Mol Des 23: 195-198.

93. Welchman R (2010) Advances and Progress in Drug Design - SMi's ninth annual meeting. IDrugs 13: 239-242.

94. Prado-Prado FJ, Ubeira FM, Borges F, González-Díaz H (2010) Unified QSAR & network-based computational chemistry approach to antimicrobials. II. Multiple distance and triadic census analysis of antiparasitic drugs complex networks. J Comput Chem 31: 164-173.

95. Prado-Prado FJ, Martinez de la Vega O, Uriarte E, Ubeira FM, Chou KC, et al. (2009) Unified QSAR approach to antimicrobials. 4. Multi-target QSAR modeling and comparative multi-distance study of the giant components of antiviral drug-drug complex networks. Bioorg Med Chem 17: 569-575.

96. Prasanna S, Daga PR, Xie A, Doerksen RJ (2009) Glycogen synthase kinase-3 inhibition by 3-anilino-4-phenylmaleimides: insights from 3D-QSAR and docking. J Comput Aided Mol Des 23: 113-127.

97. Saitoh M (2009) Design, synthesis and structure–activity relationships of 1,3,4-oxadiazole derivatives as novel inhibitors of glycogen synthase kinase-3beta. Bioorganic & Medicinal Chemistry 17: 2017-2029.

98. Freitas MP, M Goodarzi, Jensen R (2009) Feature Selection and Linear/Nonlinear Regression Methods for the Accurate Prediction of Glycogen Synthase Kinase-3ß Inhibitory Activities. J Chem Inf Model 49: 824-832.

99. Kim KH, Gaisina I, Gallier F, Holzle D, Blond SY, et al. (2009) Use of molecular modeling, docking, and 3D-QSAR studies for the determination of the binding mode of benzofuran-3-yl-(indol-3-yl)maleimides as GSK-3beta inhibitors. J Mol Model 15: 1463-1479.

100. Ryzhova EA, Koryakova AG, Bulanova EA, Mikitas OV, Karapetyan RN (2009) Syntheis, Molecular Docking, and Biological Testing of New Selective Inhibitors of Glycogen Synthase Kinase 3beta. Pharmaceutical Chemistry Journal 43: 148-153.

101. Osolodkin DI, Shulga DA, Tsareva DA, Oliferenko AA, Palyulin VA, et al. (2010) The choice of atomic charges calculation scheme in 3D-QSAR modelling of GSK-3β inhibition by paullones. Dokl Biochem Biophys 434: 274-278.

102. Zou H, Zhou L, Li Y, Cui Y, Zhong H, et al. (2010) Benzo[e]isoindole-1,3-diones as potential inhibitors of glycogen synthase kinase-3 (GSK-3). Synthesis, kinase inhibitory activity, zebrafish phenotype, and modeling of binding mode. J Med Chem 53: 994-1003.

103. Todeschini R, Consonni V (2000) Handbook of Molecular Descriptors. Wiley VCH.

104. StatSoft.Inc, Statistica (2002) (data analysis software system) version 6.0, www.statsoft.com.Statsoft, Inc.

105. Melagraki G, Afantitis A, Sarimveis H, Igglessi-Markopoulou O, Alexandridis A (2006) A novel RBF neural network training methodology to predict toxicity to Vibrio fischeri. Mol Divers 10: 213-221.

106. Concu R, Podda G, Ubeira FM, González-Díaz H (2010) Review of QSAR models for enzyme classes of drug targets: Theoretical background and applications in parasites, hosts, and other organisms. Curr Pharm Des 16: 2710-2723.

107. Roy K, Mandal AS (2008) Development of linear and nonlinear predictive QSAR models and their external validation using molecular similarity principle for anti-HIV indolyl aryl sulfones. J Enzyme Inhib Med Chem 23: 980-995.

108. Roy K, Mandal AS (2009) Predictive QSAR modeling of CCR5 antagonist piperidine derivatives using chemometric tools. J Enzyme Inhib Med Chem 24: 205-223.

109. Roy K, Pratim Roy P (2009) Comparative chemometric modeling of cytochrome 3A4 inhibitory activity of structurally diverse compounds using stepwise MLR, FA-MLR, PLS, GFA, G/PLS and ANN techniques. Eur J Med Chem 44: 2913-2922.

110. Patra JC, Singh O (2009) Artificial neural networks-based approach to design ARIs using QSAR for diabetes mellitus. J Comput Chem 30: 2494-2508.

111. Hanley JA, McNeil BJ (1982) The meaning and use of the area under a receiver operating characteristic (ROC) curve. Radiology 143: 29-36.

112. González-Díaz H, Bonet I, Terán C, De Clercq E, Bello R, et al. (2007) ANN-QSAR model for selection of anticancer leads from structurally heterogeneous series of compounds. Eur J Med Chem 42: 580-585.

113. Agüero-Chapin G, Varona-Santos J, de la Riva GA, Antunes A, González-Vlla T, et al. (2009) Alignment-free prediction of polygalacturonases with pseudofolding topological indices: experimental isolation from Coffea arabica and prediction of a new sequence. J Proteome Res 8: 2122-2128.

114. Fernandez MJ, Caballero J, Tundidor-Camba A (2006) Linear and nonlinear QSAR study of N-hydroxy-2-[(phenylsulfonyl)amino]acetamide derivatives as matrix metalloproteinase inhibitors. Bioorg Med Chem 14: 4137-4150.

24

Statins Downregulate the Constitutive Expression of HLA-DR and Reduce Intracellular CD74 in the Monocyte Cell Line Mono Mac 6

Stefan U Weber[1]*, Lutz E Lehmann[2], Makbule Kobilay[1], Frank Stüber[2] and Andreas Hoeft[1]

[1]Department of Anesthesiology and Intensive Care Medicine, University Bonn Medical Center, Germany
[2]Department of Anaesthesiology and Pain Medicine, University Hospital Bern "Inselspital", Bern, Switzerland

Abstract

Background: Statins exert immune effects and have been shown to strongly inhibit the interferon-γ induced expression of the human leukocyte antigen (HLA) DR. Monocyte HLA-DR is decreased severe in sepsis and indicates hypo inflammatory and immunosuppressive phases. The aim of the study was to investigate the statin-induced regulation of constitutive HLA-DR expression on monocytes.

Method: Monocytes and the monocyte cell line Mono Mac 6 were incubated with simvastatin, mevastatin, pravastatin and fluvastatin. HMG-Coenzyme A reductase was inhibited by l-mevalonate. Protein expression of HLA-DR, Major histocompatibility complex, invariant CD74 and apoptosis were measured by flow-cytometry. mRNA expression was assessed by PCR.

Results: Simvastatin dose dependently reduced the constitutive HLA-DR expression on monocytes starting from 500 nM. Bypassing statin-induced inhibition of HMG- Coenzyme A reductase reversed this effect. HLA-DR was also decreased in response to mevastatin, pravastatin, lovastatin and fluvastatin after 24 h. Simvastatin induced caspase-3 activation and DNA-fragmentation in a small subpopulation of Mono Mac 6 cells. HLA-DR expression was lower on apoptotic cells, but simvastatin also reduced HLA-DR on non-apoptotic cells. Simvastatin did no repress HLA-DR mRNA. For transferring HLA-DR to endosomes the chaperon CD74 is required. Intracellular CD74 was decreased by simvastatin and fluvastatin.

Conclusion: Statins decrease the constitutive expression of MHC II on monocytes and Mono Mac 6 independently of apoptosis. Reduced intracellular levels of the chaperon CD74 by statins may potentially impede HLA-DR surface expression.

Keywords: HLA-DR; MHC II; Statin; Sepsis; CD74; Monocyte

Introduction

Evidence from large observational studies indicated that statins may have benefits in the prevention of sepsis [1], acute respiratory distress syndrome [2] of patients with cardiovascular diseases [3] or kidney failure [4], as well as in ICU patients [5]. In animal models statins increase survival administered prior to and even after the experimental induction of sepsis [6]. Instead, a recent meta analysis of randomized clinical trials failed to reveal a survival benefit of *de novo* statin therapy in sepsis and acute respiratory distress syndrome [7,8]. Statin use prior to sepsis however improved survival of sepsis [9].

Statins are inhibitors of 3-hydroxy-3-methyl-glutaryl-coenzyme A reductase (HMG-CoA reductase) [10]. Apart from their mere cholesterol-lowering activity they display pleiotropic immune effects [10], for example they inhibit the interaction of antigen presenting cells and T-cells [11] and induce apoptosis in several cell types [12,13]. In endothelial cells, however, they inhibit apoptosis [14].

The interaction of antigen presenting cells and T-cells is a crucial step in the activation of the adaptive immune system and depends on the presentation of the target antigen by the major histocompatibility complex II (MHC II) [11]. The human leukocyte antigen (HLA) DR is a part of MHC II. The transport of HLA-DR from the Golgi system to endosomes, where antigen loading takes place, depends on the presence of its chaperone CD74 (invariant chain) [15,16].

Statins have been shown to strongly inhibit the interferon-γ induced expression of HLA-DR, a main component of MHC II [11]. However, in severe sepsis due to a shift from TH1 to TH2 T-cell profile [17], interferon-γ concentrations are relatively low [17-19]. Furthermore, HLA-DR expression is downregulated in severe sepsis [20,21]. A long lasting low HLA-DR expression (6 days) correlated with

sepsis severity scores and death [22]. HLA-DR in severe sepsis is down regulated on a transcriptional level [22]. Low HLA-DR is a predictor of increased mortality [23,24]. However, sepsis scores showed a better discriminatory power in the prediction of mortality [25].

The aims of this study were to investigate, (1) if different statins also inhibit the constitutive expression of HLA-DR without prior activation by interferon-γ, (2) whether this effect could be attributed to accelerated apoptosis, and whether (3) statins also affect the expression of the HLA-DR chaperone CD74.

Methods

Cell culture

Heparinized blood (Sarstedt, Frankfurt, Germany) was obtained from healthy human volunteers after informed consent with approval of the local ethics committee. The mononuclear fraction was obtained using a Ficoll gradient (Sigma-Aldrich, Steinheim, Germany). Monocytes were isolated by negative magnetic bead

*Corresponding author: Stefan U Weber, Department of Anesthesiology and Intensive Care Medicine, University Bonn Medical Center, Sigmund-Freud-Str. 25, 53105 Bonn, Germany, E-mail: stefan.weber@ukb.uni-bonn.de

separation according to manufacturer's recommendations (IMag Human Monocyte Enrichment Set, BD Biosciences, Heidelberg, Germany). Purity of monocytes after separation was monitored using flow cytometry. Monocytes were identified by double positive staining for CD14 (allophycocyanin labelled, clone M5E2, BD Biosciences, Heidelberg, Germany) and CD33 (fluorescein isothyocyanate labelled, clone HIM3-4, BD Biosciences, Heidelberg, Germany) resulting in a purity of 78% to 85%. After washing in phosphate buffered saline (PBS, Sigma-Aldrich, Steinheim, Germany), cells were placed in cell culture medium (90% RPMI 1640+10% FBS+2 mM L-glutamine (Invitrogen [GIBCO], Karlsruhe, Germany) with 100 U/mL penicillin and 100 μg/ml streptomycin at 37°C with 5% CO_2) at a density of 1×10^6 for further treatment. The Mono Mac 6 cell line (Leibnitz Institute DSMZ-German Collection of Microorganisms and Cell Cultures, Braunschweig, Germany) [26] was used as a model of monocytes to further study statin induced regulation of HLA-DR. Cultures were monitored to exclude mycoplasma contamination according to manufacturer's instructions (Venor GeM Mycoplasma Detection Kit, Sigma-Aldrich, Steinheim, Germany). Cells were cultured in 90% RPMI 1640+10% FBS+2 mM L-glutamine+non-essential amino acids+1 mM sodium pyruvate+9 μg/ml bovine insulin (Invitrogen [GIBCO], Karlsruhe, Germany) at 0.3-1.0×10^6 cells/ml in 24 well-plates (Greiner-bio-one, Solingen, Germany) at 37°C with 5% CO_2. For experiments passages 25-45 were used. The identity of the cell line was authenticated by surface staining and flowcytometric detection. The cell line expressed CD14 (BD Biosciences, Heidelberg, Germany) but not CD3 (CD3-12 AlexaFluor 488, AbD Serotec, Puchheim, Germany). For experiments, cells were placed in 24 well plates in fresh medium at a density of 1.0×10^6 cells/mL.

Cell treatments

Simvastatin, mevastatin, pravastatin, lovastatin and fluvastatin were obtained from Merck, (Darmstadt, Germany). Simvastatin and mevastatin were solved in a stock solution (20 nM) in ethanol, while the other statins were prepared in deionised water. Cells were incubated with statins in concentrations of 0.1-20 μM for 24 hours in a cell culture incubator at 37°C in an atmosphere containing 5% CO_2. To bypass the inhibition of the 3-hydroxy-3-methyl-glutaryl-Co-enzyme A reductase (HMG-CoA reductase) L-mevalonate (100 μM, Sigma Aldrich, Steinheim, Germany) was added prior to statin treatment. This concentration of L-mevalonate is sufficient to prevent the atorvastatin-induced depletion of cholesterol [27].

Apoptosis was induced by incubation with the activating monoclonal antibody anti-Fas IgM (clone CH11, Immunotech, Marseille, France) at a final concentration of 200 ng/ml containing protein G for 8 hours or by staurosporine (2 μM for 4 hours). In certain experiments lipopolysaccharide (LPS, 2 ng/mL, Escherichia coli 055:B5, Sigma Aldrich, Steinheim, Germany) or interferon-γ (IFN-γ, 400 U/ml Biomol, Hamburg, Germany) were used as controls.

Quantification of protein expression

Staining of surface proteins was carried out essentially as published earlier [21] and adapted for cell culture. 5×10^5 cells were incubated with phycoerythrin (PE) or fluorescein isothyocyanate (FITC) labelled antibodies against a non-polymorphic epitope of HLA-DR (MHC class II, clone L243, BD Biosciences, Heidelberg, Germany), HLA ABC (MHC class I, clone G 46-2.6, BD Biosciences, Heidelberg, Germany) and CD74 (clone M-B741, BD Biosciences, Heidelberg, Germany) for 30 minutes at room temperature after which the samples were fixed with FACS-Lysis-Solution (Becton Dickinson, Heidelberg, Germany),

washed twice and stored in the dark at 4°C until analysis.

For intracellular staining of proteins cells were permeabilized after blocking surface bound antigens with unlabelled antibodies against HLA-DR (clone L243, BD Biosciences, Heidelberg, Germany) or CD74 (clone M-B741, BD Biosciences, Heidelberg, Germany) respectively for one hour at 4°C. Cells were washed with PBS, (Sigma-Aldrich, Steinheim, Germany) and fixed with 750 μl PBS containing 4% paraformaldehyde (Sigma-Aldrich, Steinheim, Germany). After fixation, cells were permeabilized with 1ml PBS containing 0.5% Saponin (Sigma-Aldrich, Steinheim, Germany) and 1% bovine serum albumin (Sigma-Aldrich, Steinheim, Germany). Then, cells were incubated with PE-labeled antibodies against HLA-DR or CD74 in PBS containing 0.5% saponin/1% BSA, followed by washing.

Detection of apoptosis

The activation of caspase-3 was assessed by intracellular staining of the active fragment and evaluation by flow cytometry as described [28]. For mono-stained cells a PE-labeled antibody and for dual-staining a FITC- labeled antibody was used. DNA-fragmentation was monitored as the subdiploid DNA peak using flow cytometry according to Nicoletti et al. [29] modified as described [28].

Flow cytometry

Ten thousand events of interest were acquired by flow cytometry (FACSCalibur, Becton Dickinson, Heidelberg, Germany) and analyzed with CellQuest Pro software (CellQuest Pro, Version 4.0.2, Becton Dickinson, Heidelberg, Germany). Isotype controls were used for exclusion of background fluorescence. Mean fluorescence intensity (MFI) expressed as linear fluorescence units (LFU) and percentage of positive cells were recorded.

mRNA expression

RNA-extraction, cDNA synthesis and quantification of gene expression by real-time PCR were carried out essentially as described [30]. PCR reactions were performed under the following conditions: initial denaturation at 95°C for 15 minutes followed by 45 amplification cycles: 95°C for 15 seconds, 55°C for 35 seconds, 72°C for 30 seconds followed by an additional heating to 95°C for melting curve detection. Hypoxanthine phosphoribosyltransferase-1 (HPRT-1) was used as a housekeeping gene. It had been selected by the laboratory previously for the study of human leukocytes in the context of sepsis [30,31]. Also, in comparative studies HRPT-1 has been found suitable for gene expression studies in peripheral blood of septic patients [32]. It has also been selected for the study of HLA-DR on monocytes [33]. For specific genes the following primers were purchased: HPRT 5'-TGACCTTGATTTATTTTGCATACC, 5'-CGAGCAAGACGTTCAGTCCT (Operon, Cologne, Germany); HLA-DR α-chain Refseq No. NM_019111.3 Band Size: 97 bp Reference Positions: 712-733 (SuperArray, Frederick, MD, USA). For quantification the crossing point method was employed. Concentrations were calculated as "normalized ratio" with Relative Quantification Software (Roche, Mannheim, Germany).

Statistics

ANOVA analysis was applied to evaluate differences between different treatments. For post hoc testing the Bonferroni test was employed, when appropriate. Values were given as mean +/- SEM (standard error of the mean). Analysis was done with GraphPad for Windows (Version 3.02, San Diego, CA, USA). Experiments were carried out in duplicates and were reproduced at least twice. Significance was accepted at p<0.05.

Results

Human monocytes were exposed to varying concentrations of simvastatin and the expression of HLA-DR was recorded by flow cytometry (Figure 1a). Starting at a concentration of 500 nM simvastatin reduced the surface expression of HLA-DR (p<0.05) with a maximal effect of 28% reduction at 20 µM (p<0.01, Figure 1b). However, simvastatin did not influence the expression of MHC class I on Mono Mac 6 cells (ethanol control 765 ± 14 vs. 704 ± 26.5 LFU).

The observed effect was not restricted to simvastatin. The influence of simvastatin, mevastatin, pravastatin, lovastatin and fluvastatin on HLA-DR expression was tested in the Mono Mac 6 cell culture model at a concentration of 20 µM. All tested statins significantly lowered the expression of HLA-DR, simvastatin and fluvastatin showing the highest potencies (Table 1). Down-regulation was compared to respective solvent controls (ethanol for simvastatin and mevastatin, H₂O for the others).

To investigate whether statins inhibit HLA-DR expression in an HMG-CoA reductase dependent way, mevalonate was used to bypass statin-induced inhibition of HMG-CoA reductase. Mevalonate (100 µM, 24 h) did not downregulate HLA-DR but it reversed the statin-induced inhibition of HLA-DR expression on Mono Mac 6 cells (p<0.01, Figure 1b).

Simvastatin (20 µM, 24 h) consistently induced apoptosis only in a small proportion of Mono Mac 6 cells. It activated caspase-3 in a small proportion of cells (4.38 ± 0.02% vs. solvent control 2.33 ± 0.1% p<0.01) and caused a small but statistically significant increase in DNA-fragmentation (7.88 ± 0.23% vs. 6.1 ± 0.15%, p<0.05). Induction of apoptosis using an activating antibody to Fas or staurosporine caused a reduction of HLA-DR expression in cells with active caspase-3 (p<0.001, Figure 2a). Thus, if apoptosis induction per se decreases HLA-DR expression, simvastatin potentially could reduce HLA-DR via a mechanism of apoptosis induction. Therefore, Mono Mac 6 cells were double stained for HLA-DR and active caspase-3 after incubation with simvastatin (20 µM for 24 h). In this model simvastatin decreased HLA-DR expression both in non-apoptotic cells (p<0.001) and cells positive for caspase-3 (p<0.001 vs. ethanol control, not significant vs. active caspase-3 negative population, Figure 2a). Staining for lowered DNA-content (sub-G1 population) was used to detect late apoptotic cells. In response to simvastatin (20 µM, 24 h) HLA-DR was decreased in the subpopulation with normal DNA-content (p<0.001), but was significantly lower in cells of the sub G1 population (p<0.001, Figure 2b). When apoptosis was induced with an activating antibody against Fas or staurosporine, reduction of HLA-DR was observed in the apoptotic cell populations. In the absence of statin in cells with intact DNA, HLA-DR expression was not affected, while it decreased in the sub G1 population after incubation with aFas (p<0.001, Figures 2a and 2b).

To investigate whether lowered HLA-DR expression in response to simvastatin is regulated by inhibition of respective mRNA-expression, we quantified HLA-DR α-chain mRNA. However, Simvastatin did not change HLA-DR α-chain mRNA-expression after incubation for 3 h (1208 ± 156.6 AU; solvent control 1305 ± 502.3), 12h (1303 ± 443 AU), or 24 h (1250 ± 449.4 AU), while a positive control with interferon-γ massively increased mRNA expression (7268 ± 1699 AU, p<0.001). Correspondingly, we evaluated the intracellular HLA-

DR protein content. In contrast to the findings regarding surface expression, intracellular HLA-DR content did not decrease in response to simvastatin but showed a tendency to increase (65.55 ± 0.46 vs. 56.45 ± 2.40, p<0.05).

Intracellular HLA-DR is sorted from the golgi apparatus to late endosomes in the presence of its chaperone CD74. This step is necessary for later transfer of HLA-DR to the cell surface. Surface CD74 expression was not affected by simvastatin (97.48% + -9.2% vs. solvent control 98.7 ± 1.99% relative MFI). Regarding intracellular CD74 protein content in Mono Mac 6 cells, we observed that simvastatin as well as fluvastatin dose-dependently decreased the expression of CD74 (p<0.001 vs. ethanol control, Figure 3). 20 µM simvastatin was as effective as LPS 2 ng/ml in Mono Mac 6 cells. As a positive control, interferon-γ induced CD74 expression.

Discussion

The study shows that the constitutive HLA-DR expression on monocytes and Mono Mac 6 cells is downregulated by statins. This process does not depend on apoptosis induction by statins. Furthermore, statins also inhibit the intracellular expression of CD74, the invariant chain.

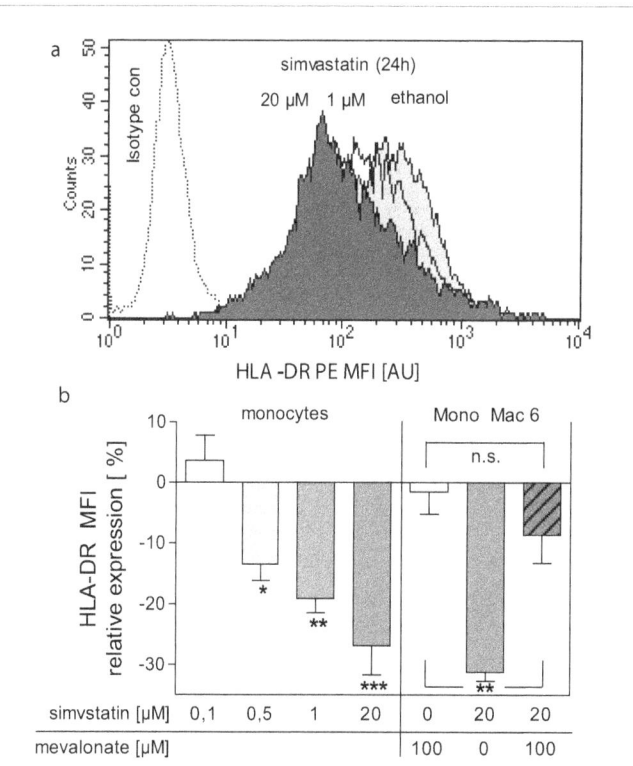

Figure 1: MHC II surface expression in response to simvastatin. Human monocytes from healthy volunteers were exposed to simvastatin ranging from 100 nM to 20 µM or respective solvent controls for 24 h.
a) Overlay histograms of HLA-DR PE fluorescence after exposure to simvastatin 1 µM and 20 µM compared to ethanol only are shown. The dotted line represents the isotype control (isotype con).
b) The relative decrease of surface HLA-DR mean fluorescence intensity (MFI) is displayed in relation to respective ethanol controls [%]. To test the influence of HMG-CoA inhibition on HLA-DR expression Mono Mac cells were incubated with simvastatin (20 µM, 24 h) or ethanol as a control. In certain experiments also the intermediate mevalonate (100 µM, 24 h) was added to restore the mevalonate pathway by supplementation of the HMG-CoA product. The results of this experiment are displayed in the three columns to the right; n.s. not significant, *p<0.05, **p<0.01, ***p<0.001.

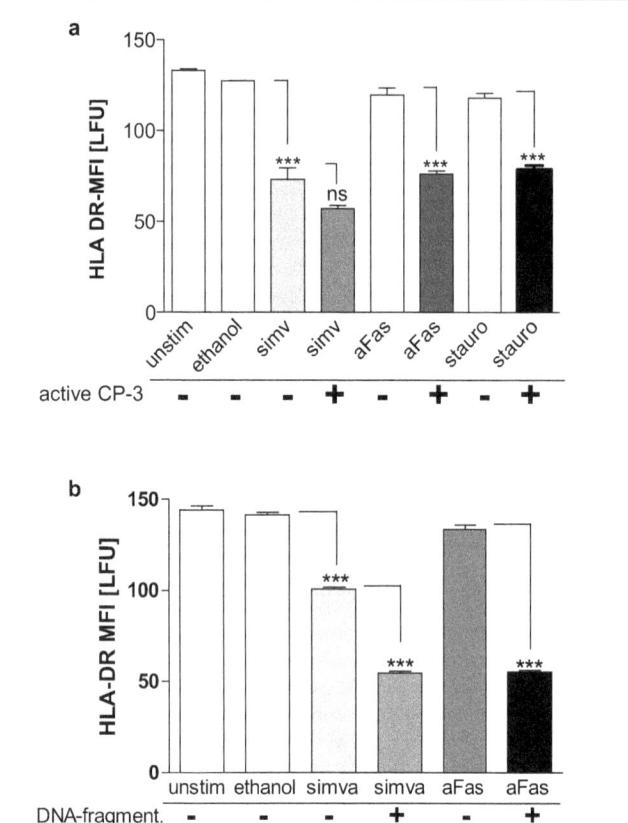

Figure 2: HLA-DR expression on apoptotic and non-apoptotic cells. Mono Mac 6 cells were incubated with simvastatin (20 µM, 24 h). Alternatively, apoptosis was induced by treatment with an activating antibody against Fas (aFas, clone CH11) or staurosporine (stauro, 2 µM for 4 h). Cells were dually stained for intracellular active caspase 3 (CP-3) and HLA-DR.
a) HLA-DR surface expression was evaluated in the non-apoptotic (active CP-3 negative) and apoptotic (active CP-3 positive) subpopulations; ns not significant, ***p<0.001.
b) Cells were dually stained for DNA-fragmentation and surface HLA-DR expression and HLA-DR expression was monitored in non-apoptotic (G1 peak) and apoptotic (sub-G1 region) cells; ***p<0.001.

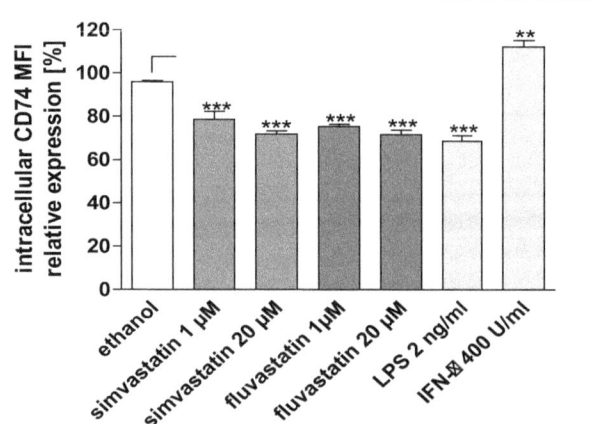

Figure 3: Modulation of CD74 (invariant chain) expression by statins. Simvastatin and fluvastatin at concentrations of 1-20 µM were incubated with Mono Mac 6 cells for 24 h. LPS (2 ng/ml) and Interferon-γ (400 U/ml) were used as control. Intracellular expression of CD74 was analyzed by flow cytometry. The graph displays the intracellular CD74 expression relative to untreated controls [%]; **p<0.01, ***p<0.001.

Initially, statins have been shown to strongly inhibit the interferon-γ mediated induction of HLA-DR on macrophages and endothelial cells [11], while the constitutive expression of MHC II on dendritic cells was not affected by atorvastatin [11]. In phytohemagglutinin-stimulated T- and B-cells simvastatin repressed MHC II without prior interferon-γ treatment. In sepsis, due to a shift from TH1 to TH2 cytokine profile, interferon-γ concentrations are relatively low [17-19]. Therefore, analysis of constitutive MHC II expression in resting monocytes may better reflect the situation in sepsis than after interferon-γ stimulation. Our studies indicate that also the constitutive MHC II expression on resting monocytes and Mono Mac 6 cells is repressed by statins. The extent of inhibition is comparable to the effect of simvastatin observed in unstimulated dendritic cells in another study [34].

Significant repression of surface HLA-DR in our experiments was observed starting at a concentration of 500 nM. In human liver microsomes the half maximal inhibitory concentrations (IC50) for simvastatin regarding HMG-CoA reductase activity is 100-300 nM [35]. In studies downregulation of interferon-gamma induced HLA-DR by atorvastatin [11] and induction of macrophage apoptosis by lovastatin [13] were observed at statin concentration of 10 µM. In endothelial cells simvastatin inhibited apoptosis at 1 µM. Thus, the statin concentrations causing HLA-DR reduction observed in the current study are in accordance with other described immune effects of statins.

Thus, the effect on HLA-DR appears at physiologically relevant concentrations. Statins exhibit several effects independent of HMG-CoA inhibition such as inhibition of P-glycoprotein [36]. The observed effect in our study however could be attributed to the inhibition of HMG-CoA reductase since bypassing HMG-CoA reductase by addition of mevalonate reversed the action of statin.

In our experimental setting simvastatin and fluvastatin were the most efficient statins in regard to decrease in HLA-DR surface expression followed by pravastatin, lovastatin and mevastatin. While statins are taken up actively in liver cells, in other cell types passive diffusion across membranes occurs [37]. Fluvastatin and simvastatin are more lipophilic than pravastatin which results for example in a lower potency of pravastatin to inhibit vascular smooth muscle proliferation [37]. Similarly, differences in lipophilicity may account for the different potencies of statins to repress constitutive HLA-DR expression in our study.

Apart from other anti-inflammatory actions, statins have been demonstrated to induce apoptosis in RAW264.7 macrophages [12], murine bone marrow cells [13] and resting T-cells [38]. Mechanisms included activation of the Rac1/Cdc42/JNK pathway [13] and an increase of the Bax/Bcl-2 ratio [38]. In our model system Mono Mac 6 simvastatin induced apoptosis only in a small subpopulation of cells. We were able to demonstrate that induction of apoptosis by activation of the receptor mediated extrinsic pathway or by staurosporine also decreases HLA-DR surface expression. Therefore, statins in principle could decrease HLA-DR already by induction of apoptosis. However, dual staining in flow cytometry revealed that HLA-DR is clearly downregulated by simvastatin in non-apoptotic cells. Thus, the MHC II lowering action of statins cannot only be attributed to induction of apoptosis in our model but occurs independently of apoptosis. Yet, in other cell types, where statins induce apoptosis more potently, this mechanism could become more important and may distort findings if experiments are not controlled for apoptosis.

Statin	Δ MFI [%] +/- SEM	p
Mevastatin	-7.27+/-0.66	<0.05
Pravastatin	-14.07+/-1.44	<0.01
Lovastatin	-14.39+/-1.22	<0.01
Simvastatin	-26.98+/-2.12	<0.001
Fluvastatin	-29.50+/-3.09	<0.001

Mono Mac 6, statins at 20 μM for 24 h. Δ MFI [%]: reduction of fluorescence in relation to untreated cells [%], SEM: Standard Error of the Mean, ANOVA with Bonferroni post-test, p versus control treatment.

Table 1: Modulation of HLA-DR expression by different statins.

The transcription of HLA-DR and other proteins of the MHC II group is controlled by the class II transactivator (CIITA) [39]. In interferon-γ treated human vascular endothelial cells statins inhibited HLA-DR expression on a transcriptional level via decreased expression of CIITA and its promoter pIV-CTA [11]. Yet, in U937 monocytes, HeLa cervical carcinoma cells and human activated primary T-cells the statin effect on interferon-γ induced MHC II regulation is regulated on a post-transcriptional level [39]. Due to the fact that the mevalonate pathway produces both cholesterol and isoprenoids, post-transcriptional activities of statins include disruption of cholesterol microdomains [40] and inhibition of small G-proteins that need isoprenoid modifications for proper targeting within the cell [41]. In unstimulated Mono Mac 6 cells we did not observe inhibition of HLA-DR α-chain mRNA expression by simvastatin. Therefore, post-transcriptional mechanisms are likely to be involved.

In the endoplasmatic reticulum (ER) MHC II heterodimers associate with the invariant chain CD74, which assists egress from the ER and directs MHC II complexes into the endocytic pathway where further processing and antigen loading take place [15]. Mice lacking invariant chain expression show a marked reduction in surface MHC class II expression [42]. While interferon-γ upregulates CD74, LPS-priming reduces intracellular CD74, which has been shown to inhibit HLA-DR expression on monocytes in response [43]. In Mono Mac 6 cells we could show that both simvastatin and fluvastatin decreased intracellular CD74. Reduced availability of the invariant chain in response to statin treatment may contribute to reduced HLA-DR surface expression by impeding HLA-DR transport. This finding may reflect the results of a clinical study where CD74 gene expression increased and correlated with HLA-DR expression during the recovery phase from septic shock [44]. Decreased CD74 expression in whole blood predicted mortality after septic shock [45]. In further studies the mechanism of statin-induced CD74 regulation and its effect on HLA-DR expression should be explored.

Evidence points towards a protective effect of statin use prior to sepsis [2]. However, it is still a matter of debate whether inhibition of HLA-DR expression by statins is beneficial in sepsis [46], since monocytes are deactivated in sepsis by reduction of HLA-DR [20,21,47], and since low HLA-DR expression during sepsis is associated with increased mortality [23,24]. During sepsis and LPS-tolerance, HLA-DR is downregulated on a transcriptional level [48,49]. Thus, post-transcriptional effects by statins could result in additive HLA-DR decrease. Large observational studies have shown a sepsis-preventing effect of statin intake [3,4]. Potentially, attenuation of the initial pro-inflammatory phase in early sepsis by chronic HLA-DR downregulation may mitigate the ensuing dangerous immune dysregulation. On the other hand downregulation of monocyte HLA-DR with ensuing monocyte deactivation may contribute to failure of statins in the treatment of sepsis, [7,8] when started after the onset of sepsis.

In conclusion, statins reduce the constitutive expression of HLA-DR on monocytes via a mechanism that does not depend on apoptosis induction but may be associated with reduced expression of the chaperon invariant chain CD74. Further studies should analyze the statin-induced down regulation of the invariant chain CD74 in the context of HLA-DR downregulation in patients with sepsis.

Acknowledgement

The authors would like to thank Caroline von dem Bussche for excellent technical assistance. The authors declare that they have no conflict of interest. The work was supported by intramural funding from BONFOR (Bonn University research grant organisation).

References

1. Terblanche M, Almog Y, Rosenson RS, Smith TS, Hackam DG (2007) Statins and sepsis: multiple modifications at multiple levels. Lancet Infect Dis 7: 358-368.

2. Mansur A, Steinau M, Popov AF, Ghadimi M, Beissbarth T, et al. (2016) Impact of statin therapy on mortality in patients with sepsis-associated acute respiratory distress syndrome (ARDS) depends on ARDS severity: a prospective observational cohort study. BMC Med 13: 128.

3. Hackam DG, Mamdani M, Li P, Redelmeier DA (2006) Statins and sepsis in patients with cardiovascular disease: a population-based cohort analysis. Lancet 367: 413-418.

4. Gupta R, Plantinga LC, Fink NE, Melamed ML, Coresh J, et al. (2007) Statin use and sepsis events [corrected] in patients with chronic kidney disease. JAMA 297: 1455-1464.

5. Schmidt H, Hennen R, Keller A, Russ M, Muller -Werdan U, et al. (2006) Association of statin therapy and increased survival in patients with multiple organ dysfunction syndrome. Intensive Care Med 32: 1248-1251.

6. Merx MW, Liehn EA, Graf J, van de Sandt A, Schaltenbrand M, et al. (2005) Statin treatment after onset of sepsis in a murine model improves survival. Circulation 112: 117-124.

7. Thomas G, Hraiech S, Loundou A, Truwit J, Kruger P, et al. (2016) Statin therapy in critically-ill patients with severe sepsis: a review and meta-analysis of randomized clinical trials. Minerva Anestesiol 81: 921-930.

8. National Heart, Lung and Blood Institute ARDS Clinical Trials Network, Truwit JD, Bernard GR, et al. (2014) Rosuvastatin for sepsis-associated acute respiratory distress syndrome. N Engl J Med 370: 2191-2200.

9. Kruger P, Bailey M, Bellomo R, Cooper DJ, Harward M, et al. (2013) A multicenter randomized trial of atorvastatin therapy in intensive care patients with severe sepsis. Am J Respir Crit Care Med 187: 743-750.

10. Gao F, Linhartova L, Johnston AM, Thickett DR (2008) Statins and sepsis. Br J Anaesth 100: 288-298.

11. Kwak B, Mulhaupt F, Myit S, Mach F (2000) Statins as a newly recognized type of immunomodulator. Nat Med 6: 1399-1402.

12. Kim YC, Song SB, Lee MH, Kang KI, Lee H, et al. (2006) Simvastatin induces caspase-independent apoptosis in LPS-activated RAW264.7 macrophage cells. Biochem Biophys Res Commun 339: 1007-1014.

13. Liang SL, Liu H, Zhou A (2006) Lovastatin-induced apoptosis in macrophages through the Rac1/Cdc42/JNK pathway. J Immunol 177: 651-656.

14. Kureishi Y, Luo Z, Shiojima I, Bialik A, Fulton D, et al. (2000) The HMG-CoA reductase inhibitor simvastatin activates the protein kinase Akt and promotes angiogenesis in normocholesterolemic animals. Nat Med 6: 1004-1010.

15. Rocha N, Neefjes J (2008) MHC class II molecules on the move for successful antigen presentation. EMBO J 27: 1-5.

16. Karakikes I, Morrison IE, O'Toole P, Metodieva G, Navarrete CV, et al. (2012) Interaction of HLA-DR and CD74 at the cell surface of antigen-presenting cells by single particle image analysis. FASEB J 26: 4886-4896.

17. Hotchkiss RS, Karl IE (2003) The pathophysiology and treatment of sepsis. N Engl J Med 348: 138-150.

18. Hotchkiss RS, Chang KC, Grayson MH, Tinsley KW, Dunne BS, et al. (2003) Adoptive transfer of apoptotic splenocytes worsens survival, whereas adoptive transfer of necrotic splenocytes improves survival in sepsis. Proc Natl Acad Sci USA 100: 6724-6729.

19. Kox WJ, Volk T, Kox SN, Volk HD (2000) Immunomodulatory therapies in sepsis. Intensive Care Med 26 Suppl 1: S124-128.

20. Docke WD, Randow F, Syrbe U, Krausch D, Asadullah K, et al. (1997) Monocyte deactivation in septic patients: restoration by IFN-gamma treatment. Nat Med 3: 678-681.

21. Docke WD, Hoflich C, Davis KA, Rottgers K, Meisel C, et al. (2005) Monitoring temporary immunodepression by flow cytometric measurement of monocytic HLA-DR expression: a multicenter standardized study. Clin Chem 51: 2341-2347.

22. Le Tulzo Y, Pangault C, Amiot L, Guilloux V, Tribut O, et al. (2004) Monocyte human leukocyte antigen-DR transcriptional downregulation by cortisol during septic shock. Am J Respir Crit Care Med 169: 1144-1151.

23. Monneret G, Lepape A, Voirin N, Bohe J, Venet F, et al. (2006) Persisting low monocyte human leukocyte antigen-DR expression predicts mortality in septic shock. Intensive Care Med 32: 1175-1183.

24. Caille V, Chiche JD, Nciri N, Berton C, Gibot S, et al. (2004) Histocompatibility leukocyte antigen-D related expression is specifically altered and predicts mortality in septic shock but not in other causes of shock. Shock 22: 521-526.

25. Hynninen M, Pettila V, Takkunen O, Orko R, Jansson SE, et al. (2003) Predictive value of monocyte histocompatibility leukocyte antigen-DR expression and plasma interleukin-4 and -10 levels in critically ill patients with sepsis. Shock 20: 1-4.

26. Ziegler-Heitbrock HW, Thiel E, Futterer A, Herzog V, Wirtz A, et al. (1988) Establishment of a human cell line (Mono Mac 6) with characteristics of mature monocytes. Int J Cancer 41: 456-461.

27. Warita K, Warita T, Beckwitt CH, Schurdak ME, Vazquez A, et al. (2014) Statin-induced mevalonate pathway inhibition attenuates the growth of mesenchymal-like cancer cells that lack functional E-cadherin mediated cell cohesion. Sci Rep 4: 7593.

28. Weber SU, Koch A, Kankeleit J, Schewe JC, Siekmann U, et al. (2009) Hyperbaric oxygen induces apoptosis via a mitochondrial mechanism. Apoptosis 14: 97-107.

29. Nicoletti I, Migliorati G, Pagliacci MC, Grignani F, Riccardi C (1991) A rapid and simple method for measuring thymocyte apoptosis by propidium iodide staining and flow cytometry. J Immunol Methods 139: 271-279.

30. Weber SU, Schewe JC, Lehmann LE, Muller S, Book M, et al. (2008) Induction of Bim and Bid gene expression during accelerated apoptosis in severe sepsis. Crit Care 12: R128.

31. Book M, Chen Q, Lehmann LE, Klaschik S, Weber S, et al. (2007) Inducibility of the endogenous antibiotic peptide beta-defensin 2 is impaired in patients with severe sepsis. Crit Care 11: R19.

32. Cummings M, Sarveswaran J, Homer-Vanniasinkam S, Burke D, Orsi NM (2014) Glyceraldehyde-3-phosphate dehydrogenase is an inappropriate housekeeping gene for normalising gene expression in sepsis. Inflammation 37: 1889-1894.

33. Wolk K, Kunz S, Crompton NE, Volk HD, Sabat R (2003) Multiple mechanisms of reduced major histocompatibility complex class II expression in endotoxin tolerance. J Biol Chem 278: 18030-18036.

34. Yilmaz A, Reiss C, Weng A, Cicha I, Stumpf C, et al. (2006) Differential effects of statins on relevant functions of human monocyte-derived dendritic cells. J Leukoc Biol 79: 529-538.

35. Dansette PM, Jaoen M, Pons C (2000) HMG-CoA reductase activity in human liver microsomes: comparative inhibition by statins. Exp Toxicol Pathol 52: 145-148.

36. Wang E, Casciano CN, Clement RP, Johnson WW (2001) HMG-CoA reductase inhibitors (statins) characterized as direct inhibitors of P-glycoprotein. Pharm Res 18: 800-806.

37. White CM (2002) A review of the pharmacologic and pharmacokinetic aspects of rosuvastatin. J Clin Pharmacol 42: 963-970.

38. Samson KT, Minoguchi K, Tanaka A, Oda N, Yokoe T, et al. (2005) Effect of fluvastatin on apoptosis in human CD4+ T cells. Cell Immunol 235: 136-144.

39. Kuipers HF, van den Elsen PJ (2005) Statins and control of MHC2TA gene transcription. Nat Med 11: 365-366.

40. Kuipers HF, Biesta PJ, Groothuis TA, Neefjes JJ, Mommaas AM, et al. (2005) Statins affect cell-surface expression of major histocompatibility complex class II molecules by disrupting cholesterol-containing microdomains. Hum Immunol 66: 653-665.

41. Kuipers HF, van den Elsen PJ (2007) Immunomodulation by statins: inhibition of cholesterol vs. isoprenoid biosynthesis. Biomed Pharmacother 61: 400-407.

42. Bikoff EK, Huang LY, Episkopou V, van Meerwijk J, Germain RN, et al. (1993) Defective major histocompatibility complex class II assembly, transport, peptide acquisition, and CD4+ T cell selection in mice lacking invariant chain expression. J Exp Med 177: 1699-1712.

43. Wolk K, Kunz S, Crompton NE, Volk HD, Sabat R (2003) Multiple mechanisms of reduced major histocompatibility complex class II expression in endotoxin tolerance. J Biol Chem 278: 18030-18036.

44. Payen D, Lukaszewicz AC, Belikova I, Faivre V, Gelin C, et al. (2008) Gene profiling in human blood leucocytes during recovery from septic shock. Intensive Care Med 34: 1371-1376.

45. Cazalis MA, Friggeri A, Cave L, Demaret J, Barbalat V, et al. (2013) Decreased HLA-DR antigen-associated invariant chain (CD74) mRNA expression predicts mortality after septic shock. Crit Care 17: R287.

46. Monneret G, Venet F (2007) Statins and sepsis: do we really need to further decrease monocyte HLA-DR expression to treat septic patients? Lancet Infect Dis 7: 697-699.

47. Nierhaus A, Montag B, Timmler N, Frings DP, Gutensohn K, et al. (2003) Reversal of immunoparalysis by recombinant human granulocyte-macrophage colony-stimulating factor in patients with severe sepsis. Intensive Care Med 29: 646-651.

48. Wolk K, Docke WD, von Baehr V, Volk HD, Sabat R (2000) Impaired antigen presentation by human monocytes during endotoxin tolerance. Blood 96: 218-223.

49. Pachot A, Monneret G, Brion A, Venet F, Bohe J, et al. (2005) Messenger RNA expression of major histocompatibility complex class II genes in whole blood from septic shock patients. Crit Care Med 33: 31-38.

25

Structure-Activity Relationship Study and Function-Based Petidomimetic Design of Human Opiorphin with Improved Bioavailability Property and Unaltered Analgesic Activity

Alexandra Bogeas[1], Evelyne Dufour[1], Jean-François Bisson[2], Michael Messaoudi[2] and C Rougeot[1]*

[1]Institut Pasteur, Laboratoire de Pharmacologie de la Douleur, Département de Biologie Structurale et Chimie, 25 rue du Dr. Roux 75724. Paris cedex 15, France
[2]ETAP-Ethologie Appliqué-Technopôle de Nancy-Brabois-13, rue du Bois de la Champelle, 54500 Vandoeuvre-lès-Nancy, France

Abstract

Human opiorphin inhibits enkephalin-inactivating ectopeptidases to produce analgesic and antidepressant-like effects in standard murine models *via* activation of μ and/or δ opioid pathways. It is an endogenous peptide regulator of enkephalin bioavailability. Opiorphin molecule, a QRFSR-peptide, is thus a promising prototype for the design of an improved class of analgesics. The major limitation on the clinical use of peptide drugs is their rapid degradation by circulating peptidases. Our goal was, therefore, to search for functional derivatives of opiorphin with improved metabolic stability. In order to identify the functional amino acid groups required for opiorphin inhibitory potency toward both AP-N and NEP human ectopeptidases, we used the Structure-Activity Relationship (SAR) method. From this data, a series of opiorphin derivatives was designed and selected. The best performing compound then underwent a complete metabolic profile using *in vitro* kinetic models. Finally, its safety profile relative to the native peptide as well as its efficacy in an *in vivo* rat model was evaluated.

We demonstrated a tight structural selectivity in the functional interaction of opiorphin with both human NEP and AP-N targets by SAR studies. Nevertheless, we found that the addition of an N-terminal Zn-chelating group, a Cys-thiol group and the replacement of the first labile peptide bond by a polyethylene surrogate, a $[CH_2]_6$ linker, and, finally, the substitution of Ser[4] by Ser-O-$[CH_2]_8$, results in a high performing C-$[(CH_2)_6]$-QRF[S-O-$[CH_2]_8$]-R peptidomimetic product. This designed opiorphin analog shows reinforced inhibitory potency toward human AP-N activity (more than 10-fold increase) and NEP activities (more than 40-fold increase) relative to the QRFSR native peptide. It also has increased metabolic stability in human plasma and yet retains full analgesic activity in the behavioral formalin-induced rat pain model. C-$[(CH_2)_6]$-QRF[S-O-$[CH_2]_8$]-R thus represents a very attractive and promising analgesic drug-candidate.

Keywords: Opiorphin; Inhibitor of enkephalin-inactivating peptidases; Functional peptidomimetics; Analgesic effect; Human opioid pathway

Introduction

Opiorphin QRFSR-peptide is an endogenous human regulator that was discovered using a functional biochemical approach [1,2]. Its characterization demonstrated that it is an authentic physiological dual inhibitor of Zn-dependent metallo-ectopeptidases, neutral endopeptidase (NEP EC3.4.21.11) and aminopeptidase N (AP-N EC3.4.11.2). These enzymes are implicated in the rapid inactivation of endogenous circulating opioid agonists, namely the enkephalins. As a consequence, opiorphin improves the specific binding and affinity of enkephalin-related peptides to membrane opioid receptors [3]. The enkephalin neuropeptides play key roles in the control of nociceptive transmission and in the modulation of the activity of cerebral structures governing the motivation and the adaptive balance of emotional states [4-8]. By increasing the half-life of circulating enkephalins, opiorphin, at systemically or centrally active doses (1-2 mg/kg I.V. or 5-10 µg/kg I.C.V.), produces analgesia in various murine models of pain [1,9,10]. At equivalent doses, opiorphin also exerts antidepressant-like effects in the standard model of depression, the forced swim test [11,12]. All opiorphin-induced effects are specifically mediated *via* endogenous enkephalin-related activation of μ and/or δ opioid pathways.

The discovery of opiorphin is the first demonstration of the existence of a physiological regulator of enkephalin bioavailability in humans. As an upstream modulator of opioid pathways in humans, it is thus of major interest from a therapeutic points of view. Indeed, endogenous human opiorphin appears to intervene in the process of adaptation mediated by enkephalins that is associated with nociception. As a consequence, opiorphin is a promising template for the design of a new class of drug-candidates able to efficiently alleviate a number of severe and chronic pain syndromes, without morphine side effects. The actions of opiorphin could be induced at a specific opioid receptor restricted pathway dynamically stimulated by natural effectors, such as enkephalins, that are recruited according to the nature, duration and intensity of the stimulus. This mechanism of action avoids excessive stimulation of ubiquitously distributed opioid receptors and prevents serious side effects such as respiratory depression, sedation, constipation, physical and psychic dependence and tolerance that have been reported in the case of μ-opioid agonists. We previously demonstrated that opiorphin subchronic intake does not develop significant abuse liability or antinociceptive drug tolerance. In addition, anti-peristalsis is not observed [10].

A major limitation to the clinical use of peptide drugs, however,

*Corresponding author: C Rougeot, Institut Pasteur, Laboratoire de Pharmacologie de la Douleur, Département de Biologie Structurale et Chimie 25 rue du Dr. Roux 75724. Paris cedex 15, France, E-mail: catherine.rougeot@pasteur.fr

is their rapid degradation by circulating peptidases and the limited permeation of peptides across biological barriers. In order to search for functional derivatives of opiorphin endowed with improved half-life stability and bioavailability properties a Structure-Activity Relationship (SAR) study on opiorphin was first carried out. Then opiorphin analogs were tested for their inhibitory potency against the two membrane-anchored human ectoenzymes, NEP that has both endopeptidase and carboxydipeptidase activities and AP-N, by using selective fluorescence-based enzyme *in vitro* assays [13-15]. Comparative degradation kinetics were done using experimental *in vitro* systems to evaluate metabolic half-life in human plasma, which is a reliable prediction model for *in vivo* stability. Metabolic stability parameters in human liver microsomes were also determined.

The final aim of the research described here was to design and analyze functional analogs of opiorphin that display *in vivo* bioavailability properties superior to the native peptide, in particular, an increase in circulating peptidase resistance and in permeation across epithelial and endo-epithelial membrane barriers, without affecting *in vitro* and *in vivo* biological properties, namely, selective inhibition of human NEP and AP-N ectoenkephalinases and potent inhibition of pain behavioral responses in rat model.

Materials and Methods

Chemicals

All peptides, human opiorphin and opiorphin derivatives, were synthesized by Genosphere Biotechnologies (Paris-France). Analytical RP-HPLC and electrospray MS confirmed the purity (≥ 95%) and molecular mass of the synthesized peptides.

FRET-based Enzyme *In Vitro* assays

Formal kinetic analysis was performed for each assay using real-time fluorescence monitoring of specific substrate hydrolysis.

Sources of the human ectopeptidases: Human recombinant NEP and human recombinant AP-N (devoid of their respective N-terminal cytosol and transmembrane segment) were purchased from R&D Systems (France) and used as a pure source of peptidases. Membrane-anchored NEP and AP-N expressed by a human cell line in culture (serum-free medium), namely, LNCaP epithelial prostate cells, were also used as a source of native ectopeptidases. Human recombinant DPPIV (dipeptidyl amino peptidase IV) and human recombinant ECE-1 (endothelin converting enzyme), purchased from R&D Systems, were used to assess compound specificity.

Substrates and inhibitors: *In vitro*, CarboxyDi- and Endo-Peptidase NEP activities were assayed by measuring the breakdown of the following synthetic selective substrates: i, Abz-dR-G-L-EDDnp FRET-peptide, an internally quenched fluorescent substrate specific for NEP-EndoPeptidase activity, was synthesized by Thermo-Fisher Scientific (Germany); ii, Abz-R-G-F-K-DnpOH FRET-peptide, an internally quenched fluorescent substrate specific for NEP-CarboxyDiPeptidase activity, was synthesized by Thermo-Fisher Scientific (Germany) [13]; iii, Mca-R-P-P-G-F-S-A-F-K-(Dnp)-OH FRET-peptide (Mca-BK2), an intramolecularly quenched fluorogenic peptide structurally related to bradykinin, which is a selective substrate for measuring NEP and ECE activity, was purchased from R&D Systems; iv, G-P-7amido-4-Mca (G-P-Mca), a selective substrate for measuring DPPIV activity, was purchased from Sigma-Aldrich (France).

FRET is the distance-dependent transfer of energy from a donor fluorophore (Abz=ortho-aminobenzoyl or Mca=7-methoxycoumarin-4-yl-acetyl) to an acceptor fluorophore (DnpOH=2,4-dinitrophenyl or EDDnp=2,4-dinitrophenyl ethylenediamine).

The modified tritiated substance P ([(3,4,3H)Pro^2-Sar9-Met(O$_2$)^{11}]-SP, NEN-PerkinElmer) was also used to assess for the specific endopeptidase activity of membrane-bound human NEP under relevant biological conditions of measurement [1,16].

H-alanine-AMC (AMC=amino-methyl-coumarin), Ala-AMC, a fluorogenic substrate for measuring aminopeptidase activity was purchased from Bachem (Switzerland).

Measurement of Ectopeptidase Activities using 96-well fluorimetric assays: Under conditions of initial velocity measurement (steady state), hydrolysis of substrates was measured by real-time monitoring of their metabolism rate by the respective recombinant and membrane-bound peptidases, in the presence and absence of tested inhibitory compound (concentrations ranging from 0.01 to 100 µM).

Measurement of NEP-endopeptidase activity using FRET specific peptide-substrate, Abz-dR-G-L-EDDnp: Using the black half-area 96 well micro-plate, the standard reaction consisted of enzyme (12 ng) in 100 mM Tris-HCl pH 7 containing 200 mM NaCl and 0.05% Brij 35 (100 µl final volume). The substrate (15 µM final concentration) was added after preincubation for 10 min at 28°C and the kinetics of appearance of the fluorescent signal (RFU) was directly analyzed for 20-40 min at 28°C (2 to 3 min interval successive measures) by using a fluorimeter micro-plate reader (monochromator Infinite 200-Tecan) at 320 nm and 420 nm excitation and emission wavelengths, respectively.

Measurement of NEP-Carboxy DiPept idase activity using FRET specific peptide-substrate Abz-R-G-F-K-DnpOH: Using the black half-area 96 well microplate, the standard reaction consisted of enzyme (2.5 ng) in 100 mM Tris-HCl pH 6.5 containing 50 mM NaCl and 0.05% Brij 35 (100 µl final volume). The substrate (4 µM final concentration) was added after pre incubation for 10 min and the kinetics of appearance of the fluorescent signal (RFU) was directly analyzed for 20-40 min at 28°C (2 to 3 min-interval successive measures) using the fluorimeter reader at 320 nm excitation and 420 nm emission wavelengths.

In addition, the intra-molecularly quenched fluorogenic peptide, Mca-BK2 (2.5 µM final concentration), was submitted to hydrolysis by 2 ng rhNEP under the same experimental conditions as those described above. Under these conditions the hNEP-enzyme acted upon Mca-R-P-P-G-F-S-A-F-K-(Dnp)-OH as a CarboxyDiPeptidase preferentially cleaving the A-F bond but also as an EndoPeptidase cleaving the G-F bond.

To measure ECE1-ectopeptidase activity, the same protocol described previously was applied except that Mca-BK2 substrate was used at 7.5 µM final concentration and rhECE1 at 5 ng final concentration.

Measurement of DPPIV activity using FRET specific peptide-substrate G-P-7amido-4-Mca: Using the black half-area 96 well microplate, the standard reaction consisted of enzyme (7 ng) in 100 mM Tris-HCl pH 8 (100 µl final volume). The substrate (5 µM final concentration) was added after preincubation for 10 min and the kinetics of appearance of the fluorescent signal (RFU) was directly analyzed for 20-40 min at 28°C (2.3 min-interval successive measures) using the fluorimeter reader at 380 nm excitation and 460 nm emission wavelengths.

Measurement of AP-N-ectopeptidase activity using Ala-AMC substrate: Using the black half-area 96 well microplate the standard reaction consisted of enzyme (3.5 ng) in 100mM Tris-HCl pH 7.0 (100 µl final volume). The Ala-AMC substrate (20 µM final concentrations) was added after preincubation for 10 min at 28°C and the kinetics of appearance of the signal was monitored for 20-40 min at 28°C using the fluorimeter reader at 380 nm excitation and 460 nm emission wavelengths.

Measurement of membrane human NEP-endopeptidase activity using tritiated substance P substrate: the method used was previously described in Wisner et al. and Rougeot et al. [1,16].

The background rate of substrate autolysis, representing the fluorescent signal obtained in the absence of enzyme, was subtracted to calculate the initial velocities in RFU (Relative Fluorescent Unit)/min. Data were analyzed using Magellan 6.0 software to evaluate initial velocities and with Excel Microsoft software. IC_{50} estimates were obtained from a sigmoidal curve fit to a plot of % inhibitory activity *versus* log inhibitor concentration, using Prism software. For each curve, inhibitors were tested across a range of concentrations differing in half log unit increments.

In vitro **pharmacokinetic and metabolic studies:** Human blood was collected in pre-chilled tubes containing 1% sodium citrate (buffered at pH 7) and kept at 4°C. The plasma was collected after centrifugation at 400 × g for 30 min at 4°C, then aliquoted and stored at -80°C.

Pharmacokinetic (PK) experiments: After thawing, plasma were again centrifuged for 30 min at 4000 rpm and +4°C, filtered (0.45 µm), and distributed at 4°C in Minisorb tubes (Nunc, Dutscher, France) at 500 µl aliquots for each kinetic point.

Peptide solutions were extemporaneously prepared in order to add the appropriate concentration of peptidein a volume of 10 µl, thus avoiding dilution of the plasma. The plasma peptide solutions were then mixed and incubated in a shaking water bath at 37°C with a continuous and slight shaking for the preset kinetic time period. The reaction was stopped by cooling the tubes simultaneously in ice and by the addition of 0.1N final concentration of HCl. For opiorphin PK experiments, a mixture of 1 µg or 40 µg QRFSR-peptide, containing 100 or 500.10^3 cpm QR [³H-F] SR (3.6 Ci/mmole, CEA-Saclay), was used. Controls, in which protease free human plasma (Methanol/TFA extract) is substituted for fresh plasma, were included. For certain experiments, different inhibitors of plasma peptidases were added immediately prior to the addition of opiorphin-peptide, bestatin, an inhibitor of aminopeptidases or GEMSA and an inhibitor of carboxypeptidase B.

All samples were stored at -80°C until subjected to Sep-Pak extraction and RP-HPLC chromatography.

C18 Solid-phase extraction: Acidified (HCl 0.1N final concentration) and clarified biological samples were applied to C18-SepPak cartridges (Waters, France) preconditioned with three successive cycles of methanol (Lichrosolv, Merck) and pure water and ultimately maintained in 0.1% TFA-water. After applying the samples to the top of the cartridge and washing with 0.1%TFA-water (5 ml), the analytes were eluted with 100% methanol containing 0.1% TFA (5 ml). The fractions were collected at 4°C, frozen at -80°C and then lyophilized at -110°C for 48 h. Under these conditions, recovery of the marker QR [³H-F] SR-opiorphin, added to plasma samples, was 76 ± 5 % (mean ± SD for n=20).

Finally, dried extracts were re-suspended in 250 µl pyrolyzed water at 4°C then centrifuged 30 min at 4000 rpm and +4°C to quantify opiorphin-related components by radioactivity measurement

(radiometer Wallac, PerkinElmer) and RP-HPLC in conjunction with PDA and radiometer analyses and/or ELISA-Opiorphin immunoassays.

Reverse phase C18-HPLC Chromatography: RP-HPLC, coupled with online PDA (224 nm) and radiometric (150-TR PerkinElmer) detection, was used to separate, identify and semi-quantify the different opiorphin-related molecular forms contained in human plasma extracts from *in vitro* PK experiments. Reversed Phase-High Performance Liquid Chromatography (RP-HPLC) used a C18-bonded stationary phase and an acetonitrile mobile phase in the presence of 0.1% trifluoroacetic acid (TFA, Sigma-France).

The re-suspended extracts (equivalent to 100 µl initial plasma volume), obtained during the above-described procedures, and were applied to the top of the C18/RP-HPLC analytical column (150×4.5 mm Luna 5 µ Phenomenex-France) under TFA 0.1%-water solvent equilibrium conditions. The various components were eluted and isolated according to their hydrophobic characteristics, in a 25-min linear gradient from 0% to 50% acetonitrile (Lichrosol, Merck), containing 0.1% TFA at a 1 ml/min flow rate (Surveyor HPLC system, Thermo Scientific-France). The entire HPLC system was thermo-regulated at 12°C. Each fraction (1 ml) was collected and lyophilized at -110°C for 48 h. Each chromatographic profile was driven, integrated and analyzed by the ChromQuest software. The peak height values of each peak of interest as well as those for a defined inner standard peak were calculated. Eluted fractions were collected at a 1 min time-interval. Each fraction was lyophilized at -110°C for 48 h. In opiorphin PK experiments, the content of radioactivity of each sample, i.e., crude plasma, plasma extracts, HPLC fractions, was determined to evaluate the recovery of each processing step.

The opiorphin-like content of samples (SepPak extracts and/or HPLC fractions) was also measured using a quantitative and specific immunoassay (competitive-ELISA) developed in the laboratory [17].

Immunoassay for opiorphin: The recently published protocol was used to assess the opiorphin-like content of samples [17]. Optimized assay conditions are summarized as follows: For the coating, 40 ng of the Y-[(CH$_2$)$_{12}$]-QRFSR peptide per 200 µl coating buffer (100 mM potassium phosphate, P^H 7.1) were added to individual wells on a 96-well micro-titration plate and incubated overnight at +4°C with light shaking. In parallel, 100 µl of standard or samples, that were serially diluted 2-fold with incubation buffer (200 mM Tris-HCl, pH 7.5+150 mM NaCl+0.1% Tween 20+0.1% bovine serum albumin), were pre-incubated in Screen Mates tubes (Matrix, Thermo Scientific-France) overnight at 10°C, in the presence of 100 µl anti-opiorphin antibody diluted at 1/80 000. The following day, after washing 5 times with washing buffer (1 tablet PBS-Sigma in 200 ml pure pyrolyzed water + 0.1% tween 20), 250 µl of saturation buffer (20 mM Tris-HCl, pH 7.5+150 mM NaCl+0.1% Tween 20+0.5% gelatin) were added to the individual coated-wells and incubated for at least 1 h at 20°C. Then, after washing, 100 µl of the pre-incubated immunological reaction were transferred onto the coated and saturated micro-titration plates and incubated 1.30 h at 10°C in a humid atmosphere. After washing, 100 µl of the anti-rabbit IgG conjugated to HRP (Pierce, ThermoScientific-France), diluted in Tris buffer (20 mM Tris-HCl, pH 7.5+150 mM NaCl+0.1% Tween 20+0.1% BSA) at 1/3 000, were added to each well and incubated for 1 h at 20°C. After incubation an ultimate wash was performed and 100 µl of the HRP chromogenic substrate (StepUltraTMB-ELISA, ThermoScientific-France) were added and incubated for 30-45 min at 20°C. Finally, the reaction was stopped by adding 100 µl 4N H$_2$SO$_4$. Plates were read at 450 mm with a micro-plate spectrophotometer (Infinite M200, Tecan-France) and the results were successively analyzed with Magellan (Tecan), Prism GraphPad (La Jolia, USA) and Excel Microsoft softwares.

In vivo studies using a rat pain model

Animals: Male Wistar rats (Harlan, France) weighing 250-280 g were used in this study. After a 7-day acclimatization period, they were weighed and randomly housed according to the treatment groups in a room with a 12 h alternating light/dark cycle (9:00 pm/9:00 am) and controlled temperature (21 ± 1°C) and hygrometry (50 ± 5%). Food and water were available ad libidum. They were experimentally only tested once.

Behavioral tests, care and euthanasia of study animals were in accordance with guidelines of the European Communities Directive 86/609/EEC and the ASAB Ethical Committee for the use of laboratory animals in behavioral research (Animal Behaviour, 2006; 71:245-53). The study protocol was approved by the local ethics committee (Comité d'Ethique Lorrain en Matière d'Expérimentation Animale) with the agreement no. CELMEA-2012-0021 obtained on December 6, 2012.

Chemicals: Opiorphin analog (Genosphere Biotechnologies, France) was dissolved in vehicle solution (55% of PBS 100 mM-45% of Acetic acid 0.01N) and systemically (I.V.) injected, 10 to 15 min prior to the behavioral tests, at doses ranging from 0.5 to 2 mg/kg body weight. Morphine HCl (Francopia, France) was dissolved in saline (0.9% sodium chloride in distilled water) and injected I.V. 15 min before the behavioral test, at 2 mg/kg dose. All drugs were administered in a volume of 1 ml/kg body weight.

The Formalin Test: The previously prescribed protocol [1,10,16] was used to assess the analgesic potency of opiorphin analog in a chemical-induced inflammatory pain model. Groups of 8 rats were used for each experiment. 50 µl of a 2.5% formalin solution was injected under the surface of the left hind paw 10-15 min after I.V. injection of opiorphin analogs, morphine or vehicle. The duration of formalin-injected paw licking and the number of inflamed paw flinches and body tremors were recorded for a period of 60 min after formalin administration. The behavioral scores were expressed as means ± standard error of the mean (SEM) for n=8 rats.

Statistical Evaluation: The significance of differences between groups was evaluated using the Kruskal-Wallis one-way analysis of variance (KWT, a non-parametric method) for comparison between several independent variables across the experimental conditions. When a significant difference among the treatments was obtained, the Mann-Whitney post hoc test (MWT) was applied to compare each treated group to the control one. For all statistical evaluations, the level of significance was set at $P < 0.05$. All statistical analyses were carried out using the software StatView$^\circledR$5 statistical package (SAS, Institute, Inc., USA).

Results and Discussion

Structure-activity relationship study

In order to identify the amino acid residues or functional groups required for opiorphin inhibitory potency toward both AP-N and NEP human ectopeptidases, the molecular relationship of structure to activity, namely Structure-Activity Relationship (SAR), of opiorphin native peptide was first investigated. The inhibiting activity of each modified compound was evaluated toward human recombinant NEP (rh-NEP) and AP-N (rh-AP-N), the residual enzyme activity was measured by continuous fluorimetric assays in the presence of specific fluorescent substrate.

Our findings, associated with a previously reported Ala substitution scanning study [18] show:

The importance of the N-terminal amine group of the NH_2-QRFSR peptide in the inhibitory potency of opiorphin toward rhAP-N. Indeed, the acetylation (Ac-QRFSR) or pyroglutamylation (pGlu^1-RFSR), the octanoylation $((CH_2)_8$-QRFSR) or biotinylation (biotine-$[(CH_2)_6]$-QRFSR) led to compounds displaying diminished inhibitory potency towards hap-N. On the other hand, pGlu^1-RFSR and $[(CH_2)_8]$-QRFSR peptides displayed at least equivalent inhibitory potency for rhNEP compared to opiorphin native peptide.

The importance of the free C-terminal carboxyl group of the QRFSR-COOH peptide in inhibitory potency toward rhNEP, in particular, rhNEP CarboxyDiPeptidase activity. Indeed, the amidation of the C terminal (QRFSR-CONH$_2$) gives rise to a compound displaying diminished inhibitory potency toward rhNEP.

The key role played by the aromatic side chain of Phe ^{3} residue (QRFSR) in the inhibitory potency of opiorphin toward rhNEP and rhAP-N activities. Indeed, substitution with a Tyr residue (QRYSR) led to a compound displaying up to an 8-fold decrease in rhAP-N inhibition potency and a slight decrease in rhNEP inhibition potency. Substitution by an Ala residue led to a compound with completely diminished inhibitory potency toward both rhNEP and rhAP-N [18].

The importance of the RFS central residues of the QRFSR peptide in the inhibitory potency of opiorphin toward rhNEP. The compounds QRGPR – QHNPR – QRFPR displayed equivalent inhibitory potency toward rhAP-N but a low or totally diminished inhibitory potential for rhNEP.

The importance of the guanidium side chains of the Arg^2 (R^2) and Arg^5 (R^5) residues in the inhibitory potency of opiorphin toward rhAPN. Indeed, their respective substitution by the ε- amine side chain of Lys residue (QKFSR and QRFSK) led to compounds displaying more than a 10-fold decrease in rhAP-N inhibitory potency while showing equivalent rhNEP inhibitory potency. Their respective substitution by an Ala residue confirmed these results [18].

In summary, there is a clear structural selectivity in the functional interaction of opiorphin with both human NEP and AP-N ectoenkephalinases. The aromatic residue of Phe^3 plays a critical role in the interactions of opiorphin with both targets. In addition, the C-terminal FSR tri-amino acids constitute the minimal active sequence for NEP inhibition; moreover, FSR-peptide is 10 times more active than the natural QRFSR-peptide in its inhibition potency toward rhNEP. Conversely, it seems that the entire amino acid sequence of opiorphin is required for full rhAP-N inhibition. In general, our results demonstrate that any change in the intra-peptide sequence inhibits or even abolishes at least one of the two inhibitory activities. In contrast, addition of an amide link with a Tyr residue at the N-terminal position of the peptide ([Y]-QRFSR) does not reduce the inhibitory potency of the peptide toward either human target and does not affect its antinociceptive potency in a pain rat model [1].

Metabolism of the native opiorphin peptide

In order to evaluate the half-life of circulating opiorphin in the human bloodstream, the fate of the natural peptide was analyzed using *in vitro* kinetic models. The metabolic profile of opiorphin native peptide in human plasma as a function of incubation time at 37°C is shown in Figure 1A. The major metabolism products, generated following a 60-min incubation period of 1 µg QRFSR/QR [^{3}H-F] SR per500 µl

Structure-Activity Relationship Study and Function-Based Petidomimetic Design of Human Opiorphin...

165

human fresh plasma, were isolated by RP-HPLC in conjunction with PDA (224 nm) and radiometric detections and semi-quantified using Chromquest software. The data are expressed by relative peak height. The addition of tracer quantity of tritiated opiorphin established the drug plasma concentration with high precision even for small amounts of compound not usually detected using standard PDA detection. Finally, analyses with Kinetica software were used to predict from the concentration-time course the metabolic half-life of the native compound, either from plasma-induced hydrolysis and/or chemical changes.

Native QRFSR-peptide disappears from human plasma with a metabolic half-life evaluated at 5 min (R^2=0.88, n=5 time points over the 8 min time course of incubation). One metabolite appeared as early as 1 min after incubation, reaching maximum relative levels after 30 min incubation. Its appearance inversely correlated with the disappearance of Gln^1-RFSR native peptide (Figure 1A). The maximal appearance after 30 min incubation was blocked in the presence of150 µM bestatin, a selective inhibitor of amino peptidases (Figure 1B). In contrast, its appearance was not affected by 150 µM GEMSA, a selective carboxy peptidase B inhibitor (Figure 1B). This result suggests that opiorphinis primarily hydrolyzed to an RFSR-peptide metabolite resulting from the activity of a plasma exo-aminopeptidase, potentially a glutamyl peptidase. Interestingly, the RFSR-peptide is about 3 fold less inhibitory than the native QRFSR-peptide toward both rhNEP and rhAP-N. To increase the 5 minutes half-life of native opiorphin, changes were designed at the level of this sensitive site.

Two additional radioactive molecular populations were distinguished on the RP-HPLC chromatograms during the time course

of incubation of QR [^{3}H-F] SR-opiorphin in human plasma. The $pGlu^1$-RFSR-peptide was observed, peaking to a maximum of 16% at 1 min time-point then disappearing with a similar metabolic half-life ($T_{1/2}$-life=6 min, R^2=0.83 for n=4 time points over the 6 min time course of incubation (Figure 1A), to the parent Gln^1-RFSR-peptide. This result does not concur with a previous report indicating that pGlu formation (in enzymatic or non-enzymatic processes) minimizes susceptibility to degradation by aminopeptidase [19]. It is also interesting to point out that $pGlu^1$-RFSR peptide is an efficient NEP inhibitor. To a lesser extent, a more hydrophilic molecular population was also observed on the HPLC profile, reaching a maximum from the 2 min time-point and remaining stable at about 12% over the 30 min incubation period. The chromatographic and kinetic behaviors of this population lead us to suggest that it could result from an opiorphin-related product binding to a human plasma component.

Selection of potent bioactive opiorphin peptidomimetics: The peptidomimetic strategy consists of altering the physical characteristics of a peptide without changing its biological activity. Here we wished to design and select functional derivatives of opiorphin that would display *in vivo* bioavailability properties superior to the native peptide, in particular increased resistance against proteolytic degradation. Several modifications are known to improve the metabolic stability of peptides. Conventional modifications consist of protecting the NH_2-and COOH-terminal ends by N-acetylation and C-amidation, respectively. However, SAR studies (see above) reveal that these modifications inhibit or even abolish opiorphin inhibitory potencies. Alternatively, amino acids can be selectively substituted with non-natural amino acids, most notably by a D-enantiomer or β-amino acid [20]. However, as previously reported, ⇓ changes on the structural conformation of N- and C- terminal amino acids (N- and C-terminally homologated opiorphin, ß$_2$hGln-Arg-Phe-Ser-ß$_3$hArg),while increasing by about 7-fold the metabolic half-life of the modified opiorphin in human plasma, reduced by up to 10-fold its inhibitory potency toward both targets. This indicated that the relocation of the terminal carboxy and/ or amino groups has an impact on opiorphin interaction with the enkephalin-inactivating NEP and AP-N [21].

A third possibility to increase the enzymatic stability of peptides is to reduce their peptide character (pseudo peptides), substituting peptide bonds with isosteric surrogates. The isosters most frequently used are the reduced peptide bond (methyl-amino, CH_2-NH), the retro-inverso link, the aza group or polyethylene chain spacers such as $(CH_2)_6$ or $(CH_2)_{12}$. Depending on the chemical residue in corporated, the most direct consequences are increased resistance to the lytic action of circulating peptidases and an increase in lipophilicity that serves to facilitate transport across biological barriers [20,22]. However, such chemically stabilized peptides can lose some, if not all, of their biological activity, such as the retro-inverso D-amino acid opiorphin analog that lost its ability to inhibit NEP (unpublished observations by Rougeot C).

Consistent with the above, most of the QRFSR-peptide changes failed to reproduce the biological activity of the natural peptide. However, a series of opiorphin derivatives were screened and selected step by step on the basis of their dual inhibitory potency for hNEP and/ or hAP-N. To test for specificity, hit compounds were further tested with respect to other members of the metallo-ectopeptidase family, such as DPPIV and ECE. Here we present only functional opiorphin derivatives displaying significant *in vitro* inhibitory activity toward human NEP and AP-N.

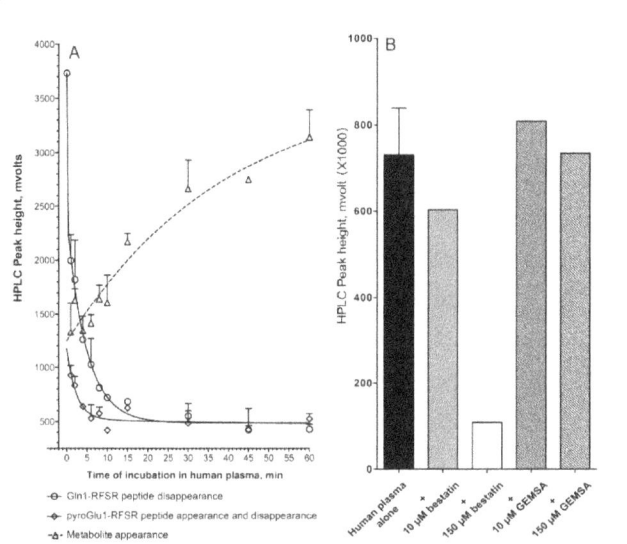

Figure 1: Opiorphin stability profile in human plasma. A. Time course of opiorphin-QR[3H-F]SR peptide disappearance (open circles: Gln1 form and open lozenges: pGlu1 form) and of the appearance of the major opiorphin metabolite (open triangles) over a 60-min incubation period at 37°C, in the presence of fresh human plasma. Samples were withdrawn at different times and analyzed by RP-HPLC together with online PDA (224nm) and radiometer detectors and semi quantified using Chromquest software. A human plasma molecule, serving as an internal standard, was used to calculate the relative peak height, represented in volts, of each identified peak. B. Representative histogram of the relative levels of radioactive opiorphin metabolite generated after 30 min incubation of 40 µg opiorphin-QR[3H-F]SR peptide in the absence (control, black bar) or presence of a specific inhibitor of plasma peptidases, bestatin (grey bar,10 µM and open bar, 150 µM) and GEMSA (diagonal-striped bars, 150 µM).

QRF-[S-O-Octanoyl]-R peptide

Comparative conformational analyses of the opiorphin peptide revealed that the hydroxyl group of the Ser[4] residue does not seem to play a critical role in its bioactive conformation for hNEP [18]. Therefore, initially we tested the product resulting from esterification by octanoic acid, $[CH_2]8$, of the serine hydroxyl group of the QRFSR peptide.

As shown in Figure 2, QRF-[S-O-$(CH_2)_8$]-R peptide prevented, in a concentration dependent manner, the Abz-dR-G-L-EDDnp cleavage, mediated by recombinant hNEP-Endopeptidase (rhNEP-endo) activity, with a half inhibitory potency (IC_{50}) at 2.1 ± 0.2 μM (r^2=0.99, n=30 determination points). It also prevented, in a concentration dependent manner, the Abz-R-G-F-K-DnpOH cleavage, mediated by recombinant hNEP-Carboxy DiPeptidase (rhNEP-CDP) activity, with an IC_{50} at 13 ± 3 μM (r^2=0.98, n=30 determination points) and also the Mca-R-P-P-G-F-S-A-F-K-(Dnp)-OH FRET-peptide (Mca-BK2) cleavage with an IC_{50} at 14 ± 4 μM (r^2=0.99, n=18 determination points). In addition, QRF-[S-O-$(CH_2)_8$]-R peptide inhibited, in a dose dependent manner, the Ala-AMC cleavage, mediated by recombinant hAP-N (rhAP-N) activity, with an IC_{50} at 12 ± 1 μM (r^2=0.99, n=27 determination points).

QRF[S-O-$(CH_2)_8$] R peptide was an essentially equipotent inhibitor compound toward AP-N compared to opiorphin natural peptide. The Ser[4] octanoylation of opiorphin-peptide reinforces, by up to 10-fold, the inhibitory potency for rhNEP-Endopeptidase and CarboxyDipeptidase activity, suggesting that the addition of a hydrophobic moiety on the Ser[4] side chain induces more favorable contacts with the hydrophobic pocket of the NEP catalytic site.

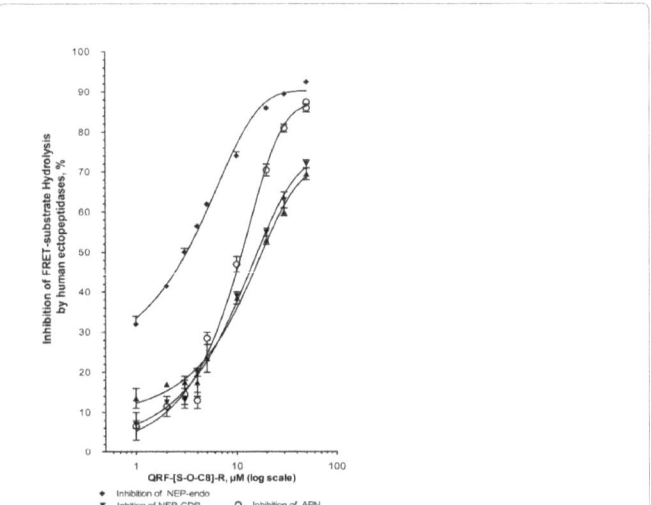

Figure 2: % Inhibition of FRET-substrate hydrolysis by human ectopeptidases in the presence of the QRF-[S-O-$(CH_2)8$]-R opiorphin analog. The graph illustrates the *in vitro* functional assay for QRF-[S-O-$(CH_2)8$]-R opiorphin analog designed in this study. Concentration-dependent inhibition by QRF-[S-O-$(CH_2)8$]-R peptide of the hydrolysis of corresponding FRET-peptide substrates by pure human recombinant hNEP (black lozenges, NEP-endo; black triangles, NEP-CDP and NEP/McaBK2) and hAP-N (open circles) is observed. Abbreviations are explained in Materials & Methods. Each point represents the percentage of intact substrate recovered and calculated as a percentage of velocity without inhibitor minus velocity in the presence of inhibitor / velocity without inhibitor. Measurements were taken in the absence or in the presence of various concentrations of QRF-[S-O-(CH2)8]-R-peptide, plotted in μM (log scale).

[C]-QRFSR peptide

We previously showed that addition of a Tyr residue at the N-terminal position of the opiorphin-peptide does not affect its *in vitro* inhibitory potency or its *in vivo* antinociceptive properties [1]. Potent NEP and AP-N inhibitors were designed on the basis that the molecules contain a strong metal-coordinating group [23]. These observations were also used to design an opiorphin peptidomimetic carrying at the N-terminal moiety a Cys-thiol functional group that is a strong Zn atom-coordinating group.

As shown in Figure 3, the [C]-QRFSR peptide inhibited, in a concentration dependent manner, the rhNEP-endo activity with an IC_{50} at 7 ± 1 μM (r^2=0.96, n=28 determination points), the rhNEP-CDP with an IC_{50} at 7 ± 1 μM (r^2=0.96, n=31 determination points) and the NEP-dependent Mca-BK2 cleavage with an IC_{50} at 17 ± 2 μM (r^2=0.99, n=16 determination points). It also prevented, in a dose dependent manner, the Ala-AMC cleavage mediated by rhAP-N activity, with an IC_{50} at 0.8 ± 0.1 μM (r^2=0.99, n=30 determination points).

Thus, the NH_2-[C]-QRFSR-COOH peptide, containing a thiol coordinating group with the Zn atom, displays reinforced inhibitory potency toward hAP-N and hNEP Zn-dependent metalloectopeptidases, 10-fold and 5-fold compared to QRFSR natural peptide, respectively.

[C]-[amino-hexanoic-acid spacer]-QRFSR peptide

In an attempt to protect the opiorphin derivative against degradation by circulating amino peptidases and thus increase its metabolic stability, a $[CH_2]_6$ polyethylene bridge [amino-hexanoic-acid spacer] was substituted for the peptide bond joining the Zn-chelating Cys[0] and the Glu[1] amino acids.

The resulting [C]-$[CH_2]_6$-QRFSR peptide showed a dose-dependent inhibition of rhNEP- ndo activity with an IC_{50} at 40 ± 5 μM (r^2=0.97, n=24 determination points), of rhNEP-CDP activity with an IC_{50} evaluated at about 158 μM (r^2=0.89, n=25 determination points), and rhAP-N activity with an IC_{50} at 0.8 ± 0.1 μM (r^2=0.99, n=16 determination points).

Surprisingly, the additional polyethylene bridge between the Cys[0] and Glu[1] residues of the [C]-QRFSR peptide was caused a decrease in inhibitory potency, of more than one order of magnitude relative to [C]-QRFSR peptide, toward NEP enzyme and particularly toward NEP-carboxypeptidase activity, whereas no difference in affinity towards AP-N was detected relative to [C]-QRFSR peptide.

[C]-[amino-hexanoic-acid spacer]-QRF-[S-O-Octanoyl]-R peptide

The [C]-$[(CH_2)_6]$-QRF-[S-O-$(CH_2)_8$]-R derivative, resulting from the combination of the three modifications above, was tested for its inhibitory potency toward rhNEP and rhAP-N. As shown in Figure 4, it inhibited, in a concentration dependent manner, rhNEP-Endo activity with an IC_{50} at 0.83 ± 0.08 μM (r^2=0.99, n=48 determination points), rhNEP-CDP activity with an IC_{50} at 0.85 ± 0.06 μM (r^2=0.99, n=27 determination points) and Mca-BK2 cleavage mediated by the rhNEP with an IC_{50} at about 2.1 ± 0.1 μM (r^2=0.99, n=18 determination points). The [C]-$[(CH_2)_6]$-QRF-[S-O-$(CH_2)_8$]-R peptide had equipotent inhibitory capacity towards rhAP-N activity with an IC_{50} at 0.95 ± 0.10 μM (r^2=0.99, n=24 determination points). Thus the combination of a well-balanced bioactive profile with equipotent inhibitory capacity encouraged us to retain [C]-$[(CH_2)_6]$-QRF-[S-O-$(CH_2)_8$]-R as the best performing opiorphin peptidomimetic and it was submitted to further

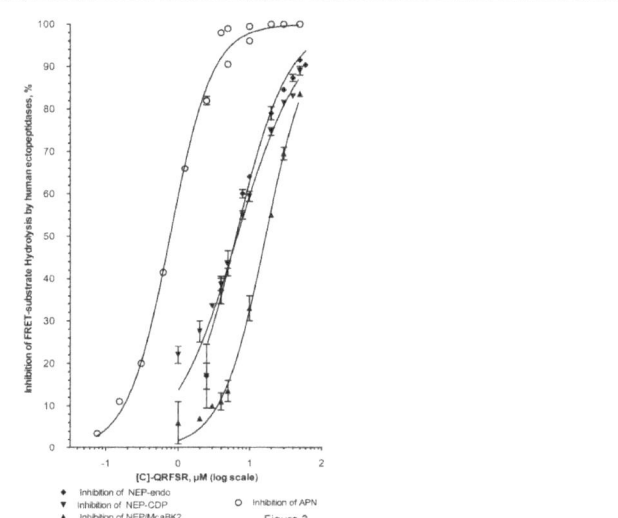

Figure 3: % Inhibition of FRET-substrate hydrolysis by human ectopeptidases in the presence of the [C]-QRFSR opiorphin analog. The graph illustrates the *in vitro* functional assay for [C]-QRFSR opiorphin analog designed in this study. Concentration-dependent Inhibition by [C]-QRFSR peptide of the hydrolysis of corresponding FRET-peptide substrates by pure human recombinant hNEP (black lozenges, NEP-endo; black triangles, NEP-CDP and NEP/McaBK2) and hAP-N (open circles) is observed. Abbreviations are explained in Materials & Methods.

Each point represents the percentage of intact substrate recovered and calculated as a percentage of velocity without inhibitor minus velocity in the presence of inhibitor / velocity without inhibitor. Measurements were taken in the absence or in the presence of various concentrations of [C]-RFSR-peptide, plotted in µM (log-scale).

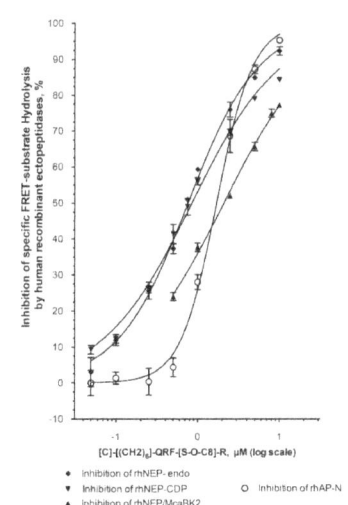

Figure 4: % Inhibition of FRET-substrate hydrolysis by human ectopeptidases in the presence of the [C]-[(CH$_2$)6]-QRF-[S-O-(CH$_2$)8]-R opiorphin analog. The graph illustrates the *in vitro* functional assay for [C]-[(CH$_2$)6]-QRF-[S-O-(CH$_2$)8]-R opiorphin analog designed in this study. Concentration-dependent Inhibition by [C]-[(CH$_2$)6]-QRF-[S-O-(CH$_2$)8]-R peptide of the hydrolysis of corresponding FRET-peptide substrates by pure human recombinant hNEP (black lozenges, NEP-endo; black triangles, NEP-CDP and NEP/McaBK2) and AP-N (open circles) is observed. Abbreviations are explained in Materials & Methods. Each point represents the percentage of intact substrate recovered and calculated as a percentage of velocity without inhibitor minus velocity in presence of inhibitor/velocity without inhibitor. Measurements were taken in the absence or in the presence of various concentrations of [C]-[(CH$_2$)6]-QRF-[S-O-(CH$_2$)8]-R-peptide, plotted in µM (log scale).

exploration.

In the biologically relevant *in vitro* assay, using substance P, the physiological NEP substrate and human cell membranes as sources of native human NEP, the [C]-[(CH$_2$)$_6$]-QRF-[S-O-(CH$_2$)$_8$]-R peptide prevented, in a concentration dependent manner, substance P cleavage mediated by membrane-bound hNEP-Endopeptidase (mhNEP-Endo) activity with an IC$_{50}$ at 1.6 ± 0.4 µM (r^2=0.95, n=13 determination points) (Figure 5). Under the same assay conditions, it appears to be at least five times more potent than opiorphin natural peptide toward hNEP [1]. In addition using fluorescent substrates with human cell membranes as sources of native hNEP, the [C]-[(CH$_2$)$_6$]-QRF-[S-O-(CH$_2$)$_8$]-R peptide inhibited in a concentration dependent manner the mhNEP-Endo activity with an IC$_{50}$ at 1.6 ± 0.4 µM, and mhAP-N activity with an IC$_{50}$ at 0.9 ± 0.1 µM (Figure 5). Thus, the designed analog presents similar affinity towards human NEP and AP-N, whether they are in a native membrane-anchored or recombinant soluble conformation.

In vitro assays using human recombinant DPP4 or ECE-1 revealed that the [C]-[(CH$_2$)$_6$]-QRF-[S-O-(CH$_2$)$_8$]-R compound did not inhibit rhECE1 and rhDPPIV-ectopeptidase activities even at 100 µM final concentration. These results indicate that, similarly to opiorphin, the opiorphin analog shows excellent selectivity with respect to related zinc-metallo peptidases, such as ECE1 (closely structurally related to NEP with 40% sequence identity) and DPPIV that is involved among other endopeptidases, including NEP, in the inactivation of the substance Pandbradykinin.

Di-peptide analogs can be metabolically more resistant to peptidase degradation. We tested the cystine-dipeptide (single disulfide bond connecting the Cys^1 residue of each peptide chain) of [C]-[(CH$_2$)$_6$]-QRF-[S-O-(CH$_2$)$_8$]-R for its inhibitory potency towards human NEP and AP-N. The resulting [C-[(CH$_2$)$_6$]-QRF-[S-O-(CH$_2$)$_8$]-R] 2cystine-dipeptideanalog showed a dose dependent inhibition of the rhNEP-Endo activity with an IC$_{50}$ at 0.99 ± 0.07 µM (r^2=0.99, n=16 determination points), and of the rhAP-N activity with an IC$_{50}$ at 0.58 ± 0.05 µM (r^2=0.99, *n*=15 determination points). Thus, *in vitro* the di-peptide demonstrates similar inhibitory potency towards hNEP and hAP-N when compared to the monomer.

[dCys]-QRF-[Ser-O-octanoyl]-[dArg]

Another strategy to protect peptide compounds against degradation by circulating peptidases is the replacement of the N-term and C-term amino acid residues, which are major targets for degradation by circulating exopeptidases, by their respective D-enantiomer.

As shown in Figure 6, [dC]-QRF-[S-O-(CH$_2$)$_8$]-[dR] derivative peptide inhibited, in a concentration dependent manner, rhNEP-Endo activity with an IC$_{50}$ at 4 ± 1 µM (r^2=0.97, *n*=30 determination points) and rhNEP-CDP activity with an IC$_{50}$ at 21 ± 1 µM (r^2=0.99, *n*=30 determination points). Strikingly, this derivative was at least 200 times more potent against rhAP-N activity than against rhNEP with an IC$_{50}$ at 0.022 ± 0.002 µM (r^2=0.98, *n*=43 determination points). We also used human cell membranes as a source of native membrane-bound hNEP and hAP-N and confirmed that the [dC]-QRF-[S-O-(CH$_2$)$_8$]-[dR] peptide displays an unbalanced inhibitory profile. Indeed, it showed a dose-dependent inhibition of mhNEP-Endo activity with an IC$_{50}$ at 9 ± 1 µM (r^2=0.98, *n*=21 determination points) and of mhNEP-CDP activity with an IC$_{50}$ at 37 ± 5 µM (r^2=0.95, *n*=21 determination points). In addition, it appeared to be 30-100 times more potent toward mhAP-N activity than toward mhNEP(IC$_{50}$ at 0.3 ± 0.1 µM, r^2=0.95,

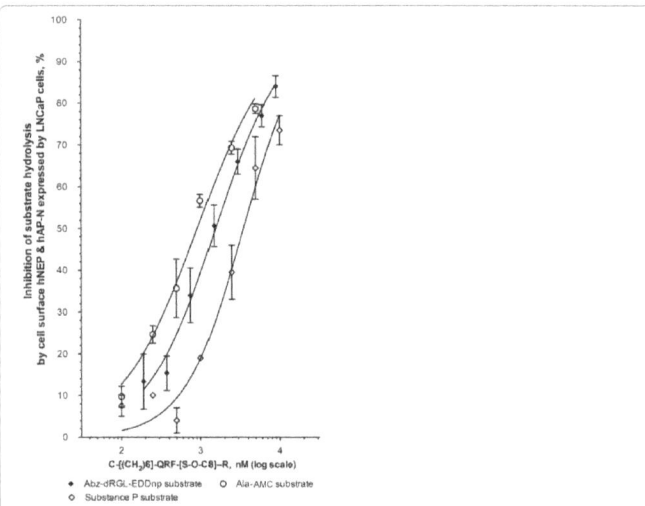

Figure 5: % Inhibition of substrate hydrolysis by cell surface hNEP & hAP-N, expressed by LNCaP cells, in the presence of the [C]-[(CH$_2$)6]-QRF-[S-O-(CH$_2$)8]-R opiorphin analog. Substance P, the physiological NEP-substrate, and human epithelial LNCaP cell membranes as a source of membrane bound human NEP and AP-N were used in an *in vitro* functional assay for [C]-[(CH$_2$)6]-QRF-[S-O-(CH$_2$)8]-R opiorphin analog. Concentration-dependent Inhibition by [C]-[(CH$_2$)6]-QRF-[S-O-(CH$_2$)8]-R peptide of the hydrolysis of substance P (open lozenges) by membrane-bound human NEP and AP-N is observed. Fluorescent synthetic substrates (black lozenges, Abz-dRGL-EDDnp for hNEP-endo activity and open circles, Ala-AMC for hAP-N activity) were also tested with human cell membranes and have similar profiles to Substance P. Abbreviations are explained in Materials & Methods. Each point represents the percentage of intact substrate recovered and calculated as a percentage of velocity without inhibitor minus velocity in the presence of inhibitor / velocity without inhibitor. Measurements were taken in the absence or in the presence of various concentrations of [C]-[(CH$_2$)6]-QRF-[S-O-(CH$_2$)8]-Rpeptide, plotted in nM (log scale).

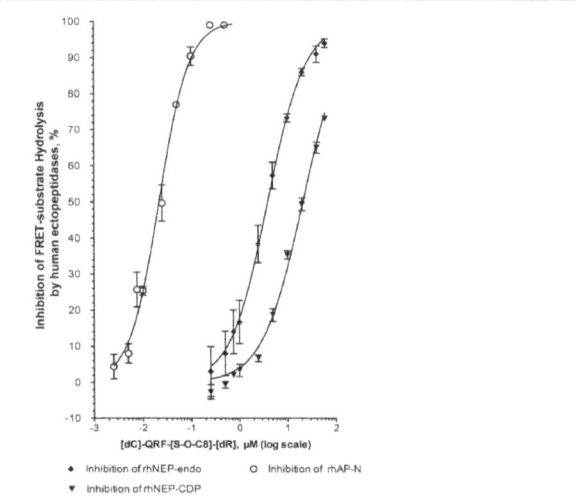

Figure 6: % Inhibition of FRET-substrate hydrolysis by human ectopeptidases in the presence of the [dC]-QRF-[S-O-(CH2)8]-[dR] opiorphin analog. The graph illustrates the *in vitro* functional assay for [dC]-QRF-[S-O-(CH2)8]-[dR] opiorphin analog designed in this study. Concentration dependent Inhibition by [dC]-QRF-[S-O-(CH2)8]-[dR] peptide of the hydrolysis of corresponding FRET-peptide substrates by pure human recombinant hNEP (black lozenges, NEP-endo; black triangles, NEP-CDP or AP-N (open circles) is observed. Abbreviations are explained in Materials & Methods. Each point represents the percentage of intact substrate recovered and calculated as a percentage of velocity without inhibitor minus velocity in presence of inhibitor /velocity without inhibitor, which was measured in the absence or in the presence of various concentrations of [dC]-QRF-[S-O-(CH2)8]-[dR]-peptide, plotted in µM (log scale).

n=21 determination points).

Furthermore, substitution of the L-Arg[5] by its respective D-enantiomer clearly affected the inhibitory potency of the compound toward hNEP-carboxydipeptidase. The related [dC]-QRF-[S-O-(CH$_2$)$_8$]-R peptide inhibited mhNEP-CDP activity with an IC[50] at 2.6 ± 0.3 µM (r^2=0.98, *n*=30 determination points), about ten times more potent than the D-Arg[5] counterpart. Such a difference leads us to propose the existence of a stereo-chemical requirement for optimal interaction of the peptide with the catalytic site of NEP. Conversely, the substitution of the L-Cys[0] by its respective D-enantiomer clearly enhanced the inhibitory potency of the compound toward hAP-N (about 50 times more potent than the L-Cys[0] counterpart) and may be due to the fact that its spatial conformation provides tight binding to the AP-N target.

The [dC]-QRF-[S-O-(CH$_2$)$_8$]-[dR] derivative probably displays some superior *in vivo* bioavailability properties compared to native opiorphin peptide, such as a possible gain in circulating amino- and carboxy-peptidase resistance. However, it's very modest gain in hNEP inhibitory potency, combined with a distinctly unbalanced bioactive profile eliminated it as a suitable candidate molecule. Therefore, only the C-[(CH$_2$)$_6$]-QRF-[S-O-(CH$_2$)$_8$]-R derivative was retained for further exploration.

Metabolism and Toxicity profile of the best performing opiorphin functional derivative

Metabolism in fresh human plasma: We established overall *in vitro* pharmacokinetic and metabolic parameters, based on an *in vitro* time-dependent system, using opiorphin or its derivative incubated in human plasma. Kinetica software, which is used to predict the metabolic half-life (T½) of the parent peptide from the concentration-time course, was used in this study.

As shown above, *in vitro* kinetic analyses in human plasma revealed that the native QRFSR-peptide disappears with a half-life evaluated at 5 min. Its disappearance results in part from the cyclization of Gln[1] (16% maximum) but mainly from the hydrolytic removal of both Gln[1]- and pGlu[1]-peptides by plasma amino peptidases (reaching a maximum of 84% of the parent peptide at 60 min incubation) and also, to a small extent (12%), from potential complex formation.

The *in vitro* kinetic change experiments in human plasma of the [C]-[(CH$_2$)$_6$]-QRF[S-O-(CH$_2$)$_8$]-R derivative, were done with 50 µg peptide/500 µl human plasma by RP-HPLC relative quantification and ELISA quantitative assay. The concentration-time profile was analyzed by Prism (Figure 7) and Kinetica softwares. The half-time disappearance of [C]-[(CH$_2$)$_6$]-QRF[S-O-(CH$_2$)$_8$]-R was evaluated at 4.5 min (R2=0.89, n=5 time points over 5 min time course of incubation). Its disappearance results primarily from the dimerization (36% maximum of [[C]-[(CH$_2$)$_6$]-QRF-[S-O-(CH$_2$)$_8$]-R]2-dimer which has a T½ disappearance of 41 min; R^2=0.87, n=7 time points over the 60 min time course of incubation). ELISA and HPLC analyses showed that 40% of the parent peptide remains stable in the human plasma even after 60 min incubation (14% for the QRFSR-peptide), indicating that the [C]-[(CH$_2$)$_6$]-QRF[S-O-(CH$_2$)$_8$]-R derivative is more metabolically stable in human plasma than opiorphin native peptide. In addition, it is important to point out that the major biotransformation product of the parent derivative, the cystine-dipeptide, is as active as the parent peptide in fluorescence-based NEP and AP-N assays.

All together, the data showed that, as expected, opiorphin derivative [C]-[(CH$_2$)$_6$-spacer]-QRF[S-O-(CH$_2$)$_8$]-R demonstrates much greater

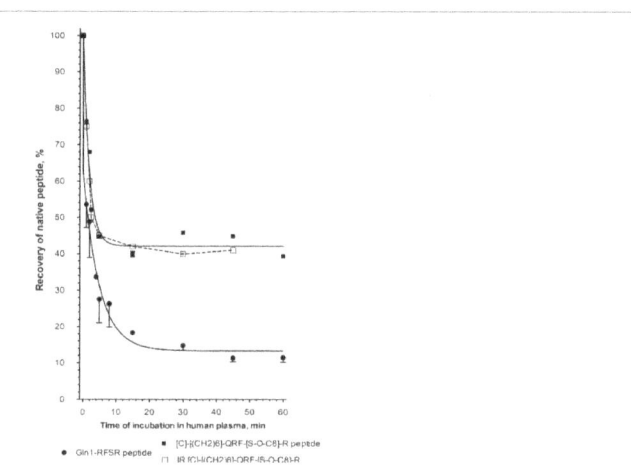

Figure 7: Stability profile of [C]-[(CH₂)6]-QRF-[S-O-(CH₂)8]-R best performing opiorphin derivative in human plasma. The time course of disappearance of [C]-[(CH₂)6]-QRF-[S-O-(CH₂)8]-R peptide (black squares, HPLC measurement; open squares, ELISA measurement) compared to native QRFSR opiorphin peptide (black circles) over a 60-min incubation period at 37°C, in the presence of fresh human plasma. Samples were withdrawn at different times and analyzed by RP-HPLC together with an online PDA detector (224nm) and semi-quantified using

Chromquest software and by ELISA immune assay. The peptide amounts at 0 min were considered as 100%. Each point represents the percentage of peptide remaining.

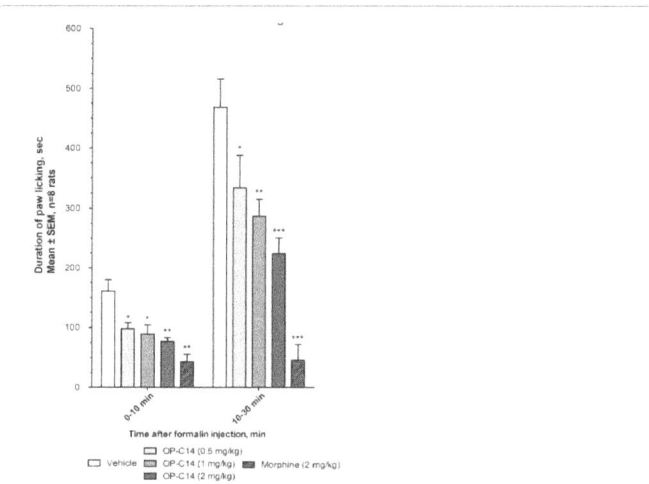

Figure 8: *In vivo* functional test for [C]-[(CH₂)6]-QRF-[S-O-(CH₂)8]-R opiorphin analog, using the formalin pain model. Representative histogram of dose-dependent anti-nociceptive effects of [C]-[(CH₂)6]-QRF-[S-O-(CH₂)8]-R peptide (gray bars, 05, 1 and 2 mg/kg I.V.) compared to vehicle negative control (open bar) and morphine (diagonal-striped bar, 2 mg/kg I.V.). Hind paws were injected with formalin and the duration of formalin-injected paw licking over successive 0-10 min and 10-30 min periods was measured. Results are expressed as means ± SEM of 8 rats. Asterisk indicates *$P<0.05$, ** $P<0.01$ and *** $P<0.001$ versus control-vehicle by MWT.

metabolic stability with respect to human plasma aminopeptidases compared to the native opiorphin peptide.

Drug Absorption and *in vitro* Cytotoxicity: A range of *in vitro* ADME-Tox assays provided by Cerep Laboratories (Celle L'Evescault-France) allowed us to evaluate a number of factors including drug absorption and membrane permeability with the A-B permeability and P-glycoprotein ATPase efflux system [24]. The Caco-2/TC7 (pH 6.5/7.4) human cell line gives an indication of the intestinal epithelial

transport potential of compounds [24]. Metabolic stability, using human liver microsomes and *in vitro* cytotoxicity in cell-based assays that measure cellular parameters such as cell viability, nuclear size and mitochondrial membrane potential using the HepG2 human cell line can also be evaluated.

Our data demonstrate that, compared to the reference positive and negative controls, no apparent *in vitro* human cell toxicityis observed for either QRFSR native peptide or [C]-[(CH₂)₆]-QRF-[S-O-(CH₂)₈]-R derivative peptide, incubated at 10, 30 and 100 µM final concentrations for 72 h at 37°C. For example, relative to controls at 100 µM, the peptides increased cell proliferation by 1and 12%, respectively and reduced nuclear size and mitochondrial membrane potential only by 1 and 5%, respectively. However, there is a clear decrease in the metabolic stability of the opiorphin derivative in the presence of human liver microsomes compared with the native opiorphin peptide: at 10 µM final concentration and after 60 min incubation, 2.5% of the parent [C]-[(CH₂)₆]-QRF-[S-O-(CH₂)₈]-R compound remains versus 47% remaining in the case of opiorphin. Surprisingly, the opiorphin derivative, although endowed with higher lipophilicity than opiorphin native peptide, did not display significantly increased trans-membrane cell permeability over the 60 min incubation-period at 37°C, as the apparent permeability coefficient of both tested compounds was <0.2×10-6 cm/s (10 µM test concentration and HPLC-MS/MS detection method). However, this result is probably due to the cellular model used, namely, TC7 human epithelial intestinal cells derived from the CaCO2 cell line, and known to express membrane-bound NEP and AP-N ectoenzymes. The cell line, therefore, is not an appropriate model for permeability studies of NEP and/or AP-N- inhibitor-ligands. Indeed, the mean recovery of the compounds in donor samples was dramatically low (0% for QRFSR and 14% for the derivative) due mainly to binding to TC7 cell membranes.

We then tested *in vivo* acute toxicity using a rat model provided by CERB (Centre de Recherches Biologiques, Baugy-France). CERB experimental conditions are based on a stepwise procedure, each step uses 3 male rats for each compound. No mortality occurred among the animals treated with QRFSR natural peptide at 100 mg/kg maximum dose, administered as a bolus in the caudal vein. This dose is a 100-fold the effective I.V. dose in the rat pain model. In contrast, the rat treated with a 100 mg/kg dose of [C]-[(CH₂)₆]-QRF-[S-O-(CH₂)₈]-R analog died 3 minutes after treatment; however, no mortality occurred among the 3 animals treated at 30 mg/kg I.V. These animals were further observed for general clinical and neurobehavioral signs, based on the Irwin method, for 14 days [25]. No clinical signs were observed during the course of the study of both peptides. Body weight gain was normal and no gross organ or tissue changes were detected by necropsy.

In conclusion, under the experimental conditions adopted by CERB, opiorphin natural QRFSR peptide administered intravenously at 100 mg/kg and [C]-[(CH₂)₆]-QRF-[S-O-(CH₂)₈]-R derivative peptide administered at 30 mg/kg did not induce signs of toxicity.

Antinociceptive effect in the rat formalin pain model: The exciting *in vitro* results from FRET-based NEP and AP-N assays prompted us to study the analgesic efficacy of the [C]-[(CH₂)₆]-QRF-[S-O-(CH₂)₈]-R analog, in terms of delay of action-both potency and duration of action, in a rat model.

Using the behavioral formalin-induced pain model, known as the Formalin Test, we investigated the anti-nociceptive potency of the [C]-[(CH₂)₆]-QRF-[S-O-(CH₂)₈]-R analog. The duration of formalin-injected paw licking (sec) and the total number of inflamed paw flinches and body tremors were recorded over the 60 min-test period. The formalin test measures the behavioral response to a chemical-induced inflammatory nociception, which induces two distinct nociceptive phases separated a stationary interphase: a early acute phase (first 10 min after formalin injection) followed by a late phase in which a more tonic pain is elicited.

Here, we demonstrate that the [C]-[(CH$_2$)6]-QRF-[S-O-(CH$_2$)$_8$]-R functional opiorphin analog inhibits, in a dose-dependent manner, the pain behavior induced by long-acting chemical stimuli with significant antinociceptive effect at 0.5, 1 and 2 mg/kg I.V. doses over early and later phases of the test (Figure 8). Thus, compared to the control vehicle rats, the opiorphin analog-treated rats at 1 and 2 mg/kg dose spent significantly less time in paw licking over the first 10 min-test period, from 161 ± 19 sec (vehicle) to 89 ± 15 sec (1 mg/kg) and 77 ± 6 sec (2 mg/kg) (P<0.05 and 0.01 vs vehicle by Mann-Whitney U-test, MWT, n=8 rats/group) as morphine-treated rats at 2 mg/kg I.V. dose (43 ± 13 sec, P<0.01 by MWT). The 1 and 2 mg-treated rats also spent significant less time in paw licking over the second 10-30 min period, from 468 ± 48 sec (vehicle) to 287 ± 28 sec (1 mg/kg) and 224 ± 27 sec (2 mg/kg) (P<0.01 and 0.001 vs vehicle by MWT, n=8 rats/group). The 0.5 mg/kg-treated rats also spent at least 30% less time in inflamed paw licking over pain periods: 98 ± 10 sec (early phase) and 334 ± 54 sec (late phase) compared to vehicle-treated rats 161 ± 19 sec and 468 ± 48 sec, respectively (P<0.05 vs vehicle by MWT, n=8 rats/group). From 30 min post-formalin injection, the duration of paw licking decreased in a parallel manner in both vehicle-and opiorphin analog-treated rats and their behavioral responses to the test compound as well as to morphine were not significant. Conversely, during this 30-60 min period, the control vehicle rats exhibited an important increase in the total number of formalin-injected paw flinches and body tremors. And systemic administration of opiorphin analog at 2 mg/kg significantly reduced this pain behavioral score throughout the 30 to 60 min time-period, from 300 ± 31 (vehicle) to 218 ± 15 (P ≤ 0.05 vs vehicle by MWT, n=8 rats/group).

This model was previously used for testing native opiorphin activity and we demonstrated that opiorphin, at 1 and 2 mg/kg I.V. doses inhibits nociception in both acute early and tonic late phases of the test by primarily activating µ-opioid pathways [1,10].

Conversely, under the same experimental conditions, we observed that the [C]-[(CH$_2$)$_6$]-QRF-[S-O-(CH$_2$)$_8$]-R cystine-dipeptide failed to significantly inhibit pain behavioral responses at 1 and 2 mg/kg tested doses (data not shown).

Thus, our data clearly indicate that the [C]-[(CH$_2$)$_6$]-QRF-[S-O-(CH$_2$)$_8$]-R opiorphin analog inhibits nociception induced by acute and long-acting chemical stimuli in the rat model. Strikingly, although metabolically more resistant and more potent in its ability to inhibit enkephalin-degrading ectopeptidases, the opiorphin analog-induced pain reduction in the formalin test is similar to the opiorphin natural peptide, in terms of dose effect, delay and duration of action. This could be due to the loss of a significant proportion of active derivative by dimerization and/or by hepatic metabolism *in vivo* in rats.

Conclusion

The goal of the study described here was to design and characterize functional analogs of opiorphin that display *in vivo* bioavailability properties superior to the native peptide. The inhibitory potency of the main functional derivatives toward human NEP and AP-N is summarized in Table 1. A close structural selectivity in the functional

Opiorphin derivatives	IC50, µM toward hAP-N	IC50, µM toward hNEP-Endopeptidase	IC50, µM toward hNEP-CarboxyDiPeptidase
Native opiorphin QRFSR	10 ± 2 (rAPN)	46 ± 5 (rNEP) 29 ± 3 (rmNEP) 11 ± 3 (mNEP/SP)	57 ± 4 (rNEP) 33 ± 6 (rmNEP)
QRF-[S-O-(CH2)8]-R	12 ± 1	2.1 ± 0.2	13 ± 3
[C]-QRFSR	0.8 ± 0.1	7 ± 1	7 ± 1
[C]-[(CH2)6]-QRFSR	0.8 ± 0.1	40 ± 5	# 158
C-[(CH2)6]-QRF-[S-O-(CH2)8]-R	0.9 ± 0.1 (rAPN) 0.9 ± 0.1 (mAPN)	0.8 ± 0.1 (rNEP) 1.6 ± 0.4 (mNEP) 1.6 ± 0.4 (mNEP/SP)	0.9 ± 0.1 (rNEP)
[dC]-QRF-[S-O-(CH2)8]-[dR]	0.022 ± 0.002 (rAPN) 0.3 ± 0.1 (mAPN)	4 ± 1 (rNEP) 9 ± 1 (mNEP)	21 ± 1 (rNEP) 37 ± 5 (mNEP)

Table 1: Comparative inhibition potencies of Opiorphin and peptidomimetic compounds toward human NEP and AP-N. Compound concentration for 50% inhibition of hNEP and hAP-N activity is expressed as mean ± SEM of at least 13 determination points. rAP-N/rNEP: soluble recombinant ectoenzymes; mAP-N/mNEP: membrane-bound native ectoenzymes expressed by LNCaP epithelial cells; rmAP-N/rmNEP: membrane-bound recombinant ectoenzymes expressed by transfected HEK cells. Numbers in bold highlight increased inhibitory potency relative to the native peptide.

interaction of opiorphin with both human NEP and AP-N targets was first demonstrated by SAR studies, thus limiting the possibilities of chemical changes. Nevertheless, results of the study clearly demonstrate that addition of a N-terminal Zn-chelating group, a Cys-thiol group and replacement of the first labile peptide bond by a polyethylene surrogate, a [CH$_2$]$_6$ linker, and, finally, substitution of Ser$_4$ by a octanoyl-Ser, Ser-O-[CH$_2$]$_8$, to the native opiorphin amino acid sequence produced a high performing C-[(CH$_2$)$_6$]-QRF[S-O-[CH$_2$]$_8$]-R derivative. This designed analog displays reinforced inhibitory potency toward hAP-N activity (more than 10-fold increase) and toward hNEP-Endopeptidase and CarboxyDiPeptidase activities (more than 40-fold increase) relative to the QRFSR natural peptide. Moreover, the analog shows increased stability in human plasma compared to unmodified opiorphin. Finally, we demonstrate that it retains the full analgesic activity characteristic of the opiorphin native peptide, in terms of delay of action and effective doses, in the behavioral formalin-induced pain rat model. If we consider that the maximum effective analgesic dose for the two compounds is 1 mg/kg I.V., the safety-effectiveness ratio is estimated at 30 for the designed analog and at 100 for the native peptide.

C-[(CH$_2$)$_6$]-QRF[S-O-[CH$_2$]$_8$]-R, has improved opiorphin pharmacological parameters and thus could be a promising analgesic drug-candidatein a preclinical and clinical setting.

Acknowledgements

This work was in large part supported by funding sources from the "Direction de la Valorisation et des Partenariats Industriels" and "Dons et Mécénat d'entreprises" Institut Pasteur. The maunscript was edited by traduction@lefevere-laoide.net

The present address of A. Bogeas: Team Glial Plasticity, U894 Inserm, Université Paris Descartes, Paris, France

No conflicts of interest, financial or otherwise, are declared by the author(s).

References

1. Wisner A, Dufour E, Messaoudi M, Nejdi A, Marcel A, et al. (2006) Human Opiorphin, a natural antinociceptive modulator of opioid-dependent pathways. Proc Natl Acad Sci USA 103: 17979-17984.

2. Rougeot C, Messaoudi M (2007) Identification of human opiorphin, a natural antinociceptive modulator of opioid-dependent pathways. M S-Med Sci 23: 37-39.

3. Toth F, Toth G, Benyhe S, Rougeot C, Wollemann M (2012) Opiorphin highly improves the specific binding and affinity of MERF and MEGY to rat brain opioid receptors. Regul Pept 178: 71-75.

4. Konig M, Zimmer AM, Steiner H, Holmes PV, Crawley JN, et al. (1996) Pain responses, anxiety and aggression in mice deficient in pre-proenkephalin. Nature 383: 535-538.

5. Filliol D, Ghozland S, Chluba J, Martin M, Matthes HW, et al. (2000) Mice deficient for delta- and mu-opioid receptors exhibit opposing alterations of emotional responses. Nat Genet 25: 195-200.

6. Ragnauth A, Schuller A, Morgan M, Chan J, Ogawa S, et al. (2001) Female preproenkephalin-knockout mice display altered emotional responses. Proc Natl Acad Sci USA 98: 1958-1963.

7. Nieto MM, Guen SL, Kieffer BL, Roques BP, Noble F (2005) Physiological control of emotion-related behaviors by endogenous enkephalins involves essentially the delta opioid receptors. Neuroscience 135: 305-313.

8. Noble F, Roques BP (2007) Protection of endogenous enkephalin catabolism as natural approach to novel analgesic and antidepressant drugs. Expert Opin Ther Targets 11: 145-159.

9. Tian XZ, Chen J, Xiong W, He T, Chen Q (2009) Effects and underlying mechanisms of human opiorphin on colonic motility and nociception in mice. Peptides 30: 1348-1354.

10. Rougeot C, Robert F, Menz L, Bisson JF, Messaoudi M (2010) Systemically Active Human Opiorphin Is a Potent yet Non-Addictive Analgesic without Drug Tolerance Effects. J Physiol Pharmacol 61: 483-490.

11. Javelot H, Messaoudi M, Garnier S, Rougeot C (2010) Human Opiorphin Is a Naturally Occurring Antidepressant Acting Selectively on Enkephalin-Dependent Delta-Opioid Pathways. J Physiol Pharmacol 61: 355-362.

12. Yang QZ, Lu SS, Tian XZ, Yang AM, Ge WW, et al. (2011) The antidepressant-like effect of human opiorphin via opioid-dependent pathways in mice. Neurosci Lett 489: 131-135.

13. Barros NM, Campos M, Bersanetti PA, Oliveira V, Juliano MA, et al. (2007) Neprilysin carboxydipeptidase specificity studies and improvement in its detection with fluorescence energy transfer peptides. Biol Chem 388: 447-455.

14. Blackmon DL, Watson AJ, Montrose MH (1992) Assay of apical membrane enzymes based on fluorogenic substrates. Anal Biochem 200: 352-358.

15. Rougeot C (2009) Method for identifying BPLP and opiorphin agonists or antagonists.

16. Rougeot C, Messaoudi M, Hermitte V, Rigault AG, Blisnick T, et al. (2003) Sialorphin, a natural inhibitor of rat membrane-bound neutral endopeptidase that displays analgesic activity. Proc Natl Acad Sci USA 100: 8549-8554.

17. Dufour E, Villard-Saussine S, Mellon V, Leandri R, Jouannet P, at al (2013) Opiorphin secretion pattern in healthy volunteers: Gender difference and organ specificity. Biochem Anal Biochem 2: 136.

18. Rosa M, Arsequell G, Rougeot C, Calle LP, Marcelo F, et al. (2012) Structure-activity relationship study of opiorphin, a human dual ectopeptidase inhibitor with antinociceptive properties. J Med Chem 55: 1181-1188.

19. Cummins PM, O'Connor B (1998) Pyroglutamyl peptidase: an overview of the three known enzymatic forms. Biochim Biophys Acta 1429: 1-17.

20. Gentilucci L, De Marco R, Cerisoli L (2010) Chemical modifications designed to improve peptide stability: incorporation of non-natural amino acids, pseudo-peptide bonds, and cyclization. Curr Pharm Des 16: 3185-3203.

21. Seebach D, Lukaszuk A, Patora-Komisarska K, Podwysocka D, Gardiner J, et al. (2011) On the terminal homologation of physiologically active peptides as a means of increasing stability in human serum--neurotensin, opiorphin, B27-KK10 epitope, NPY. Chem Biodivers 8: 711-739.

22. Hruby VJ, Qui W, Okayama T, Soloshonok VA (2002) Design of nonpeptides from peptide ligands for peptide receptors. Methods Enzymol 343: 91-123.

23. Roques BP, Noble F, Dauge V, Fournie-Zaluski MC, Beaumont A (1993) Neutral endopeptidase 24.11: structure, inhibition, and experimental and clinical pharmacology. Pharmacol Rev 45: 87-146.

24. Hidalgo IJ, Raub TJ, Borchardt RT (1989) Characterization of the human colon carcinoma cell line (Caco-2) as a model system for intestinal epithelial permeability. Gastroenterology 96: 736-749.

25. Irwin S (1968) Comprehensive observational assessment: Ia. A systematic, quantitative procedure for assessing the behavioral and physiologic state of the mouse. Psychopharmacol 13: 222-257.

26

The Effects of Gold and Silver Nanoparticles on an Enzymatic Reaction between Horseradish Peroxidase and 3,3',5,5'-Tetramethylbenzidine

Barry Morris and Farhad Behzad*

British Institute of Technology and E-commerce, London, UK

Abstract

The purpose of this investigation was to study the effects of gold (Au) and silver (Ag) nanoparticles on a commonly used enzymatic reaction between horseradish peroxidase (HRP) and the substrate, 3,3',5,5'-tetramethylbenzidine (TMB).

Two different methodologies were used in this study. The first was the addition of small quantities of nanoparticles, directly onto a solution of streptavidin peroxidase (streptavidin bound to HRP), prior to its reaction with TMB. The second, was the addition of nanoparticles to immobilised streptavidin peroxidase, covalently bounded to wells of a microtitre plate. In both cases, reactions with TMB were measured by visible absorbance spectroscopy, using a microtitre plate-reader.

The results indicate that both gold and silver nanoparticles have a significant affect; with gold suppressing the reaction and silver enhancing it.

Keywords: Nanoparticles; Horseradish peroxidase; Tetramethylbenzidine

Introduction

The reaction between the enzyme, horseradish peroxidase (HRP), and the substrate, 3,3',5,5'-tetramethylbenzidine (TMB), is well established and frequently used in Enzyme-Linked Immunosorbent Assays (ELISAs) for detecting and measuring analytes, such as proteins and antibodies. HRP has a metal ion cofactor, known as haem, which is a prosthetic group consisting of an iron ion. When haem, in the peroxidase, is combined with TMB, it produces a one-electron oxidation product, which is a free radical cation that is responsible for the change in colour from an almost colourless solution to dark blue as explained [1]. The degree of this colour change is directly reflective of the amount and activity of the enzyme; hence its use in ELISAs as the signal generating stage. When an acid is applied to the enzyme-substrate complex, a further reaction takes place, producing a two-electron diimine product, which changes the colour from dark blue to yellow.

The purpose of the following experiments was to investigate the effects of gold and silver nanoparticles on the HRP activity, using TMB as the substrate. Visible absorption spectroscopy was used to obtain readings of the amount of light transmitted through the wells of a microtitre plate. These readings, known as transmittance data, Io, were then converted into relative absorbance, Ar, using Equation 1:

$$Ar = \frac{Aw}{Ap} \times 100\% \quad .... Equation\ 1$$

——Where,

Aw = Absorbance of the contents of a microtitre well

Ap = Absorbance of the contents of a microtitre well with a positive control reference

The absorbance, Aw or Ap, was calculated using the generic equation for absorbance, A, shown in Equation 2:

$$A = Log_{10}\left[\frac{Ii}{Io}\right] \quad ...Equation\ 2$$

Where,

Ii = Intensity of light entering a microtitre well

Io = Intensity of light leaving a microtiter well (transmittance)

Materials and Apparatus

Materials

A Hyaluronidase Assay Kit, from Razie Biotech Ltd., was purchased from AMS Biotech.com.

The following materials were purchased from Sigma-Aldrich UK: 3,3',5,5'-tetramethylbenzidine; streptavidin peroxidase (streptavidin bound to HRP; 1 mg of lypholised powder was dissolved in 1 ml of phosphate buffered saline (PBS) solution, a 100 times (v/v) in PBS was used in the procedure); gold colloid solution, 20 nm; gold colloid solution, 10 nm; gold colloid solution, 5 nm; silver nanoparticles dispersed in water, citrate stabilised, 157 nm.

Apparatus

1. Two, 96-well microtitre plates; one of them coated with biotin

2. Shaker/incubator; set at 390 r.p.m. and 37 ºC

3. Microtitre plate-reader

Experimental procedure

The experimental procedure was carried out using two methodologies, a direct method and a method using a biotin bounded

*Corresponding author: Farhad Behzad, British Institute of Technology & E-commerce, London, United Kingdom; E-mail: farhad.behzad@talk21.com

plate. Both methods required streptavidin, dilute 100 times (v/v) in PBS, which was the first task to be performed.

The direct method used six wells of a non-coated, 96-well microtitre plate. Transmittance readings, through the empty wells, were recorded using the plate-reader. A 2 μl drop of streptavidin peroxidase:PBS solution was placed in the centre of one of the wells, which was used as a positive control reference well, i.e. without the addition of any nanoparticles. A 5 μl drop of 20 nm gold nanoparticles was placed in the centre of the second well, which was used as a negative control reference well, i.e. without the addition of any streptavidin:PBS solution. A 2 μl drop of streptavidin peroxidase:PBS solution was placed in the centre of each of the four remaining wells and 5 μl of nanoparticles were added to each of these drops, using the following materials: 20 nm Au nanoparticles were added to the first drop, 10 nm Au nanoparticles were added to the second drop, 5 nm Au nanoparticles were added to the third drop and 157 nm Ag nanoparticles were added to the forth. The plate was placed in the shaker/incubator for a period of 10 minutes. It was then removed from the shaker/incubator and each of the six wells were filled with 50 μl of TMB, prior to the plate being returned to the shaker/incubator. Another set of transmittance readings were recorded after 40 minutes incubation.

The bounded method, used four biotin coated wells of a 96-well, microtitre plate. Each well was filled with 50 μl of streptavidin peroxidase:PBS solution and placed in the shaker/incubator for a period of 30 minutes. The wells were emptied, washed in distilled water and dried, prior to the addition of nanoparticles. One well was left void of nanoparticles and used as a positive control reference well. The remaining three wells were filled with 50 μl of nanoparticles. The first with 5 nm Au nanoparticles, the second with 20 nm Au nanoparticles and the third with 157 nm Ag nanoparticles. The microtitre plate was returned to the shaker/incubator for a period of 10 minutes; then, emptied, washed with distilled water and dried again. Transmittance readings, of the empty wells, were recorded using the plate reader, prior to filling each well with 50 μl of TMB. The plate was returned to the shaker/incubator for a further 30 minutes, and then another set of transmittance readings were recorded.

Both sets of transmittance readings, obtained from each of the above procedures, were used to calculate the absorbance of the contents of each well, relative to the absorbance of the positive control reference wells, using Equations 1 and 2.

The procedures were repeated a number of times to obtain mean values.

For the direct method, no colour change was detected in the negative control well, where 20 nm gold nanoparticles were added to TMB on its own.

The results, expressed for each well, are the mean values of six wells, in three sets of experiments.

Results

When the wells were observed by eye, both experiments revealed that only the positive control reference wells and those containing silver nanoparticles appeared to be dark blue in colour; the remaining wells appeared to be either transparent or a very pale blue.

Discussion

The results, obtained from the two different methodologies, indicate that gold and silver nanoparticles have a significant effect on the enzymatic reaction between HRP and TMB.

The positive control reference wells contained the enzyme-substrate complexes only, without any nanoparticles. These were expecte to produce normal reactions and the relative absorbance of these complexes was used as reference points of 100%.

In the direct method, a 5 μl drop of 20 nm gold nanoparticles was placed in the centre of the negative control reference well, without the addition of any streptavidin:PBS solution. This was expected to produce no reaction and the relative absorbance of the nanoparticle/TMB solution was used as a baseline reference (i.e. the minimum amount of relative absorbance). The results clearly show that the nanoparticles did not react with the TMB and played no part on the conversion of TMB into colour products. The addition of streptavidin:PBS solution, on the other hand, together with the same size gold nanoparticles, provides evidence that colour products were produced by the reaction between streptavidin:PBS and TMB alone, while the gold nanoparticles inhibited this reaction by almost 40% relative absorbance (Figure 1).

The direct method also provides evidence that biotin, which was coated on the microtitre plate for the bounded method, had no part to play in the reactions. The role of biotin was only to bind HRP to the walls of the microtitre wells.

In both experiments, the relative absorbance of the enzyme-substrate complex, containing silver nanoparticles, exceeded that of the complex contained in the positive control reference well. Thus, indicating that the silver nanoparticles enhanced the reaction between HRP and TMB [2]. Who demonstrated that silver nanoparticles not only enhances the activity of HRP, but also alters its structure. However, their results also indicate that this only occurred within a specific concentration range of silver nanoparticles (Figure 2).

On the other hand, the relative absorbance of the enzyme-substrate complex, containing gold nanoparticles, was less than that of the complex contained in the positive control reference well. Thus, indicating that the gold nanoparticles inhibited the reaction between HRP and TMB. Furthermore, the results also show that these reactions appear to be influenced by the relative size of the nanoparticles, with 20 nm gold nanoparticles having the least effect and the smaller nanoparticles exhibiting greater inhibition.

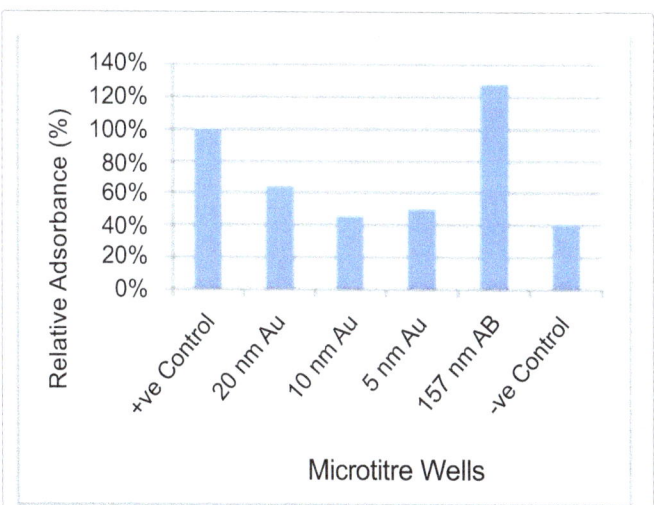

Figure 1: Results from the Direct Method- Relative Absorbance of the Wells, containing Gold (Au) and Silver (Ag) Nanoparticles using, the Direct Method

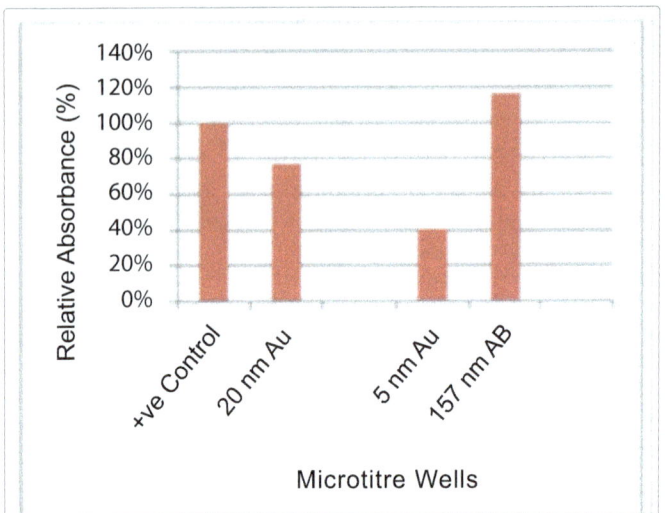

Figure 2: Results from the ELISA Method- Relative Absorbance of the Wells, containing Gold (Au) and Silver (Ag) Nanoparticles, using the Bounded Method

Considering these results, it is not unreasonable to suggest that other enzymes may also be affected by nanoparticles, and that different types of nanoparticles, of different shapes and sizes, may affect enzymatic reactions, in different ways [3], has shown that the properties of nanoparticles, such as size, shape, surface chemistry and charge, can alter the structure and function of enzymes [4], has also demonstrated that nanoparticles are able to induce protein modifications.

A great deal of research work is being carried out on the effects of nanoparticles on biological systems. It comes as no surprise that these systems are influenced by nanoparticles, since the common ground between nanoparticles and biology is the nanoscale [5], has demonstrated that gold and silver nanoparticles could enhance the radiation sensitivity of hepatocellular carcinoma cells (HCC), a common type of liver cancer. The mechanism for this is thought to be due to programmed cell death (apoptosis) or elevated DNA damage.

Veeraapandian demonstrated that protein capped gold nanoparticles have been shown to exhibit good antioxidant activity, which reduces cell damage or death, while protein capped silver nanoparticles are able to inhibit the growth of several Gram-positive and Gram-negative microorganisms [6].

Conclusion

Enzymatic reactions are influenced by nanoparticles. The mechanism of these nanoparticle-enzyme interactions are currently under investigation. This is an important area of research, since the ability to regulate enzymatic activity could potentially lead to new processes for enzyme control and modification, with possible use in new drug developments and industrial applications. It also signifies probable toxicity of nanoparticles as they become more widely present in everyday life via off-the-counter available cosmetics and household goods.

References

1. Tatzber F, Griebenow S, Wonisch W, Winkler R (2003) Dual method for the determination of peroxidase activity and total peroxides–iodide leads to a significant increase of peroxidase activity in human sera. Anal Biochem 316: 147-53.

2. Karim Z, Adnan R, Ansari MS (2012) Low Concentration of Silver Nanoparticles Not Only Enhances the Activity of Horseradish Peroxidase but Alter the Structure . PLoS ONE 7: e41422.

3. Wu ZC, Zhang B, Yan B (2009) Regulation of enzyme activity through interactions with nanoparticles. Int J Mol Sci 10: 4198-4209.

4. Sanfins E, Dairou J, Rodrigues-Lima F, Dupret JM (2011) Nanoparticle-protein interactions: from crucial plasma proteins to key enzymes. Journal of Physics: Conference Series 304: 012039.

5. Zheng Q, Yang H, Wei J, Tong JL, Shu YQ (2013) The role and mechanisms of nanoparticles to enhance radiosensivity in hepatocellular cell. Biomed Pharmacother 67: 569-575

6. Veeraapandian S, Sawant SN, Doble M (2012) Antibacterial and antioxidant activity of protein capped silver and gold nanoparticles synthesized with Escherichiacoli. J Biomed Nanotechnol 8: 140-148.

27

Therapeutic Effects of *Aloe Vera* Plant Extract Against Cyclophosphamide and Buthionine Sulfoximine Induced Toxicities in the Bladder

Kamel Rouissi[1]*[#], Soumaya Kouidhi[1#], Bechr Hamrita[1#], Slah Ouerhani[2], Mohamed Cherif[3] and Amel Benammar Elgaaied[1]

[1]*Laboratory of Genetics, Immunology, and Human Pathology, Faculty of Sciences of Tunis, University of El Manar I, 2092, Tunis, Tunisia*
[2]*Laboratory of Molecular and Cellular Hematology, Pasteur Institute of Tunis, Tunisia*
[3]*Department of Urology, Hospital of Charles Nicolle, Tunis, Tunisia*
[#]*Authors have contributed equally in this work*

Abstract

Bladder toxicity is one of the most troublesome side effects associated with chemotherapeutic treatments of cancer involving the use of cyclophosphamide (CP) and buthionine-SR-sulfoximine (BSO). The present study was undertaken to investigate the effects of pre-treatment with an *Aloe vera* plant extract (AVE) on the urotoxicity induced by acute doses of CP and BSO using a Swiss albino mice model. The modulation of toxicity was evaluated by measuring lipid peroxidation (LPO), peroxide hydrogen production (H_2O_2) and antioxidants in the urinary bladder of the animals. The findings revealed that *Aloe vera* induced remarkable protective effects in terms of both LPO and enzymatic antioxidant activities. The CP-treated mice were noted to undergo significant decreases in the activities of glutathione S-transferase (GST), glutathione reductase (GR), glutathione peroxidase (GP), and catalase (CAT) when compared to the controls. The levels of reduced glutathione (GSH) also decreased with an increase in LPO in the CP-treated animals and BSO treatment exerted an additive toxic effect in the CP-treated animals. Pre-treatment with the *Aloe vera* herbal extract restored all enzymatic activities back to normal, thus confirming its overall protective effect against the toxic effects of CP and BSO. The potential effect of AVE to prevent CP and BSO induced urotoxicity was also reflected by the histological analysis, indicative of its uroprotective effects. The restoration of GSH through treatment with *Aloe vera* may play an important role in the reversal of CP-induced apoptosis and free radical mediated LPO in urinary bladder. Due to its widespread availability in nature and relative lack of toxicity, the *Aloe vera* plant extract presented in the current study could be considered a potential strong candidate for future applications as an adjutant to cancer chemotherapies.

Introduction

Bladder cancer is one of the most frequently occurring cancers in the world. According to the current estimates by the American Cancer Society (ACS), this disease is the fourth most common cancer in men and eighth leading cause of death in women in the United States. Although several treatments and therapies, including surgery, radiation, and chemotherapy, have been used to reduce and prevent the rising death rates caused by this deadly disease, a number of serious concerns have often been voiced with respect to the troublesome side effects associated with each type of treatment.

Cyclophosphamide (CP) and buthionine-SR-sulfoximine (BSO) are two of the leading medications often prescribed for the treatment of cancer. CP is an effective alkylating agent widely used in the anti-neoplastic therapy of a variety of cancers, including lymphoma, myeloma, and chronic lymphocytic leukemia [1]. CP intake has, however, frequently been associated with a variety of troublesome side effects, including alopecia, cardiac damage, gonadotropy, hemorrhagic cystitis, hematopoetic depression, nausea, vomiting, and carcinogenicity [2] as well as lung toxicity [3]. It has also been reported to involve a number of urological side effects, such as transient irritating voiding symptoms, including dypsia, hemorrhagic cystitis, bladder fibrosis, necrosis, contracture, and vesicometral flux [4,5].

The accumulation of CP reactive metabolites in the urinary bladder has also been reported to induce reactive oxygen species (ROS) production, which cause peroxidative damage to the urinary bladder as well as to other vital organs [3]. Additionally, CP treatment has been described to bring about a decrease in the levels of reduced glutathione (GSH), which represents one of the most important organic molecules within the cell that determine its ability to suppress toxic substances, such as chemotherapeutic reactive metabolites [2,6,7].

In fact, GSH depletion is considered as an attractive strategy for

the sensitization of tumour cells to certain chemotherapeutic agents. A number of reports suggested that BSO can be used effectively to reduce the level of GSH and may help to restore the sensitivity of resistant tumours to alkylating agents. BSO is a potent inhibitor of r-glutamylcysteine synthetase, has been reported to enhance the *in vitro* antitumor efficacy of a number of drugs including CP, melphalan, adriamycin, daunomycin and mitomycin C [8]. By inhibiting this essential enzyme, BSO has the capacity to drastically reduce glutathione content and has been shown in model systems to enhance the cytotoxic effects of specific chemotherapeutic agents and radiation therapy [9]. However, CP-induced immunosuppression may incite various types of infectious agents that have serious GSH depleting effects [10]. In other words, CP treatment might decrease the GSH content itself but the secondary infections associated with it might bring additional decreases in the levels of GSH. Accordingly, a patient undergoing CP chemotherapy would need an excessive supply of GSH-restoring antioxidants or compounds that induce GSH production.

In this context, a number of GSH-inducing compounds have been reported to be effective CP and BSO toxicity reducers in animals

*Corresponding author: Dr. Kamel Rouissi, Laboratory of Genetics, Immunology, and Human Pathology, Faculty of sciences of Tunis, University of El Manar I, 2092, Tunis, Tunisia, E-mail: rouissik2000@yahoo.fr

[8]. Several extracts from plant origin have been described to exert valuable protective and/or restorative effects on BSO and CP-induced decreases of GSH [9]. Of particular interest to the aims of the present study, Aloe plants have long been used to treat a wide array of ailments and diseases. *Aloe barbadensis* Miller, commonly known as Aloe vera, is one of the most popular varieties of Aloe plants whose healing properties are immense [11]. It belongs to the Liliaceal family, of which about 360 species exist. It is a cactus-like plant that grows readily in hot, dry climates and, due to its great curative properties, has often been cultivated in large quantities. Two distinct preparations of Aloe plants are most used medicinally. The leaf exudate (Aloe latex), which is a yellow, bitter liquid derived from the skin of the Aloe leaf, has strong stimulatory and laxative properties and has, therefore, been commonly used for the treatment of diabetes, coughs, wounds, ulcers, cancer, headaches, arthritis, among various other conditions [12]. The mucilaginous gel (Aloe gel), which is a clear colourless semi-solid gel extracted from the leaf parenchyma, has attractive immunomodulatory properties, and has, therefore, been commonly used as a remedy against a variety of skin disorders [13].

Public interest in *Aloe vera* has grown quickly, and considerable research has been conducted over the past few decades to explore the various components and properties of this herbal medicine and to find out clues as to its potential cosmetic, pharmaceutical, and therapeutic applications. In fact, although scientific evidence for the cosmetic and therapeutic effectiveness of *Aloe vera* is very limited, various cosmetic and medicinal formulations have been made from Aloe latex and Aloe gel. *Aloe vera* is rich in antioxidants and various nutrients. It contains lignin, saponins, and mono and polysaccharides (including Acemannan) [14]. The consumption of *Aloe vera* leaf formulations has been shown to display anti-arthritic, anti-rheumatoid, and anti-cancer properties [15] as well as anti-diabetic benefits [16]. It has been commonly used for the topical treatment of a variety of ailments and disorders, including chronic wounds, thermal injuries, skin infections, inflammations, oral ulcers, and psoriasis [17] as well as for the prevention of ultraviolet (UV)-induced immunosuppressions [18].

Considering its widespread availability in nature, relative richness in antioxidants, and distinguished healing properties, the present study was undertaken to investigate the effects of the oral administration of an *Aloe vera* plant extract in terms of antioxidant activities, lipid peroxidation (LPO) and peroxide hydrogen ($H2O2$) production in the urinary bladder of CP and BSO treated mice that were pre-disposed or concomitantly exposed to a GSH reducing agent in the form of either an infection or antibiotic use.

Materials and Methods

Aloe vera plant extract (AVE)

The present study used a total aqueous semisolid extract of *Aloe vera* that was purchased from the Plant Extract Division of the local Central Pharmacy, Tunisia. The plant extract had moisture and ash contents of 12% and 8%, respectively. The pH of 10% aqueous solution of extract was 4.6. The authenticity of the extract was certified by the manufacturer's expert taxonomist.

Chemicals

Cyclophosphamide monohydrate (2-(bis-(2-chloroethyl) amino) tetrahydro- 2H-1 ,3,2-oxazaphosphorine 2-oxide monohydrate); CAS 6055-1 9-2; BSO (L-buthionine-SR-sulfoximine); CAS 5072-26-4 were purchased from Sigma–Aldrich Co., St. Louis, MO, USA.

Animals

The experimental essays of the present study were conducted on male Swiss albino mice (25 ± 2 g) provided by the animal service of the Pasteur Institute of Tunis, Tunisia. All care and animal handling procedures were performed in accordance with the guidelines of the Institutional Animal Ethics Committee (IAEC). The animals were bred and maintained under standard laboratory conditions (temperature 25 ± 2°C; photoperiod of 12 hrs). Commercial pellet diet and water were given *ad libitum*.

Dosage and experimental groups

BSO, CP and plant extract of *Aloe vera* (AVE) were suspended in normal saline. The animals were divided into seven groups, Groups I–VII, of six mice each. Group I (Control) referred to control mice that were administered normal saline p.o. for 10 days and a single i.p. injection on the 10th day of treatment. Group II (BSO) referred to the mice that received BSO (500 mg/kg body wt) and to which a single i.p. injection was administered on the 10th day. Group III (CP) designated the mice that received CP (50 mg/kg body wt.) and a single i.p. dose on the 10th day. Group IV (BSO + CP) referred to animals that were administered BSO i.p. 5 hrs before CP administration. Group V (CP + AVE) referred to animals that were administered plant extract for 10 days and a single i.p. injection of CP on the 10th day. Group VI (BSO + AVE) designated animals that were given plant extract treatment (100 mg/kg body wt.) p.o. for 10 days and a single i.p. injection of BSO on the 10th day. Group VII (BSO + CP + AVE) referred to the animals that were administered plant extract for 10 days and CP and BSO on the 10th day. Dosing was performed in such a way that all of the animals could be sacrificed on the same day, i.e., day 11. The selection of BSO and CP doses was based on pilot experiments that involved the assay of a wide range of doses and on data provided from previously published reports [9,19].

Biochemical investigations

Upon the completion of the treatment, the animals were sacrificed under mild anesthesia and their bladders were removed. The bladder tissue was homogenized in chilled phosphate buffer (0.1 M, pH 7.4) using a Potter homogenizer. The homogenate was centrifuged at 10,500g for 30 min at 4°C to obtain the post-mitochondrial supernatant (PMS), which was used for the biochemical measurements as described below.

Cell culture and peroxide hydrogen production:

Cell culture: The urothelial cell line T24 was employed as an *in vitro* model of the human bladder because of its ability to react to adequate stimuli, obtained from Pateur Institute of Tunis, Tunisia, was routinely grown in 75 cm² flasks (Nunc, Denmark) and maintained in minimum essential medium (MEM) (Invitrogen, Glasgow, UK) supplemented with 10% foetal bovine serum (FBS, Hyclone, Logan, UT), 100 units/ml penicillin and 100 lg/ml streptomycin. Cultures were maintained in a humidified atmosphere with 5% CO_2 at 37°C. Cell dissociation was achieved with 0.05% trypsin-0.02% EDTA. Briefly, cells were seeded on 24-well culture plates in medium at an approximate density of 10⁵ cells/cm² and, after 24 hrs stabilization, bladder urothelial cell line T24 were co-cultured with medium containing various concentrations of CP and BSO (200 and 800 μM) and *Aloe vera* plant extract (10, 50 and 100μM) for 24 hrs. The concentration of CP was selected based on previously reported cytotoxic levels in cultured cells [20]. For stock solution, CP and BSO were dissolved in MilliQ Plus sterilized water at the concentration of 800 mM and *Aloe vera* plant extract was dissolved in dimethyl sulfoxide (DMSO) to obtain a 100mM. The experimental concentrations were freshly prepared in the basal medium with a final DMSO concentration of 0.1%.

Measurement of H_2O_2: Measurement of H_2O_2 was carried out by the ferrous ion oxidation xylenol orange (FOX1) method [21]. The FOX1 reagent consisted of 25mM sulphuric acid, 250 lM ferrous ammonium sulfate, 100µM xylenol orange and 0.1 M sorbitol. Briefly, 100µl of culture medium were added to 900µl of FOX1 reagent vortexed and incubated during 30min at room temperature. Solutions were then centrifuged at 12000g for 10 min; the amount of H_2O_2 in the supernatants was determined using spectrophotometer at 560nm.

Lipid peroxidation: LPO was measured using the procedure of Uchiyama and Mihara [22]. The assay mixture consisted of 0.67% thiobarbituric acid; TBA (Sigma-Aldrich), 10 mM; butylated hydroxy toluene BHT (Sigma-Aldrich), 1%; ortho-phosphoric acid (Sigma-Aldrich); and tissue homogenate in a total volume of 3ml. The rate of LPO was expressed as nmol of TBA reactive substances (TBARS) formed/h/g of tissue using molecular extinction coefficient epsilon (ϵ) of 1.56×10^5 M^{-1} cm^{-1}.

Measurement of GSH: GSH content was measured in the PMS of urinary bladder by the method of Haque et al. [9]. PMS (1ml) was precipitated with 1ml of 4% sulfosalicylic acid (Sigma-Aldrich). The samples were incubated at 4°C for 1 hr and then centrifuged at 1200g for 15 min at 4°C. The assay mixture consisted of 0.2 ml of filtered aliquot, 2.6 ml of sodium phosphate buffer (0.1 M, pH 7.4), and 0.2 ml 100 mM DTNB (dithio-bis-2-nitrobenzoic acid, Sigma-Aldrich) in a total volume of 3 ml. The absorbance of the reaction product was measured at 412 nm, and the results were expressed as nmol GSH/g of tissue.

Antioxidant enzyme measurements: Glutathione-S-Transferase (GST) activity was assayed using the method of Haque et al. [9]. The reaction mixture consisted of 1.675 ml sodium phosphate buffer, 0.2 ml of 1 mM GSH (Sigma-Aldrich), 0.025 ml of 1 mM CDNB (1-chloro-2,4-dinitrobenzene, Sigma-Aldrich), and 0.1 ml of PMS in a total volume of 2 ml. The change in absorbance was recorded at 340 nm and the enzyme activity calculated as nmol CDNB conjugates formed/min/mg protein using epsilon (ϵ) of 9.6×10^3 M^{-1} cm^{-1}. GR (glutathione reductase) activity was assayed by the method of Sharma et al. [19]. The assay mixture consisted of 1.6 ml sodium phosphate buffer, 0.1 ml of 1 mM ethylenediamine tetra acetic acid disodium salt (EDTA, Sigma-Aldrich), 0.1 ml NADPH (nicotinamide adenine dinucleotide phosphate reduced, Sigma-Aldrich), and 0.1 ml oxidized glutathione (Sigma-Aldrich) and PMS (0.1 ml) in total volume of 2 ml.

Enzyme activity measured at 340 nm was calculated as nmol NADPH oxidized/min/mg of protein, using epsilon (ϵ) of 6.22×10^3 M^{-1} cm^{-1}. Glutathione peroxidase (GP) activity was assayed using the method of Sharma et al. [19]. The assay mixture consisted of 1.49 ml sodium phosphate buffer, 0.1 ml EDTA (1 mM), 0.1 ml sodium azide (1 mM, Central Pharmacy of Tunis, Tunisia), 0.1 ml of 1 mM GSH (Sigma–Aldrich), 0.1 ml NADPH (0.02 mM), 0.01 ml of 0.25 mM hydrogen peroxide (H_2O_2, CDH Chemicals), and 0.1 ml PMS in a total volume of 2 ml. Oxidation of NADPH was recorded spectrophotometrically at 340 nm. The enzyme activity was calculated as nmol NADPH oxidized/min/mg of protein using epsilon (ϵ) of 6.22×10^3 M^{-1} cm^{-1}. CAT (catalase) activity was assayed using the method of Haque et al. [9]. The assay mixture consisted of 1.95 ml phosphate buffer, 1 ml H2O2 (0.09 M), and 0.05 ml of PMS at a final volume of 3 ml. Change in absorbance was recorded kinetically at 240 nm. CAT activity was calculated in terms of nmol H_2O_2 consumed/min/mg of protein.

Protein measurement: Protein was measured by the method of Lowry et al. (1951).

Histological studies

Bladder urothelium tissue, extracted from the control and treated mice was fixed in 10% buffered formalin and was processed for paraffin sectioning. Sections of about 5 µm thickness were stained with hematoxylin and eosin to examine under light microscope.

Statistical analysis

Single factor one-way analysis of variance (ANOVA) was performed to determine significant differences in results of various groups. The statistical significance level was set at P values < 0.05. A Student-Newman–Keuls test was then carried out to analyze and compare the significance of the different treatment groups. The values were expressed as mean ± SE.

Results

No mortalities and significant changes in the body weight of the different groups of animals were recorded during the treatment.

Lipid peroxidation (LPO)

The findings revealed that BSO treatment brought about a significant increase (P < 0.01) in the LPO levels in the bladder over the control values (Figure 1). The administration of CP was also noted to induce LPO in significant way. Likewise, the cumulative effect of BSO + CP resulted in significant increase in the LPO as compared to Group I (control). BSO + CP group (Group IV) also underwent a significant (P < 0.01) increase in the levels of LPO when compared the CP group (Group III) alone (Figure 1). The animals pre-treated with *Aloe vera* plant extract (AVE) and subsequently exposed to BSO (BSO + AVE), on the other hand, were noted to undergo a significant (P < 0.01) reduction in terms of LPO levels in the bladder. When the values obtained for the CP + AVE group (Group V) were compared to those of the CP group (Group II), AVE treatment was also observed to significantly (P < 0.05)

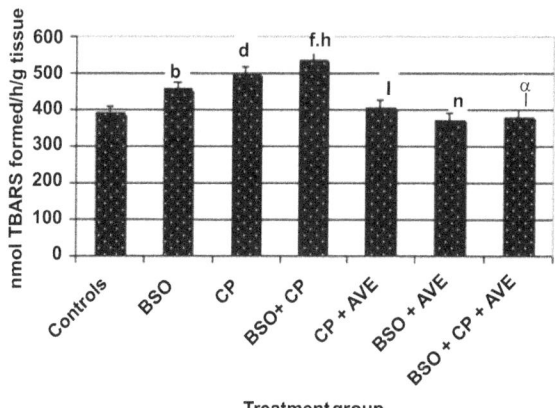

Figure 1: Effect of *Aloe vera* plant extract (AVE), BSO, and CP on the lipid peroxidation (LPO) in the urinary bladder of mice. Significant differences are indicated by $^bP < 0.01$ and $^dP < 0.01$ in Group II (BSO) and Group III (CP) treated animals, respectively and by $^fP < 0.01$ in Group IV (BSO + CP), as compared to control animals (Group I). $^hP < 0.01$ indicates significant levels for the BSO + CP group when compared to the CP group. $^iP < 0.01$ and $^nP < 0.05$ indicate significant differences of values for Group V (CP + AVE) and Group VI (BSO + AVE) when compared to Group III and Group II, respectively. $^qP < 0.01$ when values for Group IV and Group VII were compared. Values are means ± SE (n = 6).

reduce the levels of LPO in the bladder. As illustrated in Figure 1, the comparison between the LPO values obtained for the LPO of BSO + CP group (Group IV) and those of the BSO + CP + AVE group clearly shows a significant decrease (P < 0.01) in the case of the latter (Group VII).

Reduced glutathione

The findings revealed that, when compared to the control values (5.23 nmol GSH/g tissue), the BSO, CP and BSO + CP-treated groups underwent significant (P < 0.01) decreases of 2.9, 4.1 and 1.9 nmol GSH/g tissue in GSH, respectively (data generated for Cellular GSH of urinary bladder are shown in Figure 2). Likewise and when compared to the CP group (Group III), the BSO + CP group (Group IV) showed a significant (P < 0.01) decrease in terms of GSH levels. As shown in Figure 2, when the BSO and BSO + AVE groups were compared, the GSH content of the latter was noted to undergo a significant increase (P < 0.01). Similarly, the GSH content in the bladder of the CP + AVE group (Group V) showed a significant increase (P < 0.01) when compared to the group given only CP (Group III). When the GSH values obtained

for the BSO + CP (Group IV) group were compared to those of the BSO + CP + AVE group (Group VII), a significant (P < 0.01) restoration in GSH was recorded (Figure 2).

Antioxidant enzymes

BSO and CP treatments were observed to induce significant (P < 0.01) decreases in terms of GST, GR, GP and CAT activities in the bladder when compared to the control group (Table 1). The BSO + CP group also showed an additive significant (P < 0.01) decrease in the activities of GST, GR, and GP when compared to the CP or control group. However, no significant difference was observed in terms of CAT activity between the animals of group IV (BSO + CP) and group III (CP). The activities of those antioxidant enzymes increased significantly (P < 0.01) in both the BSO + AVE (Group VI) and the CP + AVE (Group V) groups when compared to their respective controls, the BSO (Group II) and CP (Group III) groups (Table 1). The animals treated with AVE and subsequently exposed to BSO + CP (Group VII, BSO + CP + AVE treatment) displayed a significant increase (P < 0.01) in the activities of all the antioxidant enzymes when compared to the BSO + CP group (Group IV).

Hydrogen peroxide (H_2O_2) production *in vitro*

Figure 3 showed the effects of CP and AVE on H_2O_2 production in urothelial cell line T24. To check if the combination of CP and AVE had any benefits, cells were treated with CP (200 and 800μM) and varying doses of AVE (10, 50 and 100μM) for 24 h. The levels of H_2O_2 generated in medium of cells were significantly (P < 0.05) increased by 159 and 241% compared to controls after exposure to CP (200 and 800μM) respectively, and were significantly (P < 0.05) deceased by (27%, 41% and 20%) cells co-culture with AVE (10, 50 and 100μM) and CP at dose (200μM) and by (40%, 49% and 25%) at dose (800μM) compared with CP alone (200 and 800μM) respectively.

Histological examination of bladder urethelium

Figure 4 illustrates the histopathological assessments of bladder urothelium tissue in experimental mice. Histopathological examination of the urothelium tissue revealed that CP treatment caused abnormal cellular arrangement with few pyknotic nucleus, vacuolated spaces and hemorrhage. However, co-administration of AVE at 100 mg/kg body weight prevented these changes and maintained normal architecture with less number of pyknotic nuclei and showed almost normal

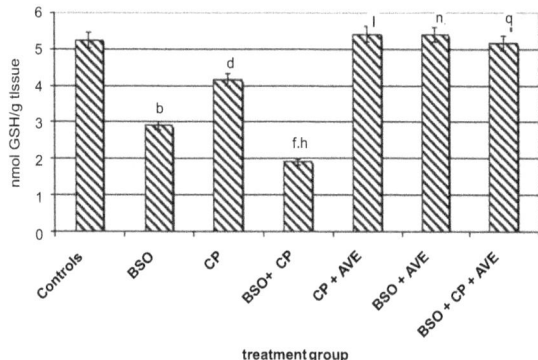

Figure 2: Effect of *Aloe vera* plant extract (AVE), BSO, and CP on GSH content in urinary bladder of mice. Significant differences are indicated by [b]P < 0.01 and [d]P < 0.01 in Group II (BSO) and Group III (CP), respectively, and [f]P < 0.01 in Group IV (BSO + CP) when compared to control animals (Group I). [h]P < 0.01 indicates significant changes in the BSO+CP group when compared to the CP group. [l]P < 0.01 and nP < 0.01 indicate significant differences in observations for Group IV (CP + AVE) and Group VI (BSO + AVE) when compared to the data obtained for the GSH levels of Groups III and II, respectively. [q]P < 0.01 when GSH data of Group IV was compared to that of Group VII. Values are means ± SE (n = 6).

Group	Activity of antioxidant enzyme			
	GST	GR	GP	CAT
I (Controls)	144 ± 3	143 ± 4	155 ± 5	104± 3
II (BSO)	100 ± 2 [b]	92 ± 4 [b]	122 ± 3 [b]	97± 2 [b]
III (CP)	115 ± 3 [d]	122 ± 5 [d]	139 ± 4 [c]	84± 3 [d]
IV (BSO+CP)	79 ± 3 [f,h]	86 ± 2 [f,h]	118 ± 3 [f,h]	82± 3 [f]
V (CP+AVE)	153 ± 5 [l]	152 ± 5 [l]	162 ± 2 [l]	107± 5 [l]
VI (BSO+AVE)	146 ± 3 [n]	149 ± 6 [n]	156 ± 4 [n]	113± 7 [n]
VII (BSO+CP+AVE)	145 ± 4 [q]	148 ± 6 [q]	154 ± 4 [q]	104± 5 [q]

CP: Cyclophosphamide; BSO: Buthionine Sulfoximine; AVE: *Aloe vera* plant extract

Values are means ± SE (n = 6). GST expressed as nmol CDNB conjugates/min/mg protein, GR as nmol NADPH oxidized/min/mg protein, and GP as nmol NADPH oxidized/min/mg protein. CAT activity is expressed as nmol H2O2 consumed/min/mg protein. Significant differences are indicated by [b]P < 0.01, [d]P < 0.01, [c]P < 0.05, and [f]P < 0.01 when compared to control animals. (Group I) [n]P < 0.01 when compared to Group II, [h]P < 0.01 and [l]P < 0.01 when compared to CP-treated animals (Group III), and [q]P < 0.01 when compared to Group IV.

Table 1: Activities of antioxidant enzymes in the urinary bladder of mice in different treatment groups.

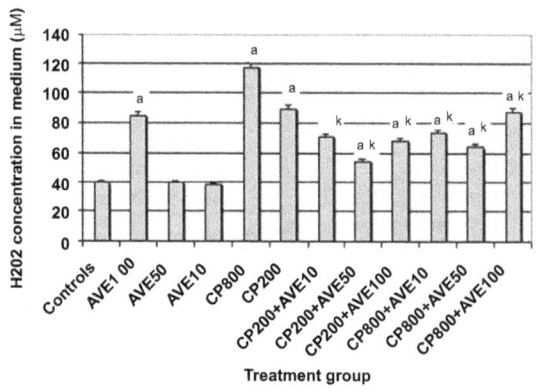

Figure 3: Effect of AVE on H_2O_2 production in the medium culture of bladder urothelium cells exposed to CP. The cells were exposed to CP or co-exposed to CP (200 and 800 IM) and AVE (10, 50 and 100 IM) for 24 h. Data represent the mean ± SD from four independent experiments. [a]P<0.05 vs. control, and [k]P<0.05 vs. CP exposed cells.

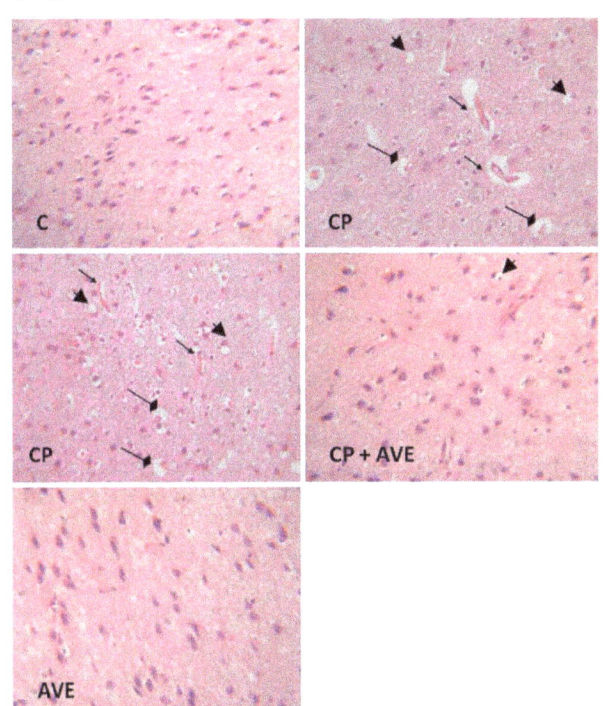

Figure 4: Photographs showing histopathological changes in bladder urothelium tissue in different groups, Control group(C), CP treated group (CP), *Aloe vera* plant extract treated group (AVE), Cyclophosphamide + plant extract treated group (CP+AVE) (hematoxylin and eosin staining, 400x).
　(↘) Haemorrhage;
　(↘) Vacuolated cytoplasm;
　(◤) Pyknotic nuclei (PN).

architecture similar to that of the untreated control. There were no histological alterations in the bladder urothelium of positive controls treated with AVE alone when compared to negative controls.

Discussion

Chemotherapeutic agents are known to influence the function of the urinary tract. Cyclophosphamide (CP) is an alkylating agent widely used in cancer chemotherapy [1]. Its cytotoxic effects are the result of chemically reactive metabolites that alkylate DNA and protein, producing cross-links [2]. It has been reported that oxidative stress mediated disruption of redox balance after CP exposure generates biochemical and physiological disruptions [11]. Several studies indicate that CP has a pro-oxidant character, and that the generation of oxidative stress after CP administration leads to a decrease in the activities of antioxidant enzymes and an increase in lipid peroxidation (LPO) in the liver, lung, and serum of mice and rats [3]. Reactive oxygen species (ROS), such as the nitric oxide radical (NO), are included in the pathogenesis of CP-induced cystitis. It has also been reported that increases in ROS, such as NO, lead to bladder oedema, inflammation, and extravasation [23].

Despite its potent antitumor activity, CP-induced urotoxicity remains the major limiting step for its clinical application. Urotoxic effects of CP can be dose limiting and have proven fatal. Since the bladder is the site for the storage of urine, the concentration of CP toxic metabolites is higher in the bladder than in any other organ. However, the mechanisms that determine the individual susceptibility to CP and the mediation of bladder toxicity remain unclear.

Treatment with buthionine sulfoximine (BSO), a potent inhibitor of r-glutamylcysteine synthetase, has been reported to enhance the *in vitro* antitumor efficacy of a number of drugs, including CP [24]. In fact, it has been shown in several animal model systems to enhance the cytotoxic effects of specific chemotherapeutic agents and radiation therapy [25]. BSO and other agents directed at modulating glutathione levels affect the content of this metabolite in normal tissues as well as in tumors. Several studies have shown that depletion of GSH after BSO treatment result in a variety of toxic effects, including cardiotoxicity, hepatic damage, and respiratory problems [26,27].

Considering the various toxic effects associated with CP treatment used alone or in combination with BSO, special attention has been given in recent research to the search for novel compositions for use as broad-spectrum chemoprotectants to help alleviate or prevent such damages. Such novel compositions could serve as adjutants to chemotherapies to protect patients' normal cells from the toxicity associated with such therapies. In this respect, folk medicine seems to be gaining increasing respect from the medical research community. More succinctly, there is a growing tendency in recent research to look for tumor-therapeutic agents of natural origins. In fact, although neither its active components nor mechanisms of action are fully understood, folk medicine has often been used with enormous success for the treatment of various diseases.

In this context, a number of natural products and compounds have been shown to reduce BSO and CP-induced toxicity mainly due to their antioxidant action [8]. Several extracts from plant origin have been described to exert valuable protective and/or restorative effects on CP-induced decreases of GSH [9]. Of particular interest, the *Aloe vera* plant has often been reported to possess attractive healing properties. Accordingly, the present study was undertaken to investigate the effects of the oral administration of an *Aloe vera* plant extract in terms of peroxide hydrogen (H_2O_2) production, antioxidant and lipid peroxidation (LPO) activities in the urinary bladder of CP and BSO treated mice that were pre-disposed or concomitantly exposed to a GSH reducing agent in the form of either an infection or antibiotic use.

The findings revealed that throughout the treatment no mortalities were recorded for the different experimental groups of animals, and that significant changes were observed in terms of their body weights. In fact, when the values pertaining to GSH reduction were compared, BSO was noted to exhibit more significant effects than CP. A difference of 42% was recorded between both agents, which, as previously reported in the literature, confirm that BSO is a more potent depletor of GSH than CP [28]. CP-induced depletion of GSH is primarily mediated by the interaction of its reactive metabolite, acrolein, with GSH (Kehrer and Biswal 2000). Acrolein not only interacts with GSH but also with cysteine, which is one of the constituent amino acids of GSH (Kehrer and Biswal 2000). Several reports in the literature have indicated that compounds containing free sulfhydryl groups may protect from the urotoxic effects of cyclophosphamide. A number of sulfhydryl (-SH) compounds, and cysteine itself; have been observed to protect experimental animals from the toxic effects of CP [28].

The intra-peritoneal administration of CP was noted to significantly induce LPO in the bladder. In fact, lipid peroxidation is widely used as an indicator to reflect oxidative stress and cell membrane damage. Free radicals, such as superoxide anion and hydroxyl radical, exert their toxic effect by acting on DNA, membrane proteins, and lipids. CP-induced LPO has been reported in different tissues of exposed animals. In CP-induced LPO, the role of acrolein has also been implied [29]. It has been suggested that by binding to nucleophilic amino acids, acrolein could directly affect transcription as well as modulate this process through its ability to deplete GSH (Kehrer and Biswal 2000).

As far as BSO treatment was concerned, the findings revealed that it resulted in the depletion of GSH and the increase of LPO in the urinary bladder. The depletion of GSH is also reported to increase the susceptibility of cells to apoptosis [30]. A depletion of intracellular GSH has been described in a number of different apoptotic systems, with several studies showing that GSH loss in cells undergoing apoptosis is the result of accelerated efflux rather than depletion by oxidation [31].

Moreover, when BSO and CP were administered together, an additive effect was observed in case of GSH and LPO among several other parameters. The purpose of using BSO along with CP was to study a likely scenario where the host is exposed to a combination of GSH depleting agents, including pathogens, and to assess whether the herbal extract treatment of *Aloe vera* has any modulatory effect on their commutative/additive effect.

In this study, pre-treatment with *Aloe vera* extract not only showed a marked protective effect with regards to CP urotoxicity but also played an efficient protective role for the animals treated with the CP + BSO combination (Group VII).

The pre-treatment with the *Aloe vera* extract was noted to restore the depleted GSH and other antioxidants and, at the same time, reduced the LPO levels in the bladder. In fact, CP-induced immunosuppression is likely to increase the incidence of infections that may deplete GSH, as many infectious agents are reported to deplete GSH [10]. Overall, the findings indicate that the herbal extract presented in the current study is a promising immunomodulatory herbal extract with powerful GSH restoring effects. This extract could, therefore, open new opportunities for the reduction of the adverse effects of CP and BSO cancer treatments.

In fact, the immunomodulatory effect of *Aloe vera* has previously been demonstrated in mice [32]. Aloe-Emodin (AE) was found to alter the expression of a number of proteins involved in oxidative stress, cell-cycle arrest, anti-metastasis, and apoptosis [33]. Moreover, AE was capable of enhancing the intracellular level of reactive oxygen species (ROS). This may not unexpected since AE has a quinone structure that is highly redox active in nature and that can form a redox cycle with their semiquinone radicals, thus leading to the formation of ROS. AE was recently found to be able to induce DNA damage through excessive production of ROS in human lung carcinoma cells [34]. This anticancer specificity further suggests that AE could be a potent chemotherapeutic agent or chemo-preventive compound. It is noteworthy that endothelial cells have recently been reported to be sensitive to AE [35]. This property was suggested to be useful for the modulation of angiogenesis as well as antitumor effects [35].

Moreover, the findings presented in the current work suggest that *Aloe vera* has a potent chemo-preventive potential for the inhibition of the toxicity processes by modulating lipid peroxidation and cellular antioxidant environments. The findings of the present study demonstrate that *Aloe vera* extract pre-treatment prevented CP urotoxicity that was primarily mediated by LPO and depleted GSH by reversing those effects.

In the present study, we have reported that exposure of urothelial cell line T24 to CP (200 and 800µM) increased significantly H_2O_2 production in extracellular medium indicating the role of ROS generation as primary mechanism for CP-induced toxicity. The ability of *Aloe vera* extract to exert great effect on CP-induced cellular injury is consistent with its increased potency in reducing ROS (e.g. H_2O_2) generation. Our results are consistent with those of Fu et al. [36] who

have found that plant extract, has an antioxidative activity and free radical scavenging properties *in vitro*, which can scavenge various oxidizing radicals such as OH•, NO_2•, O_2•, RNS•.

Furthermore, Histopathological examination of the bladder urothelium tissue reveals that CP treatment causes abnormal cellular arrangement with few pyknotic nuclei, vacuolated spaces and hemorrhage. However, co-treatment with AVE prevents these changes and also maintains normal architecture with less number of pyknotic nuclei.

In short, the present work is the first attempt to focus on the biological activities and bladder urotoxicity in Tunisia. In fact, the plant extract presented here showed a significant antioxidant potential in different assays *in vivo*. The findings provided ample support for the efficiency of the *Aloe vera* extract as a natural antioxidant agent. Due to its widespread availability in nature and relative lack of toxicity, this herbal extract could be considered a potential strong candidate for future applications as an adjutant to cancer chemotherapies. Accordingly, further studies are currently underway in our laboratories to further explore this extract in terms of cell cycle regulatory activity and antioxidant activity, to further validate its efficacy as an anti-tumor agent, and to make its use suitable for potential pharmaceutical applications as a therapeutic agent.

Acknowledgements

This study was supported by the Tunisian Ministry of Higher Education and Scientific Research and Technology and the Tunisian Ministry of Public Health. The authors would like to express their sincere gratitude to Prof. ANOUAR Smaoui from the English Section at the Sfax Faculty of Science for his valuable language polishing and proofreading services.

References

1. Baumann F, Preiss R (2001) Cyclophosphamide and related anticancer drugs. J Chromatogr B Biomed Sci Appl 764: 173-192.

2. Fleming RA (1997) An overview of cyclophosphamide and ifosfamide pharmacology. Pharmacotherapy 17: 146S-154S.

3. Patel JM, Block ER (1985) Cyclophosphamide-induced depression of the antioxidant defense mechanisms of the lung. Exp Lung Res 8: 153-165.

4. Stillwell TJ, Benson RC Jr, Burgert EO Jr (1988) Cyclophosphamide-induced hemorrhagic cystitis in Ewing's sarcoma. J Clin Oncol 6: 76-82.

5. Drake MJ, Nixon PM, Crew JP (1998) Drug-induced bladder and urinary disorders. Incidence, prevention and management. Drug Saf 19: 45-55.

6. Abd-Allah AR, Gado AM, Al-Majed AA, Al-Yahya AA, Al-Shabanah OA (2005) Protective effect of taurine against cyclophosphamide-induced urinary bladder toxicity in rats. Clin Exp Pharmacol Physiol 32: 167-172.

7. Ahmed AR, Hombal SM (1984) Cyclophosphamide (Cytoxan). A review on relevant pharmacology and clinical uses. J Am Acad Dermatol 11: 1115-1126.

8. Manesh C, Kuttan G (2005) Effect of naturally occurring isothiocyanates in the inhibition of cyclophosphamide-induced urotoxicity. Phytomedicine 12: 487-493.

9. Haque R, Bin-Hafeez B, Parvez S, Pandey S, Sayeed I, et al. (2003) Aqueous extract of walnut (Juglans regia L.) protects mice against cyclophosphamide-induced biochemical toxicity. Hum Exp Toxicol 22: 473-480.

10. Hung CR, Wang PS (2004) Gastric oxidative stress and hemorrhagic ulcer in Salmonella typhimurium-infected rats. Eur J Pharmacol 491: 61-68.

11. Moon EJ, Lee YM, Lee OH, Lee MJ, Lee SK, et al. (1999) A novel angiogenic factor derived from Aloe vera gel: beta-sitosterol, a plant sterol. Angiogenesis 3: 117-123.

12. Ghannam N, Kingston M, Al-Meshaal IA, Tariq M, Parman NS, et al. (1986) The antidiabetic activity of aloes: preliminary clinical and experimental observations. Horm Res 24: 288-294.

13. Capasso F, Gaginella TS (1997) Laxatives: a practice guide. Milan: Springer Italia.

14. Chithra P, Sajithlal BG, Chandrakasan G (1998) Influence of Aloe vera on the healing of dermal wounds in diabetic rats. J Ethnopharmacol 59:195-201.

15. Pecere T, Gazzola MV, Mucignat C, Parolin C, Vecchia FD, et al. (2000) Aloe-emodin is a new type of anticancer agent with selective activity against neuroectodermal tumors. Cancer Res 60: 2800-2804.

16. Yongchaiyudha S, Rungpitarangsi V, Bunyapraphatsara N, Chokechaijaroenporn O (1996) Antidiabetic activity of Aloe vera L juice I Clinical trial in new cases of diabetes mellitus. Phytomedicine 3: 241–243.

17. Roesler J, Steinmuller C, Kiderlen A, Emmendorffer A, Wagner H,0 ,etal. (1991) Application of purified polysaccharides from cell cultures of the plant Echinacea purpurea to mice mediates protection against systemic infections with Listeria monocytogenes and Candida albican Int J Immunopharmacol 13: 27–37.

18. Byeon SW, Pelley RP, Ullrich SE, Waller TA, Bucana CD, et al. (1998) Aloe barbadensis extracts reduce the production of interleukin-10 after exposure to ultraviolet radiation. J Invest Dermatol 110: 811-817.

19. Sharma N, Trikha P, Athar M, Raisuddin (2001) Inhibition of benzoapyrene- and cyclophoshamide-induced mutagenicity by Cinnamomum cassia. Mutat Res 481: 179–188.

20. Dadarkar SS, Fonseca LC, Thakkar AD, Mishra PB, Rangasamy AK, et al. (2010) Effect of nephrotoxicants and hepatotoxicants on gene expression profile in human peripheral blood mononuclear cells. Biochem Biophys Res Commun 401: 245-250.

21. Ou P, Wolff SP (1996) A discontinuous method for catalase determination at 'near physiological' concentrations of H_2O_2 and its application to the study of H_2O_2 fluxes within cells. J Biochem Biophys Methods 31: 59-67.

22. Uchiyama M, Mihara M (1978) Determination of malonaldehyde precursor in tissues by thiobarbituric acid test. Anal Biochem 86: 271–278.

23. Souza-Fiho MV, Lima MV, Pompeu MM, Ballejo G, Cunha FQ, et al. (1997) Involvement of nitric oxide in the pathogenesis of cyclophosphamide-induced hemorrhagic cystitis. Am J Pathol 150: 247-256.

24. Ozols RF, Louie KG, Plowman J, Behrens BC, Fine RL, et al. (1987) Enhanced melphalan cytotoxicity in human ovarian cancer in vitro and in tumor-bearing nude mice by buthionine sulfoximine depletion of glutathione. Biochem Pharmacol 36: 147-153.

25. Biaglow JE, Varnes ME, Epp ER, Clark EP, Tuttle SW, et al. (1989) Role of glutabione in the aerobic radiation response. Int J Radiat Oncol Biol Phys 16: 1311-1311.

26. Orman A, Kahraman A, Cakar H, Ellidokuz H, Serteser M (2005) Plasma malondialdehyde and erythrocyte glutathione levels in workers with cement dust-exposure [corrected]. Toxicology 207: 15-20.

27. Zhang L, Yang Y, Yu L, Wang Y, Liu L, et al. (2011) Cardioprotective effects of Glycyrrhiza uralensis extract against doxorubicin-induced toxicity. Int J Toxicol 30: 181-189.

28. Ishikawa M, Takayanagi Y, Sasaki K (1989) Modification of cyclophosphamide-induced urotoxicity by buthionine sulfoximine and disulfiram in mice. Res Commun Chem Pathol Pharmacol 65: 265–268.

29. Adams JD, Klaidrnan LK (1993) Acrolein induced oxygen radical formation. Free Radic Biol Med 15: 187–193.

30. Mirkovic N, Voehringer DW, Story MD, McConkey DJ, McDonnell TJ, et al. (1997) Resistance to radiation-induced apoptosis in Bcl-2-expressing cells is reversed by depleting cellular thiols. Oncogene 15: 1461-1470.

31. Ghibelli L, Fanelli C, Rotilio G, Lafavia E, Coppola S, et al. (1998) Rescue of cells from apoptosis by inhibition of active GSH extrusion. FASEB J 12: 479-486.

32. Davis RH, Donato JJ, Hartman GM, Haas RC (1994) Anti-inflammatory and wound healing activity of a growth substance in Aloe vera. J Am Podiatr Med Assoc 84: 77-81.

33. Lu GD, Shen HM, Ong CN, Chung MC (2007) Anticancer effects of aloe-emodin on HepG2 cells: Cellular and proteomic studies. Proteomics Clin Appl 1: 410-419.

34. Lee HZ, Lin CJ, Yang WH, Leung WC, Chang SP (2006) Aloe-emodin induced DNA damage through generation of reactive oxygen species in human lung carcinoma cells. Cancer Lett 239: 55-63.

35. CÃ¡rdenas C, Quesada AR, Medina MA (2006) Evaluation of the anti-angiogenic effect of aloe-emodin. Cell Mol Life Sci 63: 3083-3089.

36. Fu H, Lin M, Muroya Y, Hata K, Katsumura Y, et al. (2009) Free radical scavenging reactions and antioxidant activities of silybin: mechanistic aspects and pulse radiolytic studies. Free Radic Res 43: 887-897.

37. Green JA, Vistica DT, Young RC, Hamilton TC, Rogan AM, et al. (1984) Potentiation of melphalan cytotoxicity in human ovarian cancer cell lines by glutathione depletion. Cancer Res 44: 5427-5431.

38. Louie KG, Behrens BC, Kinsella TJ, Hamilton TC, Grotzinger KR, et al. (1985) Radiation survival parameters of antineoplastic drug-sensitive and -resistant human ovarian cancer cell lines and their modification by buthionine sulfoximine. Cancer Res 45: 2110-2115.

28

Antibacterial Activity and Cytotoxicity of Gold (I) and (III) Ions and Gold Nanoparticles

Shareena Dasari TP, Zhang Y and Yu H*

Department of Chemistry and Biochemistry, Jackson State University, Jackson, MS 39217, USA

Abstract

Gold nanoparticles (AuNPs) and gold ion complexes have been investigated for their antibacterial activities. However, the majority of the reports failed to disclose the concentration of free Au(I) or Au(III) present in solutions of AuNPs or gold ion complexes. The inconsistency of antibacterial activity of AuNPs may be due to the effect of the presence of Au(III). Here we report the antibacterial activity of Au(I) and Au(III) to four different bacteria: one nonpathogenic bacterium: *E. coli* and three multidrug-resistant bacteria: *E. coli, S. typhimurium DT104,* and *S. aureus.* Au(I) and Au(III) as chloride are highly toxic to all the four bacteria, with IC$_{50}$ of 0.35 - 0.49 μM for Au(III) and 0.27-0.52 μM for Au(I). The bacterial growth inhibition by both Au(I) and Au(III) increases with exposure time and is strongly affected by the use of buffers. The IC$_{50}$ values for Au(I) and Au(III) in different buffers are HEPES (0.48 and 1.55 μM) > Trizma (0.41 and 0.57 μM) > PBS (0.14 and 0.06 μM). Bacterial growth inhibition by AuNPs is gradually reduced by centrifugation-resuspension to remove residual Au(III) ion present in the crude synthetic AuNPs. After 4 centrifugations-resuspensions, AuNPs become non-toxic. In addition, both Au(I) and Au(III) are cytotoxic to skin keratinocyte and blood lymphocyte cells. These results suggest that Au(I) and Au(III) in pure or complex forms may be explored as a method to treat drug-resistant bacteria, and the test of AuNPs toxicity must consider residual Au(III), exposure time, and the use of buffers.

Keywords: Gold nanoparticle; Gold (I) and (III) ions; Antibacterial effect; Cytotoxicity

Introduction

Gold nanoparticles (AuNPs) have attracted considerable interests for fundamental and applied research. As AuNP applications continue to increase, growing human safety concerns are gaining attention [1-9]. It was pointed out that the toxic effects of AuNPs are complex due to co-existing chemicals, such as the presence of citrate and Au(III) ions during the photomutagenecity test of AuNPs [10]. Gold nanorods are toxic to human skin cells due to the surface coating chemical CTAB (cetyltrimethylammonium bromide), but not the gold nanorods [11-13]. CTAB alone is toxic to cells at sub-micromolar concentrations. The free CTAB molecules in gold nanorod solutions may be a result of inadequate purification and desorption of surface CTAB from the gold nanorods. Thus, it was suggested that proper control experiments must be carried out when studying the toxicity of AuNPs.

Studies on the antimicrobial effects of AuNPs are summarized in a recent review article [14]. Among the 70 plus reports on the antimicrobial effect of AuNPs, at least eight of them suggested that AuNPs are either not or very weakly antibacterial, while the others reported various degrees of antibacterial activity. These discrepancies in the antibacterial activities of AuNPs may be due to several factors: 1) the use of surface coating agents on AuNPs including antibiotics, 2) the test methods, and 3) residual Au(III). Since most AuNPs preparation methods involve chemical reduction of Au(III) salts in aqueous, organic, or mixed phases in the presence of reductants and surface-coating agents such as antibacterial compounds, the AuNPs solution is a mixture since some of them are used without proper purification.

Residual Au(III) ions could cause false antibacterial test results [10,14,15]. In fact, gold ions as organic complexes have been of interest as antimicrobial agents [14,16-18]. Many reported that Au(I) and Au(III) complexes with organic ligands are effective against a wide variety of microorganisms [16-23] including the review article by Gilisci and Djuran that summarized the antibacterial activity of Au(I) and Au(III) complexes [17]. Au(I) and Au(III) complexes are soluble in organic solvents, but their lack of aqueous solubility limits the potential use as antibacterial or therapeutic agents.

We hypothesize that 1) Au(I) or Au(III) is antibacterial; 2) synthetic AuNPs, if followed with proper removal of residual Au(III) ions, are weakly or not toxic to bacteria; 3) the antibacterial activity of Au(III) and Au(I) is dependent on the exposure time and the use of different buffers. Thus, we evaluated the biological activity of Au(I) and Au(III) on four bacteria: one nonpathogenic bacterium *E. coli* and three multidrug-resistant bacteria *E. coli, S. typhimurium* DT-104, and *S. aureus*; and two human cell lines: a skin keratinocyte and a blood lymphocyte cell line. The effect on the antibacterial activity by treatment time and the use of buffers (PBS, Trizma, and HEPES) were evaluated. The antibacterial effect of AuNPs was studied upon centrifugations to remove residual Au(III) from the synthesis.

Materials and Methods

Materials

Chloroauric acid (HAuCl$_4$, 99%, a form of Au(III) in solution) was purchased from Sigma-Aldrich and used without further purification. Gold (I) chloride (AuCl) was purchased from Strem Chemicals (Newburyport, MA). AuCl, due to its limited water solubility, was first suspended in nanopure water through sonication, and then the undissolved AuCl was filtered through 0.2 μm filter (Corning Incorporated, NY). The filtered solution had a final Au(I) concentration

Corresponding author: Hongtao Yu, Department of Chemistry and Biochemistry, Jackson State University, Jackson, MS 39217, USA, E-mail: hongtao.yu@jsums.edu

of 2.87 mM determined by ICP-MS (Varian Model No. 820-MS). Bacteria and cell lines used in this study include non-pathogenic *E. coli* (BAA-1431), multidrug-resistant *E. coli* (BAA-1161), multidrug-resistant *S. typhimurium* DT-104 (ATCC 700408), multidrug-resistant *S. aureus* (MRSA, BAA-44), and the blood lymphocyte cell line, TIB-152, were purchased from American Type Culture Collection (ATCC) (Manassas, VA). The HaCaT keratinocyte, a transformed human skin cell line, was obtained from Dr. Norbert Fusenig of the Germany Cancer Research Center (Heidelberg, Germany). RPMI-1640 medium was purchased from ATCC (Manassas, VA). Trypsin EDTA solutions were purchased from Cambrex Bio Science (Walkersville, MD). Tryptic Soy Broth (TSB) and Tryptic Soy Agar (TSA) used to grow the bacteria, and Trizma base (tris-(hydroxymethyl)aminomethane) and HEPES (4-(2-hydroxyethyl)-1-piperazineethanesulfonic acid) salts were purchased from Sigma-Aldrich (St. Louis, MO). Fetal bovine serum (FBS), Dulbecco's Minimum Essential Medium (DMEM), penicillin/streptomycin, dimethyl sulfoxide (DMSO), phosphate buffered saline (PBS), and CellTiter 96® AQ$_{ueous}$ One Solution Cell Proliferation Assay (MTS) were purchased from Fisher Scientific (Houston, TX).

Gold nanoparticle synthesis, purification, and characterization

AuNPs were prepared by adding 5 mL of HAuCl$_4$ (10 mM) solution and 5 mL of 38.8 mM sodium citrate (Na$_3$C$_6$H$_5$O$_7$) to 45 mL of boiling H$_2$O. Further heating (100°C) up to 20 min caused the solution to turn from yellow to wine red [24]. The solution was centrifuged at 5000 rpm for 2 h at 20°C and the resulting AuNPs pellet was washed with 5 mL of 0.1 mM sodium citrate buffer to remove residual Au(III) ions and citrate ions. This procedure was repeated 1-4 times to eliminate residual Au(III) ions. All experiments were carried out with the AuNPs ranging 15-25 nm (Figure 1). The characterization of AuNPs was carried out by UV-Vis and TEM (JEM 1011, Joel Inc.) and AuNP concentration (0.97 mM) was determined using UV-Vis as reported previously [10,13].

Bacterial growth inhibition assay with Au(I), Au(III), and synthesized AuNPs

Bacterial growth inhibition was carried out using the spread plate counting method as reported before [25]. *E. coli*, *Salmonella* DT-104, and *S. aureus* were cultured in TSB growth medium at 37°C, 200 rpm for 10-12 h in a shaker incubator. The bacterial cultures were centrifuged at 3000 rpm for 20 min, and residual bacteria were resuspended in sterilized physiological saline (0.85% NaCl). Bacterial density was adjusted to 3 × 10^8 cells/mL in PBS. The final exposure concentrations for Au(III) were 0, 0.01, 0.03, 0.1, and 0.3 µM, and for Au(I) were 0, 0.1, 0.3, 1, and 3 µM. The final concentrations of Au(III) and Au(I) for time dependent experiments were 0.1 and 1 µM, respectively. Au(III) and Au(I) solution at different concentrations were combined with the cultured bacteria and placed in a shaker incubator with continuous agitation at 200 rpm for 2 h or a designate time at 25°C. The time dependent samples (100 µL) were transferred onto TSA plates after 30, 60, 90, 120, 150 and 180 min of shaking. The transferred samples were evenly spread onto the pre-prepared agar plates, and all plates were inverted and incubated at 37°C for 24 h. For the test with different buffers, PBS (pH 7.4), Trizma (pH 7-9) and HEPES (pH 7.4) buffers were used at the final concentration of 1 mM. In addition, we tested the inhibition of bacterial growth by AuNPs with 0-4 centrifugations at 2 h exposure.

Cytotoxicity assay

HaCaT cells were grown in complete medium (DMEM, 10% FBS, and 1% Fungizone, penicillin/streptomycin) in 25 cm^2 cell culture flasks.

Cells were cultured in a humidified incubator with 5% CO$_2$ at 37°C. After the cells grew to confluence, they were detached by 25% trypsin/EDTA and diluted to 3×10^5 cells/mL by their respective complete media as reported before [26]. A 200 µL cell suspension in complete medium was added to each well of a 96-well plate and incubated under 5% CO$_2$ at 37°C for 24 h for cell adhesion. TIB-152 cells were grown in complete medium (RPMI-1640, 10% FBS) in 75 cm^2 culture flasks in the incubator until 1×10^6 cells/mL was achieved, and they were then centrifuged and resuspended in RPMI-1640 medium. After incubation, the supernatant was pipetted, and the adherent cells were washed with 1X PBS before exposed to Au(III). Then a total of 90 µL of DMEM (for HaCaT) or EMEM (for TIB-152) and 10 µL of Au(III) at desired concentrations were added to each well. A total of 3 wells were used for the test at each concentration. After 2 h or 24 h of treatment, cell viability was determined by the MTS assay: 20 µL MTS solution was added directly to each well after treatment and the absorbance was read at 490 nm using a 96-well Multiskan Ascent Plate Reader with Ascent software. The control test was performed with PBS buffer.

Statistical analysis

At least three independent experiments were carried out for each point. All statistical analyses were performed using the SAS 9.3 software. Significance was determined with Generalized Linear Model and Tukey's test to distinguish the differences between the variables for bacterial growth inhibition assays. Significance was determined with Generalized Linear Model (Duncan) for cytotoxicity assays. The significance level was defined as $p < 0.05$. IC$_{50}$ values were determined using SPSS software (IBM® SPSS® Statistics, Version 22).

Results and Discussion

Concentration and time-dependent inhibition of *Salmonella* DT-104, *E. coli* and MRSA growth by Au(I) and Au(III)

We tested bacterial growth inhibition of the four selected bacteria after exposure to Au(I) or Au(III) for 2 h. Figure 2 shows the concentration dependent inhibition of the multi-drug resistant *E. coli* (BAA-1161) growth after exposure to 0.1, 0.3, 1, and 3 µM of Au(I) or 0.01, 0.03, 0.1, 0.3, and 1 µM of Au(III). The other three bacteria show the same pattern of inhibition (data not shown). These results confirm that Au(III) and Au(I) are toxic to all the four bacteria even at very low concentrations.

From the concentration-dependent inhibition data, IC$_{50}$ values were determined by SPSS and are listed in table 1. Among the four bacteria, the Gram positive MRSA has the highest IC$_{50}$ values (0.49 µM for Au(I) and 0.52 µM for Au(III)), while the three Gram negative bacteria have

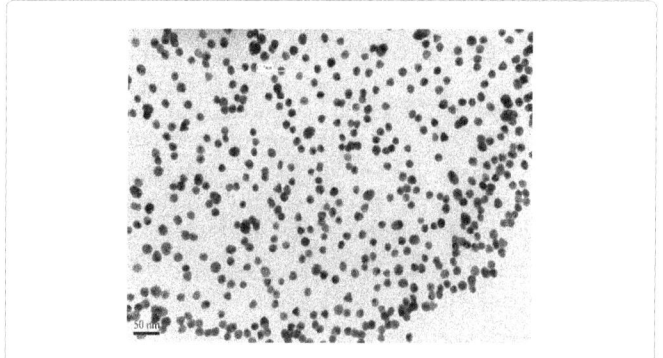

Figure 1: TEM image of the synthesized AuNPs with size range of 15-25 nm.

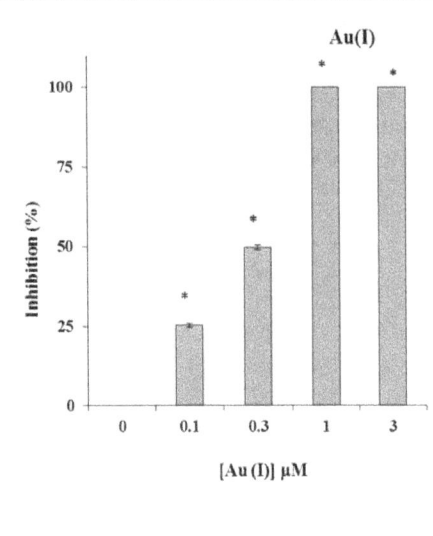

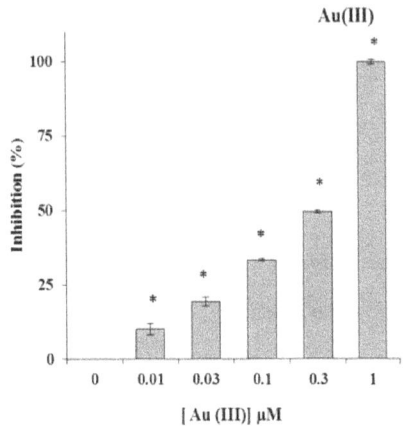

Figure 2: Concentration dependent growth inhibition by Au(I) and Au(III) ions on multi-drug resistant *E. coli* (BAA-1161). Error bars are standard deviations (n=3). * Denotes significant with p < 0.05.

	Au(I) (µM)	Au(III) (µM)
E. coli (BAA-1431)	0.38	0.34
E. coli (BAA-1161)	0.35	0.36
Salmonella DT-104 (ATCC 700408)	0.39	0.27
MRSA (BAA-44)	0.49 (*)	0.52 (*)

Table 1: IC_{50} for bacterial growth inhibition by Au(I) and Au(III). Only the IC_{50} against MRSA is significantly different against the other three bacteria (p < 0.05).

similar IC_{50} values 0.35-0.39 µM for Au(I) and 0.27-0.36 µM for Au(III). The difference in toxicity for the Gram positive and the Gram negative bacteria could be due to differences in cell wall structure. The bacterial cell wall plays a vital role in resistance or susceptibility [27]. There is very little difference in IC_{50} values between Au(I) and Au(III) for *E. coli*: 0.38 µM versus 0.34 µM for BAA-1431 and 0.35 versus 0.36 for BAA-1161, and MRSA, 0.49 µM versus 0.52 µM, respectively. However, Au(III) is more toxic to the *Salmonella* DT104 than Au(I) (IC_{50} of 0.27 µM versus 0.39 µM). The reasons for these differences in toxicity need further investigation.

Wang et al first reported the photomutagenicity of Au(III) on *S. typhimurium* TA102 and pointed out that Au(III) is also toxic to the bacterium at a concentration at 1 µM [10]. Nam et al very recently reported an extensive study of Au(III) toxicity to a variety of

microorganisms including bacteria in 2014 [15]. Due to the toxicity of Au(I) and Au(III), the tests of antibacterial activity of AuNPs as well as Au(I) and Au(III) complexes have to consider the possible presence of residual Au(I) and Au(III). Without proper purification to remove the residual Au(I) and Au(III), it may lead to erroneous results.

Time-dependent inhibition experiments were carried out to see how exposure time affects the toxicity of Au(I) and Au(III). Figure 3 shows the inhibitory effects on *E. coli* after exposure to Au(I) and Au(III) up to 3 h at two different concentrations (0.1 and 1 µM). At 1 µM, the percent of bacterial growth inhibition increases from exposure time of 30 min to 60 min, and it reaches near 100% inhibition at longer than 60 min. At 0.1 µM, the inhibition is not detectable at 30 and 60 min exposure, but continues to increase from 90 to 180 min (3 h). It seems not reaching maximum inhibition even at 3 h. Nam et al examined much longer exposure time of 72 h [15]. They found that Au(III) continues to be toxic for some bacteria at longer exposure times. This clearly shows that the toxicity of Au(I) and Au(III) to these bacteria is exposure time dependent and suggests that exposure time must be factored in when conducting similar tests.

Effect of buffers on the growth inhibition of Au(I) and Au(III) to nonpathogenic *E. coli*

PBS, Trizma, and HEPES are three commonly used buffers. The effect of using these buffers (0.01, 0.03, 0.1, 0.3, 1 and 10 µM) on the toxicity of Au(I) and Au(III) to the nonpathogenic *E. coli* was tested with 2 h exposure time (Figure 4). The IC_{50} values were determined using SPSS, and they are listed in table 2: 0.14, 0.41, and 0.48 µM for Au(I) and 0.06, 0.57 and 1.55 µM for Au(III), in PBS, Trizma, and HEPES buffers, respectively. Complete (100%) inhibition was observed for bacteria exposed to Au(III) and Au(I) at 1 µM in PBS buffer, whereas in Trizma and HEPES buffers at 10 µM of Au(III) and Au(I),

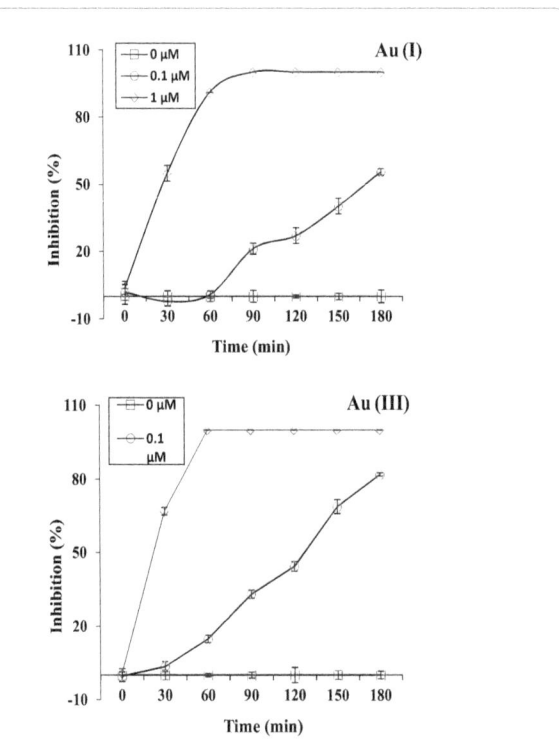

Figure 3: Time-dependent growth inhibition by Au(I) and Au(III) against nonpathogenic *E. coli* at concentrations 0, 0.1 and 1µM.

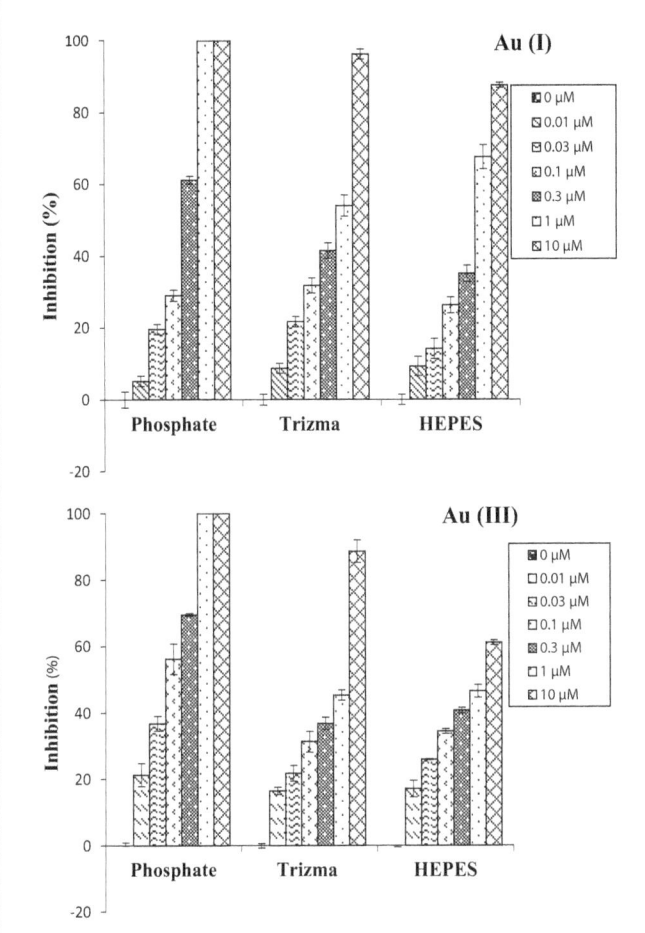

Figure 4: Growth inhibition of nonpathogenic *E. coli* by exposure to Au(I) and Au(III) at 0, 0.01, 0.03, 0.1, 0.3, 1 and 10 µM for 2 h in PBS, Trizma and HEPES.

	Au(I) (µM)	Au(III) (µM)
PBS	0.14 (*)	0.06 (*)
Trizma	0.41	0.57
HEPES	0.48	1.55

Table 2: IC$_{50}$ values for Au(I) and Au(III) against nonpathogenic *E. coli* in PBS, Trizma and HEPES buffers. Only the values in PBS are significantly different (p < 0.05).

some bacteria are still viable. Therefore, the buffers used for this type of test have a profound effect on their toxicity. It is more profound for Au(III), where the IC$_{50}$ in HEPES is 24 times of that in PBS. We believe that the use of buffers has an effect on how Au(I) and Au(III) behave in solution and how they interact with the bacterial cells. More advanced studies are needed to understand the effect of these buffers on the antibacterial effect of gold ions.

Effect of centrifugation-resuspension on the growth inhibition of AuNPs to nonpathogenic *E. coli*

E. coli growth inhibition by 50 µM of AuNPs (non-centrifuged) was compared with centrifuged (1-4 centrifugations-resuspensions) at 5000 rpm for 2 h each at 20°C. There is a 37% inhibition with non-centrifuged AuNPs, but the bacterial growth inhibition decreases to 17, 14, 10, and 1%, respectively, upon 1-4 centrifugations (Figure 5). This demonstrates that AuNPs, once the Au(III) is completely removed, do not inhibit the growth of *E. coli*. Based on figure 2 and the

calculated IC$_{50}$ values of 0.34 µM for Au(III), the percent of inhibitions of 37, 17, 14, 10 and 1% correspond to Au(III) concentrations of 0.11, 0.05, 0.04, 0.02 and 0.001 µM. This demonstrates that residual Au(III) present in AuNPs was removed through 3-4 centrifugations. Without purifications, false toxicity result could occur. We tried to obtain the accurate Au(III) concentrations in the supernatant after centrifugations, but the use of an ICP-MS, which determines total gold concentration, did not yield accurate Au(III) concentration due to the small amount of AuNPs retained in the supernatant.

Cytotoxicity of Au(III) to skin (HaCaT) and blood (TIB-152) cells

Since Au(III) is antibacterial, we want to know if it is also cytotoxic to human cells: skin keratinocyte (HaCaT) and blood lymphocyte (TIB-152) cells. The reason these two cell lines were chosen was because they are the likely targets during skin exposure and blood transport of environmental toxins. The cells (HaCaT and TIB152) were exposed to Au(III) at 1, 10 and 100 µM for 2 h and 24 h. The cell viability was determined by MTS assay (Figure 6). Au(III) is not toxic at 1 and 10 µM at both exposure times, but it is toxic at 100 µM for both cell lines with cell viabilities of 36% and 8% against HaCaT cells at 2 h and 24 h exposure times, respectively. Whereas 100 % inhibition was observed at 24 h exposure time against TIB-152 cells at 100 µM Au(III) (Figure 6).

Concluding Remarks

This work clearly demonstrates that both Au(I) and Au(III) ions are strongly antibacterial against all four tested bacteria: one nonpathogenic *E. coli* and three multidrug resistant bacteria: *E. coli*, *S. typhimurium DT104*, and *S. aureus (MRSA)*. Nonlinear dose-dependent growth inhibition is observed and the antibacterial effect of Au(I) and Au(III) ions vary slightly with the type of bacteria. The length of treatment has a significant effect on the antibacterial effect of Au(III) and Au(I). For sub-IC$_{50}$ concentrations, both Au(I) and (III) ions continue to inhibit the bacterial growth even after 3 h. The use of buffer plays a significant role in altering the antibacterial activity of both Au(III) and Au(I). The antibacterial activity is strongest in PBS, followed by Trizma and HEPES. Centrifugation of AuNPs 1-4 times to remove residual Au(III) ions reduces the antibacterial effect of "AuNPs", suggesting that AuNPs alone do not inhibit bacteria growth for the four bacteria tested. Au(III) ions are also toxic to HaCaT and

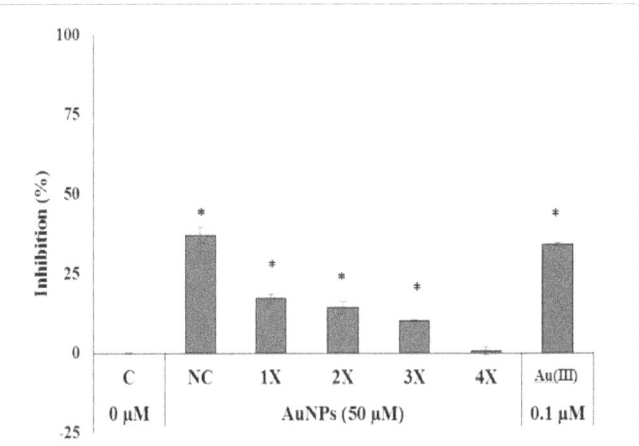

Figure 5: Effect of centrifugations of AuNPs on growth inhibition of non-pathogenic *E. coli* by AuNPs. Control (C), Non-centrifuged (NC), 1× (Centrifuge 1), 2× (Centrifuge 2), 3× (Centrifuge 3) and 4× (Centrifuge 4). * Denotes significant with p < 0.05.

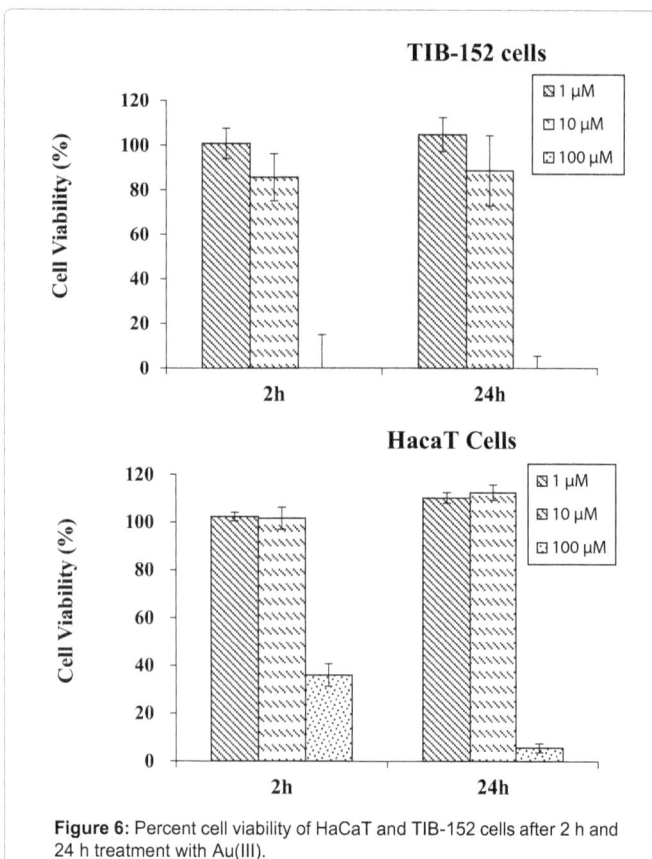

Figure 6: Percent cell viability of HaCaT and TIB-152 cells after 2 h and 24 h treatment with Au(III).

TIB152 cells at high concentrations (100 μM). The antibacterial effects of Au(III) and Au(I) may be further explored for medical purposes, especially against those three multi-drug resistant bacteria.

On the other hand, test of biological effects of nanoparticles, due to the fact that nanoparticles in solution are often a chemical mixture [26], careful controls and purifications must be carried out. Our results demonstrate that the antibacterial effect of AuNPs is strongly dependent on the number of centrifugations to remove excess Au(III), the use of buffers, the exposure time, the type of bacteria and test method. This might explain the discrepancies in the literature concerning the antibacterial effect of AuNPs since there was no mentioning about purification of the AuNPs in most of the reports. For some of the antibacterial results of the gold (I) and (III) organic complexes, one may need to investigate whether free gold ions played a role [14].

Acknowledgement

We thank National Science Foundation for grants: Partnership for Research and Education in Materials (NSF PREM DMR-1205194) and the Analytical Core Laboratory (NIH grant No. G12MD007581). We also thank Dr. Zikri Arslan, Physical Chemistry Lab at Jackson State University for providing assistance in ICP-MS analysis in the study.

References

1. Bishop P, Ashfield LJ, Berzins A, Boardman A, Buche V, et al. (2010) Printed gold for electronic applications. Gold Bulletin 43: 181-188.

2. Bond GC, Louis C, Thompson D (2006) Catalysis by gold. Gold Bull 39: 3-8.

3. Chen S, Wang Z, Ballato J, Foulger S, Carroll D (2003) Monopod, bipod, tripod, and tetrapod gold nanocrystals. J Am Chem Soc 125: 16186-16187.

4. Daniel M-C and Astruc D (2004) Gold nanoparticles: assembly, supramolecular chemistry, quantum-size-related properties, and applications toward biology, catalysis, and nanotechnology. Chem Rev 104: 293-346.

5. Fan Z, Fu P, Yu H, Ray P (2014) Theranostic nanomedicine for cancer detection and treatment. J Food Drug Anal 22: 3-17.

6. Goodman C, McCusker C, Yilmaz T, Rotello V (2004) Toxicity of gold nanoparticles functionalized with cationic and anionic side chains. Bioconjugate Chem 15: 897-900.

7. Hussain S, Warheit DB, Ng SP, Comfort KK, Grabinski CM, et al. (2015) At the Crossroads of Nanotoxicology in vitro : Past Achievements and Current Challenges. Toxicol Sci 147: 5-16.

8. Louis C, Pluchery O (2012) Gold Nanoparticles for Physics, Chemistry and Biology. World Scientific Publishing Co Pte Ltd, Pp: 1-308.

9. Van der Zande B, Böhmer M, Fokkink L, Schönenberger C (2000) Colloidal dispersions of gold rods: synthesis and optical properties. Langmuir 16: 451-458.

10. Wang S, Lawson R, Ray P, Yu H (2011) Toxic effects of gold nanoparticles on Salmonella typhimurium bacteria. Toxicol Ind Health 27: 547-554.

11. Alkilany A, Murphy C (2010) Toxicity and cellular uptake of gold nanoparticles: what we have learned so far? J Nanopart Res 12: 2313-2333.

12. Alkilany A, Nagaria PK, Hexel CR, Shaw TJ, Murphy CJ, et al. (2009) Cellular uptake and cytotoxicity of gold nanorods: molecular origin of cytotoxicity and surface effects. Small 5: 701-708.

13. Wang S, Lu W, Tovmachenko O, Rai US, Yu H, et al. (2008) Challenge in understanding size- and shape-dependent toxicity of gold nanomaterials in human skin keratinocytes. Chem Phys Lett 463: 145-149.

14. Zhang Y, Dasari T, Deng H, Yu H (2015) Antimicrobial Activity of Gold Nanoparticles and Ionic Gold. J Environ Sci Health C 3: 286-327.

15. Nam S-H, Lee WM, Shin YJ, Yoon SJ, Kim SW, et al. (2014) Derivation of guideline values for gold (III) ion toxicity limits to protect aquatic ecosystems. Water Res 48: 126-136.

16. Elsome A, Hamilton-Miller J, Brumfitt W, Noble W (1996) Antimicrobial activities in vitro and in vivo of transition element complexes containing gold(I) and osmium(VI). J Antimicrob Chemotherap 37: 911-918.

17. Glišić B, Djuran M (2014) Gold complexes as antimicrobial agents: an overview of different biological activities in relation to the oxidation state of the gold ion and the ligand structure. Dalton Trans 43: 5950-5969.

18. Ozdemir I, Temelli N, Günal S, Demir S (2010) Gold(I) Complexes of N-Heterocyclic Carbene Ligands Containing Benzimidazole: Synthesis and Antimicrobial Activity Molecules. Molecules 15: 2203-2210.

19. Elie B, Levine C, Ubarretxena-Belandia I, Varela-Ramírez A, Aguilera RJ, et al. (2009) Water-Soluble (Phosphane) gold(I) Complexes. Applications as Recyclable Catalysts in a Three-Component Coupling Reaction and as Antimicrobial and Anticancer Agents. Eur J Inorg Chem 23: 3421-3430.

20. Fernández G, Vela Gurovic M, Olivera N, Chopa A, Silbestri G (2014) Antibacterial properties of water-soluble gold(I) N-heterocyclic carbene complexes. J Inorg Biochem 135: 54-57.

21. Nomiya K, Yamamoto S, Noguchi R, Yokoyama H, Kasuga NC, et al. (2003) Ligand-exchangeability of 2-coordinate phosphine gold(I) complexes with AuSP and AuNP cores showing selective antimicrobial activities against Gram-positive bacteria. Crystal structures of [Au(2-Hmpa)(PPh3)] and [Au(6-Hmna) (PPh3)] (2-H2mpa=2-mercaptopropionic acid, 6-H2mna=6-mercaptonicotinic acid). J Inorg Biochem 95: 208-220.

22. Novelli F, Recine M, Sparatore F, Juliano C (1999) Gold(I) complexes as antimicrobial agents. II Farmaco 54: 232-236.

23. Wenzel M, Bigaeva E, Richard P, Le Gendre P, Picquet M, et al. (2014) New heteronuclear gold(I)-platinum(II) complexes with cytotoxic properties: are two metals better than one? J Inorg Biochem 141: 10-16.

24. Malcolm A, Parnis J, Vreugdenhil A (2011) Size control and characterization of Au nanoparticle agglomeration during encapsulation in sol-gel matrices. J Non-Cryst Solids 357: 1203-1208.

25. Dasari TP, Pathakoti K, Hwang H-M (2013) Determination of the mechanism of photoinduced toxicity of selected metal oxide nanoparticles (ZnO, CuO, Co3O4 and TiO2) to E. coli bacteria. J Environ Sci 25: 882-888.

26. Zhang Y, Newton B, Lewis E, Fu PP, Kafoury R, et al. (2015) Cytotoxicity of organic surface coating agents used for nanoparticles synthesis and stability. Toxicol in Vitro 29: 762-768.

27. Hajipour M, Fromm KM, Ashkarran AA, Jimenez de Aberasturi D, de Larramendi IR, et al. (2012) Antibacterial properties of nanoparticles. Trends Biotechnol 30: 499-511.

29

A Method for Purifying Native Transthyretin from Human Plasma

Aline G Santana[1,2], Paulo C Carvalho[1], Nilson IT Zanchin[1] and Tatiana ACB Souza[1]*

[1]*Laboratory of Proteomics and Proteins Engineering, Institute Carlos Chagas, Curitiba-PR, Brazil*
[2]*Universidade Federal do Paraná (UFPR), Curitiba-PR, Brazil*

Abstract

Transthyretin is a homotetrameric thyroid-hormone-transporting protein that binds to the retinol binding protein thus being involved in metabolism, growth, fertility, homeostasis of the cardiovascular and central nervous system, cell differentiation, reproduction, development and maintenance the cognitive processes during aging. Currently, there are several methodologies for natively purifying TTR from plasma, serum, tears, and amyloid fibrils; however, these procedures are laborious. Herein, a low-cost and simple protocol to purify TTR from human plasma is described. It involves the separation of plasma proteins by size exclusion and DEAE chromatography. The homogeneity was assessed by SDS-PAGE and by tandem mass spectrometry using an Orbitrap-XL (Thermo, San Jose-CA).

Keywords: Transthyretin; Plasma isolation

Introduction

Transthyretin was discovered in 1942 and originally named as pre albumin [1]; it is a highly conserved protein found in plasma and cerebrospinal fluid [1,2]. It is mainly expressed by hepatocytes [3] and epithelial cells of the choroid plexus [4]; yet it can also be expressed by the cerebral meninges [5], epithelial cells of the retina [6], pancreatic islets of Langerhans [7], visceral yolk sac [8], placenta [9], intestine [10] and at low-scale by stomach, heart muscle, and spleen [11].

The two major physiological functions of TTR are the transport of T4 hormone produced by thyroid and the transport of retinol (vitamin A) through interaction with retinol-binding protein RBP [12], thus being involved in metabolism, growth, fertility, and homeostasis of the cardiovascular and central nervous system [13], cell differentiation, reproduction, development and maintaining the cognitive processes during aging [14].

Previous reports describe evidences of TTR involvement in response to stress [15], in immunological pathways [16], metabolism of lipoproteins [17], and in neuroprotection against Alzheimer's disease by modulating the formation of β-amyloid plaques [18-20]. Paradoxically to this latter function, it is known that when some individuals inherit a mutated TTR gene, the mutated protein loses its functional structure and aggregates. This structural modification leads to formation of amyloid fibers and results in degenerative diseases that affect the nervous system, heart muscle, and other organs. Currently, the molecular mechanisms involved in the conversion of the TTR tetramer into aggregates of amyloid precursor fibers remains elusive. Although it is known that upon dissociation the TTR tetramer produces monomeric species with structural characteristics different from native monomer [21,22], the events associated with this non-native monomer in the initial process of TTR aggregation remain elusive.

The first reports for purifying TTR are from decades ago. Fex andrt Lindgren [23] purified a bovine counterpart to TTR from bovine serum by thiol-disulfide exchange chromatography on thiol-Sepharose 4B and affinity chromatography on human retinol-binding protein linked to Sepharose 4B. Berni et al. [24] purified TTR by using ammonium sulfate fractionation, followed by a hydrophobic interaction chromatography on phenyl-Sepharose and gel filtration on Sephadex G-50. Bashor et al. [25] developed a methodology for

TTR purification that involves precipitation of contaminating proteins with dilute aqueous phenol, ion-exchange chromatography on DEAE-Sephacel, and gel permeation chromatography on Sephadex G-100. Furuya et al. [26] were the first to recombinantly produce TTR fused with the *E. coli* outer membrane protein A (ompA) signal peptide. TTR has also been produced in the eukaryotic *Pichia Pastoris* system [27]. Lin et al. [28] created a method consisting of serum precipitation, anion exchange, thyroxine affinity chromatography and gel filtration. The latest methodologies for TTR purification include: 1) salting out, anion and cation exchange chromatographies, preparative electrophoresis, and size chromatography [29]; 2) ammonium sulfate fractionation followed by urea/Sephadex G-100 chromatography and a combination of two dye-affinity chromatographic steps on reactive yellow and cibacron blue coupled to agarose columns [30] and 3) extraction of TTR fibrils followed by sequential gel filtration after solubilization in a solution of guanidine hydrochloride and covalent chromatography [31]. This last method aims separating full-length TTR from C-terminal fragments found in TTR amyloid fibrils.

Aiming to establish a simple, fast and efficient method for purification of TTR, this work describes a purification strategy for TTR from blood plasma by employing two chromatographic methods in tandem. In our view, our method is one of the simplest yet for purifying TTR from a natural source; thus, ultimately aiding in studies that focus on the stabilization of the native tetramer for inhibition of their disassembly, prevention of amyloidogenic intermediates formation, inhibition of amyloidogenic intermediates aggregation or promotion of rupture of amyloid fibers [32-34]. A better understanding the TTR properties contribute to the development of more effective therapeutic strategies targeting pathologies related to this protein.

*Corresponding author: Tatiana de Arruda Campos Brasil de Souza, Instituto Carlos Chagas, ICC- FIOCRUZ-PR, Rua Prof. Algacyr Munhoz Mader, 3775, bloco C, 81350-010, Curitiba-PR, Brazil, E-mail: tatianabrasil@fiocruz.br

Material and Methods

Obtaining human plasma

Blood was collected from volunteer donors in collection tubes containing sodium citrate 3.2%. Blood samples were centrifuged at 15°C, 1500 rpm for 15 minutes. The supernatant (plasma) was collected and the pellet discarded.

Size exclusion chromatography

1 mL of human plasma obtained as described above was used as input for chromatography on Superdex 200 10/300 GL column. Sodium citrate 3.2% pH 8.0 was used as mobile phase for elution. The process was conducted on a FPLC system (Fast Performance Liquid Chromatography-GE-Healthcare). Eluted proteins were boiled in denaturant per 15 minutes and then loaded onto (15% acrylamide) as describe by [35].

Ion exchange chromatography

The fractions from gel filtration containing TTR were pooled and fractionated by ion exchange chromatography on DEAE Sepharose Fast Flow column with Sodium citrate 3.2% pH 8.0 (buffer A) and Sodium citrate 3.2% pH 8.0, 1M NaCl (Buffer B). Elution was performed with a linear gradient of 0-100% B in 10 column volumes with manual hold at each peak. The protein purification was analyzed by SDS PAGE (15% acrylamide) and by tandem mass spectrometry.

LC-MS/MS acquisition

The peptides were subjected to LC-MS/MS analysis using a Thermo Scientific Easy-nLC 1000 ultra-high performance liquid chromatography (UPLC) system coupled online to a LTQ-Orbitrap XL ETD mass spectrometer (Mass Spectrometry Facility-RPT02H PDTIS/ Carlos Chagas Institute-Fiocruz Paraná), as follows. The peptide mixtures were loaded onto a column (75 mm i.d., 15 cm long) packed in house with a 3.2 μm ReproSil-Pur C18-AQ resin (Dr. Maisch) with a flow of 500 nL/min and subsequently eluted with a flow of 250 nL/min from 5% to 40% ACN in 0.5% formic acid and 0.5% DMSO, in a 120 min gradient. The mass spectrometer was set in data-dependent mode to automatically switch between MS and MS/MS (MS2) acquisition. Survey full scan MS spectra (from m/z 300-2000) were acquired in the Orbitrap analyzer with resolution R=60,000 at m/z 400 (after accumulation to a target value of 1,000,000 in the linear trap). The ten most intense ions were sequentially isolated and fragmented in the linear ion trap. Previous target ions selected for MS/MS were dynamically excluded for 90 seconds. Total cycle time was approximately three seconds. The general mass spectrometric conditions were: spray voltage, 2.4 kV; no sheath and auxiliary gas flow; ion transfer tube temperature 100°C; collision gas pressure, 1.3 mTorr; normalized energy collision energy using wide-band activation mode; 35% for MS2. Ion selection thresholds were: 250 counts for MS2. An activation q=0.25 and activation time of 30 ms were applied in MS2 acquisitions.

Raw MS data analysis

The reviewed proteome set of Homo sapiens, composed of 20,187 sequences, was downloaded from the UniProt consortium on July 4th, 2014. PatternLab was used for generating a target-decoy database by grouping subset sequences, adding the sequences of 127 common mass spectrometry contaminants, and, for each sequence, including a reversed version of it. The final database used for PSM contained 105,551 sequences.

Peptide sequence matching

The Comet 2014 rev. 1 search engine [36], which is embedded into PatternLab for proteomics [37], was used to compare experimental tandem mass spectra against those theoretically generated from our sequence database and select the most likely peptide sequence candidate for each spectrum. Briefly, the search was limited to fully peptide candidates; we imposed carbamidomethylation of cysteine and oxidation of Methionine as fixed and variable modification, respectively. The search engine accepted peptide candidates within a 40-ppm tolerance from the measured precursor m/z and used the XCorr as the primary search engine score.

PSM validity was assessed using the search engine processor (SEPro) [38], which is embedded in PatternLab version 3.0.0.34. Briefly, identifications were grouped by charge state (+2 and > +3) resulting in two distinct subgroups. For each result, the Comet XCorr, DeltaCN, DeltaPPM, and Peaks Matched values were used to generate a Bayesian discriminator. The identifications were sorted in non-decreasing order according to the discriminator score. A cutoff score was established to accept a false-discovery rate (FDR) of 1% at the peptide level based on the number of labeled decoys. This procedure was independently performed on each data subset, resulting in an FDR that was independent of charge state. Additionally, a minimum sequence length of six amino-acid residues was required. Results were post-processed to only accept peptide spectrum matches with less than 6 ppm from the global identification average and proteins with two or more identified peptides.

Protein relative quantitation by extracted ion chromatograms

Relative quantitation by mass spectrometry describes strategies for comparing quantitative information of a same analyte between multiple samples. On the other hand, obtaining absolute quantitation values by mass spectrometry is challenging; some inherent difficulties are: a) different molecules ionize with different efficiencies in the mass spectrometer b) each protein will result in a different number of peptides after tryptic digestion. In a previous report, Zybailov et al described a strategy for normalizing spectral counting quantitation data that provides quantitation values closer to absolute values [39]. We recall that spectral counting is a label-free strategy that correlates the total number of MS/MS spectra assigned to a protein with its relative abundance. Briefly, Zybailov's normalization, the so-called Normalized Spectral Abundance Factor (NSAF), considers the fact that longer proteins tend to have more peptide identifications that shorter ones. Formally, the NSAF for a protein k is given by "the number of spectral counts (SpC) identifying a protein, k, divided by the protein's length (L), and divided by the sum of SpC / L for all N proteins in the experiment [39].

In this work, we employed a modified relative quantitation, having roots in NSAF, to assess the effectiveness of our purification approach. Briefly, instead of relying on spectral counts, or strategy, here termed Normalized Ion Abundance Factor (NIAF), replaces spectral count values by extracted ion chromatograms (XIC) values. Briefly, we recall that XICs are obtained by plotting the intensity of a particular peptide ion (m/z) over time and then integrating the area under the curve; for more on quantitative proteomic strategies we refer the reader to. XICs were obtained by using PatternLab's SEProQ module [37]. Our motivation in doing so is that protein ratios obtained by XICs yield more accurate estimates ratios than those obtained by spectral counting and therefore yielding estimates closer to the absolute values.

Results

Size exclusion chromatography (SEC), a chromatography that is widely used for purification and determination of the hydrodynamic radius of molecules [40], was the choice as first step for plasma fractionation. Human plasma, when chromatographed through Superdex 200 10/300 column is resolved into five distinct protein peaks (Figure 1).

The SDS-PAGE electrophoresis profile suggested that each peak from superdex 200 10/300 contained different blood proteins. In the fractions corresponding to the shoulder of the third peak, it was possible to verify the presence of a protein with expected size for TTR (Figure 1). Fractions containing the TTR were pooled and submitted to ion exchange chromatography on a DEAE column. IEC resulted in four distinct peaks (Figure 2A). The proteins were well separated and, in the fourth peak, it is possible to indentify TTR by mass spectroscopy with two minor contaminants detected. The active TTR in the Uniprot has ~13.9 kDa and is composed of 127 amino acids. The sequence coverage was 88% and peptides comprising 112 aminoacids out of 127 were detected. We obtained NSIAF from all proteins, as detailed in the methodology; our results showed that 92.5% of the total NSIAF from the sample was decurrently from TTR (Figure 2B). In that same fraction, 4.9% corresponded to the keratin, a common contamination that happens during sample preparation, and 2.4% refers to other proteins.

All our raw mass spectrometric data is made available at http://proteomics.fiocruz.br/tatiana/2015/. Moreover, TTR was not detected in any other fraction indicating that all TTR present in plasma is concentrated in this fraction. The yield of purification was ~0.09 mg of protein per ml of plasma. Our experimental procedure also could be helpfull to separate albumin, Serotransferrin and Antithrombin-III from other blood proteins (Figure 2).

Discussion

Several reports of plasma protein purification by size exclusion chromatography are available; but none were performed with the type of column and buffer system used in this work. By comparing the chromatographic profile of the gel filtration of human plasma presented in Figure 1 with other works, it is possible to observe that the chromatographic profile can vary widely for the same sample at the expense the column used [41,42].

Sepharose 4 FF is widely used for plasma fractionation [43], but due to its low resolution, it is most suitable in cases where the target protein and most contaminants have very distinct molecular masses. Other columns such as Superose 6, Sephadex G-200, Sephadex G-100 also appear in the literature for plasma proteins fractionation [43-46], but they all have lower resolution than Superdex 200 10/300. Sephadex G-200, the column closest to the required resolution, is capable of providing three distinct peaks when used in the first plasma fractionation step [44]. However, its use at the expense of Superdex 200 10/300, would probably require additional purification steps to obtain pure TTR due to higher amounts of remnant contaminants.

Another important aspect to be noted is that the same column and

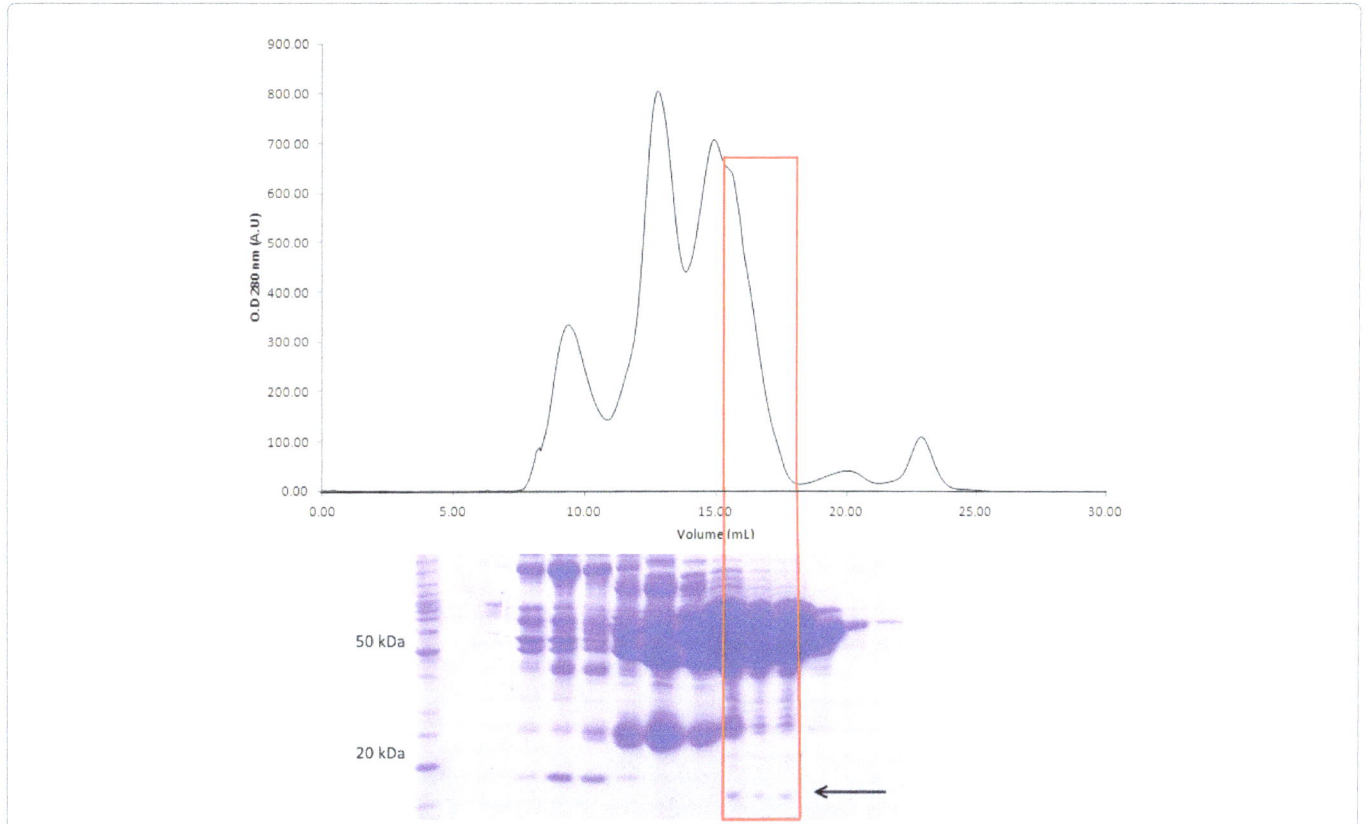

Figure 1: Chromatogram of plasma fractionation by gel filtration on a Superdex 200 10/300 column and SDS PAGE of the eluted fractions during gel filtration. The fractions containing TTR are evidenced by the red box. First lane- Molecular weight marker (Bench marker protein ladder). The arrow (←) indicates the gel bands expected to be TTR.

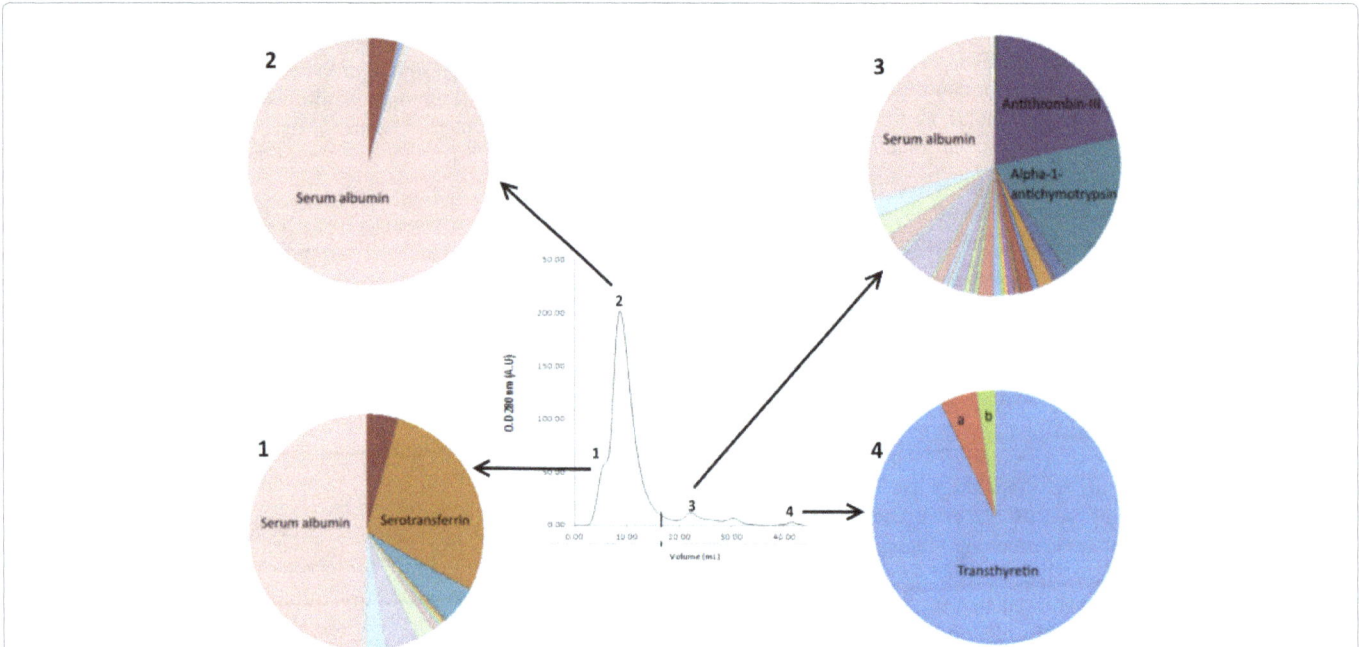

Figure 2: Identification of protein content in each DEAE peak. Chromatogram from DEAE Sepharose Fast Flow and diagram indicating protein identified by MS/MS after IEC. 1-4 corresponds to protein found in fractions 1-4, respectively. In 4, a indicate keratin contaminants and b indicate all other proteins.

sample can result in slightly different chromatographic profiles when using buffers with different pH and ionic strength. In this work, the buffer composed of 3.2% Sodium Citrate pH 8.0 was used in all steps of protein purification. The majority of the previously solutions used for plasma purification were buffered with Tris–HCl [23,41,42]. The choice of 3.2% Sodium Citrate was fundamental to better separation of plasma proteins since this buffer prevents the activation of the coagulation cascade, by sequestering calcium, and it is a good buffering at a pH close to physiological, favoring proteins to maintain the conformation found in plasma. Our experimental procedure also could be helpfull to separate albumin, Serotransferrin and Antithrombin-III from other blood proteins (Figure 2). Albumin was found in the second peak of IEC (Figure 2). This protein represents 50% -70% of all plasma proteins [45], and have a remarkable ability to bind to exogenous and endogenous components [46], making its removal important for application related to the remaining plasma proteins.

This method can also effectively be used to isolate two other important proteins: serotransferrin and antithrombin-III (Figure 2). Serotransferrin is associated with Fe^{3+} uptake, distribution and control of its quantity [47]. Antithrombin-III is an endogenous anticoagulant capable of inhibit key-factors of the coagulation cascade such as thrombin and FXa, thus, having a crucial role in homeostasis [42]. About 25% of the total NSIAF from peak 1 and peak 3 (Figures 2A and 2C) was decurrently from serotransferrin and antithrombin-III, respectively. These proteins can be further purified through additional chromatographic steps. All these results show a simple and low-cost method for chromatographic purification of human plasma TTR. The procedure is also helpfull to remove albumin and to purify two other blood proteins. TTR are often submitted to drug development screenings due to its role in important pathologies such as Senile Systemic Amyloidosis (SSA) and Familial Amyloid Polyneuropathy (FAP) [48] with some promising amyloidogenesis inhibitors [49-54] such as genistein [54,55], other flavonoids of similar structure [55], T4

analogues [49,52,53] being indentified. However all screenings for such compounds were performed with recombinant molecules.

References

1. Kabat EA, Moore DH, Landow H (1942) An Electrophoretic Study Of The Protein Components In Cerebrospinal Fluid And Their Relationship To The Serum Proteins. J Clin Invest 21: 571-577.

2. Seibert FB, Nelson JW (1942) Electrophoretic study of the blood response in tuberculosis. J Biol Chem 143: 29-38

3. Murakami T, Yasuda Y, Mita S, Maeda S, Shimada K, et al. (1987) Prealbumin gene expression during mouse development studied by in situ hybridization. Cell Differ 22: 1-9.

4. Aleshire SL, Bradley CA, Richardson LD, Parl FF (1983) Localization of human prealbumin in choroid plexus epithelium. J Histochem Cytochem 31: 608-612.

5. Herbert J, Wilcox JN, Pham KT, Fremeau RT Jr, Zeviani M, et al. (1986) Transthyretin: a choroid plexus-specific transport protein in human brain. The 1986 S. Weir Mitchell award. Neurology 36: 900-911.

6. Martone RL, Herbert J, Dwork A, Schon EA (1988) Transthyretin is synthesized in the mammalian eye. Biochem Biophys Res Commun 151: 905-912.

7. Kato M, Kato K, Blaner WS, Chertow BS, Goodman DS (1985) Plasma and cellular retinoid-binding proteins and transthyretin (prealbumin) are all localized in the islets of Langerhans in the rat. Proc Natl Acad Sci U S A 82: 2488-2492.

8. Soprano DR, Soprano KJ, Goodman DS (1986) Retinol-binding protein and transthyretin mRNA levels in visceral yolk sac and liver during fetal development in the rat. Proc Natl Acad Sci U S A 83: 7330-7334.

9. McKinnon B, Li H, Richard K, Mortimer R (2005) Synthesis of thyroid hormone binding proteins transthyretin and albumin by human trophoblast. J Clin Endocrinol Metab 90: 6714-6720.

10. Loughna S, Bennett P, Moore G (1995) Molecular analysis of the expression of transthyretin in intestine and liver from trisomy 18 fetuses. Hum Genet 95: 89-95.

11. Soprano DR, Herbert J, Soprano KJ, Schon EA, Goodman DS (1985) Demonstration of transthyretin mRNA in the brain and other extrahepatic tissues in the rat. J Biol Chem 260: 11793-11798.

12. Kanai M, Raz A, Goodman DS (1968) Retinol-binding protein: the transport protein for vitamin A in human plasma. J Clin Invest 47: 2025-2044.

13. Hulbert AJ (2000) Thyroid hormones and their effects: a new perspective. Biol Rev Camb Philos Soc 75: 519-631.

14. Brouillette J, Quirion R (2008) Transthyretin: a key gene involved in the maintenance of memory capacities during aging. Neurobiol Aging 29: 1721-1732.

15. Bernstein LH, Leukhardt-Fairfield CJ, Pleban W, Rudolph R (1989) Usefulness of data on albumin and prealbumin concentrations in determining effectiveness of nutritional support. Clin Chem 35: 271-274.

16. Burton PM, Hung P, Lin T, Lovelace C, White A (1985) The effects of homogeneous human prealbumin on in vitro and in vivo immune responses in the mouse. Int J Immunopharmacol 7: 473-481.

17. Sousa MM, Berglund L, Saraiva MJ (2000) Transthyretin in high density lipoproteins: association with apolipoprotein A-I. J Lipid Res 41: 58-65.

18. Riisøen H (1988) Reduced prealbumin (transthyretin) in CSF of severely demented patients with Alzheimer's disease. Acta Neurol Scand 78: 455-459.

19. Schwarzman AL, Gregori L, Vitek MP, Lyubski S, Strittmatter WJ, et al. (1994) Transthyretin sequesters amyloid beta protein and prevents amyloid formation. Proc Natl Acad Sci U S A 91: 8368-8372.

20. Serot JM, Christmann D, Dubost T, Couturier M (1997) Cerebrospinal fluid transthyretin: aging and late onset Alzheimer's disease. J Neurol Neurosurg Psychiatry 63: 506-508.

21. Quintas A, Vaz DC, Cardoso I, Saraiva MJ, Brito RM (2001) Tetramer dissociation and monomer partial unfolding precedes protofibril formation in amyloidogenic transthyretin variants. J Biol Chem 276: 27207-27213.

22. Lindgren M, Sörgjerd K, Hammarström P (2005) Detection and characterization of aggregates, prefibrillar amyloidogenic oligomers, and protofibrils using fluorescence spectroscopy. Biophys J 88: 4200-4212.

23. Fex G, Lindgren R (1977) Purification of a bovine counterpart to human prealbumin and its interaction with a bovine retinol-binding protein. Biochim Biophys Acta 493: 410-417.

24. Berni R, Ottonello S, Monaco HL (1985) Purification of human plasma retinol-binding protein by hydrophobic interaction chromatography. Anal Biochem 150: 273-277.

25. Bashor MM, Hewett J, Lackey A, Driskell WJ, Neese JW (1987) Purification of prealbumin from human serum. Prep Biochem 17: 209-227.

26. Furuya H, Nakazato M, Saraiva MJ, Costa SP, Sasaki H, et al. (1989) Tetramer formation of a variant type human transthyretin (prealbumin) produced by Escherichia coli expression system. Biochem Biophys Res Commun 163: 851-859.

27. Prapunpoj P, Leelawatwatana L, Schreiber G, Richardson SJ (2006) Change in structure of the N-terminal region of transthyretin produces change in affinity of transthyretin to T4 and T3. FEBS J 273: 4013-4023.

28. Lin Q, Su T, Liu G, Gu J (1996) Purification of transthyretin by high performance affinity chromatography from human plasma. Prep Biochem Biotechnol 26: 245-257.

29. Blirup-Jensen S (2013) Protein standardization I: Protein purification procedure for the purificationof human prealbumin, orosomucoid and transferrin as primary protein preparations. Clin Chem Lab Med 39: 1076-1089.

30. Raghu P, Ravinder P, Sivakumar B (2003) A new method for purification of human plasma retinol-binding protein and transthyretin. Biotechnol Appl Biochem 38: 19-24.

31. Westermark P, Westermark GT (2005) Purification of transthyretin and transthyretin fragments from amyloid-rich human tissues. Methods Mol Biol 299: 255-260.

32. Damas AM, Saraiva MJ (2000) Review: TTR amyloidosis-structural features leading to protein aggregation and their implications on therapeutic strategies. J Struct Biol 130: 290-299.

33. Saraiva MJ (2002) Hereditary transthyretin amyloidosis: molecular basis and therapeutic strategies. Expert Rev Mol Med 4: 1-11.

34. Mason JM, Kokkoni N, Stott K, Doig AJ (2003) Design strategies for anti-amyloid agents. Curr Opin Struct Biol 13: 526-532.

35. Laemmli UK (1970) Cleavage of structural proteins during the assembly of the head of bacteriophage T4. Nature 227: 680-685.

36. Eng JK, Jahan TA, Hoopmann MR (2013) Comet: an open-source MS/MS sequence database search tool. Proteomics 13: 22-24.

37. Carvalho PC, Fischer JS, Xu T, Yates JR 3rd, Barbosa VC (2012) PatternLab: from mass spectra to label-free differential shotgun proteomics. Curr Protoc Bioinformatics Chapter 13: Unit13.

38. Carvalho PC, Fischer JS, Xu T, Cociorva D, Balbuena TS, et al. (2012) Search engine processor: Filtering and organizing peptide spectrum matches. Proteomics 12: 944-949.

39. Zybailov B, Mosley AL, Sardiu ME, Coleman MK, Florens L, et al. (2006) Statistical analysis of membrane proteome expression changes in Saccharomyces cerevisiae. J Proteome Res 5: 2339-2347.

40. Mory S, Barth HG (1999) Size exclusion chromatography. Springer, Berlin.

41. JosiÄ‡ D, Horn H, Schulz P, Schwinn H, Britsch L (1998) Size-exclusion chromatography of plasma proteins with high molecular masses. J Chromatogr A 796: 289-298.

42. Kaersgaard P, Barington KA (1998) Isolation of the factor VIII-von Willebrand factor complex directly from plasma by gel filtration. J Chromatogr B Biomed Sci Appl 715: 357-367.

43. Mourey L, Samama JP, Delarue M, Choay J, Lormeau JC, et al. (1990) Antithrombin III: structural and functional aspects. Biochimie 72: 599-608.

44. Perrier H, Delcroix JP, Perrier C, Gras J (1973) An attempt to classify the plasma proteins of the rainbow trout (salmo gairdnerii richardson) using disc electrophoresis, gel filtration and salt solubility fractionation. Comp. Biochem. Physiol 46: 475-482.

45. Silverlight JJ, Prysor-Jones RA, Jenkins JS (1985) Growth hormone in normal female rat plasma appears on gel filtration as a large molecular weight form. Life Sci 36: 1927-1932.

46. Hu T, Liu Y (2015) Probing the interaction of cefodizime with human serum albumin using multi-spectroscopic and molecular docking techniques. J Pharm Biomed Anal 107: 325-332.

47. Fanali G, di Masi A, Trezza V, Marino M, Fasano M, et al. (2012) Human serum albumin: from bench to bedside. Mol Aspects Med 33: 209-290.

48. Chasteen DN (1977) Human serotrasferrin: Structure and Function. Coord Chem Rev 22: 1-36.

49. Mourey L, Samama JP, Delarue M, Choay J, Lormeau JC, et al. (1990) Antithrombin III: structural and functional aspects. Biochimie 72: 599-608.

50. Palmieri Lde C, Lima LM, Freire JB, Bleicher L, Polikarpov I, et al. (2010) Novel Zn2+-binding sites in human transthyretin: implications for amyloidogenesis and retinol-binding protein recognition. J Biol Chem 285: 31731-31741.

51. Miroy GJ, Lai Z, Lashuel HA, Peterson SA, Strang C, et al. (1996) Inhibiting transthyretin amyloid fibril formation via protein stabilization. Proc Natl Acad Sci U S A 93: 15051-15056.

52. Peterson SA, Klabunde T, Lashuel HA, Purkey H, Sacchettini JC, et al. (1998) Inhibiting transthyretin conformational changes that lead to amyloid fibril formation. Proc Natl Acad Sci U S A 95: 12956-12960.

53. Baures PW, Oza VB, Peterson SA, Kelly JW (1999) Synthesis and evaluation of inhibitors of transthyretin amyloid formation based on the non-steroidal anti-inflammatory drug, flufenamic acid. Bioorg Med Chem 7: 1339-1347.

54. Klabunde T, Petrassi HM, Oza VB, Raman P, Kelly JW, et al. (2000) Rational design of potent human transthyretin amyloid disease inhibitors. Nat Struct Biol 7: 312-321.

55. Petrassi HM, Johnson SM, Purkey HE, Chiang KP, Walkup T, et al. (2005) Potent and selective structure-based dibenzofuran inhibitors of transthyretin amyloidogenesis: kinetic stabilization of the native state. J Amer Chem Soc 127: 6662-6671.

56. Green NS, Foss TR, Kelly JW (2005) Genistein, a natural product from soy, is a potent inhibitor of transthyretin amyloidosis. Proc Natl Acad Sci U S A 102: 14545-14550.

57. Trivella DBB, Bleicher L, Palmiere LC, Wiggers HJ, Montanari CA, et al. (2010) Conformation differences between the wild type and V30M mutant transthyretin modulate its binding to genistein: implications to tetramer stability and ligand-binding. J Struct Biol 170: 522-531.

30

Adrenergic Regulation of Somatolactin Gene Expression in Tilapia Pituitary Cells

Quan Jiang[1]*, Tianqiang Liu[1,2] and Anji Lian[1]

[1]*Key Laboratory of Bio-resources and Eco-environment of Ministry of Education, College of Life Sciences, 610065, Sichuan University, Chengdu, PR China*
[2]*The Animal Health Research Institute, Tongwei Co., Ltd, China*

Abstract

Epinephrine is an important neuroendocrine regulator to control growth hormone (GH) secretion in vertebrates. Somatolactin (SL), the latest member of the GH family, is a novel pituitary hormone with diverse functions in fish. In a previous report it was shown that epinephrine had a potent inhibitory effect on SL release in fish. However, very little is known about the mechanisms responsible for epinephrine inhibition of SL gene expression. In primary cultures of tilapia neurointermediate lobe (NIL) cells, epinephrine not only reduced SL mRNA levels, but could also abolish pituitary adenylate cyclase-activating polypeptide (PACAP)-stimulated SL gene expression. The inhibitory effects of epinephrine on SL gene expression were mimicked by additions of α2-adrenergic agonists clonidine and UK14304, whereas similar treatments with the α1-agonist cirazoline or the β-agonist isoproterenol had no effects in this regard. In parallel experiments, the SL response to epinephrine was significantly abolished by co-incubations with the α2-antagonist yohimbine, but the α1- or β-antagonist was not effective in this regard. In tilapia NIL cells, the α2-adrenergic agonist clonidine suppressed cAMP production and blocked forskolin and PACAP induction of total cAMP production. By using a pharmacological approach, the adenylate cyclase (AC) activator- and cAMP analog-stimulated SL responses were blocked treatment with clonidine. Furthermore, adrenergic inhibition of SL gene expression was also mimicked by inhibiting AC and blocking protein kinase A (PKA). These results, as a whole, suggest that α2-adrenergic stimulation can downregulate SL gene transcription by inhibiting the AC/cAMP-dependent mechanism at the tilapia pituitary level.

Keywords: Epinephrine; Somatolactin; Tilapia; Pituitary cells; Signaling pathways

Abbreviations

EP: Epinephrine; SL: Somatolactin; GH: Growth Hormone; PACAP: Pituitary Adenylate Cyclase-activating Polypeptide; NIL: Neurointermediate Lobe; cAMP: Cyclic Adenosine Monophosphate; AC: Adenylate Cyclase; PKA: Protein Kinase A

Introduction

In vertebrates, the adrenergic system is known to be involved in the regulation of growth hormone (GH) secretion and gene expression at the hypothalamic and pituitary levels. The adrenergic receptors (or adrenoceptors) mediating central and peripheral actions of epinephrine are typically subdivided into three main families (α1, α2, and β) based on their pharmacology, structure, and signaling mechanisms [1,2]. The α1-adrenoceptors increase levels of intracellular calcium, whereas α2- and β-adrenoceptors inhibit and stimulate adenylyl cyclase (AC), respectively [1]. In mammals, the influences of epinephrine on GH secretion are selective for one type of adrenoceptors at the hypothalamic or pituitary cells levels. Results of studies in both primates and rodents have shown that α2-adrenoceptors play an important role in stimulating GH secretion in the central nervous system [3]. In contrast, α2-adrenoceptors are not involved in GH secretion [4] and GH gene expression [5] at the pituitary cell level. Although still controversial, β-adrenergic activation is also involved in regulation of GH secretion. In the baboon, central action of norepinephrine was mediated by β-adrenergic receptors to inhibit GH release [6], whereas β-adrenergic receptor agonists can stimulate rat GH secretion in rat pituitary cells [7] and increase GH gene expression in ovine pituitary cells [5]. Similar to mammals, the role of adrenergic as a GH-releasing factor has also been confirmed in lower vertebrates including fish. In goldfish, intraperitoneal injection of norepinephrine resulted in decreased serum GH levels, whereas intraventricular injection of norepinephrine has no effects on GH secretion *in vivo* [8]. Since the pituitary lies outside of the blood-brain barrier, these results suggest that norepinephrine may directly act on the pituitary to inhibit GH secretion. This idea is further corroborated by *in vitro* studies showing that norepinephrine is effective in suppressing goldfish GH secretion [9] and grass carp GH gene [10] in pituitary cells via α2-adrenoceptors.

Somatolactin (SL), the latest member of GH family, is a pituitary hormone unique to fish species. SL is derived from GH during early stages of gnathostome evolution [11], but lost secondarily in the lineage leading to land vertebrates after the lungfish branched off [12]. SL appears to have significant roles in chromatophore regulation and lipid metabolism [13,14], maturation [15], stress response [16], ion transport [17] and acid-base balance [18]. Among the known SL inhibitors in fish, somatostatin can inhibit SL gene expression through coupling of AC/cAMP and PLC/IP3/PKC cascades [19]. In addition to somatostatin, epinephrine has been implicated as a SL-releasing inhibitor. A previous *in vitro* study had demonstrated that epinephrine dose-dependently inhibited SL release in the organ-cultured pituitary of rainbow trout [20]. However, no information is available regarding the mechanisms responsible for epinephrine inhibition of SL gene expression at the pituitary level.

*Corresponding author: Dr. Quan Jiang, Key Laboratory of Bio-resources and Eco-environment of Ministry of Education, College of Life Sciences, 610065, Sichuan University, Chengdu, PR China, E-mail: jiangqua@gmail.com

In the present study, using primary cultures of tilapia neurointermediate lobe (NIL) cells as a model, the effects of epinephrine on the SL mRNA expression were investigated at the pituitary level. The receptor specificity was further characterized using adrenergic analogs for α1-, α2-, and β-adrenoceptors. The post-receptor signaling mechanisms for SL gene expression were also investigated. In this study, we have demonstrated for the first time that epinephrine can act at the pituitary level via α2-adrenoceptors to regulate SL gene expression through the AC/cAMP-dependent mechanism.

Materials and Methods

Animals

Sexually mature male tilapia (*Oreochromis mossambicus*) (standard length: 11 ± 0.5 cm, body weight: 50 ± 5.0 g) were maintained in freshwater aquaria at 28°C under 10 hr dark/14 hr light photoperiod. The fish were fed commercial diet (40% protein, 12% fat, 2% fiber, 8.5% moisture, 8% ash, Tongwei, China) to satiety twice a day at 10:00 and 16:00. During the process of tissue sampling, the fish were sacrificed by spinosectomy after anesthesia with 0.05% MS222 (Sigma, St Louis, MO) according to the procedures approved by the Animal Ethics Committee of Sichuan University.

Pharmacological agents

Epinephrine and Ovine PACAP38 were obtained from Sigma (St. Louis, Mo). Adrenergic analogs including clonidine, UK 14304, cirazoline, isoproterenol, propranolol, 2-{[β-(4-Hydroxyphenyl) ethyl] aminomethyl}-1-tetralone hydrochloride (HEAT), and yohimbine were obtained from Tocris (Bristol, UK). These pharmacological compounds have been previously used in goldfish [9], grass carp [10], tilapia [21] and zebrafish [22], confirming that they are highly selective for respective targets in fish models. 3-isobutyl-1-methylxanthine (IBMX), 8-(4-chloro-phenylthio)-cAMP (CPT-cAMP), forskolin, H89, MDL12330A and actinomycin D were obtained from Calbiochem (San Diego, CA). Stock solution of PACAP was dissolved in double-distilled deionized water and stored frozen in small aliquots at -80°C. Epinephrine and clonidine were dissolved freshly in culture medium right before drug treatment to avoid oxidation caused by prolonged storage. Other test agents were first dissolved in dimethyl sulfoxide (DMSO). Stock solutions of test substances were diluted with prewarmed (28°C) culture medium to appropriate concentrations 15 min prior to drug treatment. The final dilutions of DMSO were less than 0.1% and had no effects on SL gene expression in tilapia NIL cells.

Primary culture of tilapia NIL cells

Tilapia pituitary cells were prepared by trypsin/DNase II digestion method as described previously [23]. Briefly, The NIL of individual pituitaries was isolated by manual dissection under a stereomicroscope, diced into 0.6 mm fragments using a McILwain tissue chopper (Brinkmann, Mississauga, Ont.), and digested in type II trypsin (4 mg/ml, GIBCO) for 30 min at 28°C with constant shaking. After that, the reaction was terminated by adding trypsin inhibitor (2.5 mg/ml, Sigma) and pituitary fragments were dispersed in Ca²⁺- free MEM [S-MEM with 26 mM NaHCO3, 25 mM HEPES, 1% antibiotic-antimycotic, and 0.1% BSA; pH 7.7] with DNase II (0.01 mg/ml, Sigma). After that, total cell yield and percentage viability were estimated by cell counting in the presence of trypan blue using a hemocytometer. NIL cells were cultured in 48-well culture plates (Costar, Corning Inc., N.Y.) at a seeding density of ~1 × 10⁶ cells/well in M199 (Invitrogen). NIL cells were incubated overnight at 28°C under 5% CO_2 and saturated humidity to allow for the recovery of membrane receptors after trypsin digestion. On the following day, culture medium was replaced with serum-free M199 and drug treatment was initiated for the duration as indicated in individual experiments.

Real-time PCR measurement of SL

Tilapia NIL cells were seeded at a density of ~1 × 10⁶ cells/ml/well in 48-well culture plates and treated with hormones or drugs for the duration as indicated in individual experiments. After that, total RNA was isolated using RNAzol (MRC, Cincinnati, OH, USA), digested with RNase-free DNase I to remove genomic DNA contamination, and reversely transcribed using M-MLV (TaKaRa, Dalian, China). After that, real-time PCR assays were performed on the CFX96 Real-Time PCR Detection System (Bio-Rad Laboratories, CA, USA). PCR reaction were conducted with a SYBR Select Master Mix kit (Applied Biosystems) using the primers specific for tilapia SL (GenBank No: AB442015) [SL forward primer: 5' CCCACTCCCTTTGCGACTT 3' and SL reverse primer: 5' TAGCGGTCCAGTGTCGTCT 3']. Real-time PCR for the SL were performed with initial denaturation at 94°C for 3 min followed by 35 cycles of amplification with denaturation at 94°C for 30 sec, annealing at 56°C for 30 sec, and extension at 72°C for 30 sec and then fluorescent signal collection at 80°C for 1 sec. For data calibration, serial dilutions of plasmid DNA containing the ORF of SL was used as the standards for these real-time PCR assay. As an internal control, real-time PCR for 18S rRNA was conducted using the primers specific for 18S rRNA [forward primer: 5' GGACACGGAAAGGATTGACAG 3' and reverse primer: 5' GTTCGTTATCGGAATTAACCAGAC 3']. In these experiments, no significant changes were observed for 18S rRNA expression. The quantitative results were normalized as a ratio of the target gene/18S rRNA expression level.

Measurement of cAMP production

The NIL cells were seeded at a density of ~1 × 10⁶ cells/2 ml/dish in poly-D-lysine precoated 35-mm dishes and cultured overnight at 28°C as previously described [19]. On the following day, culture medium was replaced with 0.9 ml HEPES-buffered Hanks' balanced salt solution with 0.1% BSA and 0.1 mM IBMX. IBMX, the inhibitor for phospho-diesterases, was included to prevent cAMP degradation in NIL cells. Drug treatment was initiated with various combinations of drugs at appropriate concentrations and the cells were allowed to incubate at 28°C for 30 min. After that, culture medium was harvested for the measurement of cAMP release whereas cellular cAMP content was extracted from NIL cells with 1 ml PBS. These cAMP samples were quantified by using a cAMP ELISA kit (Wuhan EIAab Science Co., Ltd).

Data transformation and statistics

All of the experiments were performed at least twice, and all of the treatments in each experiment were tested in quadruplicate from 40 individual fish. For real-time PCR of SL transcripts, standard curves with a dynamic range of 10⁵ and correlation coefficient of ≥ 0.95 were used for data calibration with Bio-rad CFX 3.0 software. The quantitative results were normalized as a ratio of the target gene/18S rRNA expression level. Data of SL gene expression were transformed as a percentage of the mean value in the control group without drug treatment (referred to as "% Ctrl"). Data presented (as means ± SEM, N = 4) were analyzed using ANOVA followed by Duncan's test using Prism 6.0. Differences between groups were considered as significant at $P < 0.05$.

Results

Adrenergic regulation of SL gene expression in tilapia NIL Cells

To examine adrenergic regulation of SL gene expression at the pituitary level, we used a tilapia NIL cells as a model to test the direct effects of epinephrine on SL mRNA expression. As shown in Figure 1A, treatment with epinephrine (1 μM) could time-dependently inhibit SL mRNA expression, and the maximal inhibition on SL mRNA expression was observed at 48 h. The duration of drug treatment was fixed at 48 h unless stated otherwise in subsequent experiments. In parallel experiments, increasing concentrations (0.01-10 μM) of epinephrine were effective in triggering a dose-dependent decrease in SL mRNA levels (Figure 1B). The minimal effective dose for epinephrine to inhibit SL gene expression was 10 nM, and SL transcripts were reduced to 45% of control levels at maximal effective doses of 1 μM.

Effects of adrenergic agonists on SL gene expression

To clarify the receptor specificity for epinephrine action, the effects of adrenergic agonists on SL gene expression were examined in tilapia NIL cells. As shown in Figure 2A, the inhibitory effects of epinephrine on SL gene expression were mimicked by the increasing levels of α2-agonist clonidine (0.01-10 μM) and UK14304 (0.01-10 μM), whereas α1-agonist cirazoline (0.01-10 μM) or β-agonist isoproterenol (0.01-10 μM) was not effective in altering SL mRNA expression (Figure 2B).

Effects of adrenergic antagonists on epinephrine inhibition of SL gene expression

To further characterize the receptor specificity of epinephrine inhibition on SL gene, tilapia NIL cells were exposed to adrenergic antagonists specific for different subtypes of adrenoceptors. In these experiments, the inhibitory effect of epinephrine was tested in the presence or absence the α2-antagonist yohimbine, or α1-antagonist HEAT, or β-antagonist propranolol. In this case, epinephrine consistently suppressed SL gene expression and this inhibitory action was blocked by simultaneous treatment with α2-antagonist yohimbine (5 μM, Figure 3A), but not affected by treatment with the α1-antagonist HEAT (Figure 3B) and β-antagonist propranolol (Figure 3C). To further examine the specificity of α2 receptor activation on SL gene expression, the effects of α2-antagonist yohimbine on the SL response to the α2-agonists clonidine and UK14304 were studied in tilapia NIL cells. In the present study, α2-agonist clonidine- and UK14304-inhibited SL gene expression were prevented in the presence of the α2-antagonist yohimbine (Figures 3D and 3E).

α2-adrenergic regulation of SL transcript stability

To shed light on the mechanisms for α2-adrenergic inhibition of SL mRNA expression, the effects of α2-agonist clonidine treatment on SL mRNA stability were also tested. Clearance analysis of SL transcript was performed in NIL cells pretreated with the transcription inhibitor actinomycin D (8 μM). In this case, the clearance rate of SL transcripts expressed as the time required for half of the original amount of SL mRNA to degrade (i.e., $T_{1/2}$) was used as an index to monitor SL transcript stability. As shown in Figure 4, SL mRNA levels were reduced gradually in a time-dependent manner with a $T_{1/2}$ value of ~ 31 h. However, the clearance profile or $T_{1/2}$ value for SL transcripts was not affected by the co-treatment with clonidine (1 μM).

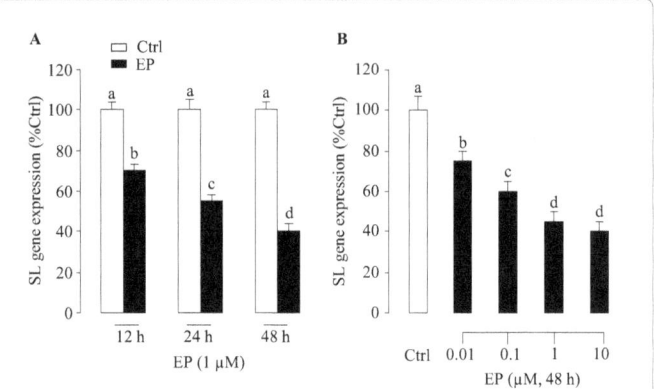

Figure 1: Adrenergic regulation of SL mRNA expression in tilapia NIL cells. (A) Time-course and (B) dose-dependency of epinephrine (EP) on SL mRNA expression. NIL cells were incubated with EP (1 μM) for 12, 24, 48 h or with increasing doses of EP (0.01-10 μM) for 48 h. SL mRNA data are expressed as mean ± SEM and groups denoted by different letters represent a significant difference at P < 0.05 (ANOVA followed by Duncan's test).

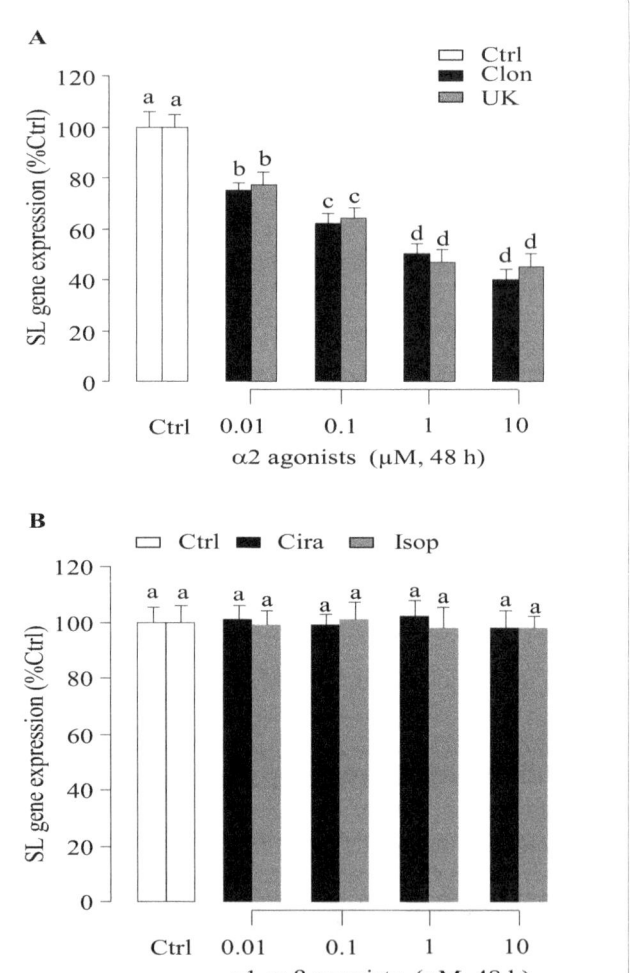

Figure 2: Effects of adrenergic agonists on SL gene expression. Tilapia NIL cells were incubated with increasing doses of α2 agonist clonidine (Clon, 0.01-10 μM) and UK14304 (UK, 0.01-10 μM) (A), or incubated with α1-agonist cirazoline (Cira, 0.01-10 μM) or β agonist isoproterenol (Isop, 0.01-10 μM) (B) for 48 h. SL mRNA data are expressed as mean ± SEM and groups denoted by different letters represent a significant difference at P < 0.05 (ANOVA followed by Duncan's test).

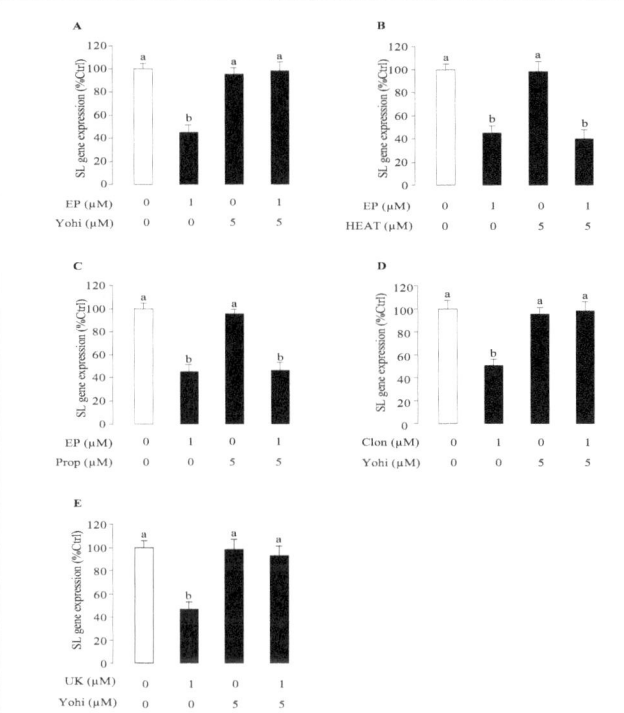

Figure 3: Effects of adrenergic antagonists on SL gene expression. Pituitary NIL cells were incubated with epinephrine (EP, 1 μM) in presence or absence of α2-antagonist yohimbine (Yohi, 5 Mm, A) or α1-antagonist HEAT (5 μM, B), or β-antagonist propranolol (Prop, 5 μM, C) for 48 h. In parallel experiments, the inhibitory effects of α2-agonist clonidine (Clon, 1 μM, D) and UK14304 (UK, 1 μM, E) on SL gene expression could be blocked by α2-antagonist yohimbine (Yohi, 5 μM) for 48 h. SL mRNA data are expressed as mean ± SEM and groups denoted by different letters represent a significant difference at $P < 0.05$ (ANOVA followed by Duncan's test).

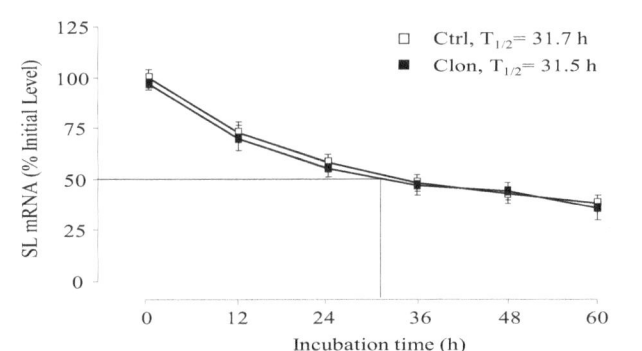

Figure 4: Effects of α2-agonist clonidine on SL mRNA stability. Tilapia NIL cells were incubated with actinomycin D (8 μM) in the presence or absence of α2-agonist clonidine (Clon, 1 μM) for 12, 24, 36, 48 and 60 h, respectively. The half-life of SL transcript was defined as the time required for SL mRNA levels to drop to 50% of its original values and was deduced based on the one-phase exponential decay model using GraphPad Prism.

Adrenergic regulation of basal and PACAP-stimulated SL mRNA expression

The role of PACAP as a novel SL regulator has received increasing attention in teleosts [24-28]. To test the functional interactions between PACAP and epinephrine in regulating SL gene expression, tilapia NIL cells were challenged with PACAP (10 nM) for 48 h in the presence or absence of epinephrine. In this study, basal levels of SL mRNA were elevated by PACAP treatment, and this stimulatory action could be

blocked by simultaneous incubation with epinephrine (1 μM, Figure 5). Similarly, this stimulatory effect was also blocked by simultaneous treatment with the α2-agonist clonidine (1 μM).

α2-adrenergic inhibition of cAMP production

Given that is known to inhibit cAMP synthesis via activation of α2-adrenergic receptor at the pituitary level in fish [10], the effects of α2-adrenergic receptor agonist clonidine on cAMP production were tested in tilapia NIL cells. As shown in Figure 6A, forskolin was effective in elevating total cAMP production. In contrast, basal levels and forskolin-induced increases in cAMP production were significantly attenuated by application of clonidine (Figure 6A). In tilapia NIL cells, cAMP contents were also significantly elevated by PACAP treatment (10 nM), and this stimulatory action could be alleviated by simultaneous incubation with clonidine (Figure 6A). In parallel studies, increasing levels (0.01-10 μM) of the AC inhibitor MDL12330A (Figure 6B) and the PKA inhibitor H89 (Figure 6C) could mimic the dose dependence of clonidine inhibition on SL gene expression. To further evaluate the functional role of the cAMP-dependent pathway in clonidine-induced inhibition of SL gene expression, tilapia NIL cells were exposed to clonidine (1 μM) in the presence of the AC activator forskolin (1 μM) and cAMP analog CPT-cAMP (100 μM), respectively. In this case, addition of clonidine (1 μM) inhibited not only basal SL gene expression but also forskolin- and CPT-cAMP-stimulated SL gene expression (Figure 6D).

Discussion

Based on the studies in rainbow trout, epinephrine dose-dependently inhibited SL release in the organ-cultured pituitary [20]. Since epinephrine does not readily cross the blood brain barrier [29], this catecholamine must directly act at the level of pituitary gland to inhibit SL secretion. This idea was further corroborated by our present studies that showed epinephrine could inhibit SL gene expression in a time- and dose-dependent manner, suggesting that SL response to epinephrine may represent a common phenomenon in fish models. To shed light on the receptor specificity for SL response to epinephrine at the pituitary level, we clarified the receptor specificity using a pharmacological approach. In the present study, epinephrine-induced inhibitory actions were mimicked by the α2-agonist clonidine and UK14304 but not by the α1-agonist cirazoline or β-agonist isoproterenol. Furthermore, epinephrine inhibition on SL gene expression could be prevented by the α2-antagonist yohimbine, whereas the α1-antagonist HEAT and the β antagonist propranolol were not effective in this regard. Apparently, α2 inhibition of SL gene expression could not be due to SL mRNA degradation as clonidine treatment did not alter the half-life of SL transcripts. These results, as a whole, provide evidence for the first time that the inhibitory action of epinephrine on SL gene expression is mediated by α2-adrenoceptors in tilapia NIL cells.

To further evaluate the functional role of epinephrine as a SL inhibitor in fish, we also examined functional interactions between PACAP and epinephrine in regulating SL gene expression. PACAP is a member of the secretin/glucagon/vasoactive intestinal polypeptide (VIP) family [30]. This peptide was first isolated in ovine hypothalamus based on its ability to stimulate AC activity in rat pituitary cells [31]. The mature peptide of PACAP reported in other vertebrate species, including fish, amphibians, and birds, exhibits more than 90% sequence homology when compared to the mammalian counterpart [32]. The role of PACAP as a hypophysiotropic factor is supported by the findings that: 1) PACAP nerve fibers are present in the median eminence and 2)

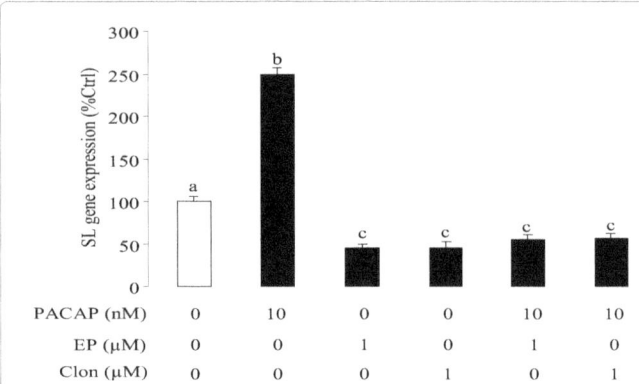

Figure 5: Effects of epinephrine and clonidine on PACAP-stimulated SL mRNA expression. NIL cells were incubated with PACAP (10 nM) in presence or absence of epinephrine (EP, 1 μM) or clonidine (Clon, 1 μM) for 48 h. SL mRNA data are expressed as mean ± SEM and groups denoted by different letters represent a significant difference at $P < 0.05$ (ANOVA followed by Duncan's test).

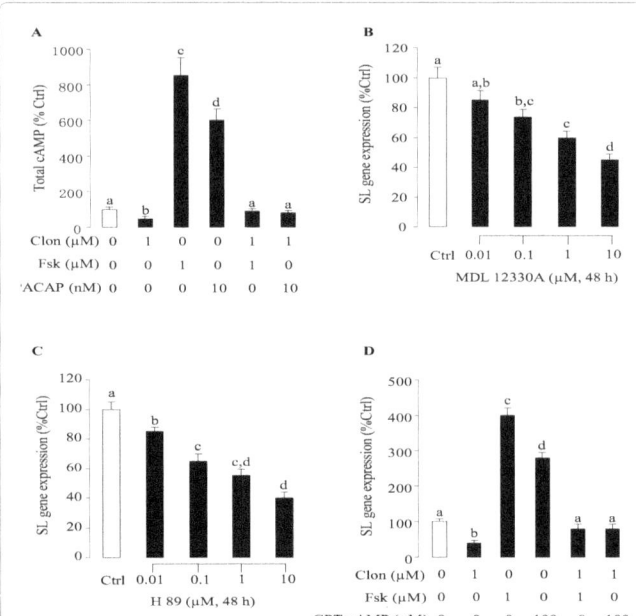

Figure 6: Functional role of cAMP-dependent mechanisms in epinephrine-inhibited SL gene expression. (A) Tilapia NIL cells were incubated for 30 min with α2 agonist clonidine (Clon, 1 μM) in the presence or absence of the AC activator forskolin (FSK, 1 M) or PACAP (10 nM). cAMP values are expressed as a percentage of control without drug treatment. In parallel experiments, NIL cells were exposed to increasing doses of the AC inhibitor MDL12330A (0.01-10 μM, B) or protein kinase A inhibitor H89 (0.01-10 μM, C) for 48 h. (D) Tilapia NIL cells were incubated for 48 h with α2 agonist clonidine (Clon, 1 μM) in the presence or absence of the AC activator forskolin (FSK, 1 M) or cAMP analog CPT-cAMP (100 μM). SL mRNA data are expressed as mean ± SEM and groups denoted by different letters represent a significant difference at $P < 0.05$ (ANOVA followed by Duncan's test).

PACAP can elevate basal secretion of GH, gonadotopin, prolactin, SL and adrenocorticotropic hormone [33]. In the present study, PACAP consistently stimulated SL mRNA expression in tilapia NIL cells, and these stimulatory actions could be blocked by epinephrine or the α2-agonist clonidine. Therefore, it would be logical to postulate that epinephrine may act as a negative regulator for PACAP induction of SL gene expression by acting through α2-adrenoceptors in the tilapia pituitary.

In general, α2-adrenoceptors are functionally coupled to G_i/G_o G-proteins [34], which are negatively coupled with AC. However, the post-receptor signaling mechanisms for epinephrine-induced inhibition of SL gene expression are largely unknown. In tilapia NIL cells, α2-agonist clonidine treatment could inhibit total cAMP production and the ability of forskolin to increase cAMP production was also inhibited by clonidine. In our previous studies, PACAP-induced stimulation of SL mRNA expression can be attributed to the coupling of the AC/cAMP/PKA system [26]. These findings have prompted us to speculate that epinephrine may interfere with these signaling pathways to inhibit the stimulatory actions of PACAP on SL gene expression. This hypothesis was supported by the results of direct measurement of cAMP production in tilapia NIL cells. In the present study, PACAP consistently elevated cAMP levels in tilapia NIL cells, and these stimulatory actions could be blocked by simultaneous treatment with the α2-agonist clonidine. In parallel experiments, clonidine inhibition on SL mRNA expression could be mimicked by blocking cAMP-dependent pathway with the AC inhibitor MDL12330A and the PKA inhibitor H89. Furthermore, the α2-agonist clonidine was effective in abolishing the SL responses to CPT-cAMP and forskolin, suggesting that epinephrine may interfere with the AC/cAMP pathways to inhibit SL gene expression. These results, as a whole, suggest that α2-adrenergic stimulation can downregulate SL gene transcription by inhibiting the AC/cAMP/PKA pathway in tilapia NIL cells.

Conclusion

In summary, we have demonstrated for the first time that epinephrine can suppress SL gene expression by acting directly at the pituitary cell level. These inhibitory actions are mediate through α2-adrenoceptors negatively coupled to the cAMP-dependent pathway. This adrenergic inhibition not only affects basal SL gene transcripts but also attenuates the SL response to PACAP. Since PACAP is an important physiological SL-releasing factor in fish, the present findings may suggest that the α2 inhibitory influence at the pituitary level is an integral component of the neuroendocrine control of SL gene expression.

Acknowledgement

The project was supported by grants from the National Natural Science Foundation of China (31302165). We are grateful to Dr. Yajun Wang (Sichuan University) for providing technical assistance.

References

1. Najafi A, Sequeira V, Kuster DW, van der Velden J, et al. (2016) β-adrenergic receptor signalling and its functional consequences in the diseased heart. Eur J Clin Invest.

2. Cotecchia S, Del Vescovo CD, Colella M, Caso S, Diviani D (2015) The alpha1-adrenergic receptors in cardiac hypertrophy: signaling mechanisms and functional implications. Cell Signal 27: 1984-1993.

3. Devesa J, Arce V, Lois N, Tresguerres JA, Lima L (1990) Alpha 2-adrenergic agonism enhances the growth hormone (GH) response to GH-releasing hormone through an inhibition of hypothalamic somatostatin release in normal men. J Clin Endocrinol Metab 71: 1581-1588.

4. Gaynor PJ, Simmons CR, Lookingland KJ, Tucker HA (1996) 5-hydroxytryptaminergic receptor-mediated regulation of growth hormone secretion in Holstein steers occurs via alpha 2-adrenergic-dependent and -independent mechanisms. Proc Soc Exp Biol Med 212: 355-361.

5. Soyoola EO, Burgess MF, Bird RC, Kemppainen RJ, Williams JC, et al. (1994) Neurotransmitter receptor agonists regulate growth hormone gene expression in cultured ovine pituitary cells. Proc Soc Exp Biol Med 207: 26-33.

6. McWilliam JR, Meldrum BS (1983) Noradrenergic regulation of growth hormone secretion in the baboon. Endocrinology 112: 254-259.

7. Gabriel SM, Milbury CM, Alexander SM, Nathanson JA, Martin JB (1989) Iso stimulation of GH and cAMP: comparison of beta-adrenergic- to GRF-stimulated GH release and cAMP accumulation in monolayer cultures of anterior pituitary cells in vitro. Neuroendocrinology 50: 170-176.

8. Chang JP, Marchant TA, Cook AF, Nahorniak CS, Peter RE (1985) Influences of catecholamines on growth hormone release in female goldfish, Carassius auratus. Neuroendocrinology 40: 463-470.

9. Lee EK, Chan VC, Chang JP, Yunker WK, Wong AO (2000) Norepinephrine regulation of growth hormone release from goldfish pituitary cells. I. Involvement of alpha2 adrenoreceptor and interactions with dopamine and salmon gonadotropin-releasing hormone. J Neuroendocrinol 12: 311-322.

10. Wang X, Chu MM, Wong AO (2007) Signaling mechanisms for alpha2-adrenergic inhibition of PACAP-induced growth hormone secretion and gene expression grass carp pituitary cells. Am J Physiol Endocrinol Metab 292: E1750-1762.

11. Kawauchi H, Sower SA (2006) The dawn and evolution of hormones in the adenohypophysis. Gen Comp Endocrinol 148: 3-14.

12. Fukamachi S, Meyer A (2007) Evolution of receptors for growth hormone and somatolactin in fish and land vertebrates: lessons from the lungfish and sturgeon orthologues. J Mol Evol 65: 359-372.

13. Fukamachi S, Sugimoto M, Mitani H, Shima A (2004) Somatolactin selectively regulates proliferation and morphogenesis of neural-crest derived pigment cells in medaka. Proc Natl Acad Sci USA 101: 10661-10666.

14. Fukamachi S, Yada T Mitani H (2005) Medaka receptors for somatolactin and growth hormone: phylogenetic paradox among fish growth hormone receptors. Genetics 171: 1875-1883.

15. Rand-Weaver M, Swanson P, Kawauchi H, Dickhoff WW (1992) Somatolactin, a novel pituitary protein: purification and plasma levels during reproductive maturation of coho salmon. J Endocrinol 133: 393-403.

16. Rand-Weaver M, Pottinger TG, Sumpter JP (1993) Plasma somatolactin concentrations in salmonid fish are elevated by stress. J Endocrinol 138: 509-515.

17. Lu M, Swanson P, Renfro JL (1995) Effect of somatolactin and related hormones on phosphate transport by flounder renal tubule primary cultures. Am J Physiol 268: R577-582.

18. Kakizawa S, Kaneko T, Hirano T (1996) Elevation of plasma somatolactin concentrations during acidosis in rainbow trout (Oncorhynchus mykiss). J Exp Biol 199: 1043-1051.

19. Jiang Q, Wong AO (2014) Somatostatin-28 inhibitory action on somatolactin-Iα and -Iβ gene expression in goldfish. Am J Physiol Regul Integr Comp Physiol 307: R755-768.

20. Kakizawa S, Kaneko T, Hirano T (1997) Effects of hypothalamic factors on somatolactin secretion from the organ-cultured pituitary of rainbow trout. Gen Comp Endocrinol 105: 71-78.

21. Vianen GJ, Obels PP, van den Thillart GE, Zaagsma J (2002) Beta-adrenoceptors mediate inhibition of lipolysis in adipocytes of tilapia (Oreochromis mossambicus). Am J Physiol Endocrinol Metab 282: E318-325.

22. Kumai Y, Ward MA, Perry SF (2012) Iβ-Adrenergic regulation of Na+ uptake by larval zebrafish Danio rerio in acidic and ion-poor environments. Am J Physiol Regul Integr Comp Physiol 303: R1031-1041.

23. Jiang Q, Ko WK, Wong AO (2011) Insulin-like growth factor as a novel stimulator for somatolactin secretion and synthesis in carp pituitary cells via activation of MAPK cascades. Am J Physiol Endocrinol Metab 301: E1208-1219.

24. Azuma M, Suzuki T, Mochida H, Tanaka S, Matsuda K (2013) Pituitary adenylate cyclase-activating polypeptide (PACAP) stimulates release of somatolactin (SL)-alpha and SL-beta from cultured goldfish pituitary cells via the PAC(1) receptor-signaling pathway, and affects the expression of SL-alpha and SL-beta mRNAs. Peptides 43: 40-47.

25. Jiang Q, Ko WK, Lerner EA, Chan KM, Wong AO (2008) Grass carp somatolactin: I. Evidence for PACAP induction of somatolactin-alpha and -beta gene expression via activation of pituitary PAC-I receptors. Am J Physiol Endocrinol Metab 295: E463-476.

26. Jiang Q, He M, Wang X, Wong AO (2008) Grass carp somatolactin: II. Pharmacological study on postreceptor signaling mechanisms for PACAP-induced somatolactin-alpha and -beta gene expression. Am J Physiol Endocrinol Metab 295: E477-490.

27. Matsuda K, Nejigaki Y, Satoh M, Shimaura C, Tanaka M, et al. (2008) Effect of pituitary adenylate cyclase-activating polypeptide (PACAP) on prolactin and somatolactin release from the goldfish pituitary in vitro. Regul Pept 145: 72-79.

28. Azuma M, Tanaka M, Nejigaki Y, Uchiyama M, Takahashi A, et al. (2009) Pituitary adenylate cyclase-activating polypeptide induces somatolactin release from cultured goldfish pituitary cells. Peptides 30: 1260-1266.

29. Gerstberger R, Muller AR, Simon-Oppermann C (1992) Functional hypothalamic angiotensin II and catecholamine receptor systems inside and outside the blood-brain barrier. Prog Brain Res 91: 423-433.

30. Rawlings SR, Hezareh M (1996) Pituitary adenylate cyclase-activating polypeptide (PACAP) and PACAP/vasoactive intestinal polypeptide receptors: actions on the anterior pituitary gland. Endocr Rev 17: 4-29.

31. Miyata A, Arimura A, Dahl RR, Minamino N, Uehara A, et al. (1989) Isolation of a novel 38 residue-hypothalamic polypeptide which stimulates adenylate cyclase in pituitary cells. Biochem Biophys Res Commun 164: 567-574.

32. Sherwood NM, Krueckl SL, McRory JE (2000) The origin and function of the pituitary adenylate cyclase-activating polypeptide (PACAP)/glucagon superfamily. Endocr Rev 21: 619-670.

33. Vaudry D, Falluel-Morel A, Bourgault S, Basille M, Burel D, et al. (2009) Pituitary adenylate cyclase-activating polypeptide and its receptors: 20 years after the discovery. Pharmacol Rev 61: 283-357.

34. Kuroda R, Shintani-Ishida K, Unuma K, Yoshida K (2015) Immobilization Stress With alpha2-Adrenergic Stimulation Induces Regional and Transient Reduction of Cardiac Contraction Through Gi Coupling in Rats. Int Heart J 56: 537-543.

31

Activity of *Panax ginseng* C.A. Meyer on Energy Production in Mammals

Marilou Pannacci[1], Valeria Lucini[1], Silvana Dugnani[1], Rocco Ciracì[1], Andrea Zangara[2] and Francesco Scaglione*[1]

[1]*Department of Medical Biotechnology and Translational Medicine, University of Milan, Italy*
[2]*Centre for Human Psychopharmacology, Swinburne University of Technology, Hawthorn, Australia*

Abstract

Panax ginseng is traditionally used for enhancement of physical capacities, especially in condition of severe fatigue. To evaluate the ability of ginseng in enhancing performance, we focused on the gene expression of AMPK, PGC-1α and SIRT1 genes, involved in energy balance. Gene expression was evaluated in C_2C_{12} myotubes, using *P. ginseng* C.A. Meyer standardized extract G115, at various concentrations (10-50-100-200 mg/L) for 24, 48, 72 h of incubation. G115 increased significantly expression of AMPK and PGC-1α in dose and time-dependent manner: at the concentration of 10 mg/L there is an increase after 72 h of incubation while at 50 mg/L after 48 h and maintained for 72 h. G115 increased expression of SIRT1 at 10 mg/L after 24 h, while at 50 mg/L after 24 and 48 h. The treatment enhanced cellular ATP levels and O_2 consumption only at 50 mg/L.

We investigated AMPK, PGC-1α and SIRT1 expression in gastrocnemius muscle during acute and prolonged exercise in mice treated with G115. G115 showed no effect on acute exercise compared to untreated mice, but after prolonged exercise there were significant increases of AMPK and PGC-1α. Expression of SIRT1 was also significant in treated animals' undergone prolonged exercise.

Our data indicate that treatment with G115 increases AMPK and SIRT1 expression that may be related to the induction of PGC-1α expression which improves the energy balance, as demonstrated by increased production of ATP and oxygen consumption. In addition, G115 is able to counteract the inhibition of gene expression of AMPK and PGC-1α due to the prolonged exercise.

Keywords: *Panax ginseng;* Energy; Gene expression; G115

Introduction

Panax ginseng (P. ginseng C.A. Meyer, Araliaceae) has been used in oriental medicine for over 2000 years having a long history as a general tonic promoting health and it is believed to be a panacea and to promote longevity [1]. The bioactive compounds of *P. ginseng* consist mainly of ginsenosides, polysaccharides, phenolics and polyacetylenes [2]. It is generally believed that ginsenosides and their metabolites are the major active principles of *P. ginseng*. These are saponins derived from the triterpenedammarane structure and are of two different types of derivatives of two major aglycones: protopanaxatriol and protopanaxadiol.

All ginsenosides have been reported to exhibit various biological activities such as anti-cancer, anti-diabetic, anti-obesity, neuroprotective, radioprotective, antiamnestic and antiageing effects [2]. Extensive scientific research has documented and reviewed the useful effects of *P. ginseng* C.A. Meyer. However, as the ginsenosides content of ginseng extracts can vary depending on a number of factors including the species, the age and part of the plant used, and the time of year of harvest, there is a high variability in composition of products in the market; this variability has affected the results of the studies, often confounding a clear interpretation of data generated with different extracts. In addition, the use of non-standardized products leads to a poor reproducibility of results, and lack of batch-to-batch uniformity. To address these issues, the compound used in our study was the G115 extract (Ginsana Products, Lugano, Switzerland), standardized to an invariable 4% ginsenosides content. This extract is produced in Switzerland under the control of Swissmedic, the Swiss agency for the authorisation and market supervision of all therapeutic products, and constantly controlled for appropriate standardization and microbiological quality, as well as for the possible presence of impurities. After the optimal standardization of G115 was achieved, in 1984 Dr. Soldati and Prof. Tanaka documented a relationship between the age of the plant and the content of ginsenosides [3,4]. Since then, only roots harvested after 5 years of growth are used for the extract. In the last 30 years, extensive analytical, preclinical and clinical research has been carried out to study the quality, efficacy and safety of G115, which has consequently attracted widespread research interest, and made it possible to generate reproducible results. Several clinical studies have been conducted with this extract, particularly in the area of performance enhancement [5-9]. In our previous study, we developed a murine model of stressful exercise in which mice were subjected to chronic swimming exercise, in order to examine the effects of ginseng extract on immune function, focusing in particular on Toll like receptor gene expression after G115 extract administration [10]. It was therefore deemed relevant to further investigate G115 activity and mechanism of action in respect of energy production. Ginseng is considered as an adaptogen, which is a substance assisting normalization of body system functions altered by stress. Studies with animals show that ginseng, or its active components, may prolong survival to physical or chemical stress [4]. Then, since exercise is considered a form of stress, people subject to exercise frequently make use of adaptogens. The ability of ginseng to improve an individual's strength, endurance and speed of recovery has been investigated in many studies [11-13], however,

*Corresponding author:** Francesco Scaglione, Professor, Department of Medical Biotechnology and Translational Medicine, University of Milan, Via Vanvitelli 32, 20129- Milan, Italy, E-mail: francesco.scaglione@unimi.it

with some criticisms [14]. Various methodological problems such as inadequate sample size and lack of double-blind control and placebo paradigms may have contributed to conflicting results. Enhancement of physical work capacity was selectively observed in studies with larger subjects' number, where ginseng was taken with sufficient dosage (200–400 g/day of standardized *P. ginseng* root extracts containing 4% ginsenosides) and for not less than 8 weeks; age and physical condition of the subjects seems also relevant for the identification of ergogenic effects [15]. Ginseng has been also traditionally used to enhance well-being, energy and recovery of physical strength and the potential for recovery is corroborated by studies with animal models of severe fatigue [16,17]. Anti-mental fatigue effects of ginseng extract G115 have been reported in clinical trials on healthy volunteers [18]. Although to date, there are not many information about the anti-fatigue effects of ginseng polysaccharide, they seem to play a relevant role for these therapeutic properties possibly related to prevention of oxidative stress [19]. In animal studies the G115 extract exerted a dose dependent inhibition of the formation of free radicals in rats subjected to physical stress exercise on a treadmill [20]. A clinical study [21] suggests that the beneficial effect of 4 weeks ginseng administration observed in patients with idiopathic chronic fatigue (ICF) may be partly attributed to its antioxidant properties, and oxidative stress is considered as a main contributor to the pathology of chronic fatigue [22]. Moreover, animal studies with the extract G115 show enhancement of glucose transportation in the cells [23], and its pre-treatment increased the production of the Toll like receptor 4 in mice during physical stress [10].

While each individual study mentioned here cannot on its own be taken as a proof of efficacy, these investigations, taken together provide, albeit weak, a support for a beneficial effect of ginseng in these indications.

To evaluate the possible mechanism of action of ginseng in enhancing performance, we focused our attention on the expression of AMPK, PGC-1α and SIRT1 genes, which are involved in the energy balance, acting as a coordinated system that controls energy intake.

AMPK activation plays a relevant role in the transcriptional adaptation to physiological condition of energy expenditure and in the maintenance of intracellular energetic equilibrium under ATP-depleting energetic stresses like exercise, [24]. AMPK regulates metabolic enzymes, increasing the expression of those genes related to mitochondrial respiration, glucose transport and glycolysis [25,26].

Furthermore, AMPK is a modulator of the transcription factor coactivator peroxisome proliferator-activated receptor γ coactivator-1α (PGC-1α) [27]. PGC-1α is a critical regulator of mitochondrial biogenesis, cellular respiration and energy substrate utilization in skeletal muscle, under acute contraction [28,29] or exercise training [30], by activation of transcription factors modulating a transcriptional pathway that regulates energy homeostasis [31].

PGC-1α activity is also regulated by Silent Information Regulator T1 (SIRT1) that directly interacts and deacetylates PGC-1α. SIRT1-mediated regulation of PGC-1α activity has a major role in the metabolic adaptations to energy metabolism in different tissues [32]. A number of articles were published to demonstrate that the pharmacological or physiological activities of ginsenosides are associated with AMPK [33-39].

In this study, we tested the hypothesis that *P. ginseng* extract G115 influences the production of energy through the activation of AMPK. Since SIRT1 can also directly interact with PGC-1α [40,41], additionally we evaluated the effect of *P. ginseng* on the expression of SIRT1.

Materials and Methods

P. ginseng C.A. Meyer (G115) powder was provided by Ginsana SA. (Bioggio-Switzerland). This root extract has been standardized at 4% of ginsenosides and characterized by HPLC (Figure 1).

Ginseng preparation

Since ginsenosides are activated by deglycosylation by colonic bacteria in large intestine, before the transit to the circulation [42], the *in vitro* experiments were performed after degradation and bioconversion of G115 at acidic (gastric) conditions and in the presence of intestinal microbiota. 100 mg of G115 was incubated with 10 mL of an artificial gastric fluid (37 mM NaCl, 0.03 M HCl, 3.2 mg/mL pepsin, pH 1.6) at 37°C for 2 h. After incubation, the acidity was neutralized by adding 0.5 mL of 2.2 M NaOH. Then, 10 mL of an artificial intestinal fluid (30 mM K_2HPO_4, 160 mM NaH_2PO_4, 20 mg/mL pancreatin) were added, and the pH was adjusted to 7.4 using 0.6 M NaOH and 0.2 M HCl. The mixture was shaken in a 37°C incubator for an additional 2 h, centrifuged at 3000 × g for 30 min at 4°C and filtered. Five millilitres of the filtrate were applied to a Sep-Pak® Vac C18 column (Waters) to remove the polar compounds, such as proteins and ions. The loading sample was washed with 30 mL of water and then eluted with 15 mL of methanol. The methanol was removed, and the residue was dissolved in water and then freeze-dried.

Cell culture

C_2C_{12} mouse skeletal muscle cell line was maintained in DMEM (Euroclone, Pero, Italy) with 10% calf serum. Differentiation was induced at 80-90% confluence by switching the cell media with DMEM with 2% horse serum (Euroclone, Pero, Italy). Experimental treatments were started after 96 h by which time the myoblasts were differentiated to form myotubes.

Digested G115 was added to the medium at concentration of 10-50-100-200 mg/L for 24, 48 and 72 h. After this time, to minimize the possible effects of nutrient deprivation on the cells, they will be washed once in drug-free, fresh culture medium and equilibrated in it for an additional 3 h at 37°C. Cells were then collected and washed twice in PBS.

For the O_2-consumption, the cells were suspended (10^7 cells per mL) in a buffer containing 118 mM NaCl, 4.8 mM KCl, 1.2 mM KH_2PO_4, 1.2 mM $MgSO_4$, 1 mM $CaCl_2$, 10 mM glucose, and 25 mM Hepes (pH 7.2). For the remaining experimental procedures, the cells were sedimented by centrifugation and kept at 80°C until use.

Animals

Male 6-weeks-old BALB/c pathogen-free mice (Charles River Laboratories, Calco, Italy) were housed in the Pathogen-Free Facility. Animals were treated in accordance with European Community Guidelines and the protocol was approved by the Institutional Animal Care and Use Committee of the Ministry of Healthy- Italy; mice were sacrificed under anaesthesia with urethane (1.6 g/kg).

Mice were subjected to exercise, using a swimming model in which were kept swimming daily for 60 min in a plastic tank filled with water at a temperature of 25(± 2)°C.

Animals (10 animals per group) were divided in: control group, control ginseng group, swimming group and swimming ginseng group. Ginseng groups were treated daily with 25 mg kg⁻¹ day⁻¹ of extract G115 by oral gavage. Swimming exercise was performed every day for two

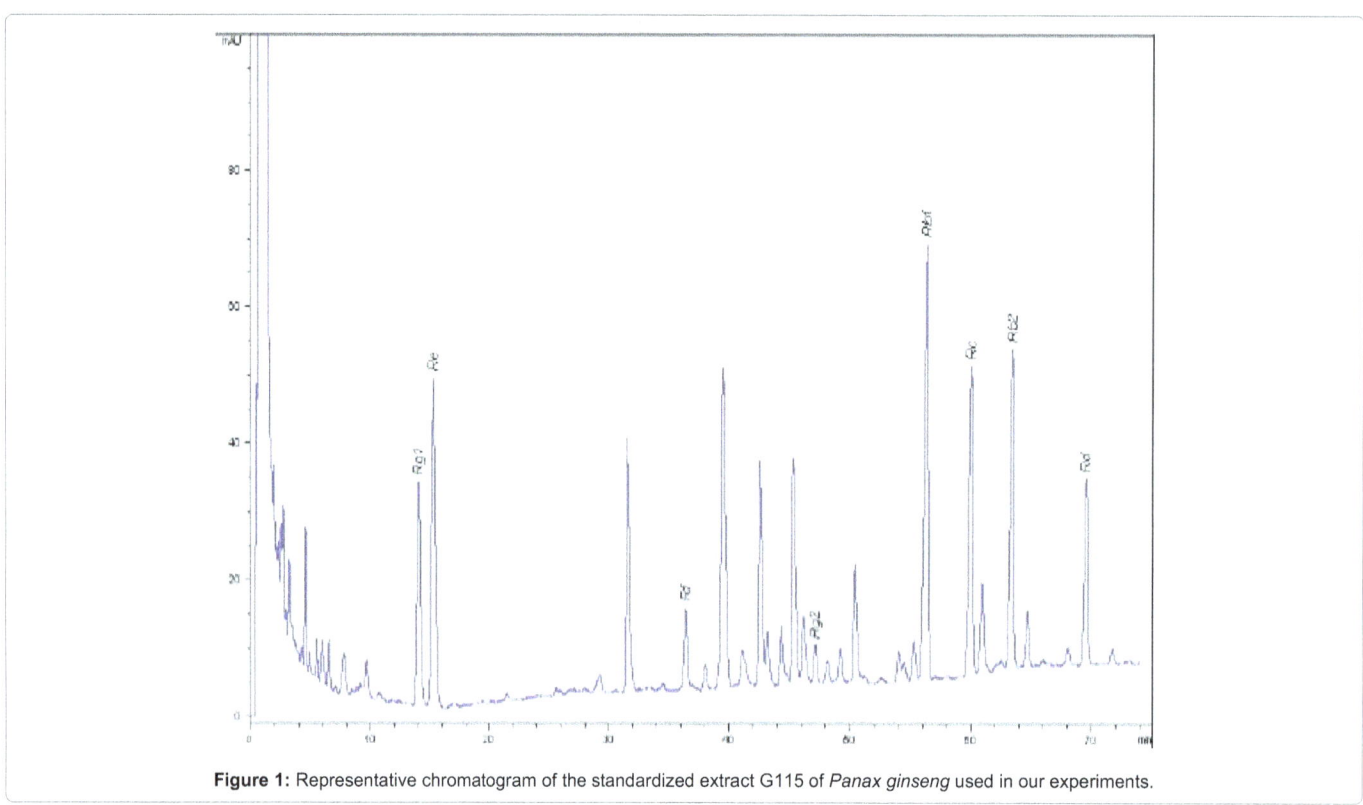

Figure 1: Representative chromatogram of the standardized extract G115 of *Panax ginseng* used in our experiments.

weeks. After the first session (acute) or after last session of prolonged exercise, animals were anesthetized and sacrificed; gastrocnemius muscles were isolated and snap frozen in liquid nitrogen for Real time PCR analysis.

Gene expression analysis

RNA was extracted from cells using the Trizol reagent (Invitrogen-Life Technologies, Carlsbad, CA) and treated with Dnase (Dna-freeTM, Ambion Inc.- Life Technologies, Carlsbad, CA) to avoid false-positive results due to amplification of contaminating genomic DNA. Concentrations of RNA were determined by the absorbance value of the sample at 260 nm. First-strand cDNA was synthesized from 1 µg total RNA, using an High-capacity cDNA Archive Kit (Applied Biosystems, Forster City, CA) and then analyzed by Real Time PCR, using Stepone Plus Real Time Systems (Applied Biosystems, Forster City, CA). TaqMan PCR was performed using an TaqMan' Universal PCR Master Mix (Applied Biosystems, Forster City, CA); TaqMan probe/primers specific for 18S (code number: Hs99999901_s1), SIRT1 (code number: Mm00490758_m1), PGC-1α (code number: Mm01208835_m1) and AMPK (code number: Mm01296700_m1) were purchased from Taqman' Assays-on-Demand™ Gene Expression Products (Applied Biosystems, Forster City, CA).

All data were normalized to 18S expression and quantification was performed using the $\Delta\Delta_{CT}$ method. The amount of target, normalized to an endogenous reference and relative to a calibrator, is given by $2^{-\Delta\Delta CT}$.

Measurement of O_2 consumption.

1-mL cell or tissue sample was incubated at 37°C in a gas-tight vessel that is equipped with a Clark-type O_2 electrode (Rank Brothers, Bottisham, U.K.) connected to a chart recorder. Cellular O_2 consumption was measured as described [80]. Protein content in both cell and tissue samples was determined by the bicinchoninic acid protein assay.

ATP measurements in cultured cells

The ATP content in myotubes was determined in 2.5% perchloric acid extracts neutralized with K_2CO_3, by reversed-phase HPLC. Lactate will be measured in the culture medium after deproteinization by using Ultra-4 centrifugal filter devices (cut-off, 10,000; Amicon) as well as in cells after extraction in cold perchloric acid.

ATP measurements in gastrocnemius muscle tissue

Frozen muscles were treated with perchloric acid and neutralized with K_2CO_3 on ice, and then levels were assayed by HPLC. ATP was quantified based on peak area compared with a standard curve and normalized to frozen tissue weight.

Statistical analysis

Data were analyzed using GraphPad Prism statistical software (GraphPad Software Inc., San Diego, CA). Data were analyzed using the univariate analysis of variance (One-Way ANOVA), followed by Bonferroni's t-test for multiple comparisons. Statistical significance was accepted when P<0.05. All data are reported as mean ± standard error of the mean.

Results

Gene expression of AMPK and PGC-1α and SIRT-1, in the C_2C_{12} myotubes

To determine whether G115 affects gene expression in muscle cells, C_2C_{12} myotubes were incubated in absence (control) or in presence of G115 at 10-50-100-200 mg/L for 24, 48 and 72 h.

G115, at concentration of 10 mg/L, significantly increased AMPK gene expression in myotubes after 72 h of incubation (p<0.001 vs controls). At concentration of 50 mg/L G115 significantly enhanced gene expression of AMPK at 24, 48 and 72 h (p<0.05, p<0.001 and p<0.001 vs controls, respectively) (Figure 2A). At concentration of 100 and 200 mg/L there was no observed effect: while at these concentrations not clear toxicity showed, the cells did not grow and showed morphological signs of apoptosis, suggesting a possible limiting toxicity at very high concentrations. We next examined the effect of G115 on gene expression of PGC-1α in myotubes. Unlike AMPK, G115 significantly increases the gene expression of PGC-1α only at a concentration of 50 mg/L after 48 and 72 h of incubation (Figure 2B). Also in this case it was not observed any effect at concentrations of 100 and 200 mg/L.

Since the expression and activity of muscle PGC-1α is increased by the activation of SIRT1, we examined whether G115 may increase the gene expression of SIRT1. G115 significantly increased the expression of SIRT1 earlier. An increase was observed, at the concentration of 10 mg/L, after 24 h only, while at 50 mg/L concentration there was an increase after 24 and 48 h, returning to basal value after 72 h of incubation (Figure 2C).

Measurements of ATP production and O$_2$ consumption

To examine whether the AMPK and PGC-1α gene expression was associated with an increased respiration and ATP synthesis, we measured the O$_2$ consumption and the ATP production.

The treatment with G115 increased significantly cellular ATP levels (Figure 3) and O$_2$ consumption (Figure 4) at the concentration of 50 mg/L only.

In vivo studies

Previous studies have indicated that *P. ginseng* may increase physical potency, especially in patients having medical conditions producing severe fatigue. Therefore, we have investigated whether AMPK, PGC-1α and SIRT1 are expressed in gastrocnemius muscle during acute and chronic physical stress in mice treated or untreated with G115. The gene expression of AMPK and PGC-1α shows the same behaviour. After acute stress exercise there is an increase of gene expression (p<0.001) while after chronic stress exercise there is a decrease of gene expression of both AMPK and PGC-1α (p<0.005 and p<0.01, respectively). The treatment with G115 shows no effect on acute stress exercise compared to stressed untreated mice, but after chronic stress exercise there is a significant increase of both AMPK and PGC-1α compared to both controls and chronic stressed mice (p<0.001 and p<0.01, respectively) (Figures 5A and B). The expression of SIRT1 shows a different pattern. A significant increase was observed in the gastrocnemius of treated animals' undergone chronic exercises (Figure 5C). The O$_2$ consumption and the ATP production measured in the gastrocnemius of mice have shown the same pattern observed for AMPK and PGC-1α (Figure 6).

Discussion

Many investigators have found that ginseng may increase the duration of exercise to exhaustion during forced exercise trials [14,21]. In absence of experimental data, this was believed to be due to a general adaptogenic activity of ginseng supplementation [43]. *P. ginseng* has been investigated extensively for its stress-attenuating activity [44] and it is believed that this adaptation to stress may increase exercise time to exhaustion [45,46].

In untrained adults, it has been reported that consumption of 1,350 mg ginseng per day for 30 days improved their endurance time by more than 7 min and lowered their maximal mean blood pressure and maximal oxygen consumption (VO$_2$max) at the 24th minute during endurance cycling exercise [47]. In another placebo controlled cross-over study [48], in which the subjects were administered with *P. ginseng*, Siberian ginseng or placebo supplements (1 g/day for 6 weeks for each supplement), it was reported that *P. ginseng* significantly increased maximal oxygen consumption, post-exercise recovery and pectoral and quadriceps strength. Furthermore, it has been shown that a single dose of 200 mg extract of *P. ginseng* standardized at 4%

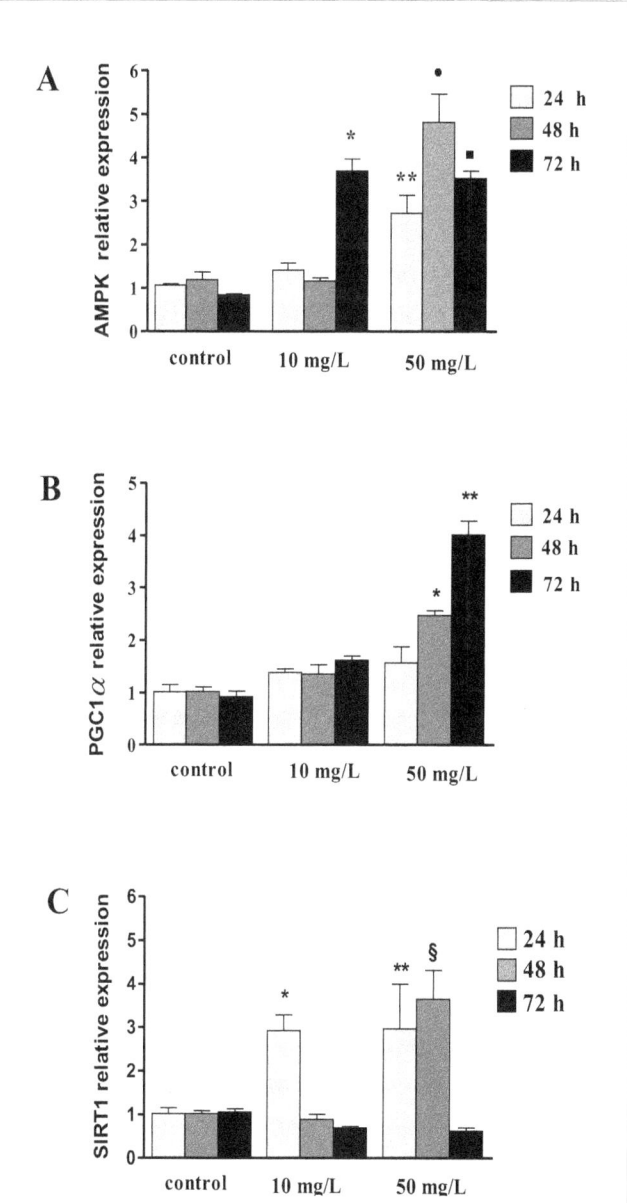

A: *P<0.001 VS. CONTROL; **P<0.05 VS. CONTROL; •P<0.001 VS. CONTROL; ▪P<0.001 VS. CONTROL;
B: * P<0.001 VS. CONTROL; **P<0.001 VS. CONTROL
C: *P<0.05 VS. CONTROL; **P<0.05 VS. CONTROL; §P< 0.001 VS. CONTROL.

Figure 2: AMPK (A), PGC1α (B), and SIRT1 (C) mRNA expression in C$_2$C$_{12}$ myotubes was determined by RealTime PCR analysis. After differentiation in myotubes, cells were incubated in presence or absence of digested G115 at 10-50-100-200 mg/L for 24, 48 and 72 h.

of ginsenosides, can modulate circulating blood glucose level, enhance cognitive performance on a mental arithmetic task and ameliorate the increase in subjective feeling of mental fatigue during sustained intense cognitive processing [49].

The results of many studies using ginseng in animal models showed improvements in exercise performance, but the use of large doses or parenteral administration (bioconversion of ginsenosides is known to occur in stomach acid and gut microbial actions before uptake) and the various methods of preparation weakens extrapolation of these data to humans [14].

In our study we used a *P. ginseng* standardized extract from ginseng roots that are harvested after 5 years of growth, containing invariably 4% ginsenosides (G115; Ginsana Products, Lugano, Switzerland). This extract is well characterised and supported by robust published data, obtained through rigorous quality steps starting from good agricultural and collection practices (GACP). In *in vitro* studies, the extract was

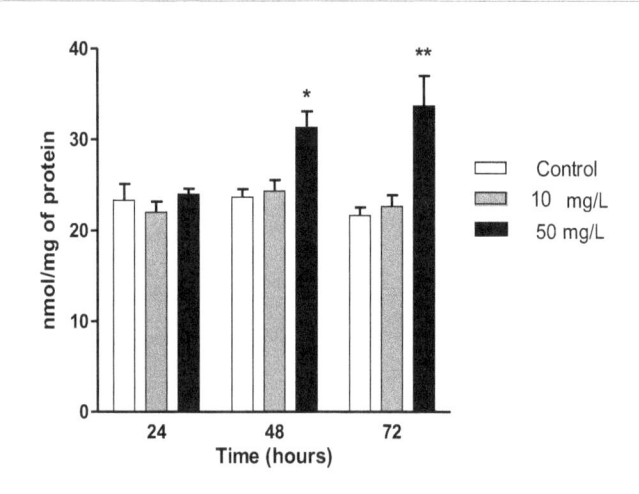

Figure 3: ATP production after treatment of digested G115 at 10-50-100-200 mg/L for 24, 48 and 72 h. *p<0.01 vs. control; **p<0.001.

Figure 4: O$_2$ consumption after treatment of digested G115 at 10-50-100-200 mg/L for 24, 48 and 72 h. *vs. control p<0.05; **vs. control p<0.01; §vs. control p<0.001.

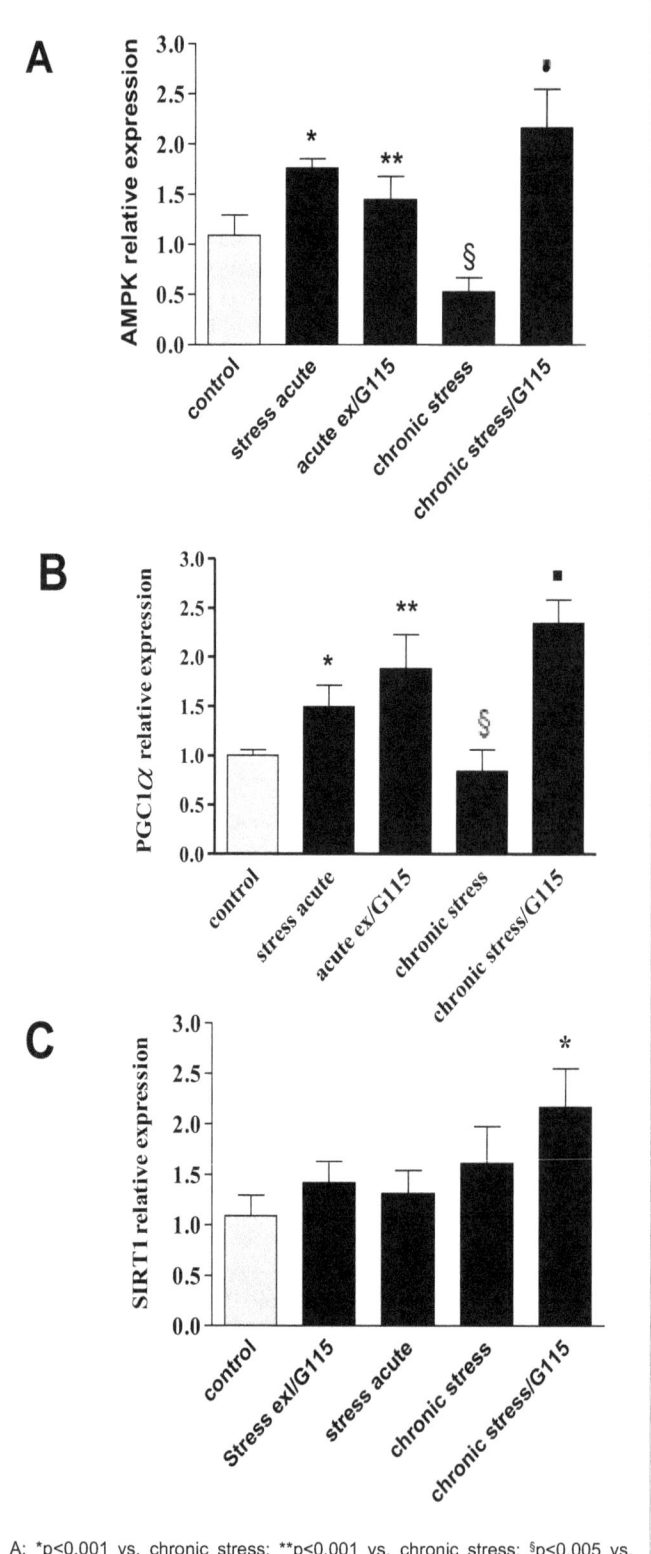

A: *p<0.001 vs. chronic stress; **p<0.001 vs. chronic stress; §p<0.005 vs. controls; ■p<0.001 vs. chronic stress/G115.
B: *p<0.001 vs. chronic stress; **p<0.05 vs. chronic stress; §p<0.01 vs. controls; ■p<0.01 vs. chronic stress/G115.
C: *p<0.01 vs. controls.

Figure 5: AMPK (A), PGC1α (B), and SIRT1 (C) mRNA expression in gastrocnemius muscle, determined by RealTime PCR analysis, after acute and chronic session of physical stress.

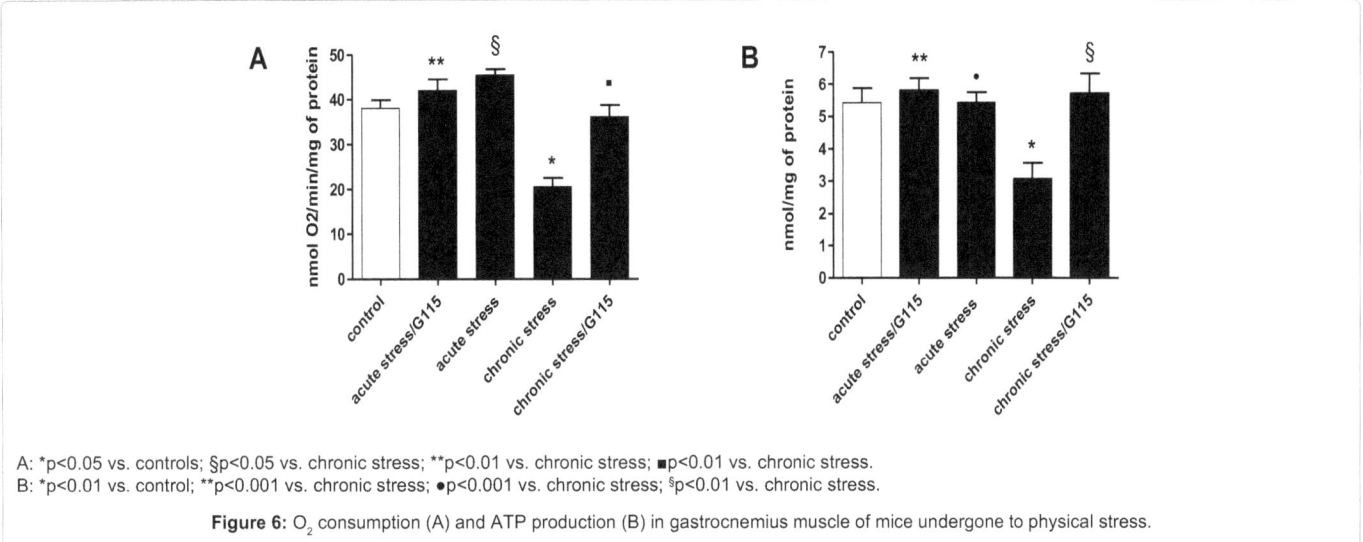

A: *p<0.05 vs. controls; §p<0.05 vs. chronic stress; **p<0.01 vs. chronic stress; ■p<0.01 vs. chronic stress.
B: *p<0.01 vs. control; **p<0.001 vs. chronic stress; ●p<0.001 vs. chronic stress; §p<0.01 vs. chronic stress.

Figure 6: O_2 consumption (A) and ATP production (B) in gastrocnemius muscle of mice undergone to physical stress.

previously digested in order to obtain active ingredients while in *in vivo* studies the extract was administered by oral route. Considering the support, albeit weak, that ginseng studies taken together provide in increasing physical performance, it appears relevant to highlight that our study identified clear indications that this specific extract has an important role in improving energy balance. Our findings provide an interpretation for previous clinical evidences of G115, potentially unlocking an important mechanism of action of ginseng extract.

The effectiveness of *P. ginseng* in increasing physical performance can be due to its effect on some key determinants of energy metabolism, rather than to a general "adaptogen" effect.

In this study, *P. ginseng* increased gene expression of AMPK in C_2C_{12} myotubes in a dose and time-dependent manner. At 10 mg/L concentration the effect appears significant after 72 h incubation while at 50 mg/L concentrations the increase appears significant after 24 h, maintained for 72 h. Higher concentrations of 100 and 200 mg/L did not show any effect, probably because of cellular toxicity (the viability of cells appeared reduced- data not shown).

The gene expression of PGC-1α shows the same behaviour of AMPK. Previous studies have demonstrated that there is a strong overlap in the genes transcriptionally regulated by AMPK and those by PGC-1α, hence suggesting that PGC-1α might be an important mediator of AMPK-induced gene expression [50,51]. Supporting this hypothesis, we may assume that components of the ginseng extract are able to induce the gene expression of AMPK that leads to increased PGC-1α expression.

In this context SIRT1 could play an important role. Several lines of evidence indicate that SIRT1-mediated regulation of PGC-1α activity may play a major role in the metabolic adaptations to energy metabolism in different tissues [52-55].

Our results show, for the first time, that the expression of SIRT1 is early induced by G115 in C_2C_{12} myotubes: either at 10 and 50 mg/L concentration of G115, the gene expression of SIRT1 significantly increased after 24 h of incubation and fell at basal value after 48 and 72 h respectively, indicating that SIRT1 could be an early target of *P. ginseng* action. It is possible to speculate that the increased expression of SIRT1 and AMPK induced by G115 increases expression of PGC-1α [32].

In any case, the induction by G115 on PGC-1α by AMPK and or SIRT1 may positively control energy production and expenditure.

The action of G115 on the gene expression of SIRT1, AMPK and PGC-1α appears more interesting in *in vivo* study. In exercise and sports science, ginseng is believed to be a physical performance enhancer; moreover, ginseng has been touted as possessing a stimulant effect and thus improves alertness and decreases fatigue and stress [15,43]. Nevertheless, it has been reported that its benefits were best seen in individuals in poor physical condition [14].

Based on these observations, we evaluated the effect of G115 on gene expression of AMPK, SIRT1 and PGC-1α in the gastrocnemius muscle of mice subjected to intensive acute exercise or to strenuous chronic physical exercise. Acute exercise significantly increases gene expression of AMPK and PGC-1α as reported by previous studies [56,57].

Treatment with G115 showed no change compared to untreated animals subjected to acute exercise. This result, apparently in contrast with the *in vitro* data, is agreement with a number of previous papers demonstrating that the requirements that ginseng root extracts must have to increase muscular strength and aerobic work capacity are sufficient daily dose (≥ 2000 mg *P. ginseng* root powder or an equivalent amount of 200 mg of root extract with standardized ginsenoside content), sufficient duration for effects to develop (≥ 8 weeks), and sufficient intensity of physical activity (especially in untrained or older subjects) [58-59]. Interesting results were observed in mice subjected to chronic strenuous exercise in which the expression of AMPK and PGC-1α was significantly depressed compared to the controls while the chronic treatment with G115 induced a significant increase of expression compared to animals untreated as well as to the controls. This result appears in contrast with previous studies demonstrating that PGC-1α as well as AMPK mRNA content was shown to be up-regulated in rodent skeletal muscle after a single swimming exercise bout [59] as well as in humans even in prolonged exercise [60-63].

The gene expression of SIRT1 shows a different pattern with a little non-significant increase after acute exercise both in treated and untreated animals. After strenuous chronic exercise there is an increase (not statistically significant) rather than a decrease, as observed for AMPK and PGC-1α in untreated animals, while in treated animals there is a significant increase compared to controls but not compared to untreated stressed animals.

There is an evident discrepancy in the different behaviour of AMPK, PGC-1α and SIRT1, that we cannot currently fully address. Clearly,

AMPK, SIRT1 and PGC-1α do not function independently or linearly; also in previous study, following chronic exercise (multiple bouts of prolonged exercise) in rats, a negative correlation between SIRT1 and PGC-1α expression was identified [64]. In contrast, other studies have shown an increase in SIRT1 expression with exercise in old [65] or adult [66] rat skeletal muscle. Interestingly, one study [60] showed that SIRT1 expression decreased with age and recovered following a single, acute bout of intense exercise, while, in direct contrast, another [67] examined the same muscle in Wistar rats and found that there were elevated amounts of SIRT1 protein with aging, which were then reduced with chronic exercise training.

However, in humans, both an acute bout of sprint exercise [68], and high intensity training for 2 weeks [69] resulted in elevated SIRT1 protein content.

These different results may be consequent to the type of exercise in terms of strength and duration as well as how much stressful is the exercise. We must also consider that in almost all studies that have investigated the expression/activity of AMPK, PGC-1α and SIRT1 in muscle after exercise, were used physiological models of acute or prolonged exercise training not particularly stressful. Our model of stressful exercise [10] has never been used in other similar studies. Therefore, other factors involved in regulation of gene expression may be involved.

Thus, it is apparent from this diverse set of results that more clear evidence is required to understand the relationship between SIRT1 expression/activity, and exercise using standardized models.

Conclusions

Our data suggest that treatment with ginseng extract G115 results in induction of PGC-1α expression that could be related to the observed increase of AMPK and SIRT1. This translates into an improvement of the energy balance as demonstrated by increased production of ATP and by the increase in oxygen consumption. In addition, G115 is able to counteract the inhibition of gene expression of AMPK and PGC-1α due to the prolonged strenuous exercise. These results further support the consistency and effectiveness of the standardized ginseng extract G115, and help to explain the effects of *P. ginseng* in improving physical performance. We believe our findings are relevant to the many health conditions where energy balance is compromised such as Chronic Fatigue Syndrome, metabolic diseases and cancer, and deserve further scientific and clinical interest.

Acknowledgements

The work was supported by funds from the Department of Medical Biotechnology and Translational Medicine.

References

1. Attele AS, Wu JA, Yuan CS (1999) Ginseng pharmacology: multiple constituents and multiple actions. Biochem Pharmacol I58: 1685-1693.

2. Liang Y, Zhao S (2008) Progress in understanding of ginsenoside biosynthesis. Plant Biol (Stuttg) 10: 415-421.

3. Soldati F, Tanaka O (1984) Panax ginseng C.A. Meyer-relation between age of plant and content of ginsenosides. Planta Med 51: 351-352.

4. Soldati F (2000) Panax ginseng; standardization and biological activity. In: Cutler SJ, Cutler HG editor. Biologically active natural products, CRC Press, New York, pp 209-232.

5. Doerling E, Kirchdorfer AM, Rueckert KH (1980) Do ginsenosides influence the performance? Results of a double - blind study. Not Med 10: 241-246.

6. Forgo I, Kayasseh L, Staub JJ (1981) Effect of standardized ginseng extract on general well-being, reaction capacity, pulmonary function and gonadal hormones. Med Welt 32: 751-756.

7. Forgo I, G. Schimert (1985) The duration of effect of the standardized ginseng extract G115® in healthy competitive athletes. Notab Med 15: 636-640.

8. Van Schepdael P (1993) The effects of ginseng G115 on physical performance of endurance athletes. Acta Ther 19: 337-347.

9. Pujol P (1996) Effects of ginseng extract (G115) alone and combined with other elements on free radical production and haemoglobin reoxygenation following a maximal stress test. Int Pre-Olympic Sci Cong: Dallas.

10. Pannacci M, Lucini V, Colleoni F, Martucci C, Grosso S, et al. (2006) Panax ginseng C.A. Mayer G115 modulates pro-inflammatory cytokine production in mice throughout the increase of macrophage toll-like receptor 4 expression during physical stress. Brain Behav Immun 20: 546-551.

11. Jung HL, Kwak HE, Kim SS, Kim YC, Lee CD, et al. (2011) Effects of Panax ginseng supplementation on muscle damage and inflammation after uphill treadmill running in humans. Am J Chin Med 39: 441-450.

12. Hwang HJ, Kwak YS, Yoon GA, Kang MH, Park JH, et al. (2007) Combined effects of swim training and ginseng supplementation on exercise performance time, ROS, lymphocyte proliferation, and DNA damage following exhaustive exercise stress. Int J Vitam Nutr Res 77: 289-296.

13. Liang MT, Podolka TD, Chuang WJ (2005) Panax notoginseng supplementation enhances physical performance during endurance exercise. J Strength Cond Res 19: 108-114.

14. Bahrke MS, Morgan WP, Stegner A (2009) Is ginseng an ergogenic aid? Int J Sport Nutr Exerc Metab 19: 298-322.

15. Bucci LR (2000) Selected herbals and human exercise performance. Am J Clin Nutr 72: 624S-636S.

16. Saito H, Yoshida Y, Takagi K (1974) Effect of Panax Ginseng root on exhaustive exercise in mice. Jpn J Pharmacol 24: 119-127.

17. Tang W, Zhang Y, Gao J, Ding X, Gao S (2008) The anti-fatigue effect of 20(R)-ginsenoside Rg3 in mice by intranasally administration. Biol Pharm Bull 31: 2024-2027.

18. Neale C, Camfield D, Reay J, Stough C, Scholey A (2013) Cognitive effects of two nutraceuticals Ginseng and Bacopa benchmarked against modafinil: a review and comparison of effect sizes. Br J Clin Pharmacol 75: 728-737.

19. Wang J, Sun C, Zheng Y, Pan H, Zhou Y, et al. (2013) The effective mechanism of the polysaccharides from *Panax ginseng* on chronic fatigue syndrome. Arch Pharm Res 37: 530-538.

20. Voces J, Alvarez AI, Vila L, Ferrando A, Cabral de Oliveira C, et al. (1999) Effects of administration of the standardized *Panax ginseng* extract G115 on hepatic antioxidant function after exhaustive exercise. Comp Biochem Physiol C Pharmacol Toxicol Endocrinol 123: 175-184.

21. Kim HG, Cho JH, Yoo SR, Lee JS, Han JM, et al. (2013) Antifatigue effects of *Panax ginseng* C.A. Meyer: a randomised, double-blind, placebo-controlled trial. PLoS ONE 8: e61271.

22. Richards RS, Roberts TK, McGregor NR, Dunstan RH, Butt HL (2000) Blood parameters indicative of oxidative stress are associated with symptom expression in chronic fatigue syndrome. Redox Rep 5: 35-41.

23. Yamasaki K, Murakami C, Ohtani K, Kasai R, Kurokawa T, et al. (1993) Effects of the standardized *Panax ginseng* extract g115 on the D-glucose transport by Ehrlich ascites tumour cells. Phytotherapy Research 7: 200-202.

24. Mihaylova MM, Shaw RJ (2011) The AMPK signalling pathway coordinates cell growth, autophagy and metabolism. Nat Cell Biol 13: 1016-1023.

25. Hardie DG (2011) AMP-activated protein kinase: an energy sensor that regulates all aspects of cell function Genes Dev 25: 1895-1908.

26. Ojuka EO, Nolte LA, Holloszy JO (2000) Increased expression of GLUT-4 and hexokinase in rat epitrochlearis muscles exposed to AICAR in vitro. J Appl Physiol 88: 1072-1075.

27. Jäger S, Handschin C, St-Pierre J, Spiegelman BM (2007) AMP-activated protein kinase (AMPK) action in skeletal muscle via direct phosphorylation of PGC-1alpha. Proc Natl Acad Sci 104: 12017-12022.

28. Lira VA, Brown DL, Lira AK, Kavazis AN, Soltow QA, et al. (2010) Nitric oxide and AMPK cooperatively regulate PGC-1α in skeletal muscle cells. J Physiol 588: 3551-3566.

29. Pilegaard H, Saltin B, Neufer PD (2003) Exercise induces transient transcriptional activation of the PGC-1alpha gene inhuman skeletal muscle. J Physiol 546: 851-858.

30. Russell AP, Hesselink MK, Lo SK, Schrauwen P (2005) Regulation of metabolic transcriptional co-activators and transcriptionfactors with acute exercise. FASEB J 19: 986-988.

31. Burgomaster KA, Howarth KR, Phillips SM, Rakobowchuk M, Macdonald MJ, et al. (2008) Similar metabolic adaptations during exercise after low volume sprint interval and traditional endurance training in humans. J Physiol 586: 151-160.

32. Cantó C, Auwerx J (2009) PGC-1alpha, SIRT1 and AMPK, an energy sensing network that controls energy expenditure. Curr Opin Lipidol 20: 98-105.

33. Nag SA, Qin JJ, Wang W, Wang MH, Wang H, et al. (2012) Ginsenosides as Anticancer Agents: In vitro and in vivo Activities, Structure-Activity Relationships, and Molecular Mechanisms of Action. Front Pharmacol 3: 25

34. Yuan HD, Kim do Y, Quan HY, Kim SJ, Jung MS, et al. (2012) Ginsenoside Rg2 induces orphan nuclear receptor SHP gene expression and inactivates GSK3β via AMP-activated protein kinase to inhibit hepatic glucose production in HepG2 cells. Chem Biol Interact 195: 35-42.

35. Kim do Y, Park YG, Quan HY, Kim SJ, Jung MS, et al. (2012) Ginsenoside Rd stimulates the differentiation and mineralization of osteoblastic MC3T3-E1 cells by activating AMP-activated protein kinase via the BMP-2 signaling pathway. Fitoterapia 83: 215-22.

36. Quan HY, Yuan HD, Jung MS, Ko SK, Park YG, et al. (2012) Ginsenoside Re lowers blood glucose and lipid levels via activation of AMP-activated protein kinase in HepG2 cells and high-fat diet fed mice. Int J Mol Med 29: 73-80.

37. Lee KT, Jung TW, Lee HJ, Kim SG, Shin YS, et al. (2011) The antidiabetic effect of ginsenoside Rb2 via activation of AMPK. Arch Pharm Res 34: 1201-1208.

38. Jung MS, Chung SH (2011) AMP-activated protein kinase: a potential target for ginsenosides? Arch Pharm Res 34: 1037-1040.

39. Kim do Y, Park KH, Jung MS, Huang B, Yuan HD, et al. (2011) Ginsenoside Rh2(S) induces differentiation and mineralization of MC3T3-E1 cells through activation of the PKD/AMPK signaling pathways. Int J Mol Med 28: 753-759.

40. Rodgers JT, Lerin C, Haas W, Gygi SP, Spiegelman BM, et al. (2005) Nutrient control of glucose homeostasis through a complex of PGC-1alpha and SIRT1. Nature 434: 113-118.

41. Houtkooper RH, Pirinen E, Auwerx J (2012) Sirtuins as regulators of metabolism and healthspan. Nat Rev Mol Cell Biol 13: 225-238.

42. Clementi E, Brown GC, Feelisch M, Moncada S (1998) Persistent inhibition of cell respiration by nitric oxide: crucial role of S-nitrosylation of mitochondrial complex I and protective action of glutathione Proc. Natl Acad Sci 95: 7631-7636.

43. Kim SH, Park KS, Chang MJ, Sung JH (2005) Effects of Panax ginseng extract on exercise-induced oxidative stress. J Sports Med Phys Fitness 45: 178-182.

44. Gaffney BT, Hugel HM, Rich PA (2001) The effects of Eleutherococcussenticosus and Panax ginseng on steroidal hormone indices of stress and lymphocyte subset numbers in endurance athletes. Life Sci 70: 431-442.

45. Kennedy DO, Scholey AB (2003) Ginseng: potential for the enhancement of cognitive performance and mood. Pharmacol Biochem Behav 75: 687-700.

46. Popov IM, Goldwag WJ (1973) A review of the properties of clinical effects of ginseng. Am J Chin Med 1: 263-270

47. Liang MTC, Podolka TD, Chuang WJ (2005) Panax notoginseng supplementation enhances physical performance during endurance exercise. J Strength Cond Res 19: 108-114.

48. McNaughton L, Egan G, Caelli G (1989) A comparison of Chinese and Russian ginseng as ergogenic aids to improve various effects of physical fitness. Int Clin Nutr Rev 90: 32-35.

49. Reay JL, Kennedy DO, Scholey AB (2006) Effects of Panax ginseng, consumed with and without glucose, on blood glucose levels and cognitive performance during sustained 'mentally demanding' tasks. J Psychopharmacol 20: 771-781.

50. Suwa M, Nakano H, Kumagai S (2003) Effects of chronic AICAR treatment on fiber composition, enzyme activity, UCP3, and PGC-1 in rat muscles. J Appl Physiol 95: 960-968.

51. Terada S, Goto M, Kato M, Kawanaka K, Shimokawa T, et al. (2002) Effects of low-intensity prolonged exercise on PGC-1 mRNA expression in rat epitrochlearis muscle. Biochem Biophys Res Commun 296: 350-354.

52. Rodgers JT, Lerin C, Haas W, Gygi SP, Spiegelman BM, et al. (2005) Nutrient control of glucose homeostasis through a complex of PGC-1alpha and SIRT1. Nature 434: 113-118.

53. Nemoto S, Fergusson MM, Finkel T (2005) SIRT1 functionally interacts with the metabolic regulator and transcriptional coactivator PGC-1{alpha}. J Biol Chem 280: 16456-16460.

54. Lagouge M, Argmann C, Gerhart-Hines Z, Meziane H, Lerin C, et al. (2006) Resveratrol improves mitochondrial function and protects against metabolic disease by activating SIRT1 and PGC-1alpha. Cell 127: 1109-1122.

55. Gerhart-Hines Z, Rodgers JT, Bare O, Lerin C, Kim SH, et al. (2007) Metabolic control of muscle mitochondrial function and fatty acid oxidation through SIRT1/PGC-1alpha. Embo J 26: 1913-1923.

56. Irrcher I, Ljubicic V, Kirwan AF, Hood DA (2008) AMP-activated protein kinase-regulated activation of the PGC-1α promoter in skeletal muscle cells. PLoS ONE 3: e3614.

57. Egan B, Carson BP, Garcia-Roves PM, Chibalin AV, Sarsfield FM, et al. (2010) Exercise intensity-dependent regulation of peroxisome proliferator-activated receptor coactivator-1 mRNA abundance is associated with differential activation of upstream signalling kinases in human skeletal muscle. J Physiol 588: 1779-1790.

58. D'Angelo L, Grimaldi R, Caravaggi M, Marcoli M, Perucca E, et al. (1986) A double-blind, placebo-controlled clinical study on the effect of a standardized ginseng extract on psychomotor performance in healthy volunteers. J Ethnopharmacol 16: 15-22.

59. Jager S, Handschin C, St-Pierre J, Spiegelman BM (2007) AMP-activated protein kinase (AMPK) action in skeletal muscle via direct phosphorylation of PGC-1alpha. PNAS 104: 12017-12022.

60. Baar K, Wende AR, Jones TE, Marison M, Nolte LA, et al. (2002) Adaptations of skeletal muscle to exercise: rapid increase in the transcriptional coactivator PGC-1. FASEB J 16: 1879-1886.

61. Pilegaard H, Saltin B, Neufer PD (2003) Exercise induces transient transcriptional activation of the PGC-1alpha gene in human skeletal muscle. J Physiol 546: 851-858.

62. Friedrichsen M, Mortensen B, Pehmøller C, Birk JB, Wojtaszewski JF (2013) Exercise-induced AMPK activity in skeletal muscle: role in glucose uptake and insulin sensitivity. Mol Cell Endocrinol 366: 204-214.

63. Gurd BJ, Yoshida Y, Lally J, Holloway GP, Bonen A (2009) The deacetylase enzyme SIRT1 is not associated with oxidative capacity in rat heart and skeletal muscle and its overexpression reduces mitochondrial biogenesis. J Physiol 587: 1817-1828.

64. Pauli JR, Ropelle ER, Cintra DE, De Souza CT, da Silva AS, et al. (2010) Acute exercise reverses aged-induced impairments in insulin signaling in rodent skeletal muscle. Mech Ageing Dev 131: 323-329.

65. Suwa M, Nakano H, Radak,Z, Kumagai S (2008) Endurance exercise increases the SIRT1 and peroxisome proliferator-activated receptor gamma coactivator-1alpha protein expressions in rat skeletal muscle. Metabolism 57: 986-998.

66. Koltai E, Szabo Z, Atalay M, Boldogh I, Naito H, et al. (2010) Exercise alters SIRT1, SIRT6, NAD and NAMPT levels in skeletal muscle of aged rats. Mech Ageing Dev 131: 21-28.

67. Guerra B, Guadalupe-Grau A, Fuentes T, Ponce-González JG, Morales-Alamo D, et al. (2010) SIRT1, AMP-activated protein kinase phosphorylation and downstream kinases in response to a single bout of sprint exercise: influence of glucose ingestion. Eur J Appl Physiol 109: 731-743.

68. Little JP, Safdar A, Wilkin GP, Tarnopolsky MA, Gibala MJ (2010) A practical model of low-volume high-intensity interval training induces mitochondrial biogenesis in human skeletal muscle: potential mechanisms. J Physiol 588: 1011-1022.

69. Kong H, Wang M, Venema K, Maathuis A, van der Heijden R, et al. (2009) Bioconversion of red ginseng saponins in the gastro-intestinal tract in vitro model studied by high-performance liquid chromatography-high resolution Fourier transform ion cyclotron resonance mass spectrometry. J Chromatogr A 1216: 2195-2203.

Permissions

All chapters in this book were first published in BP, by OMICS International; hereby published with permission under the Creative Commons Attribution License or equivalent. Every chapter published in this book has been scrutinized by our experts. Their significance has been extensively debated. The topics covered herein carry significant findings which will fuel the growth of the discipline. They may even be implemented as practical applications or may be referred to as a beginning point for another development.

The contributors of this book come from diverse backgrounds, making this book a truly international effort. This book will bring forth new frontiers with its revolutionizing research information and detailed analysis of the nascent developments around the world.

We would like to thank all the contributing authors for lending their expertise to make the book truly unique. They have played a crucial role in the development of this book. Without their invaluable contributions this book wouldn't have been possible. They have made vital efforts to compile up to date information on the varied aspects of this subject to make this book a valuable addition to the collection of many professionals and students.

This book was conceptualized with the vision of imparting up-to-date information and advanced data in this field. To ensure the same, a matchless editorial board was set up. Every individual on the board went through rigorous rounds of assessment to prove their worth. After which they invested a large part of their time researching and compiling the most relevant data for our readers.

The editorial board has been involved in producing this book since its inception. They have spent rigorous hours researching and exploring the diverse topics which have resulted in the successful publishing of this book. They have passed on their knowledge of decades through this book. To expedite this challenging task, the publisher supported the team at every step. A small team of assistant editors was also appointed to further simplify the editing procedure and attain best results for the readers.

Apart from the editorial board, the designing team has also invested a significant amount of their time in understanding the subject and creating the most relevant covers. They scrutinized every image to scout for the most suitable representation of the subject and create an appropriate cover for the book.

The publishing team has been an ardent support to the editorial, designing and production team. Their endless efforts to recruit the best for this project, has resulted in the accomplishment of this book. They are a veteran in the field of academics and their pool of knowledge is as vast as their experience in printing. Their expertise and guidance has proved useful at every step. Their uncompromising quality standards have made this book an exceptional effort. Their encouragement from time to time has been an inspiration for everyone.

The publisher and the editorial board hope that this book will prove to be a valuable piece of knowledge for researchers, students, practitioners and scholars across the globe.

List of Contributors

Shaimaa GA and Mahmoud MS
Functional Food and Nutrition Department, Food Technology Research Institute, Agricultural Research Center, Giza 12613, Egypt

Mohamed MR and Emam AA
Biochemistry Department, Cairo University, Giza 12613, Egypt

Kathryn Leake, Jyotsana Singhal and Sharad S Singhal
Department of Diabetes, Endocrinology & Metabolism, California, USA

Sanjay Awasthi
Department of Diabetes, Endocrinology & Metabolism, California, USA
Department of Medical Oncology and Experimental Therapeutics, City of Hope Comprehensive Cancer Center, Duarte, California, USA

Harkness Troy AA and Arnason Terra G
Departments of Anatomy and Cell Biology, and College of Medicine, University of Saskatchewan, Saskatoon, Canada

Hoda Boushehri, Shahnaz Khaghani and Hossein Mirmiranpour
Department of Biochemistry, Tehran University of Medical Sciences, Tehran, Iran

Sedigheh Shams
Medicine Department, Pathology division, Tehran University of Medical Sciences, Tehran, Iran

Mohammad Zangooei
Department of Biochemistry, Tehran University of Medical Sciences, Tehran, Iran

Esameldin E Elgorashi, Babatunde B Samuel, Vinasan Naidoo and Jacobus N Eloff
Phytomedicine Programme, Department of Paraclinical Sciences, Faculty of Veterinary Science, University of Pretoria, Private Bag X04, Onderstepoort, 0110, South Africa

Mohammed M Suleiman
Phytomedicine Programme, Department of Paraclinical Sciences, Faculty of Veterinary Science, University of Pretoria, Private Bag X04, Onderstepoort, 0110, SouthAfrica

Department of Pharmacology and Toxicology, Faculty of Veterinary Medicine, Ahmadu Bello University, Zaria, Nigeria

Mengmeng Li, Xiaofan Xu, Yuanyuan Yue, Zhenyin Chen, Huinan Zhang and Zhongli Luo
The College of Basic Medical Sciences, Chongqing Medical University, Chongqing 400016, China
Molecular Medicine and Cancer Research Center, Chongqing Medical University, Chongqing 400016, China

Ran Wang, Feng Li and Lifeng Jin
China Tobacco Gene Research Center, Zhengzhou Tobacco Research Institute, Zhengzhou, 450001, China

Duanhua Li, Kanran Wang, Xinyuan Li, Mao Tan and Shanshan Zhang
Sichuan Industrial Institute of Antibiotics, Chengdu University, Chengdu, 610051, China

Yuelin Sun and Tianxin Zhao
The College of Clinical Pediatrics, Chongqing Medical University, Chongqing 400016, China

Nan Liu
China National Tobacco Quality Supervision and Test Centre, Zhengzhou, 450001, China

Jianping Gong
The College of Clinical Medicine, The First Affiliated hospital of Chongqing Medical university, Chongqing Medical University, Chongqing 400016, China

Kunyue Tan
The College of Clinical Medicine, The Second Affiliated hospital of Chongqing Medical university, Chongqing Medical University, Chongqing 400016, China

Pierre Mugabo and Mercy I Abaniwonda
School of Pharmacy, University of the Western Cape, Private Bag X17, 7535. Bellville, South Africa

Danie Theron and Leonie Van Zyl
Brewelskloof Hospital, Department of Health, Province of Western Cape, South Africa

Shafick M Hassan
Department of Nursing and Radiology, Cape Peninsula University of Technology, Bellville, South Africa

Marietjie Stander
Department of Biochemistry, University of Stellenbosch, South Africa

Helen McIlleron
Department of Medicine, Division of Clinical Pharmacology, University of Cape Town, South Africa

Richard Madsen
Department of Statistics, University of Missouri, USA

Oukkache N and Ghalim N
Laboratory of Venoms and Toxins, Institut Pasteur du Maroc, 1- Place Louis Pasteur, Casablanca 20360, Morocco

Chgoury F
Laboratory of Venoms and Toxins, Institut Pasteur du Maroc, 1- Place Louis Pasteur, Casablanca 20360, Morocco
Laboratory of Biology and Health, URAC 34, Hassan II University Casablanca, Faculty of Science Ben M'sik, Morocco

Benabderrazek R, Hmila I and Ayeb ME
Laboratory of Venoms and Therapeutic Molecules, Pasteur Institute of Tunis/University of Tunis El Manar, 13 Place Pasteur, BP74, 1002 - Tunis, Tunisia

Bouhaouala-Zahar B
Laboratory of Venoms and Therapeutic Molecules, Pasteur Institute of Tunis/University of Tunis El Manar, 13 Place Pasteur, BP74, 1002 - Tunis, Tunisia
Medical School of Tunis, 15 Rue Djebel Lakhdhar, La Rabta 1007, Tunis-Tunisia-University of Tunis El Manar

Tounsi H and Boubaker
Laboratory of Human and Experimental Pathology, Pasteur Institute of Tunis/University of Tunis El Manar, 13 Place Pasteur, BP74, 1002 - Tunis, Tunisia

Saïle R
Laboratory of Biology and Health, URAC 34, Hassan II University Casablanca, Faculty of Science Ben M'sik, Morocco

Dixit V and Yadav RA
Laser and Spectroscopy Laboratory, Department of Physics, Banaras Hindu University, Varanasi -221005, India

Yeh TY, Peng YP and Chen KF
Department of Civil and Environmental Engineering, National University of Kaohsiung, Taiwan

Raghunandan S Nathawat, Preeti Mishra and Vidya Patni
Plant Pathology, Tissue Culture and Biotechnology Laboratory, Department of Botany, University of Rajasthan, Jaipur, India

Anil P Bidkar, Krishan K Thakur, Nityanand B Bolshette and Jyotibon Dutta
Laboratory of Biotechnology, Department of Biotechnology, National Institute of Pharmaceutical Education and Research (NIPER), Guwahati Medical College, Guwahati-781032, Assam, India

Ranadeep Gogoi
Department of Biotechnology & Bioengineering, Institute of Science and Technology, Guwahati University, Guwahati-781014, Assam, India

Katsutoshi Shoda, Hirotaka Konishi, Daisuke Ichikawa, Yuji Fujita, Hidekazu Hiramoto, Junichi Hamada, Tomohiro Arita, Toshiyuki Kosuga, Shuhei Komatsu, Atsushi Shiozaki, Kazuma Okamoto and Eigo Otsuji
Division of Digestive Surgery, Department of Surgery, Kyoto Prefectural University of Medicine, 465 Kajii-cho, Kamigyo-ku, Kyoto 6028566, Japan

Katiucha KHR Rocha, Rodrigo P Ureshino, Janaína Peixoto and Soraya S Smaili
Department of Pharmacology, Institute of Pharmacology, Federal University of São Paulo, São Paulo, Brazil

Fernanda Mani
Department of Chemistry and Biochemistry, Institute of Biological Sciences, São Paulo State University, Botucatu, São Paulo, Brazil

Chieko Ihoriya, Minoru Satoh, Norio Komai, Tamaki Sasaki and Naoki Kashihara
Department of Nephrology and Hypertension, Kawasaki Medical School, Kurashiki, Okayama, Japan

Hong-ling Wang, Mao-wu Guo, Qin Liao, Hui Wang, Wei-juan Zhang, Yun-xia Sun and Conglin Zuo
Beijing Key Laboratory of Bio-products Safety Assessment, JOINN Laboratories, Beijing, China

Li Han and Tomoko Tsuji
Nippon Suisan Kaisha, Ltd., Tokyo, Japan

Mahendra Kumar Trivedi, Alice Branton, Dahryn Trivedi and Gopal Nayak
Trivedi Global Inc., 10624 S Eastern Avenue Suite A-969, Henderson, NV 89052, USA

Ragini Singh and Snehasis Jana
Trivedi Science Research Laboratory Pvt. Ltd., Hall-A, Chinar Mega Mall, Chinar Fortune City, Hoshangabad Rd, Bhopal- 462026, Madhya Pradesh, India

Tabin S and Gupta RC
Department of Botany, Punjabi University Patiala, Punjab, India

Kamili AN
Centre of Research for Development, University of Kashmir, Srinagar, India

Bansal G
Department of Pharmaceutical Sciences and Drug Research, Punjabi University Patiala, Punjab, India

Spencer Swarts, Theresa Carlson and Peter van der Geer
Department of Chemistry and Biochemistry, San Diego State University, San Diego, CA, USA

Pal A
Department of Biochemistry, PGIMER, Chandigarh 160012, India

Ana Martins
Grupo de Micobacterias, UEI Microbiology, Medical Microbiology and Parasitology Unidade de (UPMM), Instituto de Medicina Tropical and Higiene, Universidade Nova de Lisboa, Portugal
Institute of Medical Microbiology and Immunobiology, Faculty of Medicine, University of Szeged, Hungary
Institute of Pharmacognosy, Faculty of Pharmacy, University of Szeged, Hungary

Gabriella Spengler and Joseph Molnar
Institute of Medical Microbiology and Immunobiology, Faculty of Medicine, University of Szeged, Hungary

Leonard Amaral
Grupo de Micobacterias, UEI Microbiology, Medical Microbiology and Parasitology Unidade de (UPMM), Instituto de Medicina Tropical and Higiene, Universidade Nova de Lisboa, Portugal
Institute of Medical Microbiology and Immunobiology, Faculty of Medicine, University of Szeged, Hungary
Grupo de Micobacterias, UEI Microbiology, Centro de Malaria and Outras doenças Tropicais (CMDT), Instituto de Medicina Tropical and Higiene, Universidade Nova de Lisboa, Portugal

Abdul-Wahab R Hamad
Department of Medical Allied Sciences, Zarka University College, Al-Balqa Applied University, Zarka13115, Jordan

Hala I Al-Daghistani and Walid D Shquirat
Department of Medical Allied Sciences; Al-Salt College for Humanitarian Sciences, Al-Balqa Applied University, Al-Salt 19117, Jordan

Muna Abdel-Dayem and Mohammad Al-Swaifi
Medical Al-Hussein City Hospital, Amman 11855, Jordan

García I
Department of Organic Chemistry, University of Vigo, 36200, Spain

Prado-Prado F
Biomedical Sciences Department, Health Sciences Division, University of Quintana Roo, 77039, Mexico

Stefan U Weber, Makbule Kobilay and Andreas Hoeft
Department of Anesthesiology and Intensive Care Medicine, University Bonn Medical Center, Germany

Lutz E Lehmann and Frank Stüber
Department of Anaesthesiology and Pain Medicine, University Hospital Bern "Inselspital", Bern, Switzerland

Alexandra Bogeas, Evelyne Dufour and C Rougeot
Institut Pasteur, Laboratoire de Pharmacologie de la Douleur, Département de Biologie Structurale et Chimie, 25 rue du Dr. Roux 75724. Paris cedex 15, France

Jean-François Bisson and Michael Messaoudi
ETAP-Ethologie Appliqué-Technopôle de Nancy-Brabois-13, rue du Bois de la Champelle, 54500 Vandoeuvre-lès-Nancy, France

Barry Morris and Farhad Behzad
British Institute of Technology and E-commerce, London, UK

Kamel Rouissi, Soumaya Kouidhi, Bechr Hamrita and Amel Benammar Elgaaied
Laboratory of Genetics, Immunology, and Human Pathology, Faculty of Sciences of Tunis, University of El Manar I, 2092, Tunis, Tunisia

Slah Ouerhani
Laboratory of Molecular and Cellular Hematology, Pasteur Institute of Tunis, Tunisia

Mohamed Cherif
Department of Urology, Hospital of Charles Nicolle, Tunis, Tunisia

Shareena Dasari TP, Zhang Y and Yu H
Department of Chemistry and Biochemistry, Jackson State University, Jackson, MS 39217, USA

Paulo C Carvalh, Nilson IT Zanchin and Tatiana ACB Souza
Laboratory of Proteomics and Proteins Engineering, Institute Carlos Chagas, Curitiba-PR, Brazil

Aline G Santana
Laboratory of Proteomics and Proteins Engineering, Institute Carlos Chagas, Curitiba-PR, Brazil
Universidade Federal do Paraná (UFPR), Curitiba-PR, Brazil

Quan Jiang and Anji Lian
Key Laboratory of Bio-resources and Eco-environment of Ministry of Education, College of Life Sciences, 610065, Sichuan University, Chengdu, PR China

Tianqiang Liu
Key Laboratory of Bio-resources and Eco-environment of Ministry of Education, College of Life Sciences, 610065, Sichuan University, Chengdu, PR China
The Animal Health Research Institute, Tongwei Co., Ltd, China

Marilou Pannacci, Valeria Lucini, Silvana Dugnani, Rocco Ciracì and Francesco Scaglione
Department of Medical Biotechnology and Translational Medicine, University of Milan, Italy

Andrea Zangara
Centre for Human Psychopharmacology, Swinburne University of Technology, Hawthorn, Australia

Index

www.ingramcontent.com/pod-product-compliance
Lightning Source LLC
Chambersburg PA
CBHW080414190526
45161CB00003B/234